Myocarditis

Alida L. P. Caforio
Editor

Myocarditis

Pathogenesis, Diagnosis and Treatment

Springer

Editor
Alida L. P. Caforio
Cardiology, Department of Cardiac
Thoracic Vascular Science and Public Health
University of Padova, Policlinico Universitario
Padova, Italy

ISBN 978-3-030-35275-2 ISBN 978-3-030-35276-9 (eBook)
https://doi.org/10.1007/978-3-030-35276-9

This Springer imprint is published by the registered company Springer Nature Switzerland AG
The registered company address is: Gewerbestrasse 11, 6330 Cham, Switzerland

Preface

There are three phases to treatment: diagnosis, diagnosis and diagnosis. William Osler W. (1892) *Principles and Practice of Medicine*

William Osler, with this serendipitous sentence, stated, back in 1892, in his Medicine textbook: "There are three phases to treatment: diagnosis, diagnosis and diagnosis." This sentence clearly applies to modern medicine, pointing out that, even nowadays, with the wide armamentarium of sophisticated imaging and molecular diagnostic tools, optimal, personalized clinical management is based upon an accurate etiopathogenetic diagnosis. Traditionally, myocarditis has been considered a rare and poorly understood condition and a diagnostic challenge for the clinician. There has been also wide skepticism in the cardiology community on the possibility to cure the disease. As a matter of fact, myocarditis is not rare and does not have a pathognomonic presentation, mimicking many noninflammatory cardiac diseases. Prognosis is also very heterogeneous, ranging from spontaneous resolution to progressive heart failure, development of burned-out dilated cardiomyopathy, and death or heart transplantation. Typically myocarditis affects the young with a predilection for male gender, although it may occur at any age. The first comprehensive studies with a modern approach to etiopathogenesis were published in 1980 by Woodroof JF, who highlighted the etiological role of Coxsackieviruses and of the immune system in the progression of cardiac damage, with possible evolution to a dilated cardiomyopathy. A major advance in diagnosis was the development of the endomyocardial biopsy technique using the King's bioptome by Richardson. Another fundamental advance was the publication of a consensus histopathological classification and definition of myocarditis by endomyocardial biopsy findings, known as the Dallas criteria. Meanwhile, the first experimental observations were made, suggesting the involvement of autoimmunity to cardiac self-antigens; a mouse model for myosin-induced autoimmune myocarditis was described by Neu et al. Subsequently, various groups in the late 1980s and early 1990s reported the presence of circulating anti-heart autoantibodies against myosin as well as other self-antigens in acute and chronic myocarditis or dilated cardiomyopathy, in keeping with the hypothesis of autoimmunity being involved in a substantial proportion of patients. A retrospective multicenter registry from the USA by Cooper et al. reported for the first time the efficacy of combined immunosuppressive therapy in a rare but lethal form of myocarditis, e.g., giant cell myocarditis, that is currently considered the prototype of autoimmune myocarditis and that currently, if a biopsy-proven diagnosis is achieved early, has better prognosis on immunosuppression. The multicenter Myocarditis Treatment Trial was designed using the Dallas criteria to recruit myocarditis patients to 6 months immunosuppression; the therapy with azathioprine and prednisone or cyclosporine A and prednisone was well tolerated, and no significant effect on survival was observed, although the study was not powered to detect differences in survival. The results of the trial strongly discouraged cardiologists in the next decades on the use of endomyocardial biopsy to detect and treat myocarditis. However, researchers developed new diagnostic tools to be added to standard histology, in particular immunohistochemistry, to increase sensitivity of endomyocardial biopsy and characterize the number and type of infiltrating inflammatory cells, and molecular detection of genomic material of infectious agents mainly by polymerase chain reaction (PCR), to diagnose infectious, particularly viral myocarditis. This work led to another major step forward, e.g., the 1995 WHO classification of cardiomyopathies, with the acknowledgment that myocarditis is diagnosed on endomyocardial biopsy by established histological, immunological, and immunohistochemical criteria; molecular techniques on EMB were recommended to identify viral etiology. In the WHO classification, infectious, autoimmune, and idiopathic forms of myocarditis are recognized that may lead to dilated cardiomyopathy. Using serum cardiac autoantibody testing as well as histology, immunohistology, and viral PCR on endomyocardial biopsy, it is nowadays possible to define distinct etiopathogenetic subsets of myocarditis, in particular infectious versus immune-mediated, e.g., infection-negative forms. This characterization is key to define who are the infection-negative cases in which immunosuppression and immunomodulation may be beneficial. Conversely, immunosuppression and immunomodulation are contraindicated in patients with active myocardial infection. In this regard, we propose here, for the first time, a patient safety checklist before the introduction of immunosuppressive therapy in autoimmune biopsy-proven myocarditis. In the last years, another advance has been the development of cardiovascular magnetic resonance imaging (CMR) as a noninvasive imaging tool in inflammatory heart muscle disease. CMR does not replace endomyocardial biopsy; it is currently unable to differentiate between infectious and immune-mediated forms, but is valuable to refine the clinical suspicion of myocarditis and for noninvasive follow-up. These concepts were summarized by the 2013 European Myocarditis Task Force that produced the first consensus document on myocarditis, helping in the design of future multicenter trials of etiology-directed treatment, according to homogeneous consensus criteria.

It has been a privilege to coordinate in this book worldwide recognized expert groups on myocarditis who, in the last 20 years, provided and are still providing major insights into the pathogenesis, diagnosis, and treatment of myocarditis. I gratefully thank all of them for their precious and enthusiastic contributions. This book was aimed at providing the current cutting edge between knowledge and ignorance. Myocarditis is no longer a neglected disease; it is currently a hot issue. There are suggestions that immune-mediated pathogenesis may be a final common pathway of heart dysfunction and arrhythmia not only in "idiopathic" myocarditis but also in genetic cardiomyopathies and nonischemic heart failure. It is hoped that this book will provide a useful reference for new young researchers who would like to work on this fascinating disease.

This book would not have been possible without the serendipity and support of Dr. Donatella Rizza, Editor at Springer Italy, who suggested dedicating a book to a generally neglected cause of heart failure. The book is addressed to cardiologists, internists, rheumatologists, clinical immunologists, cardiac pathologists as well as basic scientists with an interest in myocarditis, since myocarditis is a multidisciplinary challenge. Last but not least, I would like to dedicate this book to our patients, the lucky ones, who were cured with specific therapies or underwent cardiac transplantation, but especially to those, the unlucky ones, who died because of sudden cardiac death or waiting for a new heart. We are confident that we are on the right path and will rapidly progress in finding new and effective tailored treatments for myocarditis.

Padova, Italy Alida L. P. Caforio

Contents

1 Classification, Histopathology, Immunohistology, and Molecular Diagnosis of Myocarditis

Stefania Rizzo, Elisa Carturan, Gaetano Thiene, and Cristina Basso

1.1 Definition and Classification

In the 1995 WHO Classification of Cardiomyopathies [1], myocarditis, also named inflammatory cardiomyopathy, is listed among specific cardiomyopathies and is defined as an "inflammatory disease of the myocardium associated with cardiac dysfunction." The diagnosis of myocarditis is based on endomyocardial biopsy (EMB) according to established histological, immunological, immunohistochemical, and molecular criteria. Different causes of myocarditis, including infectious, autoimmune, and idiopathic forms, are recognized and they may progress along the clinical course toward dilated cardiomyopathy, a disease frequently requiring cardiac transplantation [2].

New definitions and classifications of cardiomyopathies have been advanced by the American Heart Association (AHA) in 2006 [3] and the European Society of Cardiology (ESC) in 2008 [4]. In the 2006 AHA document, myocarditis is classified among the primary cardiomyopathies, in the acquired subgroup (with infectious, autoimmune, and toxic causes), but also in the mixed subgroup, as inflammatory dilated cardiomyopathy (i.e., predominantly non-genetic, with infectious, autoimmune, and toxic causes). In the 2008 ESC document [4], specific morphofunctional categories of cardiomyopathies are recognized, subclassified into familial and non-familial forms. Myocarditis forms are grouped among the dilated cardiomyopathies, thus possibly excluding acute/fulminant myocarditis or those forms presenting in the setting of an almost preserved ventricular function with arrhythmias and/or chest pain.

S. Rizzo
Department of Cardiac, Thoracic, Vascular Sciences and Public Health, Padua University Hospital, Padua, Italy
e-mail: stefania.rizzo_01@aopd.veneto.it, stefania.rizzo75@gmail.com

E. Carturan · G. Thiene · C. Basso (✉)
Cardiovascular Pathology, University of Padua, Padua, Italy
e-mail: elisa.carturan@unipd.it; gaetano.thiene@unipd.it; cristina.basso@unipd.it

A. L. P. Caforio (ed.), *Myocarditis*, https://doi.org/10.1007/978-3-030-35276-9_1

In the 2013 ESC Working Group of Myocardial and Pericardial diseases report [5], the disease is defined histologically as an inflammatory disease of the myocardium diagnosed on EMB, based upon histological, immunological, immunohistochemical, and molecular findings to detect possible infectious causes. Inflammatory cardiomyopathy is defined as myocarditis associated with cardiac dysfunction.

Finally, the MOGE(S) classification system published in 2013 reflects the rapidly growing knowledge on genetic and acquired causes (i.e., intramyocardial inflammation, viral infections) and further conditions involved in the induction of cardiomyopathies (e.g., toxicity) [6].

Myocarditis is a broad term and can be classified based upon several parameters, such as etiology, stage, and histopathology.

Based on etiology, several agents may lead to development of myocarditis, including infectious agents (with viruses showing the higher incidence and prevalence, Table 1.1 [7]), physical (radiation), pharmacologic (like anthracyclines, 5-fluorouracil, alcohol, tricyclic antidepressants, immune check point inhibitors [8]), hematologic (essentially the eosinophilic myocarditis, either associated or not with hypereosinophilic conditions), and autoimmune disorders. Unfortunately, different etiologies might lead to similar histopathological characteristics. For example, viral, toxic, radiation-associated, and autoimmune myocarditis might lead to acute lymphocytic myocarditis with similar pathologic findings.

Based on the disease stage, the inflammation may be acute (and then might spontaneously resolve or progress), subacute, and chronic, with tissue remodeling and fibrosis that are eventually similar regardless of the initial subtype of myocarditis [9, 10]. It is possible that, with disease progression, several etiologic subtypes merge into a common pathogenic process, characterized by tissue remodeling with chronic inflammation, fibrosis, myocyte damage, and eventually leading to a dilated cardiomyopathy phenotype. Although the incidence of dilated cardiomyopathy as a sequela of previous myocarditis is not known, retrospective studies report that up to 50% of dilated cardiomyopathy cases have histological evidence of myocarditis, suggesting a persistent inflammatory process

Table 1.1 Myocarditis: infective agents

DNA viruses: Adenovirus, herpes virus (cytomegalovirus, Epstein–Barr virus, varicella-zoster virus, human herpes virus 6), hepatitis B, parvovirus B19
RNA viruses: Arbovirus, hepatitis C virus, picornavirus (entero, rhino), orthomyxovirus (influenza A and B), paramyxovirus (rubella, mumps, respiratory syncytial virus), retrovirus, HIV
Bacteria: Staphylococcus, Streptococcus, Pneumococcus, Meningococcus, Gonococcus, Salmonella, Corynebacterium diphtheriae, Haemophilus influenzae, Mycoplasma pneumoniae, Brucella species
Mycobacteria: Tuberculosis, Avium intracellulare, Leprae
Fungi: Aspergillus, Candida, Actinomyces, Blastomyces, Cryptococcus, Histoplasma
Protozoa: Toxoplasma gondii, Trypanosoma cruzi
Rickettsiae: Coxiella burnetii (Q fever), Rickettsia rickettsii, Rickettsia tsutsugamushi
Chlamydiae: Trachomatis, Psittaci
Parasitic: Trichinella spiralis

[2, 11, 12]. The progression rate of myocarditis to irreversible tissue damage varies depending on the etiology. Ongoing disease may be due to either persistence of virus in the myocardium or an autoimmune process.

EMB is essential not only for the definitive diagnosis of myocarditis but also to reach a classification of myocarditis based on histological criteria, that is, lymphocytic, eosinophilic, polymorphous, granulomatous, giant cell, which might reflect a different etiopathogenesis of the myocardial inflammatory process and may have treatment implications. Moreover, molecular techniques may allow us to specify the etiology of the inflammatory disease.

1.2 Histopathological Diagnosis

The gold standard for the diagnosis of myocarditis remains EMB. However, this diagnostic tool has limitations due to the patchy involvement of the myocardium and therefore a negative biopsy may not exclude disease, due to EMB sampling error [13–19]. Appropriate timing of the procedure close to symptom onset, the number of EMB samples, the serial sectioning technique with multiple-level examination of specimens [20], and possibly biventricular EMB [21] are all important factors to increase diagnostic sensitivity of EMB in the setting of suspected myocarditis. Moreover, there is controversy whether or not to perform EMB, being an invasive procedure with possible associated complications, such as arrhythmias and perforation. If EMB is performed by experienced teams, the complication rate is low and similar to that of standard coronary angiography [22–24]. The reason to proceed with EMB is that it allows a certain diagnosis and may guide therapy. In patients with clinically suspected myocarditis, the ESC Working Group recommended selective coronary angiography and EMB, including conventional histology, immunohistochemistry, and molecular detection of infectious agents for an etiology-specific strategy [5, 25].

Diagnostic guidelines for the histopathological classification of myocarditis (the so-called Dallas criteria) were published for the first time in 1986, in order to standardize the pathology reports (Table 1.2) [26, 27]. Myocarditis is defined as an "inflammatory infiltrate of the myocardium with necrosis and/or degeneration of adjacent myocytes, not typical of ischemic damage associated with coronary artery disease." At that time, it was based on conventional staining procedures (hematoxylin-eosin) and not immunohistochemistry. According to the histologic features, myocarditis was categorized as follows:

Table 1.2 Dallas criteria: morphological diagnosis of myocarditis

First biopsy
Myocarditis with/without fibrosis
Borderline myocarditis (repeat biopsy may be indicated)
No myocarditis
Subsequent biopsy
Ongoing (persistent) myocarditis with/without fibrosis
Resolving (healing) myocarditis with/without fibrosis
Resolved (healed) myocarditis with/without fibrosis

(a) Myocarditis with/without fibrosis, if routine light microscopy reveals infiltrating lymphocytes and myocyte necrosis
(b) Borderline myocarditis, with lymphocytic infiltration in the absence of myocytolysis
(c) No myocarditis, if both lymphocytic infiltration and myocytolysis are absent

Follow-up biopsies should be reported as persistent, healing, or healed myocarditis [26, 27].

Further description of the variant of myocarditis can be made based on the quality of the inflammatory cell infiltrate, e.g., eosinophilic, polymorphous, lymphocytic, or granulomatous [27].

When the diagnosis was only based upon the histological Dallas diagnostic criteria, myocarditis was considered to be a relatively rare cause of heart failure and/or of sudden cardiac death [10, 28]. Moreover, Dallas criteria are not particularly useful to understand the pathophysiologic and immunologic aspects, and their usefulness has decayed over time. Several limitations of the Dallas criteria have been raised: (a) inflammatory cell characterization by immunohistochemistry and fibrosis amount have not been considered; (b) the type and extent of myocyte damage have not been further specified; (c) inflammatory infiltrates other than lymphocytes were just mentioned (i.e., lymphocytic, eosinophilic, polymorphous, giant cell, and granulomatous myocarditis); (d) a diagnosis of healing or healed myocarditis was not feasible on the first biopsy, but only when unequivocal myocarditis had been previously diagnosed; (e) the term borderline myocarditis, including also chronic forms, remains equivocal and does not help in the clinical setting; (f) any reference to etiological agents was lacking; and (g) finally, interobserver variability was evident in pathologic interpretation [29, 30].

We previously put forward a proposal for a classification of myocarditis based upon a semiquantitative histological criteria, including, besides the inflammatory cell type, a system of grading (i.e., semiquantitative assessment of myocyte damage/inflammation) and staging (i.e., semiquantitative assessment of fibrosis), as it is currently applied in extracardiac inflammatory diseases and in graft rejection [30, 31]. Grading might be used in myocarditis to describe the intensity of necroinflammatory activity. Staging, on the other hand, may be a measure of fibrosis and architectural changes, which are the consequence of tissue injury and repair.

1.3 Immunohistopathological Diagnosis

An increase in sensitivity of EMB has now been reached by using immunohistochemistry [IHC] together with histology, thus overcoming some limitations of the Dallas criteria. Many interstitial cells such as mast cells, fibroblast nuclei cut in cross section, pericytes, histiocytes, and endothelial cells may be difficult to characterize on routine hematoxylin eosin-stained sections and may resemble lymphocytes [32–35]. Moreover, a small number of inflammatory cells, including lymphocytes, may be found in the normal myocardium.

Table 1.3 Proposed common definition/nomenclature of inflammatory myocardial disease by histology/immunohistochemistry

Acute (active) myocarditis
>14 leukocytes/mm^2 with the presence of CD3 T lymphocytes >7 cells/mm^2
Necrosis or degeneration of the cardiomyocytes present
Fibrosis may be either absent or present[a]
Chronic myocarditis
>14 leukocytes/mm^2 with the presence of CD3 T lymphocytes >7 cells/mm^2
Necrosis or degeneration of the cardiomyocytes absent
Fibrosis usually present[a]
Inflammatory cardiomyopathy (or dilated cardiomyopathy with inflammation)
>14 leukocytes/mm^2 with the presence of CD3 T lymphocytes >7 cells/mm^2
Cardiomyopathic changes
Fibrosis may be either absent or present[a]

[a]The pathology report should always specify whether fibrosis is absent or present for prognostic implications

A large panel of specific antibodies is now mandatory, besides routine histology, for the identification, localization, and characterization of mononuclear cell infiltrates as well as the activated immunological processes. The main antibodies used for immunophenotype cell characterization are CD45 (leukocyte antigen common), CD43 (T lymphocytes), CD3 (T cell marker), CD4 (helper T cell marker), CD8 (cytotoxic T cell marker), CD45RO (memory subset of CD8+ T cell marker, expressed on activated T cells), CD20 (B lymphocytes), and CD68 (macrophages). A value of >14 leukocytes/mm^2 with the presence of CD3 T lymphocytes >7 cells/mm^2 has been considered a cutoff to reach a diagnosis of myocarditis. Additional stains relevant to immune activation include HLA-ABC and HLA-DR to assess HLA class II expression in antigen-presenting immune cells. Recently, it has also been suggested that the use of the more common leukocyte marker CD45 may increase the diagnostic sensitivity of EMB [36].

Based on the immunopathology findings, we will discuss the various forms of inflammatory myocardial diseases (Table 1.3).

1.4 Acute (Active) Myocarditis

It is the most common form of myocarditis, usually lymphocytic. It is a nonspecific and variable form of inflammatory cardiomyopathy, often associated with viral infections [37], autoimmune/connective tissue diseases, or toxic myocarditis/catecholamine-induced myocardial injury. It is characterized by a predominant myocardial patchy infiltration of T lymphocytes, typically identified in IHC by CD3 expression. Areas of lymphocyte infiltration colocalize with CD68+ macrophages. Necrosis or degeneration of the cardiomyocytes is compulsory, while fibrosis may be either absent or present (Figs. 1.1 and 1.2).

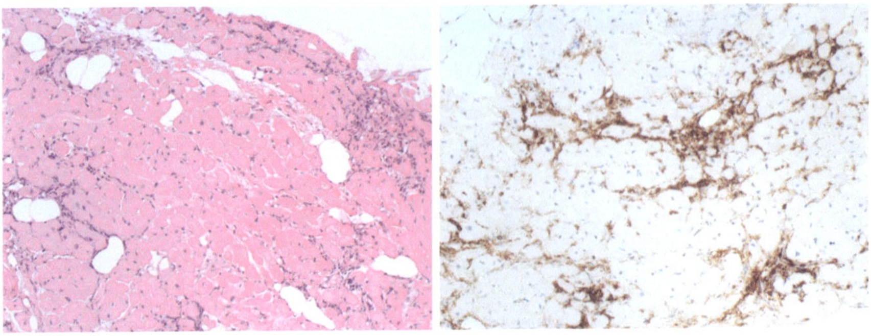

Fig. 1.1 Acute (active) myocarditis: Lymphocytic myocarditis with plurifocal interstitial inflammation and diffuse necrosis of the myocardium. Immunophenotypic characterization of inflammatory cells shows that the infiltrate mainly comprised active T lymphocytes (CD3+ > 7/mm^2)

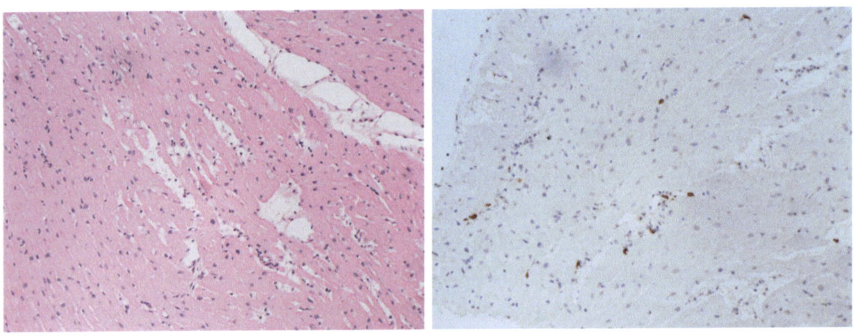

Fig. 1.2 Acute (active) myocarditis: Lymphocytic myocarditis with signs of edema, mild lymphomonocyte interstitial infiltration, and foci of myocardial necrosis. At immunohistochemistry, clear-cut evidence of CD3+ T lymphocytes >7/mm^2

1.5 Chronic Myocarditis

It is thought to be a chronic stage of acute lymphocytic myocarditis; this entity is pathologically characterized by the presence of replacement-type fibrosis in the myocardium, still accompanied by leukocyte infiltration. Necrosis or degeneration of the cardiomyocytes is usually non-evident. The timing for such progression from acute to chronic inflammation is variable and currently unpredictable. The areas of fibrosis, when present, are the consequence of the evolution of the myocardial inflammatory process (Fig. 1.3).

According to some authors, the presence of chronic inflammatory cells by histology and immunohistochemistry, in association with cardiomyopathic changes, could define a category called *dilated cardiomyopathy with inflammation* or *inflammatory cardiomyopathy* [38] (Fig. 1.4).

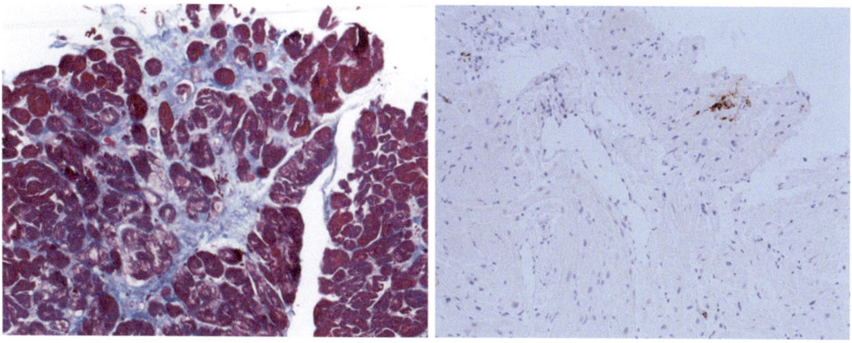

Fig. 1.3 Chronic myocarditis: Replacement type fibrosis with patchy lymphomonocytic infiltrate (CD3+ > 7/mm^2) in the absence of myocardial necrosis

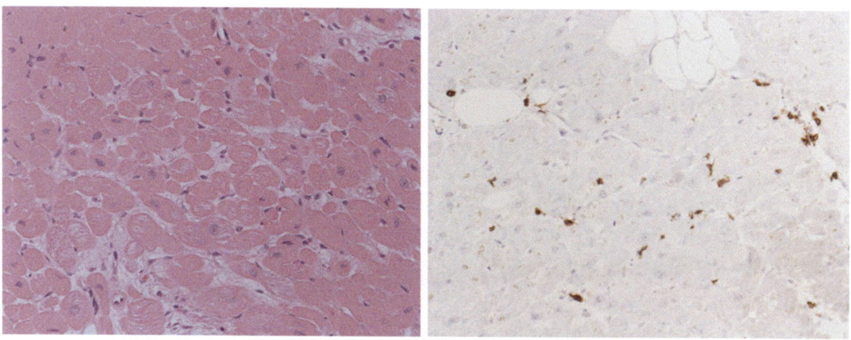

Fig. 1.4 Inflammatory cardiomyopathy: Cardiomyopathic changes of the myocytes with increased diameter, perinuclear halo, and dysmetric nuclei. There are sparse lymphocytic T cells CD3+ not associated with myocardial necrosis

1.6 Giant Cell Myocarditis

Giant cell myocarditis is characterized by the unique histological features and particular aggressiveness. More frequently it presents clinically as fulminant myocarditis with progression to chronic life-threatening complications like dilated cardiomyopathy in up to 80% of cases [9]. Giant cell myocarditis is thought to be a consequence of autoimmunity, a view supported by the association of giant cell myocarditis with several autoimmune diseases and the not so rare posttransplantation recurrence of giant cells in heart grafts [39]. Myocardial involvement is diffuse, which explains the high sensitivity of EMB [40–43]. Histologically, giant cell myocarditis is characterized by a prominent and extensive leukocyte infiltration with myeloid cell predominance (mainly CD68+ macrophages) as compared with T cell infiltration and massive myocyte necrosis, without well-formed granulomas. Interestingly, eosinophils are also often present within the cellular infiltrates (Fig. 1.5).

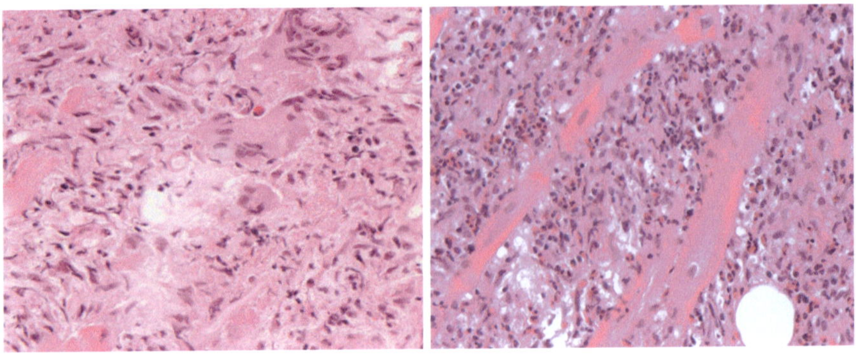

Fig. 1.5 Giant cell myocarditis showing the presence of diffuse inflammatory infiltration of the myocardium with lymphocytes, eosinophils, and multinucleated giant cells in the absence of granulomas associated with diffuse myocardial necrosis

1.7 Sarcoidosis

This is a systemic "idiopathic" disorder characterized by an antigen-presenting cells dysfunction, generating chronic tissue inflammation and granulomatous lesions in organs like the lung, lymph nodes, and heart. Sarcoidotic myocarditis displays extensive infiltration by activated macrophages, leading to chronic inflammation and tissue damage with non-necrotizing granulomas and fibrotic replacement, in the absence of infection. Eosinophils and necrosis are rare or absent [40]. The macrophages within sarcoid granulomas tend to become epithelioid and form multinucleated giant cells. The giant cells may contain cytoplasmic inclusions, particularly Schaumann bodies or asteroid bodies. The latter are stellate-shaped inclusion bodies, generally within a cytoplasmic clearing (Fig. 1.6). Both Schaumann and asteroid bodies are suggestive but not specific for sarcoid. As cardiac sarcoidosis progresses, the granulomatous inflammation elicits a repair response with scarring. Sarcoidosis affects the heart nonuniformly, with the ventricular septum and left ventricle basal free wall most commonly affected. As a result, EMB has only 20% to 30% sensitivity, if not guided by imaging [40]. Granulomatous forms of myocarditis are also likely due to autoimmunity, mycobacterial infection, or fungal infection and these should enter in differential diagnosis.

1.8 Eosinophilic Myocarditis

This form of myocarditis is often observed in conditions associated with peripheral eosinophilia (e.g., primary idiopathic hypereosinophilia, hypersensitivity reaction to drugs or parasitic infections, allergic diseases, and autoimmune disorders), but

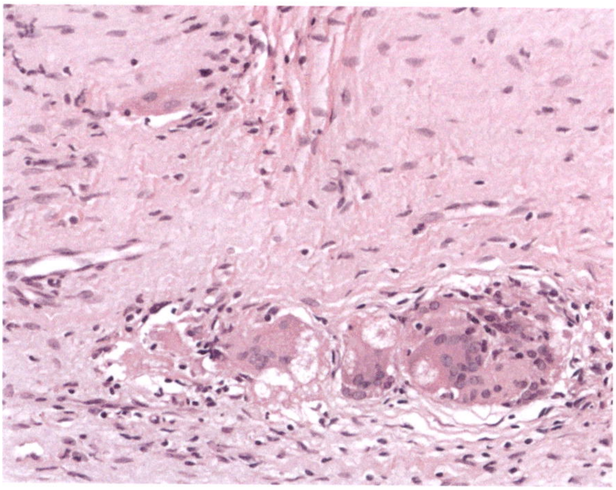

Fig. 1.6 Cardiac sarcoidosis showing noncaseating granuloma with epithelioid histiocytes, multinucleated giant cells with asteroid bodies, and lymphocytes embedded in a collagenous stroma

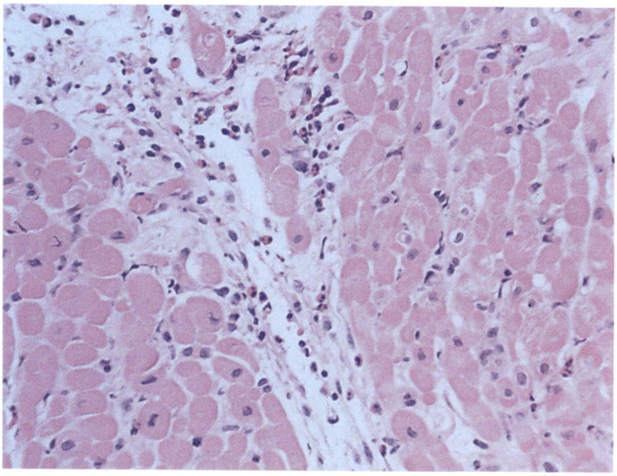

Fig. 1.7 Eosinophilic myocarditis with interstitial inflammation within the myocardium mainly represented by eosinophilic leukocytes

may also appear as a primary isolated disease. Its landmark is the presence of patchy, interstitial eosinophils, in significant numbers, in myocardial infiltrates (Fig. 1.7). This entity, similar to giant cell myocarditis, also shows a poor long-term prognosis despite broad immunosuppressive treatment [9]. Eosinophils release toxic granules, cationic proteins, pro-inflammatory cytokines, and oxygen free radicals that will cause myocyte injury and necrosis. There is a spectrum of disease, ranging from hypersensitivity myocarditis to hypereosinophilic syndrome [44], which is defined as persistent (>6 months) blood eosinophilia >1500/μL and evidence of eosinophil-mediated organ damage. Hypereosinophilic syndrome is characterized by three stages, the acute stage with inflammation and necrosis, thrombosis of damaged myocardium, and finally the fibrotic stage characterized by both severe atrioventricular regurgitation and restrictive cardiomyopathy. End-stage disease is termed Loeffler's endocarditis.

1.9 Myocarditis and Sudden Death

A special issue is the diagnosis of myocarditis at postmortem in full specimens [30, 45]. Myocarditis has been traditionally considered an important cause not only of heart failure-related death but also of sudden death, particularly in young individuals [46–48]. However, patchy inflammatory infiltrate (<14 leukocytes/mm^2), not necessarily associated with myocyte necrosis, is frequently observed in sudden death cases. Thus, the prevalence of myocarditis may have been exaggerated because of over-interpretation of histological data and lack of standardized morphologic criteria. For these reasons, the Association for European Cardiovascular Pathology (AECVP) put forward guidelines which represent the minimum standard that is required in the routine autopsy practice for adequate assessment of sudden cardiac death, including a protocol not only for heart examination and histological sampling but also for toxicology and molecular investigation [45]. Accordingly, scattered inflammatory foci with or without small foci of fibrosis ("physiological" changes) should be distinguished from borderline/focal myocarditis ("pathological" changes). In this document, it has been clearly emphasized that, in the absence of myocyte necrosis, small foci of inflammatory cells (even after immunohistochemistry) are not sufficient evidence of myocarditis; scattered small foci of fibrosis are also insignificant. Both findings should prompt examination of additional blocks and viral infection should be excluded by molecular techniques.

1.10 Molecular Diagnosis

Lymphocytic myocarditis is the most common form of myocarditis in Western countries, and most of the cases are viral in origin (Table 1.1) [49]. Non-viral infectious agents may be identified by routine histology including special stains, although microbiologic cultures are essential for precise isolation [49, 50]. Conversely, classical morphological analysis has great limitations in the detection of viral agents and usually lacks specific cytopathic features, with the rare exception of some forms of cytomegalovirus myocarditis.

Serological studies and peripheral viral cultures lack sensitivity and specificity [29]. Thanks to the advent of molecular biological techniques, including in situ hybridization [51, 52], but particularly amplification methods, e.g., polymerase chain reaction (PCR) or nested-PCR, it is possible to detect low copy viral genomes even from an extremely small amount of tissue such as EMB specimens.

Numerous studies on myocarditis have demonstrated the usefulness of PCR analysis for etiologic diagnosis [53–62]. Moreover, in pediatric patients with a clinical suspicion of myocarditis, since EMB may be technically difficult to be performed, it has been demonstrated that tracheal aspirates may be a useful surrogate for the identification of causative agents by PCR analysis. Previous molecular studies demonstrated high concordance of viral genome detection in EMB specimens and in tracheal aspirates [63, 64].

EMB samples from patients with lymphocytic myocarditis are evaluated by PCR, using specific primers and probes, for genome of the following cardiotropic viruses: adenovirus, enterovirus, Epstein–Barr Virus (EBV), cytomegalovirus, herpes simplex virus 1, herpes simplex virus 2, parvovirus B19 (PVB19), human herpes virus 6, H1N1 strains of influenza virus, and hepatitis C virus. In case of virus-positive EMB, blood samples, collected at the time of the EMB, are also tested for the same virus to exclude passive blood contamination; viral blood positivity requires additional investigation by quantitative PCR analysis [49, 50].

Enteroviruses, specifically Coxsackievirus group B serotypes, have traditionally been identified as the predominant viral cause [65], although adenoviruses, PVB19, and human herpes virus 6 nowadays can also cause myocarditis. In contrast, herpes simplex virus (HSV) rarely causes acute myocarditis. In subjects with chronic inflammatory cardiomyopathy, parvovirus B19 and human herpes virus 6 genomes predominate [60, 65, 66].

However, it has been underlined that the presence of viral genomes does not automatically imply a direct role of viruses in the pathogenesis of myocarditis, since an infective agent detected by PCR/nested-PCR may be just an innocent bystander. Therefore, it is recommended to use molecular techniques as diagnostic tools ancillary to other mandatory investigations, either clinical or morphological, and apply it with skilled expertise. On the other hand, while interpreting the molecular results, a limitation is still represented by the number of EMB specimens needed to obtain an acceptable sensitivity for the detection of viruses: only a positive PCR result is diagnostic, whereas a negative PCR does not exclude viral disease, particularly when a very small sample of tissue is analyzed. Moreover, the identification of an underlying organism is not usually possible or effective because viruses are often cleared by the immune system, before significant inflammation occurs, so the timing of EMB is also important.

Among the molecular biology techniques used to differentiate viral genomes, gene sequencing allows not only the precise characterization of the infective agent but can also help in assessing the molecular basis of cardiotropism as well as cardiovirulence [67, 68].

A further step in the molecular pathology investigation can be represented by the identification of the "infective status" of viruses; the detection of virus replication is useful not only for those DNA viruses known to be in the latent form [68] but also for RNA viruses [69, 70].

More recently, the need of viral genome load quantification has been advanced by means of real-time polymerase chain reaction [71]. In particular, in the last few years, several studies revealed a prevalence up to 60% of PVB19 [72]. However, PVB19 was also detected in healthy transplant donors, in autoptic samples without myocarditis or with borderline myocarditis, and in patients undergoing EMB for other reasons [73–77]. In situ hybridization revealed that endothelial cells are the principal target, even though a myocyte tropism has also been demonstrated [78]. Bock et al. [79] measured viral loads in EMB specimens obtained from 498 patients with myocarditis or chronic dilated cardiomyopathy who were positive for PVB19 on immunohistologic analysis and suggested that a viral load of more than 500 ge per microgram in EMB specimens is a clinically relevant threshold for the maintenance of myocardial inflammation.

PCR analysis should be applied on follow-up EMB of patients with viral myocarditis and may represent the best way to verify the efficacy of specific antiviral therapy and to evaluate viral clearance.

A role for laser microdissection has also been suggested in peculiar types of myocarditis. The definition of viral myocarditis requires unequivocal demonstration of the viral genome or virus gene products within the cardiomyocytes and their absence in unaffected hearts. In particular, EBV has been occasionally detected in myocardial tissue of patients with myocarditis, but may persist for life in circulating B cells after a primary infection; thus, blood contamination might be the source of the identified viral DNA. To this aim, Chimenti et al. [80] studied a series of patients with inflammatory cardiomyopathy by laser microdissection and identified intramyocyte EBV genome in up to 6.3% of them, as to suggest a cytopathic EBV role and an antiviral/immunomodulatory therapy.

In the future, panviral microarray approach could achieve a more sensitive diagnosis of viral myocarditis versus nonviral cases [71]. Microarray analysis has been recently reported by Heidecker et al. [81] as valid diagnostic tool for improving the diagnosis of inflammatory versus non-inflammatory cardiomyopathy. Given emerging treatment strategies for viral and inflammatory myocarditis, accurate diagnostic tools are of outmost importance.

Multicenter joint efforts including a large number of cases are needed to understand the different phenotypes of myocarditis, trying to distinguish self-limiting cases from those with a progressive course. Different virus- or host-related factors may influence the clinical phenotype of myocarditis. Among virus-related factors, the type of virus, viral load, or certain specific strains within the same viral family represent the most important issues, which are also largely investigated to design appropriate vaccines for prevention program planning [82]. Various host-related factors could influence the different susceptibility and disease course. Among these, specific viral receptors (CAR, DAF), transcriptional/translation factors (JAK, STAT, SOCS, NFkB), or immune mediators are the most commonly studied [83–85].

Different pro-inflammatory cytokines have a crucial role in the development and progression of myocarditis. Tumor necrosis factor alpha (TNFα) is thought to play a pivotal role in the development and progression of viral myocarditis [64]. A high level of TNFα has been detected by our group in EMBs from adult patients with myocarditis. The cytokine overexpression significantly correlated with impaired cardiac function and its persistency, as demonstrated in the follow-up EMB or in the explanted heart from patients who died or underwent heart transplantation, supporting the view that TNFα is implicated in disease progression and development of irreversible heart failure [85].

The final question whether persistent virus or reactivation of latent virus is responsible for chronic myocarditis and contributes to the development of dilated cardiomyopathy requires further research. The availability of EMB has renewed attention to the importance of persistent virus in chronic myocarditis and dilated cardiomyopathy [86].

References

1. Richardson P, McKenna WJ, Bristow M, Maisch B, Mautner B, O'Connell J, Olsen E, Thiene G, Goodwin J, Gyarfas I, Martin I, Nordet P. Report of the 1995 WHO/ISFC task force on the definition of cardiomyopathies. Circulation. 1996;93:841–2.
2. Huber S. Viral myocarditis and dilated cardiomyopathy: etiology and pathogenesis. Curr Pharm Des. 2016;22:408–26.
3. Maron BJ, Towbin JA, Thiene G, Antzelevitch C, Corrado D, Arnett D, Moss AJ, Seidman CE, Young JB. Contemporary definitions and classification of cardiomyopathies. An American heart association scientific statement from the council on clinical cardiology, heart failure and transplantation committee; quality of care and outcome research and functional genomics and translational biology interdisciplinary working groups: and council on epidemiology and prevention. Circulation. 2006;113:1807–16.
4. Elliott P, Andersson B, Arbustini E, Bilinska Z, Cecchi F, Charron P, Dubourg O, Kühl U, Maisch B, McKenna WJ, Monserrat L, Pankuweit S, Rapezzi C, Seferovic P, Tavazzi L, Keren A. Classification of the cardiomyopathies: a position statement from the European Society of Cardiology working group on myocardial and pericardial disease. Eur Heart J. 2007;29:270–6.
5. Caforio AL, Pankuweit S, Arbustini E, Basso C, Gimeno-Blanes J, Felix SB, Fu M, Helio T, Heymans S, Jahns R, Klingel K, Linhart A, Maisch B, McKenna W, Mogensen J, Pinto YM, Ristic A, Schultheiss H-P, Seggewiss H, Tavazzi L, Thiene G, Yilmaz A, Charron P, Elliott PM. Current state of knowledge on aetiology, diagnosis, management, and therapy of myocarditis: a position statement of the European Society of Cardiology Working Group on Myocardial and Pericardial Diseases. Eur Heart J. 2013;34:2636–48.
6. Arbustini E, Narula N, Dec GW, Reddy KS, Greenberg B, Kushwaha S, Marwick T, Pinney S, Bellazzi R, Favalli V, Kramer C, Roberts R, Zoghbi WA, Bonow R, Tavazzi L, Fuster V, Narula J. The MOGE(S) classification for a phenotype-genotype nomenclature of cardiomyopathy: endorsed by the World Heart Federation. J Am Coll Cardiol. 2013;62:2046–72.
7. Barbaro G. Cardiovascular manifestations of HIV infection. Circulation. 2002;106:1420–5.
8. Atallah-Yunes SA, Kadado AJ, Kaufman GP, Hernandez-Montfort J. Immune checkpoint inhibitor therapy and myocarditis: a systematic review of reported cases. J Cancer Res Clin Oncol. 2019;145:1527.
9. Kindermann I, Barth C, Mahfoud F, Ukena C, Lenski M, Yilmaz A, Klingel K, Kandolf R, Sechtem U, Cooper LT, Böhm M. Update on myocarditis. J Am Coll Cardiol. 2012;59:779–92.
10. Pollack A, Kontorovich AR, Fuster V, Dec GW. Viral myocarditis-diagnosis, treatment options, and current controversies. Nat Rev Cardiol. 2015;12:670–80.
11. Cooper LT, Baughman KL, Feldman AM, Frustaci A, Jessup M, Kuhl U, Levine GN, Narula J, Starling RC, Towbin J, Virmani R. The role of endomyocardial biopsy in the management of cardiovascular disease: a scientific statement from the American Heart Association, the American College of Cardiology, and the European Society of Cardiology. Endorsed by the Heart Failure Society of America and the Heart Failure Association of the European Society of Cardiology. J Am Coll Cardiol. 2007;50:1914–31.
12. Kindermann I, Kindermann M, Kandolf R, Klingel K, Bültmann B, Müller T, Lindinger A, Böhm M. Predictors of outcome in patients with suspected myocarditis. Circulation. 2008;118(6):639–48.
13. Billingham ME. Acute myocarditis: is sampling error a contraindication for diagnostic biopsies? J Am Coll Cardiol. 1989;14:921–2.
14. Edwards WD, Holmes DR, Reeders GS. Diagnosis of active lymphocytic myocarditis by endomyocardial biopsy: quantitative criteria for light microscopy. Mayo Clin Proc. 1982;57:419–25.
15. Edwards WD. Myocarditis and endomyocardial biopsy. Cardiol Clin. 1984;2:647–56.
16. Edwards WD. Current problems in establishing quantitative histopathologic criteria for the diagnosis of lymphocytic myocarditis by endomyocardial biopsy. Heart Vessel. 1985;1:138–42.
17. Chow LH, Radio SJ, Sears TD, McManus BM. Insensitivity of right ventricular endomyocardial biopsy in the diagnosis of myocarditis. J Am Coll Cardiol. 1989;14:915–20.

18. Hauck AJ, Kearney DL, Edwards WD. Evaluation of postmortem endomyocardial biopsy specimens from 38 patients with lymphocytic myocarditis: implications for role of sampling error. Mayo Clin Proc. 1989;64:1235–45.
19. Thiene G, Bartoloni G, Poletti A, Boffa GM. Tecniche, indicazioni ed utilità della biopsia endomiocardica. In: Baroldi G, Thiene G, editors. Biopsia endomiocardica—Testo atlante. Padova: Edizioni Piccin; 1996. p. 5–45.
20. Burke AP, Farb A, Robinowitz M, Virmani R. Serial sectioning and multiple level examination of endomyocardial biopsies for the diagnosis of myocarditis. Mod Pathol. 1991;4:690–3.
21. Frustaci A, Bellocci F, Osen EG. Results of biventricular endomyocardial biopsy in survivors of cardiac arrest with apparently normal hearts. Am J Cardiol. 1994;74:890–5.
22. Thiene G, Bruneval P, Veinot J, Leone O. Diagnostic use of the endo-myocardial biopsy: a consensus statement. Virchows Arch. 2013;463:1–5.
23. Dominguez F, Kühl U, Pieske B, Garcia-Pavia P, Tschöpe C. Update on Myocarditis and Inflammatory Cardiomyopathy: Reemergence of Endomyocardial Biopsy. Rev Esp Cardiol (Engl Ed). 2016;69:178–87A.
24. Leone O, Veinot JP, Angelini A, Baandrup UT, Basso C, Berry G, Bruneval P, Burke M, Butany J, Calabrese F, d'Amati G, Edwards WD, Fallon JT, Fishbein MC, Gallagher PJ, Halushka MK, McManus B, Pucci A, Rodriguez ER, Saffitz JE, Sheppard MN, Steenbergen C, Stone JR, Tan C, Thiene G, van der Wal AC, Winters GL. 2011 consensus statement on endomyocardial biopsy from the Association for European Cardiovascular Pathology and the Society for Cardiovascular Pathology. Cardiovasc Pathol. 2012;21:245–74.
25. Caforio AL, Marcolongo R, Basso C, Iliceto S. Clinical presentation and diagnosis of myocarditis. Heart. 2015;101:1332–44.
26. Aretz HT, Billingham ME, Edwards WD, Factor SM, Fallon JT, Fenoglio JJ, Olsen EG, Schoen FJ. Myocarditis. A histopathologic definition and classification. Am J Cardiovasc Pathol. 1987;1:3–14.
27. Aretz HT. Myocarditis: the Dallas criteria. Hum Pathol. 1987;18:619–24.
28. Cooper LT Jr. Myocarditis. N Engl J Med. 2009;360:1526–38.
29. Baughman KL. Diagnosis of myocarditis: death of Dallas criteria. Circulation. 2006;113:593–5.
30. Basso C, Calabrese F, Angelini A, Carturan E, Thiene G. Classification and histological, immunohistochemical, and molecular diagnosis of inflammatory myocardial disease. Heart Fail Rev. 2013;18:673–81.
31. Calabrese F, Angelini A, Carturan E, Thiene G. Myocarditis and inflammatory cardiomyopathy: histomorphological diagnosis. In: Schultheiss HP, Kapp JF, Grotzbach G, editors. Chronic viral and inflammatory cardiomyopathy. Berlin: Springer; 2006. p. 305–21.
32. Hauck AJ, Edwards ED. Histopathologic examination of tissues obtained by endomyocardial biopsy. In: Fowles RE, editor. Cardiac biopsy. Mount Kisco: Futura; 1992. p. 95–153.
33. Linder J, Cassling RS, Rogler WC, Wilson JE, Markin RS, Sears TD, McManus BM. Immunohistochemical characterization of lymphocytes in uninflamed ventricular myocardium. Implications for myocarditis. Arch Pathol Lab Med. 1985;109:917–20.
34. Schnitt SJ, Ciano PS, Schoen FJ. Quantitation of lymphocytes in endomyocardial biopsies: use and limitations of antibodies to leukocyte common antigen. Hum Pathol. 1987;18:796–800.
35. Tazelaar HD, Billingham ME. Myocardial lymphocytes. Fact, fancy or myocarditis? Am J Cardiovasc Pathol. 1987;1:47–50.
36. Woudstra L, Biesbroek PS, Emmens RW, Heymans S, Juffermans LJ, van der Wal AC, van Rossum AC, Niessen HWM, Krijnen PAJ. CD45 is a more sensitive marker than CD3 to diagnose lymphocytic myocarditis in the endomyocardium. Hum Pathol. 2017;62:83–90.
37. Cihakova D, Rose NR. Pathogenesis of myocarditis and dilated cardiomyopathy. Adv Immunol. 2008;99:95–114.
38. Maisch B, Portig I, Ristic A, Hufnagel G, Pankuweit S. Definition of inflammatory cardiomyopathy (myocarditis): on the way to consensus. A status report. Herz. 2000;25:200–9.
39. Okura Y, Dec GW, Hare JM, Kodama M, Berry GJ, Tazelaar HD, Bailey KR, Cooper LT. A clinical and histopathologic comparison of cardiac sarcoidosis and idiopathic giant cell myocarditis. J Am Coll Cardiol. 2003;41:322–9.

40. Blauwet LA, Cooper LT. Idiopathic giant cell myocarditis and cardiac sarcoidosis. Heart Fail Rev. 2013;18:733–46.
41. Cooper LT Jr, Berry GJ, Shabetai R. Idiopathic giant-cell myocarditis – natural history and treatment. Multicenter giant cell myocarditis study group investigators. N Engl J Med. 1997;336:1860–6.
42. Cooper LT Jr, Hare JM, Tazelaar HD, Edwards WD, Starling RC, Deng MC, Menon S, Mullen GM, Jaski B, Bailey KR, Cunningham MW, Dec GW. Usefulness of immunosuppression for giant cell myocarditis. Am J Cardiol. 2008;102(11):1535–9.
43. Maleszewski JJ, Orellana VM, Hodge DO, Kuhl U, Schultheiss HP, Cooper LT. Long-term risk of recurrence, morbidity and mortality in giant cell myocarditis. Am J Cardiol. 2015;115:1733–8.
44. Perazzolo Marra M, Thiene G, Rizzo S, De Lazzari M, Carturan E, Tona F, Caforio AL, Cacciavillani L, Marcolongo R, Tarantini G, Corbetti F, Iliceto S, Basso C. Cardiac magnetic resonance features of biopsy-proven endomyocardial diseases. JACC Cardiovasc Imaging. 2014;7:309–12.
45. Basso C, Aguilera B, Banner J, Cohle S, d'Amati G, de Gouveia RH, di Gioia C, Fabre A, Gallagher PJ, Leone O, Lucena J, Mitrofanova L, Molina P, Parsons S, Rizzo S, Sheppard MN, Mier MPS, Kim Suvarna S, Thiene G, van der Wal A, Vink A, Michaud K, Association for European Cardiovascular Pathology. Guidelines for autopsy investigation of sudden cardiac death: 2017 update from the Association for European Cardiovascular Pathology. Virchows Arch. 2017;471:691–705.
46. Basso C, Carturan E, Corrado D, Thiene G. Myocarditis and dilated cardiomyopathy in athletes: diagnosis, management, and recommendations for sport activity. Cardiol Clin. 2007;25:423–9.
47. Basso C, Calabrese F, Corrado D, Thiene G. Postmortem diagnosis in sudden cardiac death victims: macroscopic, microscopic and molecular findings. Cardiovasc Res. 2001;50:290–300.
48. Maron BJ, Udelson JE, Bonow RO, et al. Eligibility and disqualification recommendations for competitive athletes with cardiovascular abnormalities: task force 3: hypertrophic cardiomyopathy, arrhythmogenic right ventricular cardiomyopathy and other cardiomyopathies, and myocarditis: a scientific statement from the American Heart Association and American College of Cardiology. J Am Coll Cardiol. 2015;66:2362–71.
49. Calabrese F, Thiene G. Myocarditis and inflammatory cardiomyopathy: microbiological and molecular biological aspects. Cardiovasc Res. 2003;60:11–25.
50. Calabrese F, Carturan E, Thiene G. Cardiac infections: focus on molecular diagnosis. Cardiovasc Pathol. 2010;19:171–82.
51. Chapman NM, Tracy S, Gauntt CJ, Fortmueller U. Molecular detection and identification of enteroviruses using enzymatic amplification and nucleic acid hybridization. J Clin Microbiol. 1990;28:843–50.
52. Hilton DA, Variend S, Pringle JH. Demonstration of Coxsackie virus RNA in formalin-fixed tissue sections from childhood myocarditis cases by in situ hybridization and the polymerase chain reaction. J Pathol. 1993;170:45–51.
53. Jin O, Sole MJ, Butany JW, Chia WK, McLaughlin PR, Liu P, Liew CC. Detection of enterovirus RNA in myocardial biopsies from patients with myocarditis and cardiomyopathy using gene amplification by polymerase chain reaction. Circulation. 1990;82:8–16.
54. Grasso M, Arbustini E, Silini E, Diegoli M, Percivalle E, Ratti G, Bramerio M, Gavazzi A, Vigano M, Milanesi G. Search for Coxsackievirus B3 RNA in idiopathic dilated cardiomyopathy using gene amplification by polymerase chain reaction. Am J Cardiol. 1992;69:658–64.
55. Petitjean J, Kopecka H, Freymuth F, Langlard JM, Scanu P, Galateau F, Bouhour JB, Ferrière M, Charbonneau P, Komajda M. Detection of enterovirus in endomyocardial biopsy by molecular approach. J Med Virol. 1993;41:260.
56. Martin AB, Webber S, Fricker FJ, Jaffe R, Demmler G, Kearney D, Zhang YH, Bodurtha J, Gelb B, Ni J. Acute myocarditis. Rapid diagnosis by PCR in children. Circulation. 1994;90:330–9.
57. Pauschinger M, Bowles NE, Fuentes-Garcia FJ, Pham V, Kühl U, Schwimmbeck PL, Schultheiss HP, Towbin JA. Detection of adenoviral genome in the myocardium of adult patients with idiopathic left ventricular dysfunction. Circulation. 1999;99:1348–54.

58. Calabrese F, Valente M, Thiene G, Angelini A, Testolin L, Biasolo MA, Soteriou B, Livi U, Palù G. Enteroviral genome in native hearts may influence outcome of patients who undergo cardiac transplantation. Diagn Mol Pathol. 1999;8:39–46.
59. Calabrese F, Rigo E, Milanesi O, Boffa GM, Angelini A, Valente M, Thiene G. Molecular diagnosis of myocarditis and dilated cardiomyopathy in children. Clinico-pathologic features and prognostic implications. Diagn Mol Pathol. 2002;11:212–21.
60. Kuhl U, Pauschinger M, Noutsias M, Seeberg B, Bock T, Lassner D, Poller W, Kandolf R, Schultheiss HP. High prevalence of viral genomes and multiple viral infections in the myocardium of adults with "idiopathic" left ventricular dysfunction. Circulation. 2005;111:887–93.
61. Kühl U, Pauschinger M, Seeberg B, Lassner D, Noutsias M, Poller W, Schultheiss HP. Viral persistence in the myocardium is associated with progressive cardiac dysfunction. Circulation. 2005;112:1965–70.
62. Caforio AL, Calabrese F, Angelini A, Tona F, Vinci A, Bottaro S, Ramondo A, Carturan E, Iliceto S, Thiene G, Daliento L. A prospective study of biopsy-proven myocarditis: prognostic relevance of clinical and aetiopathogenetic features at diagnosis. Eur Heart J. 2007;28:1326–33.
63. Akhtar N, Ni J, Stromberg D, Rosenthal GL, Bowles NE, Towbin JA. Tracheal aspirate as a substrate for polymerase chain reaction detection of viral genome in childhood pneumonia and myocarditis. Circulation. 1999;99:2011–8.
64. Carturan E, Milanesi O, Kato Y, Giacometti C, Biffanti R, Thiene G, Calabrese F. Viral detection and tumor necrosis factor alpha profile in tracheal aspirates from children with suspicion of myocarditis. Diagn Mol Pathol. 2008;17:21–7.
65. Breinholt JP, Moulik M, Dreyer WJ, Denfield SW, Kim JJ, Jefferies JL, Rossano JW, Gates CM, Clunie SK, Bowles KR, Kearney DL, Bowles NE, Towbin JA. Viral epidemiologic shift in inflammatory heart disease: the increasing involvement of parvovirus B19 in the myocardium of pediatric cardiac transplant patients. J Heart Lung Transplant. 2010;29:739–46.
66. Heymans S, Eriksson U, Lehtonen J, Cooper LT Jr. The quest for new approaches in myocarditis and inflammatory cardiomyopathy. J Am Coll Cardiol. 2016;68:2348–64.
67. Dunn JJ, Chapman NM, Tracy S, Romero JR. Genomic determinants of cardiovirulence in coxsackievirus B3 clinical isolates: localization to the 5′ non-translated region. J Virol. 2000;74:4787–94.
68. Höfling K, Kim KS, Leser JS, Chapman NM, Willian S, Gauntt CJ, Tracy S. Progress toward vaccines against virus that cause heart disease. Herz. 2000;25:286–90.
69. Lam KM, Oldenburg N, Khan MA, Gaylore V, Mikhail GW, Strouhal PD, Middeldorp JM, Banner N, Yacoub M. Significance of reverse transcription polymerase chain reaction in the detection of human cytomegalovirus gene transcripts in thoracic organ transplant recipients. J Heart Lung Transplant. 1998;17:555–65.
70. Pauschinger M, Phan MD, Doerner A, Kuehl U, Schwimmbeck PL, Poller W, Kandolf R, Schultheiss HP. Enteroviral RNA replication in the myocardium of patients with left ventricular dysfunction and clinically suspected myocarditis. Circulation. 1999;99:889–95.
71. Katano H, Kano M, Nakamura T, Kanno T, Asanuma H, Sata T. A novel real-time PCR system for simultaneous detection of human viruses in clinical samples from patients with uncertain diagnoses. J Med Virol. 2011;83:322–30.
72. Mahrholdt H, Goedecke C, Wagner A, Meinhardt G, Athanasiadis A, Vogelsberg H, Fritz P, Klingel K, Kandolf R, Sechtem U. Cardiovascular magnetic resonance assessment of human myocarditis: a comparison to histology and molecular pathology. Circulation. 2004;109:1250–8.
73. Donoso Mantke O, Meyer R, Prösch S, Nitsche A, Leitmeyer K, Kallies R, Niedrig M. High prevalence of cardiotropic viruses in myocardial tissue from explanted hearts of heart transplant recipients and heart donors: a 3-year retrospective study from a German patients' pool. J Heart Lung Transplant. 2005;24:1632–8.
74. Schenk T, Enders M, Pollak S, Hahn R, Huzly D. High prevalence of human parvovirus B19 DNA in myocardial autopsy samples from subjects without myocarditis or dilative cardiomyopathy. J Clin Microbiol. 2009;47:106–10.

75. Wang X, Zhang G, Liu F, Han M, Xu D, Zang Y. Prevalence of human parvovirus B19 DNA in cardiac tissues of patients with congenital heart diseases indicated by nested PCR and in situ hybridization. J Clin Virol. 2004;31:20–4.
76. Stewart GC, Lopez-Molina J, Gottumukkala RV, Rosner GF, Anello MS, Hecht JL, Winters GL, Padera RF, Baughman KL, Lipes MA. Myocardial parvovirus B19 persistence: lack of association with clinicopathologic phenotype in adults with heart failure. Circ Heart Fail. 2011;4:71–8.
77. De Salvia A, De Leo D, Carturan E, Basso C. Sudden cardiac death, borderline myocarditis and molecular diagnosis: evidence or assumption? Med Sci Law. 2011;51(Suppl 1):S27–9.
78. Bültmann BD, Klingel K, Sotlar K, Bock CT, Baba HA, Sauter M, Kandolf R. Fatal parvovirus B19-associated myocarditis clinically mimicking ischemic heart disease: an endothelial cell-mediated disease. Hum Pathol. 2003;34:92–5.
79. Bock CT, Klingel K, Kandolf R. Human parvovirus B19-associated myocarditis. N Engl J Med. 2010;362:1248–9.
80. Chimenti C, Russo A, Pieroni M, Calabrese F, Verardo R, Thiene G, Russo MA, Maseri A, Frustaci A. Intramyocyte detection of Epstein-Barr virus genome by laser capture microdissection in patients with inflammatory cardiomyopathy. Circulation. 2004;110:3534–9.
81. Heidecker B, Kittleson MM, Kasper EK, Wittstein IS, Champion HC, Russell SD, Hruban RH, Rodriguez ER, Baughman KL, Hare JM. Transcriptomic biomarkers for the accurate diagnosis of myocarditis. Circulation. 2011;123:1174–84.
82. Park JH, Kim DS, Cho YJ, Kim YJ, Jeong SY, Lee SM, Cho SJ, Yun CW, Jo I, Nam JH. Attenuation of coxsackievirus B3 by VP2 mutation and its application as a vaccine against virus-induced myocarditis and pancreatitis. Vaccine. 2009;27:1974–83.
83. Pinkert S, Westermann D, Wang X, Klingel K, Dörner A, Savvatis K, Grössl T, Krohn S, Tschöpe C, Zeichhardt H, Kotsch K, Weitmann K, Hoffmann W, Schultheiss HP, Spiller OB, Poller W, Fechner H. Prevention of cardiac dysfunction in acute coxsackievirus B3 cardiomyopathy by inducible expression of a soluble coxsackievirus-adenovirus receptor. Circulation. 2009;120:2358–66.
84. Barry SP, Townsend PA, Latchman DS, Stephanou A. Role of the JAK-STAT pathway in myocardial injury. Trends Mol Med. 2007;13:82–9.
85. Calabrese F, Carturan E, Chimenti C, Pieroni M, Agostini C, Angelini A, Crosato M, Valente M, Boffa GM, Frustaci A, Thiene G. Overexpression of tumor necrosis factor (TNF) alpha and TNF alpha receptor I in human viral myocarditis: clinicopathologic correlations. Mod Pathol. 2004;17:1108–18.
86. Fung G, Luo H, Qiu Y, Yang D, Mcmanus B. Myocarditis. Circ Res. 2016;118:496–514.

2 Clinical Presentation of Myocarditis

Alida L. P. Caforio, Renzo Marcolongo, Chun-Yan Cheng, Anna Baritussio, Giuseppe Tarantini, and Sabino Iliceto

2.1 Introduction

Myocarditis has a heterogeneous spectrum of clinical presentations, ranging from mild to severe [1]. It may be paucisymptomatic, with a slow and insidious course, leading to delayed diagnosis. It may also have a distinct onset of unexplained cardiac signs and symptoms up to rapidly progressive or fulminant forms, which include life-threatening arrhythmias and aborted sudden death, cardiogenic shock and severely impaired left ventricular function (Table 2.1) [1]. Myocarditis may also mimic non-inflammatory myocardial diseases; for instance, in hyper-acute myocarditis the echocardiographic appearance of increased wall thickness may resemble hypertrophic cardiomyopathy, or in acute-coronary-syndrome like myocarditis, segmental wall motion abnormalities may be similar to those observed in an acute coronary syndrome [1–7]. Cardiac signs and symptoms lack specificity, depending on the degree of myocardial inflammation and ventricular dysfunction, and may be subtle; thus, the disease may be unrecognised [8–13]. Myocarditis is a diagnosis of exclusion. Clinical suspicion of the disease should be high if cardiac

A. L. P. Caforio (✉) · C.-Y. Cheng · A. Baritussio
Cardiology, Department of Cardiac, Thoracic, Vascular Sciences and Public Health, Padua University, Padova, Italy

Cardioimmunology Outpatient Clinic, Padua University, Padova, Italy
e-mail: alida.caforio@unipd.it; 073047chengchunyan@163.com; anna.baritussio@gmail.com

R. Marcolongo
Cardioimmunology Outpatient Clinic, Padua University, Padova, Italy

Haematology and Clinical Immunology Unit, Department of Medicine, Padua University, Padova, Italy
e-mail: renzo.marcolongo@tiscali.it

G. Tarantini · S. Iliceto
Cardiology, Department of Cardiac, Thoracic, Vascular Sciences and Public Health, Padua University, Padova, Italy
e-mail: giuseppe.tarantini.1@unipd.it; sabino.iliceto@unipd.it

A. L. P. Caforio (ed.), *Myocarditis*, https://doi.org/10.1007/978-3-030-35276-9_2

Table 2.1 Clinical presentations of patients with biopsy-proven myocarditis (modified from [1])

1. *Acute coronary syndrome-like*
(a) Acute chest pain
– Frequently starting within 1–4 weeks of a respiratory or gastrointestinal infection
– Symptoms may be severe and recurrent, similar to ischaemic pain if pericarditis is associated
– In the absence of angiographic evidence of CAD
(b) ST/T-wave changes
– ST-segment elevation or depression
– T-wave inversions
(c) With or without normal global or regional LV and/or RV dysfunction on echocardiography or CMR
(d) With or without increased TnT/TnI, that may have a time course similar to acute myocardial infarction or a prolonged and sustained release over several weeks or months
(e) Reactive C protein (RCP) most frequently within normal range, may be increased if associated pericarditis is present
(f) It may present as Takotsubo cardiomyopathy
2. *New onset or worsening heart failure* in the absence of CAD and known causes of heart failure:
(a) New onset or progressive heart failure *over 2 weeks to 3 months*
– Dyspnoea
– Peripheral oedema
– Chest discomfort
– Fatigue
(b) Impaired systolic LV and/or RV function, with or without an increase in wall thickness, with or without dilated LV and/or RV on echocardiography or CMR
(c) Symptoms possibly started after a respiratory or gastrointestinal infection, or in the peripartum period
(d) Non-specific ECG signs, bundle branch block, AV-block and/or ventricular arrhythmias
3. *Chronic heart failure* in the absence of CAD and known causes of heart failure (see point 2 above):
(a) Heart failure symptoms (with recurrent exacerbations) of >*3 months duration*
(b) Fatigue, palpitation, dyspnoea, atypical chest pain, arrhythmia in an ambulant patient
(c) Impaired systolic LV and/or RV function on echocardiography or CMR suggestive of DCM or non-ischaemic cardiomyopathy
(d) Non-specific ECG signs, sometimes bundle branch block and/or ventricular arrhythmias and/or AV-block
4. *"Life-threatening condition"*, in the absence of CAD and known causes of heart failure comprising
(a) Life-threatening arrhythmias and aborted sudden death
(b) Cardiogenic shock
(c) Severely impaired LV function
5. *Asymptomatic*, occasional finding of unexplained arrhythmia at cardiac screening (ECG, 24 h Holter monitoring), and/or impaired systolic LV and/or RV function on echocardiography and/or CMR pattern suggestive of non-ischaemic DCM or myocarditis

Table 2.1 (continued)

6. *Paucisymptomatic* (unexplained fatigue, palpitation, dyspnoea, atypical chest pain, arrhythmia, syncope, in an ambulant patient) with abnormal ECG, 24 h Holter monitoring and/or impaired systolic LV and/or RV function on echocardiography and/or CMR pattern suggestive of non-ischaemic DCM or myocarditis
7. *Mixed presentations*, e.g. (1) combined with (2) or (3)

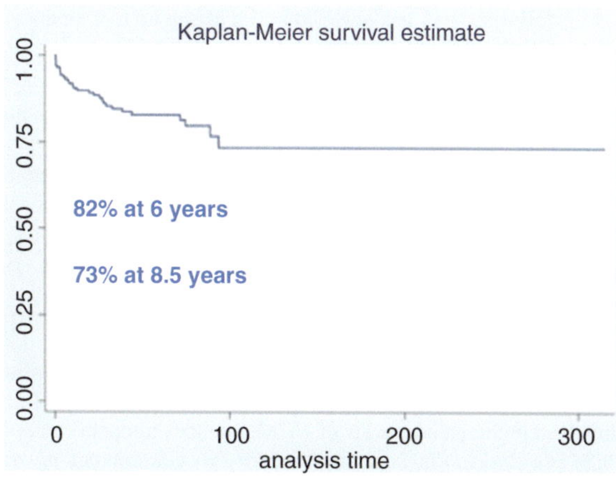

Fig. 2.1 Biopsy-proven myocarditis: actuarial survival free from death or heart transplantation in a contemporary prospective Padua cohort ($n = 214$) prior to introduction of immunosuppressive therapy (end of December, year 2010) [14]

signs and symptoms are unexplained and occurring in predominantly young or middle-aged male patients with few or no coronary artery disease risk factors, although it may be observed in the elderly. Myocarditis may resolve spontaneously, recur or progress, leading about 25% of biopsy-proven cases to dilated cardiomyopathy (DCM), sudden or heart failure-related death or heart transplantation [1–4, 9, 10]. Figure 2.1 shows an actuarial survival free from death or heart transplantation of 90% at 1 year, 82% at 6 years and 73% at 8.5 years in a contemporary prospective cohort of 214 biopsy-proven patients from the Padova Cardioimmunology Outpatient Clinic with a median follow-up of 55 (13–89.5) months (reported in December 2010, prior to introduction of immunosuppressive therapy) [14]. In keeping with expert consensus and current classifications, the diagnosis of certainty and aetiological diagnosis in myocarditis require endomyocardial biopsy (EMB); the definitions used here are those recommended by the World Health Organization/International Society and Federation of Cardiology (WHO/ISFC) and the 2013 European Society of Cardiology (ESC) myocarditis expert position statement and are summarised in Table 2.2 [1, 4, 15–19]. The various aetiological forms of myocarditis are summarised in Table 2.3 [1]. The incidence of myocarditis is difficult to assess, due to the fact that diagnostic gold standard, EMB, is not used in all cases where the disease is suspected clinically and/or at non-invasive cardiac imaging [1]. Autopsy studies on sudden cardiac death in young people report a highly variable prevalence, ranging from 2 to 42% of cases [19]. Biopsy-proven myocarditis is reported in 9–16% of adult patients with unexplained non-ischaemic dilated cardiomyopathy (DCM) [3, 6] and in 46% of children with an identified cause of DCM [8]. Most clinical studies show a higher frequency of myocarditis and DCM in males [1].

Table 2.2 Definitions

Definite (Biopsy-Proven) Myocarditis (WHO /ISFC, ESC) [1, 15–17]
Inflammatory disease of the myocardium diagnosed by (1) established histological, (2) immunohistochemical and (3) immunological criteria
(1) Established histological Dallas criteria [17] defined as follows: "histological evidence of inflammatory infiltrates within the myocardium associated with myocyte degeneration and necrosis of non-ischaemic origin"
(2) Immunohistochemical criteria, abnormal inflammatory infiltrate [1, 18, 19] defined as follows: "≥14 leucocytes/mm^2 including up to 4 monocytes/mm^2 with the presence of CD 3 positive T-lymphocytes ≥ 7 cells/mm^2"
(3) Immunological criteria and myocarditis aetiology defined as follows [1]:
– Viral: Histology (Hx) and immunoHx positive (pos), polymerase chain reaction (PCR) pos for ≥virus
– Autoimmune: Hx and immunoHx pos; viral PCR negative (neg); with or without pos cardiac autoantibodies (aabs); exclusion of other known inflammatory causes
– Viral and immune[a]: Hx and immunoHx pos; viral PCR pos; cardiac aabs pos
Inflammatory Cardiomyopathy and Dilated Cardiomyopathy (DCM) (WHO /ISFC, ESC)[b] [15–17]
Myocarditis in association with cardiac dysfunction

[a]N.B. a follow-up EMB may identify persistent viral myocarditis, resolved myocarditis (Hx and virological), or persistent virus-negative myocarditis, e.g. post-infectious autoimmune
[b]Involved in the pathogenesis of DCM, includes idiopathic, autoimmune and infectious subtypes. *DCM is a clinical diagnosis characterised by dilation and impaired contraction of the left or both ventricles that is not explained by abnormal loading conditions or coronary artery disease*. DCM includes idiopathic, familial/genetic, viral and/or immune, alcoholic/toxic subtypes

Table 2.3 Etiological forms of myocarditis (modified from reference [1])

Infectious myocarditis	
Bacterial	Staphylococcus, Streptococcus, Pneumococcus, Meningococcus, Gonococcus, Salmonella, Corynebacterium diphtheriae, Haemophilus influenzae, Mycobacterium (tuberculosis), Mycoplasma pneumoniae, Brucella
Spirochaetal	Borrelia (Lyme disease), Leptospira (Weil disease)
Fungal	Aspergillus, Actinomyces, Blastomyces, Candida, Coccidioides, Cryptococcus, Histoplasma, Mucormycosis, Nocardia, Sporothrix
Protozoal	Trypanosoma cruzi, Toxoplasma gondii, Entamoeba, Leishmania
Parasitic	Trichinella spiralis, Echinococcus granulosus, Taenia solium, Toxocara canis
Rickettsial	Coxiella burnetii (Q fever), R. rickettsii (Rocky Mountain spotted fever), R. tsutsugamuschi
Viral	RNA viruses: Coxsackieviruses A and B, echoviruses, polioviruses, influenza A and B viruses, respiratory syncytial virus, mumps virus, measles virus, rubella virus, hepatitis C virus, dengue virus, yellow fever virus, chikungunya virus, Junin virus, Lassa fever virus, rabies virus, human immunodeficiency virus-1
	DNA viruses: Adenoviruses, parvovirus B19, cytomegalovirus, human herpes virus-6, Epstein–Barr virus, varicella-zoster virus, herpes simplex virus, variola virus, vaccinia virus

Table 2.3 (continued)

Infectious myocarditis	
Immune-mediated myocarditis	
Allergens	Tetanus toxoid, vaccines, serum sickness
	Drugs: Penicillin, cefaclor, colchicine, furosemide, isoniazid, lidocaine, tetracycline, sulfonamides, phenytoin, phenylbutazone, methyldopa, thiazide diuretics, amitriptyline
Alloantigens	Heart transplant rejection
Autoantigens	Organ-specific: Infection-negative lymphocytic, giant cell
	Associated with other organ-specific or systemic immune-mediated disorders (SIDs): Systemic lupus erythematosus, rheumatoid arthritis, eosinophilic granulomatosis with polyangiitis (EGPA, formerly Churg–Strauss syndrome), Kawasaki's disease, inflammatory bowel disease, scleroderma, polymyositis, myasthenia gravis, insulin-dependent diabetes mellitus, thyrotoxicosis, sarcoidosis, granulomatosis with polyangiitis (GPA, formerly Wegener's granulomatosis), rheumatic heart disease (rheumatic fever)
Toxic myocarditis	
Drugs	Amphetamines, anthracyclines, cocaine, cyclophosphamide, ethanol, fluorouracil, lithium, catecholamines, hemetine, interleukin-2, trastuzumab, clozapine, mesalazine
Heavy metals	Copper, iron, lead (rare, more commonly cause intramyocyte accumulation)
Miscellaneous	Scorpion sting, snake, and spider bites, bee and wasp stings, carbon monoxide, inhalants, phosphorus, arsenic, sodium azide
Hormones	Phaeochromocytoma, vitamins: Beri-beri
Physical agents	Radiation, electric shock

2.2 Possible Myocarditis Presentations According to the 2013 ESC Myocarditis Expert Position Statement (Table 2.1)

2.2.1 Acute Coronary-Syndrome Like

A common clinical scenario entails a previously asymptomatic subject with few coronary artery disease risk factors who, days or weeks after a presumed viral respiratory or gastrointestinal prodromal phase, with or without increased systemic inflammatory markers and fever, develops one or more of the following features: (1) dyspnoea/orthopnoea, (2) palpitation, (3) effort intolerance/malaise, (4) heart failure, (5) chest pain (which may be pleuritic if concomitant pericarditis is present) and (6) cardiac troponin release with a time curve similar to that seen in acute myocardial infarction or prolonged over days/weeks, occasionally months, and reveals unobstructed coronary arteries [1–13, 20–23]. This scenario, dominated by pseudo-infarct presentation with normal coronary arteries, may become relapsing/recurrent with a variable level of troponin release.

2.2.2 New-Onset (Days up to 3 Months) or Worsening Heart Failure

Biopsy-proven myocarditis may be the underlying aetiology of acute or fulminant non-ischaemic unexplained heart failure with or with a DCM phenotype [1–13, 20, 24]. The fulminant presentation has been described as having (1) a viral prodromal phase within 4 weeks from the onset of cardiac symptoms, (2) a distinct onset of life-threatening unexplained heart failure, (3) haemodynamic compromise and/or cardiogenic shock and (4) good prognosis, at least in the reported series [25], which excluded specific forms with dismal prognosis, in particular giant cell myocarditis [24]. Myocarditis should be differentiated from peripartum [1, 2] or Takotsubo cardiomyopathy [26] and from arrhythmogenic right ventricular cardiomyopathy (ARVC) [27]. Non-inflammatory causes (e.g. valve heart disease, pericardial constriction, coronary artery disease) should always be excluded.

2.2.3 Subacute/Chronic (>3 Months) or Worsening Heart Failure

Biopsy-proven myocarditis may also be found in patients with a long (from >3 months to several years) symptom duration, with recurrent exacerbations, or in paucisymptomatic ambulant subjects, with a smouldering course, and a history of fatigue, palpitation, dyspnoea, atypical chest pain and arrhythmia. LV and/or RV function on echocardiography or CMR may be mildly, moderately or severely impaired, with or without increased ventricular dilation, suggesting a DCM or non-ischaemic hypokinetic non-dilated cardiomyopathy [28, 29]. Tissue characterisation by CMR may reveal normal findings, active myocardial inflammation or fibrotic changes with a non-ischaemic late gadolinium enhancement (LGE) pattern [11–13, 30, 31]. ECG findings are often abnormal, non-specific, sometimes bundle branch block and/or ventricular arrhythmias and/or AV-block may be present. Table 2.4 shows that univariate predictors of death or heart transplantation at presentation in the prospective biopsy-proven cohort from Padova Cardioimmunology Outpatient Clinic before the introduction of immunosuppressive therapy [14]. Negative predictors included young age, female gender, heart failure presentation, advanced NYHA class, giant cell myocarditis, high titre anti-nuclear antibody, lower left ventricular ejection fraction, high left ventricular end-diastolic volume and other haemodynamic or echocardiographic indexes of biventricular dysfunction.

2.2.4 Life-Threatening

Myocarditis should always be suspected, in the absence of coronary artery disease and of other known causes, in patients with:

(a) Life-threatening arrhythmias and aborted sudden death
(b) Cardiogenic shock
(c) Severely impaired LV function

Table 2.4 Univariate predictors of death/transplant in biopsy-proven myocarditis prior to introduction of immunosuppressive therapy—Prospective Padova Myocarditis Cohort December 2010 [14]

	Alive ($n = 153$)	Dead or transplanted ($n = 34$)	P
Age at presentation (years, mean ± SD)	39 ± 16	31 ± 19	0.018
Female gender (%)	51 (33)	20 (59)	0.006
History of myocarditis (yes/no)[a]	22/130	6/27	NS
Heart failure presentation (%)[b]	63 (41)	28 (82%)	0.000
NYHA class (II-IV)[b]	64 (42)	32 (79%)	0.001
Dallas class (active/borderline)[c]	77/69	16/17	NS
Giant cell myocarditis (%)[b]	2 (1.3)	4 (12%)	0.002
Viral polymerase chain reaction(positive/negative)[d]	32/86	7/13	NS
ANA (positive/negative)[e]	15/105	7/15	0.01
Left atrium dimension-Echo (mm)	40 ± 9	48 ± 15	0.04
LV EDV-Echo (mL/m^2)	86 ± 35	110 ± 52	0.04
LVEF-Echo (%)	45 ± 14	31 ± 12	0.000
LVSP (mmHg)	119 ± 20	102 ± 28	0.001
RA mean (mmHg)	4 ± 3	8 ± 6	0.006
Angiographic LVEF (%)	50 ± 17	31 ± 17	0.000
CO (L/min)	3.6 ± 1.7	2.7 ± 0.7	0.002
Angiographic LVEDV (mL/m^2)	105 ± 42	139 ± 45	0.005

Total of patients $n = 187$, lost to follow-up $n = 27$

ANA anti-nuclear autoantibody, *CO* cardiac output at cardiac catheterisation, *Echo* standard transthoracic echocardiography, *LVEDV* left ventricular end-diastolic volume, *LVEF* left ventricular ejection fraction, *LVSP* left ventricular systolic pressure at cardiac catheterisation, *RA mean* right atrial mean pressure at cardiac catheterisation

[a]Available data on 185 patients

[b]Available data on 186 patients

[c]Non diagnostic (Dallas criteria in the remainder of patients' BEM)

[d]Available data on 138 patients

[e]Available data on 142 patients

The arrhythmia presentation includes the whole clinical spectrum from mildly symptomatic brady- or tachyarrhythmia or occasional finding of significant arrhythmia at cardiac screening to syncope or aborted sudden death [1–13, 24].

Patients with one of the life-threatening presentations, particularly if haemodynamically unstable or refractory to standard cardiological therapy, should be promptly referred to centres with expertise in EMB as well as in advanced mechanical assist devices, as a bridge to recovery or to heart transplantation. In these patients, EMB is a class I indication [1, 4, 14, 19], as it may reveal forms susceptible of aetiology-directed therapy, e.g. immunosuppression for idiopathic giant cell myocarditis or idiopathic eosinophilic myocarditis.

2.2.5 Asymptomatic/Oligosymptomatic and Combined Scenarios

Myocarditis may ultimately be diagnosed in asymptomatic patients with occasional findings of unexplained arrhythmia at cardiac screening (ECG, 24 h Holter monitoring), and/or impaired systolic LV and/or RV function on echocardiography and/or CMR patterns suggestive of non-ischaemic DCM or myocarditis. Similarly, ambulant patients may have unexplained fatigue, palpitation, dyspnoea, atypical chest pain, with abnormal ECG, 24 h Holter monitoring, and/or impaired systolic LV and/or RV function on echocardiography and/or CMR pattern suggestive of non-ischaemic DCM or myocarditis.

The clinical presentation may also combine one or more scenarios (Table 2.1), for instance pseudo-myocardial infarct and arrhythmia, or heart failure [1].

2.2.6 Ancillary Features

Ancillary features in the family history include presence of DCM, other cardiomyopathy, sudden cardiac death and extra-cardiac autoimmune disease among relatives. Additional ancillary findings in the patient's history include previous clinically suspected (according to ESC 2013 criteria) or biopsy-proven myocarditis, recent (days to 2 weeks) upper respiratory or gastrointestinal suspected viral syndrome, allergy, other autoimmune diseases, heavy alcohol intake, consumption of drugs and toxic substances (e.g. cocaine), peripartum period, vaccines, travel to places where specific cardiotropic infection is possible or endemic (e.g. Brazil, Argentina and Chile for Chagas' disease), proximity with domestic animals, conventional coronary risk factors, etc. The aim is to search as well as exclude possible treatable causes (e.g. drug-related toxicity or hypersensitivity) (Table 2.3) [1]. The diagnosis of clinically suspected myocarditis according to ESC criteria may be given with or without ancillary features, although their presence strengthens the clinical suspicion [1].

2.3 Possible Myocarditis Diagnostic Findings According to the 2013 ESC Myocarditis Expert Position Statement

2.3.1 Category I: Electrocardiographic (ECG) and/or Holter and/or Stress Testing

Electrocardiographic (ECG) findings commonly lack specificity [1–13, 20, 24]. In myocarditis, ST-T segment elevation is more concave (convex in ischaemia) and diffusely present over the precordial leads, without reciprocal changes. PR depression is frequently present in pericarditis associated with myocarditis, but is rare in cardiac ischaemia. Q-waves are uncommon in myocarditis. T-wave inversion generally occurs after complete ST-T normalisation in myocarditis, but usually takes place while the ST segment is still elevated after myocardial infarction.

Possible diagnostic features include newly abnormal 12 lead ECG and/or Holter and/or stress testing, in particular any of the following:

> I to III-degree atrioventricular block, or bundle branch block, ST/T wave change, sinus arrest, ventricular tachycardia or fibrillation and asystole, atrial fibrillation, reduced R wave height, intraventricular conduction delay (widened QRS complex), abnormal Q waves, low voltage, frequent premature beats, supraventricular tachycardia [1].

2.3.2 Category II. Biomarkers of Necrosis, Inflammation, Heart Failure

Erythrocyte sedimentation rate and reactive C protein levels are not raised in the majority of patients with biopsy-proven myocarditis and conversely are a major feature in acute pericarditis [1, 2, 9]. Cardiac troponins do not differentiate ischaemic from inflammatory myocyte injury, may be raised in several other conditions and when normal do not exclude myocarditis [1, 2, 9, 23]. This also applies to brain natriuretic peptides, circulating cytokines and other markers [1]. Positive viral serology does not imply active myocardial infection [32–35] and does not correlate with EMB findings [35]. Viral serology is not generally recommended, except for hepatitis C, rickettsial phase 1 and phase 2, Lyme disease in endemic areas as well as human immunodeficiency virus serologies in high-risk patients and populations [1]. Serum anti-heart autoantibodies (AHA) contribute to the aetiological diagnosis of autoimmune myocarditis in index cases and identify relatives at risk [1, 2, 19, 28, 29, 36–41]. Some of them may have a functional and prognostic role [36, 42–61].

Possible diagnostic findings for category II include *increased cardiac troponins*.

2.3.3 Category III: Functional and Structural Abnormalities on Cardiac Imaging (Echo/Angio/CMR) and Category IV: Tissue Characterisation (CMR)

Echocardiography defines morphology and biventricular function, but it is not specific [62, 63]. Apical left ventricular aneurisms suggest Chagas's disease. In fulminant myocarditis, there may be an increase in left ventricular wall thickness and a mildly dilated severely hypokinetic ventricle [62].

Cardiac magnetic resonance (CMR) imaging defines morphology and function and provides tissue characterisation [1, 11–13, 30]. The Lake-Louise criteria [30] are used to differentiate myocarditis from non-inflammatory aetiologies and are incorporated into the 2013 ESC Task Force criteria for clinically suspected myocarditis [1]. CMR does not differentiate specific inflammatory cells (e.g. lymphocytes, giant cells) or viral from non-viral myocarditis [1, 11–13, 30, 31]. Gallium-67 scintigraphy and positron emission tomography with fluorodeoxyglucose may be of great value in the acute phase and in the follow-up of cardiac sarcoidosis [64].

Possible diagnostic findings for category III include new, otherwise unexplained left ventricular (LV) and/or right ventricular (RV) functional and structural abnormalities on cardiac imaging (echo/angio/cardiac magnetic resonance), including incidental finding in apparently asymptomatic subjects, in particular any of the following:

Regional wall motion or global systolic or diastolic abnormality, with or without ventricular dilatation, with or without increased wall thickness, with or without pericardial effusion, with or without endocavitary thrombi [1].

Possible diagnostic findings for category IV include:

Oedema and/or late gadolinium enhancement (LGE) of classical myocarditis pattern (according to Lake-Louise criteria) [20].

2.4 Clinically Suspected and Definite (Biopsy-Proven) Myocarditis: The 2013 Task Force Criteria

In 2013 ESC Myocarditis Task Force has introduced new criteria for clinically suspected myocarditis, using the combination of ≥1 plausible clinical presentation and ≥1 diagnostic criteria from different categories, as well as exclusion of known non-inflammatory causes, e.g. coronary artery disease that could explain the syndrome (Fig. 2.2) [1]. These criteria were proposed to better refine the clinical and non-invasive diagnosis of myocarditis also in centres that do not routinely perform EMB.

In clinically suspected myocarditis, it is recommended to consider selective coronary angiography and EMB, including histology, immunohistochemistry and PCR detection of infectious agents [1, 19] since:

- EMB, including conventional histology (Dallas criteria), immunohistochemistry and PCR detection of infectious agents, is the diagnostic gold standard.
- Absence of infectious agents identifies immune-mediated myocarditis, either primary or post-infectious if an infectious agent had been identified on a previous EMB and is the basis for safe (infection negative) immunosuppression [1, 65]. EMB is essential to identify specific myocarditis types (e.g. giant cell, eosinophilic, sarcoidosis) which imply different treatments and prognosis [1, 2, 10, 19, 20].

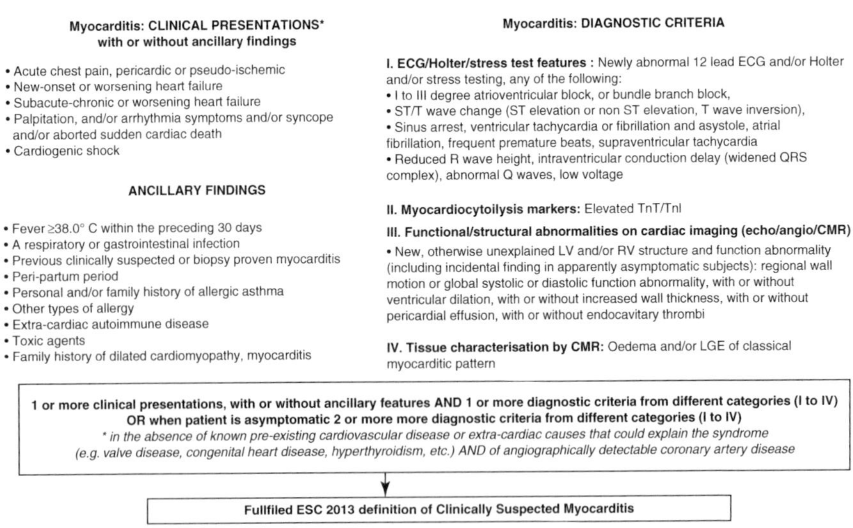

Fig. 2.2 The 2013 ESC Task Force criteria of clinically suspected myocarditis [1]

- EMB provides differential diagnosis from diseases that may mimic myocarditis (arrhythmogenic right ventricular cardiomyopathy, Takotsubo cardiomyopathy, peripartum cardiomyopathy, infiltrative/storage disorders, cardiac masses) [4, 19].
- If EMB is performed in experienced centres, its complication rate (0–0.8) is similar to that of standard coronary angiography [1, 65–67].

2.5 Clinical Presentation of Specific Forms of Myocarditis

Lyme disease, caused by the *spirochete* Borrelia burgdorferi, can result in a variety of presentations, from asymptomatic first-degree to advanced heart block or to transient life-threatening myocardial dysfunction [68]. Advanced heart block may require temporary pacing; it resolves within 1 week in most cases following appropriate antibiotic treatment.

Trypanosoma cruzi (Chagas' disease), a common cause of myocarditis/DCM in South America with a suggested post-infectious autoimmune component, has an acute phase of mild febrile course, and a prolonged (up to 30 years) symptom-free latent phase [69]. Systolic and diastolic heart failure, ventricular aneurisms, arrhythmias and cardiac autonomic dysfunction may be present.

Toxoplasma gondii associated and fungal myocarditis is mainly observed among sero-negative cardiac transplant recipients of sero-positive donors and in other immune-deficient populations with multiple opportunistic infections, in particular HIV [1].

Giant cell myocarditis, the prototype of autoimmune myocarditis, a rare but devastating disease, is characterised by a rapid and severe downhill course, despite optimal standard care [1, 2, 4, 19, 20, 24, 70]. If the diagnosis is reached early and cardiac damage is not massive, giant cell myocarditis can be stabilised on immunosuppression. It may be associated with other autoimmune disorders and with up to 25% recurrence rate in the native heart after recovery and in the donor heart following transplantation; relapse in both conditions usually responds to intensified immunosuppression [1, 2, 4, 19, 20, 24, 70]. The disease is discussed in detail in Chap. 12.

Sarcoidosis is a systemic granulomatous immune-mediated disease [64]. Heart involvement may occur at any time and does not correlate with other extra-cardiac locations. Sarcoid granulomas may involve any site of the heart, although left ventricular free wall, posterior interventricular septum, papillary muscles, the atria and the right ventricle are most frequently affected [64]. Ventricular septum and conduction system involvement can lead to brady- or tachyarrhythmia and sudden cardiac death [4, 64]. Myocarditis should be suspected if a patient with known sarcoidosis develops conduction blocks, tachyarrhythmia, congestive cardiac failure or DCM [71]. If the right ventricle is involved, cardiac sarcoid should be differentiated from ARVC. Since sarcoid lesions are focal, sensitivity of EMB may be low due to sampling error, and the definitive diagnosis of cardiac involvement is based on a multiparametric approach, often including CMR and PET [64]. If positive, EMB provides differential diagnosis from idiopathic GCM and other infectious granulomatous forms (e.g. mycobacteria, Bartonella henselae, Toxoplasma gondii and Yersinia) [19]. Myocarditis in sarcoidosis and in other immune-mediated systemic diseases is discussed in Chap. 11 [72–76].

Hypersensitivity myocarditis, probably the most common form of drug-induced cardiac toxicity, is unpredictable, and not related to drug dosage (Table 2.3). Non-specific skin rash, malaise, fever and eosinophilia may suggest the diagnosis, but are absent in many cases [19, 20, 77]. Conversely, a *direct cardiac toxicity* is dose-dependent, may be reversible and is often potentiated by other anti-neoplastic treatments, such as radiotherapy (see Chap. 12).

2.5.1 Myocarditis in Rheumatic Heart Disease

Rheumatic fever (RF) is still a leading cause of acquired cardiac disease in the world, but recent EMB-based studies are lacking, since RF is rare in Europe and North America; most of the literature on this subject dates back to the 1950s. It is unclear whether or not myocarditis in RF can be defined as infectious or post-infectious autoimmune according to the 2013 Task Force criteria [19, 20, 78–80]. Rheumatic myocarditis is thought to be a component of acute rheumatic carditis, which also includes pericarditis and valvulitis. However, in acute rheumatic myocarditis, histopathology reveals no necrosis and for this feature there are authors who have questioned that rheumatic myocarditis exists [19, 20, 78–80]. The diagnostic criteria are summarised in Table 2.5. Rheumatic myocarditis may be asymptomatic or present tachycardia or mild heart failure, a first-degree atrioventricular heart block and mild to moderate pericardial effusion (rarely pericardial tamponade) [19, 20, 78–80]. The main endocardial lesions, the rheumatic *verrucae*, are nowadays visualised by transoesophageal echocardiography as small multiple vegetations on the edge of native valves. Imaging techniques that highlight inflammation in the heart may also be useful, e.g. Gallium-67 myocardium scintigraphy [19,

Table 2.5 Rheumatic heart disease: diagnostic criteria [79, 80]

• Rheumatic fever (RF) is an inflammatory multisystem disease, occurring few weeks to 6 months following group A streptococcal (GAS) infection of the tonsillopharynx. Its diagnosis dates back to the 1992 revised Jones' criteria [80]
• Major criteria:
– Carditis, polyarthritis, chorea, erythema marginatum, subcutaneous nodules
• Minor criteria:
– Fever, arthralgia, elevated erythrocyte sedimentation rate or C-reactive protein, prolonged P-R interval on standard 12-lead ECG
• If supported by evidence of GAS, e.g. positive throat culture or rapid streptococcal antigen test, high or rising streptococcal antibody titre, the presence of two major criteria (or one major and two minor) indicates a high probability of acute RF
• The diagnosis of cardiac involvement during acute RF is based upon fulfilment of any of the following features:
– New onset of nonfunctional cardiac murmurs; cardiac enlargement; sign and symptoms of heart failure; pericardial friction rubs or pericardial effusion

20, 78]. Positron-emission scintigraphy associated with tomography (PET-CT) is being evaluated [19, 20, 78]. Acute rheumatic myocarditis is a difficult diagnosis that should be considered in any patient, including patients who have just undergone valve surgery, with rheumatic valvular heart disease who present with a sudden worsening of heart failure symptoms or rapid-onset ventricular dysfunction, particularly if the patient is not on secondary prophylaxis for RF. However, myocarditis in RF only occasionally leads to important pump dysfunction [19, 20]. Even patients with severe myocardial dysfunction seem to resolve with corticosteroid treatment [78–80]. Management of RF and rheumatic carditis is reviewed elsewhere [79, 80].

2.6 Conclusion

Clinical presentation of myocarditis lacks specificity; thus clinical suspicion needs to be supported by non-invasive diagnostic tools, including CMR with tissue characterisation. The diagnosis of certainty and of myocarditis aetiology requires EMB, after exclusion of non-inflammatory causes. The ESC 2013 Task Force recommends a systematic consideration of EMB in clinically suspected myocarditis [1]. EMB should not be limited to standard histology, but include immunohistochemistry and molecular analysis for infectious agents and should be performed by experienced teams. The rationale for this effort is the availability of a wide range of antiviral [1] (see Chap. 17), immunosuppressive [9, 20, 65, 70, 81] and immunomodulatory therapies [1, 9, 20, 59] for infection-negative patients, to stop or control the chronic immune-mediated cardiac tissue injury leading to post-inflammatory irreversible DCM (see Chaps. 14, 15, and 16) [20]. For some specific forms of myocarditis, immunosuppression is established [1, 4, 9, 18, 19, 23, 31, 67, 69–74], but more evidence-based data from multicentre-controlled trials are needed in the majority of patients with infection-negative myocarditis.

References

1. Caforio ALP, Pankuweit S, Arbustini E, et al. Current state of knowledge on aetiology, diagnosis, management and therapy of myocarditis. A position statement of the European Society of Cardiology Working Group on myocardial and pericardial diseases. Eur Heart J. 2013;34:2636–48.
2. Caforio AL, Calabrese F, Angelini A, et al. A prospective study of biopsy-proven myocarditis: prognostic relevance of clinical and aetiopathogenetic features at diagnosis. Eur Heart J. 2007;28:1326–33.
3. Mason JW, O'Connell JB, Herskowitz A, et al. A clinical trial of immunosuppressive therapy for myocarditis. N Engl J Med. 1995;333:269–75.
4. Cooper LT, Baughman KL, Feldman AM, et al. The role of endomyocardial biopsy in the management of cardiovascular disease: a scientific statement from the American Heart Association, the American College of Cardiology, and the European Society of Cardiology. Endorsed by the Heart Failure Society of America and the Heart Failure Association of the European Society of Cardiology. J Am Coll Cardiol. 2007;50:1914–31.

5. Bock CT, Klingel K, Kandolf R. Human parvovirus B19-associated myocarditis. N Engl J Med. 2010;362:1248–9.
6. Felker GM, Hu W, Hare JW, Hruban RH, Baughman KL, Kasper EK. The spectrum of dilated cardiomyopathy. The Johns Hopkins experience in 1278 patients. Medicine. 1999;78:270–83.
7. Martin AB, Webber S, Fricker FJ, et al. Acute myocarditis, rapid diagnosis by PCR in children. Circulation. 1994;90:330–9.
8. Towbin JA, Lowe AM, Colan SD, Sleeper LA, Orav EJ, Clunie S, Messere J, Cox GF, Lurie PR, Hsu D, Canter C, Wilkinson JD, Lipshultz SE. Incidence, causes, and outcomes of dilated cardiomyopathy in children. JAMA. 2006;296:1867–76.
9. Schultheiss HP, Kühl U, Cooper LT. The management of myocarditis. Eur Heart J. 2011;32:2616–25.
10. Kindermann I, Kindermann M, Kandolf R, et al. Predictors of outcome in patients with suspected myocarditis. Circulation. 2008;118:639–48.
11. Francone M, Chimenti C, Galea N, et al. CMR sensitivity varies with clinical presentation and extent of cell necrosis in biopsy-proven acute myocarditis. JACC Cardiovasc Imaging. 2014 Mar;7:254–63.
12. Röttgen R, Christiani R, Freyhardt P, et al. Magnetic resonance imaging findings in acute myocarditis and correlation with immunohistological parameters. Eur Radiol. 2011;21:1259–66.
13. Mahrholdt H, Goedecke C, Wagner A, Meinhardt G, Athanasiadis A, Vogelsberg H, Fritz P, Klingel K, Kandolf R, Sechtem U, et al. Circulation. 2004;109(10):1250–8.
14. Caforio ALP, Angelini A, Calabrese F, et al. Biopsy-proven myocarditis: young age, female gender and right ventricular dysfunction at diagnosis are independent predictors of death or transplantation in a contemporary prospective series. American Heart Association 2010 scientific sessions. Circulation. 2010;122:A17976.
15. Richardson P, McKenna WJ, Bristow M, et al. Report of the 1995 World Health Organization/International Society and Federation of Cardiology Task Force on the definition and classification of cardiomyopathies. Circulation. 1996;93:841–2.
16. Elliott P, Andersson B, Arbustini E, et al. Classification of the cardiomyopathies: a position statement from the European Society of Cardiology working group on myocardial and pericardial disease. Eur Heart J. 2007;29:270–6.
17. Aretz HT, Billingham ME, Edwards WE, et al. Myocarditis: a histopathologic definition and classification. Am J Cardiovasc Pathol. 1985;1:1–10.
18. Maisch B, Bültmann B, Factor S, Gröne H-J, Hufnagel G, Kawamura K, Kühl U, Olsen EJ, Pankuweit S, Virmani R, McKenna W, Richardson PJ, Thiene G, Schultheiss HP, Sekiguchi M. World heart federation consensus conferences's definition of inflammatory cardiomyopathy (myocarditis): report from two expert committees on histology and viral cardiomyopathy. Heartbeat. 1999;4:3–4.
19. Leone O, Veinot JP, Angelini A, et al. 2011 consensus statement on endomyocardial biopsy from the Association for European Cardiovascular Pathology and the Society for Cardiovascular Pathology. Cardiovasc Pathol. 2012;21:245–74.
20. Caforio ALP, Marcolongo R, Jahns R, et al. Immune-mediated and autoimmune myocarditis: clinical presentation, diagnosis and treatment. Heart Fail Rev. 2013;18:715–32.
21. Kuhl U, Pauschinger M, Bock T, Klingel K, Schwimmbeck CP, Seeberg B, Krautwurm L, Poller W, Schultheiss HP, Kandolf R. Parvovirus B19 infection mimicking acute myocardial infarction. Circulation. 2003;108:945–50.
22. Yilmaz A, Mahrholdt H, Athanasiadis A, Vogelsberg H, Meinhardt G, Voehringer M, Kispert EM, Deluigi C, Baccouche H, Spodarev E, Klingel K, Kandolf R, Sechtem U. Coronary vasospasm as the underlying cause of chest pain in patients with PVB19 myocarditis. Heart. 2008;94:1456–63.
23. Agewall S, Beltrame JF, Reynolds HR, Niessner A, Rosano G, Caforio AL, De Caterina R, Zimarino M, Roffi M, Kjeldsen K, Atar D, Kaski JC, Sechtem U, Tornvall P, WG on Cardiovascular Pharmacotherapy. ESC working group position paper on myocardial infarction with non-obstructive coronary arteries. Eur Heart J. 2017;38(3):143–53.
24. Kandolin R, Lehtonen J, Kupari M. Cardiac sarcoidosis and giant cell myocarditis as causes of atrioventricular block in young and middle-aged adults. Circ Arrhythm Electrophysiol. 2011;4(3):303–9.

25. McCarthy RE, Boehmer JP, Hruban RH, Hutchins GM, Kasper EK, Hare JM, Baughman KL. Long-term outcome of fulminant myocarditis as compared with acute (nonfulminant) myocarditis. N Engl J Med. 2000;342:690–5.
26. Caforio ALP, Tona F, Vinci A, Calabrese F, Ramondo A, Cacciavillani L, Corbetti F, Leoni L, Thiene G, Iliceto S, Angelini A. Acute biopsy-proven lymphocytic myocarditis mimicking Takotsubo cardiomyopathy. Eur J Heart Fail. 2009;11:428–31.
27. Basso C, Thiene G, Corrado D, Angelini A, Nava A, Valente M. Arrhythmogenic right ventricular cardiomyopathy. Dysplasia, dystrophy, or myocarditis? Circulation. 1996;94(5):983–91.
28. Pinto YM, Elliott PM, Arbustini E, Adler Y, Anastasakis A, Böhm M, Duboc D, Gimeno J, de Groote P, Imazio M, Heymans S, Klingel K, Komajda M, Limongelli G, Linhart A, Mogensen J, Moon J, Pieper PG, Seferovic PM, Schueler S, Zamorano JL, Caforio AL, Charron P. Proposal for a revised definition of dilated cardiomyopathy, hypokinetic non-dilated cardiomyopathy, and its implications for clinical practice: a position statement of the ESC working group on myocardial and pericardial diseases. Eur Heart J. 2016;37(23):1850–8.
29. Schultheiss HP, Fairweather DL, Caforio ALP, Escher F, Hershberger RE, Lipshultz SE, Liu P, Matsumori A, Mazzanti A, Mcmurray J, Priori SG. Dilated cardiomyopathy. Nat Rev Dis Primers. 2019;5:32.
30. Friedrich G, Sechtem U, Schulz-Menger J, International Consensus Group on Cardiovascular Magnetic Resonance in Myocarditis, et al. Cardiovascular magnetic resonance in myocarditis: a JACC white paper. J Am Coll Cardiol. 2009;53:1475–87.
31. Baccouche H, Mahrholdt H, Meinhardt G, Merher R, Voehringer M, Hill S, Klingel K, Kandolf R, Sechtem U, Yilmaz A. Diagnostic synergy of non-invasive cardiovascular magnetic resonance and invasive endomyocardial biopsy in troponin-positive patients without coronary artery disease. Eur Heart J. 2009. 2009;30:2869–79.
32. Bozkurt B, Colvin M, Cook J, Cooper LT, Deswal A, Fonarow GC, Francis GS, Lenihan D, Lewis EF, McNamara DM, Pahl E, Vasan RS, Ramasubbu K, Rasmusson K, Towbin JA, Yancy C, American Heart Association Committee on Heart Failure and Transplantation of the Council on Clinical Cardiology, Council on Cardiovascular Disease in the Young, Council on Cardiovascular and Stroke Nursing, Council on Epidemiology and Prevention, Council on Quality of Care and Outcomes Research. Current diagnostic and treatment strategies for specific dilated cardiomyopathies: a scientific statement from the American Heart Association. Circulation. 2016;134(23):e579–646.
33. Pankuweit S, Klingel K. Viral myocarditis: from experimental models to molecular diagnosis in patients. Heart Fail Rev. 2013;18:683–702.
34. Klingel K, Hohenadl C, Canu A, Albrecht M, Seemann M, Mall G, Kandolf R. Ongoing enterovirus-induced myocarditis is associated with persistent heart muscle infection: quantitative analysis of virus replication, tissue damage, and inflammation. Proc Natl Acad Sci U S A. 1992;89(1):314–8.
35. Mahfoud F, Gärtner B, Kindermann M, Ukena C, Gadomski K, Klingel K, Kandolf R, Böhm M, Kindermann I. Virus serology in patients with suspected myocarditis: utility or futility? Eur Heart J. 2011;32:897–903.
36. Caforio ALP, Tona F, Bottaro S, Vinci A, Daliento L, Thiene G, Iliceto S. Clinical implications of anti-heart autoantibodies in myocarditis and dilated cardiomyopathy. Autoimmunity. 2008;41(1):35–45.
37. Caforio AL, Keeling PJ, Zachara E, Mestroni L, Camerini F, Mann JM, Bottazzo GF, McKenna WJ. Evidence from family studies for autoimmunity in dilated cardiomyopathy. Lancet. 1994;344:773–7.
38. Caforio AL, Mahon NG, Baig MK, Tona F, Murphy RT, Elliott PM, McKenna WJ. Prospective familial assessment in dilated cardiomyopathy. Cardiac autoantibodies predict disease development in asymptomatic relatives. Circulation. 2007;115:76–83. https://doi.org/10.1038/s41572-019-0084-1.
39. Caforio ALP, Bonifacio E, Stewart JT, et al. Novel organ-specific circulating cardiac autoantibodies in dilated cardiomyopathy. J Am Coll Cardiol. 1990;15:1527–34.
40. Caforio ALP, Goldman JH, Haven AJ, Baig KM, Dalla Libera L, McKenna WJ. Circulating cardiac autoantibodies as markers of autoimmunity in clinical and biopsy-proven myocarditis. Eur Heart J. 1997;18:270–5.

41. Caforio ALP, Grazzini M, Mann JM, Keeling PJ, Bottazzo GF, McKenna WJ, Schiaffino S. Identification of α-and β-cardiac myosin heavy chain isoforms as major autoantigens in dilated cardiomyopathy. Circulation. 1992;85:1734–42.
42. Li Y, Heuser JS, Cunningham LC, Kosanke SD, Cunningham MW. Mimicry and antibody-mediated cell signaling in autoimmune myocarditis. J Immunol. 2006;177:8234–40.
43. Okazaki T, Honjo T. Pathogenic roles of cardiac autoantibodies in dilated cardiomyopathy. Trends Mol Med. 2005;11:322–6.
44. Warraich RS, Griffiths E, Falconar A, Pabbathi V, Bell C, Angelini G, Suleiman MS, Yacoub MH. Human cardiac myosin autoantibodies impair myocyte contractility: a cause-and-effect relationship. FASEB J. 2006;20:651–60.
45. Lauer B, Schannwell M, Kuhl U, Strauer BE, Schultheiss HP. Antimyosin autoantibodies are associated with deterioration of systolic and diastolic left ventricular function in patients with chronic myocarditis. J Am Coll Cardiol. 2000;35:11–8.
46. Wallukat G, Morwinski M, Kowal K, Förster A, Boewer V, Wollenberger A. Antibodies against the β-adrenergic receptor in human myocarditis and dilated cardiomyopathy: β-adrenergic agonism without desensitization. Eur Heart J. 1991;12(Suppl D):178–81.
47. Magnusson Y, Wallukat G, Waagstein F, Hjalmarson A, Hoebeke J. Autoimmunity in idiopathic dilated cardiomyopathy: characterization of antibodies against the beta 1-adrenoceptor with positive chronotropic effect. Circulation. 1994;89:2760–667.
48. Muller J, Wallukat G, Dandel M, Bieda H, Brandes K, Spiegelsberger S, Nissen E, Kunze R, Hetzer R. Immunoglobulin adsorption in patients with idiopathic dilated cardiomyopathy. Circulation. 2000;101:385–91.
49. Staudt A, Bohm M, Knebel F, Grosse Y, Bischoff C, Hummel A, Dahm JB, Borges A, Jochmann N, Wernecke KD, Wallukat G, Baumann G, Felix SB. Potential role of autoantibodies belonging to the immunoglobulin G-3 subclass in cardiac dysfunction among patients with dilated cardiomyopathy. Circulation. 2002;106:2448–53.
50. Nishimura H, Okazaki T, Tanaka Y, Nakatani K, Hara M, Matsumori A, Sasayama S, Mizoguchi A, Hiai H, Minato N, Honjo T. Autoimmune dilated cardiomyopathy in PD-1 receptor-deficient mice. Science. 2001;291:319–22.
51. Okazaki T, Tanaka Y, Nishio R, Mitsuiye T, Mizoguchi A, Wang J, Ishida M, Hiai H, Matsumori A, Minato N, Honjo T. Autoantibodies against cardiac troponin I are responsible for dilated cardiomyopathy in PD-1-deficient mice. Nat Med. 2003;9:1477–83.
52. Schultheiss HP, Ulrich G, Janda I, Melzner B, Ulrich G, Morad M. Antibody mediated enhancement of calcium permeability in cardiac myocytes. J Exp Med. 1988;168:2105–19.
53. Jahns R, Boivin V, Hein L, Triebel S, Angermann CE, Ertl G, Lohse MJ. Direct evidence for a β1-adrenergic receptor directed autoimmune attack as a cause of idiopathic dilated cardiomyopathy. J Clin Invest. 2004;113:1419–29.
54. Fu LX, Magnusson Y, Bergh CH, Liljeqvist JA, Waagstein F, Hjalmarson A, Hoebeke J. Localization of a functional autoimmune epitope on the muscarinic acetylcholine receptor-2 in patients with idiopathic dilated cardiomyopathy. J Clin Invest. 1993;91:1964–8.
55. Nikolaev VO, Boivin V, Störk S, Angermann CE, Ertl G, Lohse MJ, Jahns R. A novel fluorescent method for the rapid detection of functional beta1-adrenergic receptor autoantibodies in heart failure. J Am Coll Cardiol. 2007;50:423–31.
56. Maisch B, Deeg P, Liebau G, Kochsiek K. Diagnostic relevance of humoral and cytotoxic immune reactions in primary and secondary dilated cardiomyopathy. Am J Cardiol. 1983;52:1072–8.
57. Christ T, Wettwer E, Dobrev D, Adolph E, Knaut M, Wallukat G, Ravens U. Autoantibodies against the beta1 adrenoceptor from patients with dilated cardiomyopathy prolong action potential duration and enhance contractility in isolated cardiomyocytes. J Mol Cell Cardiol. 2001;33:1515–25.
58. Staudt Y, Mobini R, Fu M, Felix SB, Kühn JP, Staudt A. Beta1-adrenoceptor antibodies induce apoptosis in adult isolated cardiomyocytes. Eur J Pharmacol. 2003;466:1–6.

59. Trimpert C, Herda LR, Eckerle LG, Pohle S, Müller C, Landsberger M, Felix SB, Staudt A. Immunoadsorption in dilated cardiomyopathy: long-term reduction of cardiodepressant antibodies. Eur J Clin Investig. 2010;40:685–91.
60. Schulze K, Becker BF, Schauer R, Schultheiss HP. Antibodies to ADP-ATP carrierDOUBLEHYPHENan autoantigen in myocarditis and dilated cardiomyopathyDOUBLEHYPHENimpair cardiac function. Circulation. 1990;81:959–69.
61. Caforio AL, Angelini A, Blank M, Shani A, Kivity S, Goddard G, Doria A, Schiavo A, Testolina M, Bottaro S, Marcolongo R, Thiene G, Iliceto S, Shoenfeld Y. Passive transfer of affinity-purified anti-heart autoantibodies (AHA) from sera of patients with myocarditis induces experimental myocarditis in mice. Int J Cardiol. 2015;179:166–77.
62. Felker GM, Boehmer JP, Hruban RH, Hutchins GM, Kasper EK, Baughman KL, Hare JM. Echocardiographic findings in fulminant and acute myocarditis. J Am Coll Cardiol. 2000;36:227–32.
63. Pinamonti B, Alberti E, Cigalotto A, Dreas L, Salvi A, Silvestri F, Camerini F. Echocardiographic findings in myocarditis. Am J Cardiol. 1988;62:285–91.
64. Sekhri V, Sanal S, Delorenzo LJ, Aronow WS, Maguire GP. Cardiac sarcoidosis: a comprehensive review. Arch Med Sci. 2011;7(4):546–54.
65. Frustaci A, Russo MA, Chimenti C. Randomized study on the efficacy of immunosuppressive therapy in patients with virus-negative inflammatory cardiomyopathy: the TIMIC study. Eur Heart J. 2009;30:1995–2002.
66. Yilmaz A, Kindermann I, Kindermann M, Mahfoud F, Ukena C, Athanasiadis A, Hill S, Mahrholdt H, Voehringer M, Schieber M, Klingel K, Kandolf R, Böhm M, Sechtem U. Comparative evaluation of left and right ventricular endomyocardial biopsy: differences in complication rate and diagnostic performance. Circulation. 2010;122:900–9.
67. Holzmann M, Nicko A, Kühl U, Noutsias M, Poller W, Hoffmann W, Morguet A, Witzenbichler B, Tschöpe C, Schultheiss HP, Pauschinger M. Complication rate of right ventricular endomyocardial biopsy via the femoral approach: a retrospective and prospective study analyzing 3048 diagnostic procedures over an 11-year period. Circulation. 2008;118:1722–8.
68. Costello JM, Alexander ME, Greco KM, Perez-Atayde AR, Laussen PC. Lyme carditis in children: presentation, predictive factors, and clinical course. Pediatrics. 2009;123(5):e835–41.
69. Fernandes F, Valente Moreira CH, Barbosa-Ferreira JM, Sabino EC. Chagas cardiomyopathy. In: Nussinovitch U, editor. The heart in rheumatologic, inflammatory and autoimmune diseases. Cambridge: Academic; 2017. p. 553–74.
70. Cooper LT Jr, Hare JM, Tazelaar HD, Edwards WD, Starling RC, Deng MC, Menon S, Mullen GM, Jaski B, Bailey KR, Cunningham MW, Dec GW, Giant Cell Myocarditis Treatment Trial Investigators. Usefulness of immunosuppression for giant cell myocarditis. Am J Cardiol. 2008;102(11):1535–9.
71. Birnie DH, Sauer WH, Bogun F, Cooper JM, Culver DA, Duvernoy CS, Judson MA, Kron J, Mehta D, Cosedis Nielsen J, Patel AR, Ohe T, Raatikainen P, Soejima K. HRS expert consensus statement on the diagnosis and management of arrhythmias associated with cardiac sarcoidosis. Heart Rhythm. 2014;11:1305–23.
72. Neumann T, Manger B, Schmid M, et al. Cardiac involvement in Churg-Strauss syndrome: impact of endomyocarditis. Medicine. 2009;88:236–43.
73. Oliveira GH, Seward JB, Tsang TS, Specks U. Echocardiographic findings in patients with Wegener granulomatosis. Mayo Clin Proc. 2005;80:1435–40.
74. Frustaci A, Gentiloni N, Caldarulo M. Acute myocarditis and left ventricular aneurism as presentations of systemic lupus erythematosus. Chest. 1996;109:282–4.
75. Dankó K, Ponyi A, Constantin T, et al. Long-term survival of patients with idiopathic inflammatory myopathies according to clinical features: a longitudinal study of 162 cases. Medicine. 2004;83:35–42.
76. Courand PY, Croisille P, Khouatra C, et al. Churg-Strauss syndrome presenting with acute myocarditis and cardiogenic shock. Heart Lung Circ. 2012;21:178–81.

77. Japanese Circulation Society (JCS) Joint Working Group. Guidelines for diagnosis and treatment of myocarditis. Circ J. 2011;75:734–43.
78. Spina GS, Sampaio RO, Branco CE, Miranda GB, Rosa VE, Tarasoutchi F. Incidental histological diagnosis of acute rheumatic myocarditis: case report and review of the literature. Front Pediatr. 2014;2:126. https://doi.org/10.3389/fped.2014.00126.
79. Guilherme L, Sampaio RO, Freschi De Barros S, Köhler KF, Spina GS, Tarasoutchi F, Kalil J. Rheumatic fever and rheumatic heart disease. In: Nussinovitch U, editor. The heart in rheumatologic, inflammatory and autoimmune diseases. Cambridge: Academic; 2017. p. 529–48.
80. Dajani AS, et al. Guidelines for the diagnosis of rheumatic fever: Jones criteria, updated 1992. JAMA. 1992;268(15):2069–73.
81. Wojnicz R, Nowalany-Kozielska E, Wojciechowska C, Glanowska G, Wilczewski P, Niklewski T, Zembala M, Polonski L, Rozek MM, Wodniecki J. Randomized, placebo controlled study for immunosuppressive treatment of inflammatory dilated cardiomyopathy. Two-year follow-up results. Circulation. 2001;104:39–45.

Endomyocardial Biopsy

3

Cristina Chimenti and Andrea Frustaci

Endomyocardial biopsy (EMB) of the right ventricle (RV) and left ventricle (LV) was introduced into clinical practice in 1963 by Sekiguchi and Konno [1] and gradually became a recognized, valuable diagnostic investigation for primary myocardial diseases.

Over the years, the development of new techniques such as immunohistochemistry, in situ hybridization, and polymerase chain reaction to detect a myocardial viral infection improved the diagnostic performance on EMB tissue. On the other hand, the development of new therapies for specific myocardial diseases, administrable on the basis of histological and molecular diagnosis, has given adjunctive value to the contribution of EMB.

The role of EMB in the management of cardiovascular disease was described for the first time in a joint scientific statement from the American Heart Association (AHA), the American College of Cardiology, and the European Society of Cardiology in 2007 [2]. A group of experts identified several clinical scenarios in which the value of EMB was weighed against the procedural risks. In subsequent years, other position papers confirm the important role of this procedure, particularly in myocarditis, where it is recognized as the diagnostic gold standard [3, 4].

Nevertheless, the use of EMB procedure is still controversial because of concerns about the risk of complications due to the invasive nature of the procedure and the uncertain diagnostic contribution.

C. Chimenti · A. Frustaci (✉)
Cardiovascular, Respiratory, Nephrological, Anaesthetic and Geriatric Sciences Department, La Sapienza University, Rome, Italy

IRCCS L Spallanzani, Rome, Italy
e-mail: cristina.chimenti@uniroma1.it; biocard@inmi.it

A. L. P. Caforio (ed.), *Myocarditis*, https://doi.org/10.1007/978-3-030-35276-9_3

3.1 Techniques and Safety of Endomyocardial Biopsy

The most common approaches for EMB procedures are through the right internal jugular vein, and the femoral vein, for the EMB taken from the right ventricular site of the interventricular septum (RVEMB) and through the femoral artery, for the EMB of the left side of the interventricular septum (LVEMB) [5–7].

The right internal jugular vein is the most common percutaneous access site for RVEMB in the USA. In Germany and Italy, the femoral vein is commonly used for percutaneous access [2]. Sonographic techniques, to identify location, size, and respiratory phasic variation in size of the internal jugular vein, decrease duration of the procedure and complications. EMB via the femoral approach is safely performed under fluoroscopic guidance.

In our center from 1989 to 2008, more than 4000 patients underwent diagnostic EMB [8].

EMB was usually performed in the left, right, or both ventricles, approached with a King's bioptome until 1990 and afterward by BIPAL biopsy forceps (Cordis Corporation 430 Route 22 East Bridgewater, NJ 08807) using a 7F (501-613A Cordis Corporation 430 Route 22 East Bridgewater, NJ 08807) long sheet introduced from a right and/or left femoral access (Fig. 3.1a). A long sheath with angulated tip is introduced through the femoral vein and used for right ventricular EMB, while a long sheath with straight tip is introduced through the femoral artery and used for left ventricular EMB. The left ventricular EMB procedure starts with a 7F pigtail guiding catheter that is introduced into the long sheath and then passed retrogradely through the aortic valve into the left ventricle using a standard J tip guide wire. Once the sheath is positioned near to the segment of the left ventricle where the biopsy should be performed, the guiding catheter is withdrawn through the sheath. The bioptome is advanced through the guiding sheath into the left ventricle under biplane fluoroscopic control (30° RAO and 60° LAO) which helps to guide the tip of the catheter to the target area. The site of the biopsy is identified on a radiographic view using flashing of contrast medium. For right ventricular biopsy, a 7F pigtail guiding catheter inserted into the sheath with angulated tip is advanced over a J tip guide wire into the right ventricle. Under fluoroscopic control at 30° RAO, the tip of the guiding catheter is positioned in the septal position. Then the guiding catheter is withdrawn through the sheath, the bioptome is advanced, and the biopsies are taken from the septum. Coronary angiography is always performed before the EMB procedure. EMBs are usually performed by experienced interventionists with several years of experience in EMB procedures. For better anatomic definition of the specimen site, noninvasive techniques of cardiac imaging may usefully be associated, such as gadolinium magnetic resonance imaging in targeting bioptic specimens in suspected myocarditis [9].

Major complications of EMB included death, perforation with cardiac tamponade requiring pericardiocentesis, pericardial effusion not requiring pericardiocentesis, brain embolization with transient cerebral ischemia or stroke, pulmonary embolization, and permanent complete atrioventricular block. Minor complications included transient conduction disturbances, transient ventricular or supraventricular arrhythmias, transient chest pain, and intramyocardial hematoma. Local complications included vasovagal reaction, local nerve paresis, local hematoma, and femoral arterial-venous fistula.

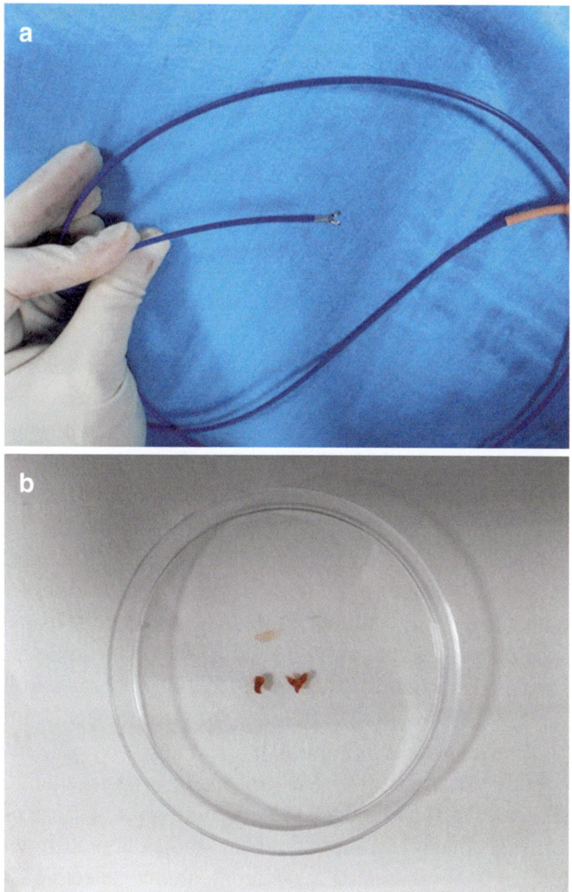

Fig. 3.1 (**a**) The BIPAL biopsy forceps (Cordis Corporation 430 Route 22 East Bridgewater, NJ 08807) used to perform left and right ventricular endomyocardial biopsies at our center. (**b**) Two endomyocardial biopsy samples taken from the left ventricle measuring 2–3 mm^3

In our experience, the incidence of major complications after LVEMB was very low (0.33%) and comparable to that of RVEMB (0.45%), suggesting that a biopsy in the LV is as safe as in the RV.

The overall major complication rate in our patient population was 0.39%. These results are at variance with another study reporting a major complication rate for LVEMB of 0.64% and for RVEMB of 0.82%, likely related to a greater operator experience obtained over a longer period of time [9].

Remarkably, no patients died. In particular, LVEMB showed a lower incidence of cardiac perforation compared with RVEMB, most likely because of the thinner RV wall. A major complication of LVEMB was brain embolization (0.24%). Importantly, this complication was associated with transient cerebral ischemia and no permanent damage and was significantly reduced when patients were pretreated with high-dose aspirin.

The low complication rate may also be related to the high level of experience of a few operators dedicated to the execution of EMB at our center. A higher rate of complications from EMB was reported in previous studies [5, 10] in which the procedure was performed in >1 center or by a high number of operators, while a lower incidence of EMB complications was present when only a small number of interventional cardiologists with extensive experience with the EMB procedure (>100 EMB procedures per year) were operating [11].

Importantly, operator performance improved significantly with experience acquired over time. Indeed, a higher number of major complications were recorded over the years that significantly and progressively reduced as experience accumulated, denoting a steep learning curve [8].

3.2 Diagnostic Contribution of Endomyocardial Biopsy

EMB is still the gold standard for in vivo diagnosis of myocarditis. The number of obtained samples is crucial to decrease sampling error and increase the diagnostic value of EMB. The number of specimens to be taken should range from five to ten and each sample should be 2–3 mm^3 in size (Fig. 3.1b). The sample must be carefully handled to minimize artifacts and transferred from the bioptome to fixative (10% neutral buffered formalin) by the use of a sterile needle. The fixative should be at room temperature to prevent contraction band artifacts. In general, at least four to five samples are submitted for light microscopic examination, one to two are fixed in 4% glutaraldehyde at room temperature for transmission electron microscopy, and additional specimens should be snap-frozen in OCT-embedding medium and stored at −80° for immunohistochemistry and flash-freezing in liquid nitrogen or preserved in RNA later for molecular biology studies and for virus molecular investigation [2, 3].

A biventricular approach is generally advisable since it does not increase the overall periprocedural risks (0.5% for biventricular EMB and 0.44% for univentricular EMB) and reduce the sampling error because of the higher number of available specimens. Moreover, recent studies demonstrated that biventricular biopsies have a higher diagnostic yield compared to selective LV or RV biopsies [8, 9].

However, when minimizing the length of the procedure is a consideration, LVEMB should be preferred to RVEMB given that LVEMB gives a higher diagnostic yield while having a lower risk of complications.

In particular, in the clinical suspicion of myocarditis, when both ventricles show echocardiographic abnormalities, EMB can be either performed in the LV or the RV, whereas in the presence of selective LV involvement, an LVEMB is advisable [8, 12]. In our study the overall diagnostic yield for LVEMB was 96.3%, while for RVEMB was 71.4%. This discrepancy was even more evident when structural or functional echocardiographic abnormalities exclusively affected the LV; the diagnostic yield of LVEMB increased to 97.8% and the diagnostic yield of RVEMB decreased to 53%. Thus, in the clinical suspicion of myocarditis omitting LVEMB would have resulted in missing 47% of the histological diagnoses. Similarly, in the study by Yilmaz et al. [9] omitting the LVEMB would have resulted in missing 18.7% of cases with myocardial inflammation, whereas leaving out the RVEMB would have missed 7.9% of patients with inflammatory disease. Considering the therapeutic and prognostic relevance of myocardial inflammation in EMBs as recently demonstrated [7–9], valuable diagnostic EMB data will be missed if biopsies are taken only from 1 ventricle and particularly if taken only from the RV.

Myocarditis is usually the most frequent diagnosis (43.6 and 49.4%, respectively) at EMB examination [8, 9]. In our study, myocardial inflammation with either diffuse or focal signs of cardiomyocyte necrosis (i.e., active myocarditis) was detected in 88% of patients and without these signs (borderline myocarditis) in 12% of patients. Most patients (95.5%) were affected by a lymphocytic myocarditis (CD45RO+, CD3+, CD20−), whereas in 3.6%, an eosinophilic inflammatory process, including necrotizing vasculitis (Churg–Strauss disease), drug hypersensitivity, and Loeffler disease, was detected. In the remaining 0.9%, granulomatous myocarditis (sarcoidosis) and giant-cell myocarditis were observed (Fig. 3.2).

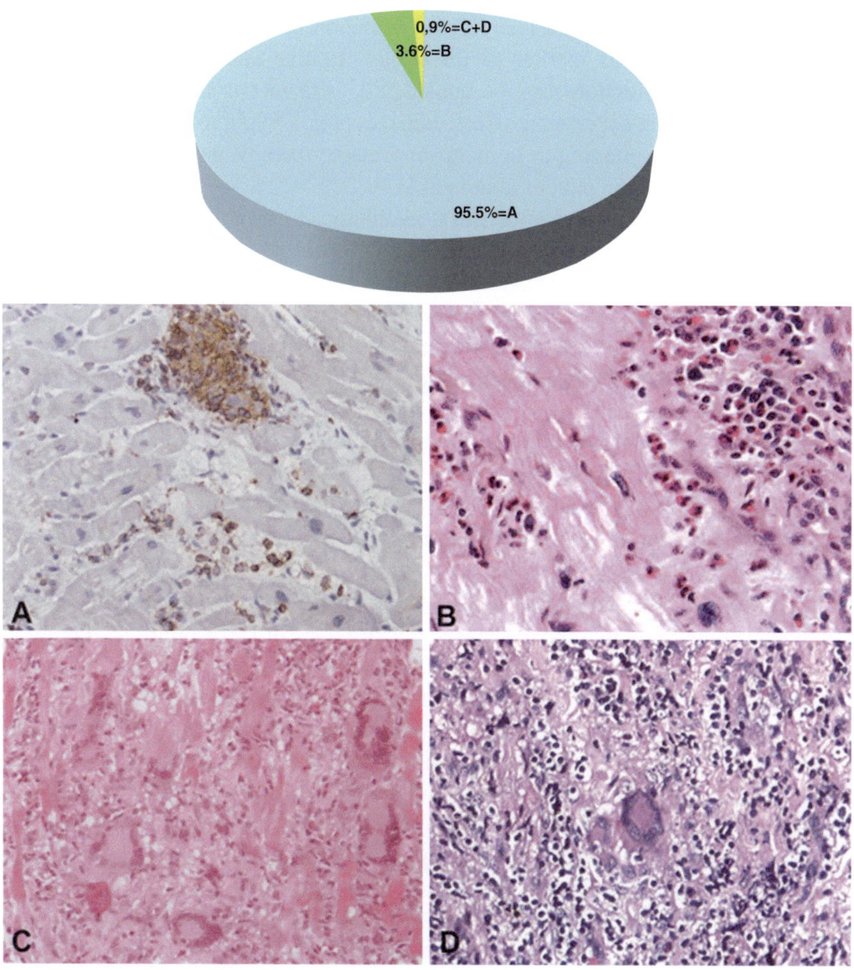

Fig. 3.2 Prevalence of different forms of myocarditis (A = lymphocytic, B = eosinophilic, C = giant cell and sarcoid) in left ventricular endomyocardial biopsy. (**a**) Immunoperoxidase for CD45RO, 200×, (**b**) H&E, 250×, (**c**) H&E, 200×, (**d**) H&E, 200×. From Chimenti C. and Frustaci A. Contribution and Risks of Left Ventricular Endomyocardial Biopsy in Patients with Cardiomyopathies, Volume: 128, Issue: 14, Pages: 1531–1541

Among the 1752 patients (49.4%) who globally received a diagnosis of myocarditis, 322 (18.4%) were diagnosed in the 7 years in which only the Dallas criteria were adopted, and 1430 (81.6%) were diagnosed in the 21 years after the introduction of immunohistochemistry, with an average of 46 cases of myocarditis per year without immunohistochemistry and 68 cases of myocarditis per year with immunohistochemistry, representing an overall 48%/y increase in the rate of diagnosis. Thus, the histologic Dallas criteria should always be implemented with immunohistochemical identification of the inflammatory infiltrate [4]. To increase the diagnostic sensitivity of immunohistochemistry, the use of a large panel of monoclonal and polyclonal antibodies (including anti-CD3, T lymphocytes; anti-CD68, macrophages; and anti-HLA-DR) is mandatory for the identification and characterization of the inflammatory infiltrate and for the detection of HLA-DR upregulation on EMB tissue sections as marker of infectious-negative autoimmune myocarditis where immunosuppression may be considered. In a recent study, immunohistochemical myocardial expression of Toll-like receptor 4 was able to identify patients with myocarditis responding to immunosuppressive therapy and can be considered a biomarker to guide the patient treatment [13].

The diagnostic contribution of EMB is enhanced by molecular analysis with DNA–RNA extraction and RT-PCR amplification of viral genomes. In a recent German study [9], polymerase chain reaction analyses revealed the presence of PVB19 in 51.2%, HHV6 in 23.3%, both PVB19 and HHV6 in 14.5%, and EBV in 4.4%, as well as other combinations and viruses (comprising mainly adenoviruses and enteroviruses) in 6.6% of patients. In our study [8], polymerase chain reaction analysis revealed the presence of a viral infection in 28% of patients consisting of adenovirus (35%), Epstein–Barr virus (30%), enterovirus (16%), influenza A virus (5.2%), parvovirus B19 (3.3%), human herpes virus 6 (1.9%), hepatitis C virus (4.4%), and a combination of viruses (4.2%), showing a different distribution of viral genomes compared with the series reported from German centers.

Cardiac magnetic resonance (CMR) has been proposed as a tool to direct EMB. A small study suggested that the diagnostic performance of EMB might be increased when biopsies were obtained from the region of late gadolinium enhancement (LGE) [14]. Most often, LGE is found either in the interventricular septum, which is best reached by the bioptome from the right side, or in the posterolateral LV wall to which the bioptome is automatically directed after its passage through the aortic valve in case of LV-EMB. Although obtaining EMBs exactly from the region of LGE could indeed result in an even higher number of positive diagnoses of myocarditis, this can be often a nonachievable goal. Indeed, a recent study from a high number of patients demonstrated that there were no substantial differences in the number of diagnostic LVEMB, RVEMB, or biventricular EMB when related to the site of LGE [9]. LGE shows a variable sensitivity to detect active or chronic inflammation and active myocarditis may not always lead to large enough regions of necrotic myocytes to be visually detectable with CMR [15]. Moreover, the sensitivity of CMR depends on the clinical presentation of myocarditis, being elevated in patients with an infarct-like clinical presentation, moderate in patients with a cardiomyopathic pattern, and low in those with an arrhythmic clinical profile [16].

Consequently, our current routine clinical approach is to preferentially take EMB in a standardized procedure from the ventricle demonstrating LGE but not necessarily from the "area" of LGE.

References

1. Sekiguchi M, Konno S. Diagnosis and classification of primary myocardial disease with the aid of endomyocardial biopsy. Jpn Circ J. 1971;35:737–54.
2. Cooper LT, Baughman KL, Feldman AM, Frustaci A, Jessup M, Kuhl U, Levine GN, Narula J, Starling RC, Towbin J, Virmani R. American Heart Association; American College of Cardiology; European Society of Cardiology. The role of endomyocardial biopsy in the management of cardiovascular disease: a scientific statement from the American Heart Association, the American College of Cardiology, and the European Society of Cardiology. Circulation. 2007;116:2216–33.
3. Leone O, Veinot JP, Angelini A, Baandrup UT, Basso C, Berry G, Bruneval P, Burke M, Butany J, Calabrese F, d'Amati G, Edwards WD, Fallon JT, Fishbein MC, Gallagher PJ, Halushka MK, McManus B, Pucci A, Rodriguez ER, Saffitz JE, Sheppard MN, Steenbergen C, Stone JR, Tan C, Thiene G, van der Wal AC, Winters GL. 2011 consensus statement on endomyocardial biopsy from the Association for European Cardiovascular Pathology and the Society for Cardiovascular Pathology. Cardiovasc Pathol. 2012;21(4):245–74.
4. Caforio AL, Pankuweit S, Arbustini E, Basso C, Gimeno-Blanes J, Felix SB, Fu M, Heliö T, Heymans S, Jahns R, Klingel K, Linhart A, Maisch B, McKenna W, Mogensen J, Pinto YM, Ristic A, Schultheiss HP, Seggewiss H, Tavazzi L, Thiene G, Yilmaz A, Charron P, Elliott PM. Current state of knowledge on aetiology, diagnosis, management and therapy of myocarditis. A Position statement of the European Society of Cardiology Working Group on myocardial and pericardial diseases. Eur Heart J. 2013;34(33):2636–48, 2648a–d.
5. Deckers JW, Hare JM, Baughman KL. Complications of transvenous right ventricular endomyocardial biopsy in adult patients with cardiomyopathy: a seven-year survey of 546 consecutive diagnostic procedures in a tertiary referral center. J Am Coll Cardiol. 1992;19:43–7.
6. Felker GM, Hu W, Hare JM, Hruban RH, Baughman KL, Kasper EK. The spectrum of dilated cardiomyopathy: the Johns Hopkins experience with 1,278 patients. Medicine (Baltimore). 1999;78:270–83.
7. Frustaci A, Pieroni M, Chimenti C. The role of endomyocardial biopsy in the diagnosis of cardiomyopathies. Ital Heart J. 2002;3:348–53.
8. Chimenti C, Frustaci A. Contribution and risks of left ventricular endomyocardial biopsy in patients with cardiomyopathies: a retrospective study over a 28-year period. Circulation. 2013 Oct 1;128(14):1531–41.
9. Yilmaz A, Kindermann I, Kindermann M, Mahfoud F, Ukena C, Athanasiadis A, Hill S, Mahrholdt H, Voehringer M, Schieber M, Klingel K, Kandolf R, Böhm M, Sechtem U. Comparative evaluation of left and right ventricular endomyocardial biopsy: differences in complication rate and diagnostic performance. Circulation. 2010;122:900–9.
10. Sekiguchi M, Take M. World survey of catheter biopsy of the heart. In: Sekiguchi M, Olsen EG, editors. Cardiomyopathy: clinical, pathological and theoretical aspects. Baltimore: University Park Press; 1988. p. 217–25.
11. Holzmann M, Nicko A, Kühl U, Noutsias M, Poller W, Hoffmann W, Morguet A, Witzenbichler B, Tschöpe C, Schultheiss HP, Pauschinger M. Complication rate of right ventricular endomyocardial biopsy via the femoral approach: a retrospective and prospective study analyzing 3048 diagnostic procedures over an 11-year period. Circulation. 2008;118(17):1722–8.
12. Escher F, Lassner D, Kühl U, Gross U, Westermann D, Poller W, Skurk C, Weitmann K, Hoffmann W, Tschöpe C, Schultheiss HP. Analysis of endomyocardial biopsies in suspected myocarditis--diagnostic value of left versus right ventricular biopsy. Int J Cardiol. 2014;177(1):76–8.

13. Chimenti C, Verardo R, Scopelliti F, Grande C, Petrosillo N, Piselli P, De Paulis R, Frustaci A. Myocardial expression of toll-like receptor 4 predicts the response to immunosuppressive therapy in patients with virus-negative chronic inflammatory cardiomyopathy. Eur J Heart Fail. 2017;19:915–25.
14. Mahrholdt H, Goedecke C, Wagner A, Meinhardt G, Athanasiadis A, Vogelsberg H, Fritz P, Klingel K, Kandolf R, Sechtem U. Cardiovascular magnetic resonance assessment of human myocarditis: a comparison to histology and molecular pathology. Circulation. 2004;109:1250–12.
15. Friedrich MG, Sechtem U, Schulz-Menger J, Holmvang G, Alakija P, Cooper LT, White JA, Abdel-Aty H, Gutberlet M, Prasad S, Aletras A, Laissy JP, Paterson I, Filipchuk NG, Kumar A, Pauschinger M, Liu P. Cardiovascular magnetic resonance in myocarditis: a JACC white paper. J Am Coll Cardiol. 2009;53:1475–87.
16. Francone M, Chimenti C, Galea N, Scopelliti F, Verardo R, Galea R, Carbone I, Catalano C, Fedele F, Frustaci A. CMR sensitivity varies with clinical presentation and extent of cell necrosis in biopsy-proven acute myocarditis. JACC Cardiovasc Imaging. 2014;7:254–63.

4 Genetic Basis of Myocarditis: Myth or Reality?

Eloisa Arbustini, Nupoor Narula, Lorenzo Giuliani, and Alessandro Di Toro

4.1 Introduction

4.1.1 Definition

The term myocarditis describes the presence of inflammatory cells in the myocardium. This descriptive diagnosis encompasses a wide spectrum of etiologically different diseases that share, as a unique criterion, the presence of myocardial inflammation [1] (Fig. 4.1). The term, however, does not specify the type of inflammation, the nature of inflammatory cells, and the cause. In clinical practice, the diagnosis of myocarditis implies that the observed phenotype is attributable to the inflammation of the myocardium or that the myocardial inflammation constitutes a "comorbidity" or "complication" of preexisting known heart disease, even of a non-inflammatory nature [2].

4.1.2 Immunocompetent Cells in Myocardial Tissue

Unlike other organs and tissues, the myocardium does not host lymphoid tissue (e.g., BALT in lung, MALT in gastrointestinal tract) and does not possess resident

E. Arbustini (✉) · L. Giuliani · A. Di Toro
Centre for Inherited Cardiovascular Diseases – IRCCS Policlinico San Matteo, Pavia, Italy
e-mail: e.arbustini@smatteo.pv.it; l.giuliani@smatteo.pv.it; a.ditoro@smatteo.pv.it

N. Narula
Centre for Inherited Cardiovascular Diseases – IRCCS Policlinico San Matteo, Pavia, Italy

Division of Cardiology, Department of Medicine, New York Presbyterian Hospital, Weill Cornell Medicine, New York, NY, USA
e-mail: nun9005@nyp.org

A. L. P. Caforio (ed.), *Myocarditis*, https://doi.org/10.1007/978-3-030-35276-9_4

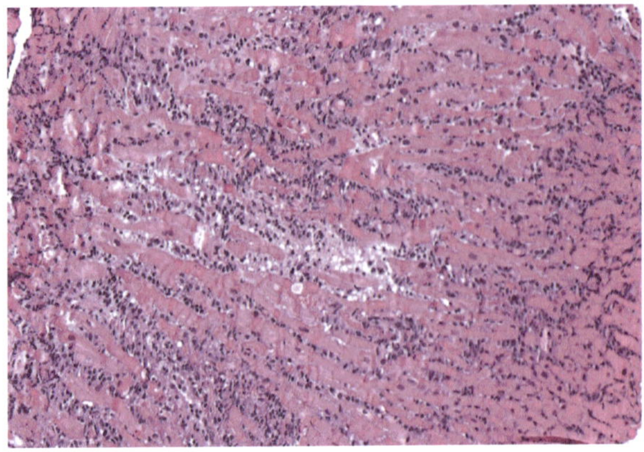

Fig. 4.1 The figure shows the typical features of acute lymphocytic myocarditis in an endomyocardial biopsy of a young male patient presenting with acute heart failure and elevated troponin levels

"reticulo-endothelial (RE)" cells (e.g., liver and spleen), such as alveolar macrophages in the lung, glia cells in the brain, or glomerular-mesangial cells in the kidney. However, a fair amount of steady-state, resident macrophages is present in myocardial tissue [3, 4]. These macrophages originate from yolk sac and fetal monocytic progenitors and are either replenished by local proliferation in infancy [3] or by blood monocytes in adulthood [4]. At birth, resident macrophages express major histocompatibility complex class II (HLA II) molecules and the CX3CR1+ Fractalkine receptor and are therefore distinct from conventional αE integrin CD103+ dendritic cells [5]. With age, the number of HLA II macrophages increases while the number of CX_3CR_1+ macrophages decreases [6]; the proliferation capacity of embryo-derived cardiac macrophages progressively declines after the perinatal period [6]. Cardiac-resident macrophages display distinct functional properties from those of monocyte-derived macrophages in cardiac tissue. Resident macrophages interweave a complex molecular dialogue with cardiac myocytes, likely mediated by cytokines; macrophages can modulate the different signals that originate from the injured cardiac tissue [7]. In cardiac inflammatory diseases, resident macrophages likely participate in attracting circulating monocytes and other inflammatory cells, depending on the local signal triggering the inflammation [8]. Therefore, the myocardial tissue is not lacking in its own immune defenses, but it does not have a structured RE system like other organs that are much more commonly the target of infections.

4.1.3 Why Does Myocardial Tissue Trigger Inflammation?

Myocardial tissue becomes a target of inflammation when it has to repair tissue damage (e.g., acute myocardial infarction or toxic necrosis), if the myocytes are infected by cardiotropic pathogens (infective myocarditis) or in an allogeneic condition (e.g., transplant), if other cardiac structures (valves or pericardium) become targets of inflammation due to self/pathogen mimicry mechanisms (e.g., rheumatic fever), or become self-reactive as in immune-mediated myocarditis, or if genetic defects induce deficiency of the immunologic system (e.g., primary immunodeficiency and auto-inflammatory diseases). The understanding of mechanisms of myocardial inflammation in infectious and non-infectious myocarditis is challenging, as it is difficult to understand whether individual constitutional gene variants can influence these mechanisms. In fact, it is noted that individuals exposed to the same pathogens may or may not develop myocarditis, even within the same environmental exposure context. This is one of the reasons why the search for predisposing genetic factors continues to attract the interest of researchers.

In this chapter, we will briefly review the main types of myocarditis and discuss individual genetic susceptibility to different types of myocarditis from both a clinical and research development perspective. Each type of myocarditis is reviewed in other chapters of this book.

4.2 Is Myocarditis a Genetic Disease?

Overall, myocarditis can be simply grouped by infectious, non-infectious (autoimmune, immune-mediated, or auto-inflammatory), and toxic etiologies (Table 4.1). Infectious myocarditis can be caused by DNA and RNA viruses, bacteria, fungi, protozoa, and helminths. The most common causes of infectious myocarditis in both children and adults are cardiotropic viruses [9]. Non-viral cardiotropic infections such as *Trypanosoma Cruzi* (Chagas disease) [10] and *Borrelia burgdorferi* (Lyme disease) [11] can affect immune-competent individuals in endemic areas. In immunocompromised patients, typically heart transplant recipients, the most common opportunistic infections include the human cytomegalovirus (HCMV) and Toxoplasma gondii. The state of knowledge on the etiology, diagnosis, management, and therapy of myocarditis and that on the diagnosis and management of myocardial involvement in systemic immune-mediated diseases are reported in two position statements of the European Society of cardiology [12, 13].

Precise rules define the criteria for the diagnosis of systemic and organ involvement [14], including the heart. Myocardial involvement is diagnosed when the infectious agent is detected in myocardial tissue by pathologic and pathogen-related genomic studies [12, 13]. Often, in clinical practice, the diagnosis of myocarditis is suspected, based more on clinical, biochemical, and imaging criteria than on the demonstration of myocardial tissue inflammation. Failure to precisely diagnose the cause can lead to overlooking a potentially toxic origin (e.g., pheochromocytoma) [15] and genetic familial diseases with similar clinical expression. Resuscitated cardiac arrest is one of the examples in which imaging-detected interstitial edema [15] can lead to incorrect diagnostic hypotheses. As expected, infectious myocarditis is not a genetic disease; in the absence of the pathogen, there is no myocarditis. However, the role of genetic susceptibility has been repeatedly raised in clinical and experimental studies in an attempt to understand why some individuals develop myocarditis, while others, perhaps exposed to the same risk, do not.

Table 4.1 Possible causes of myocarditis or diseases in which myocarditis can occur

Infectious					Non-infectious-toxic		Adaptive immunity diseases		Innate immunity Mendelian dis.	
RNA Viruses	DNA Viruses	Bacteria	Protozoa/ helminths/fungi	Heritable infectious	Medications	Toxic agents/ poisons/physical agents/drugs	Autoimmune/immune-mediated		Auto-inflammatory	Primary immunodeficiencies
• Coxsackieviruses A and B • Echoviruses • Polioviruses • Influenza A and B viruses • Respiratory syncytial virus • Mumps virus • Measles virus • Hepatitis C virus • Dengue virus • Yellow fever virus • Chikungunya virus • Junin virus • Lassa fever virus • Rabies virus • Rubella virus • Human immunodeficiency virus-1 • Coronavirus[a] (MeRS-CoV) • Cardiovirus B (Saffold virus, SAFV)	• Adenoviruses • Parvovirus B19 • Human cytomegalovirus • Human herpes virus-6 • Epstein-Barr virus • Varicella-zoster virus • Herpes simplex virus • Variola virus • Vaccinia virus • Polyoma virus • Trichodysplasia spinulosa-associated polyomavirus (TSV)[b]	• Staphylococcus • Streptococcus • Pneumococcus • Meningococcus • Gonococcus • Salmonella • Corynebacterium diphtheriae • Haemophilus influenzae • Leptospira (Weil disease) • Borrelia Burgdorferi (Lyme disease) • Neisseria • Mycobacterium (tuberculosis), • Mycoplasma pneumoniae, • Brucella • Tropheryma whipplei	• Trypanosoma cruzi (Chagas disease) • Toxoplasma gondii • Entamoeba histolytica • Leishmania • Echinococcus • Trichinella • Taenia solium • Fungal • Aspergillus, • Actinomyces, • Blastomyces, • Candida, • Coccidioides, • Cryptococcus, • Histoplasma, • Mucormycosis, • Nocardia, • Sporothrix	• Chromosomally-integrated HHV-6 (ciHHV-6): • Myocarditis • Organ and HSCT • Transplant	• Penicillin, • Phenylbutazone, • Methyldopa, • Thiazide diuretics, • Amitriptyline • Cefaclor • Colchicine • Furosemide • Isoniazid • Lidocaine • Tetracycline • Phenytoin • Sulfonamides • Phenylbutazone • Methyldopa • Thiazide diuretics • Dobutamine • Clozapine • Amitriptyline • Interleukin 2	• Lithium • Arsenic • Lead • Copper • Iron • Phosphorus • Carbon monoxide • Ethanol • Poisons by insect stings and bites • Electric shock • Heat • Radiation/ radio-therapy • Cocaine • Heroin	• Systemic lupus erythematosus, • Rheumatoid arthritis, • Churg–Strauss syndrome, • Kawasaki's disease, • Inflammatory bowel disease, • Scleroderma, • Polymyositis • Myasthenia gravis, • Insulin-dependent diabetes mellitus • Thyrotoxicosis, • Wegener's granulomatosis, • Organ-specific infectious negative lymphocytic myocarditis	• Sarcoidosis • Giant cell myocarditis • Myocardial involvement in systemic diseases with giant cells • Rheumatic heart disease • Farber's disease (lipo-granulomatosis)	• IL-1-mediated auto-inflammatory syndromes • IL-18-mediated auto-inflammation and susceptibility to *MAS* • A20 haplo-insufficiency • Interferon-mediated auto-inflammatory diseases • Immunodeficiency and immune dysregulation overlap	• Immunodeficiencies affecting cellular and humoral immunity • Combined immunodeficiencies with associated or syndromic features • Predominantly antibody deficiencies • Diseases of immune dysregulation • Congenital defects of phagocyte number, function, or both • Defects in intrinsic and innate immunity • (Auto-inflammatory diseases) • Complement deficiencies

[a]Causing the Middle East respiratory syndrome
[b]Human polyomavirus identified in 2010

4.3 Infectious Myocarditis and Genetics

Reasons to suspect a genetic susceptibility in infectious myocarditis may derive from twin studies (usually newborn or children) [16–18], familial clustering suggesting genetic determinants or predisposing genetic factors [19–21], and rare Mendelian diseases [22, 23] as well as endemic infections linked to both pathogen and population genetic make-up [24]. The topic must be discussed with caution so as not to transform infectious diseases into genetic ones, especially as the distinction between genetic susceptibility from exclusive environmental factors that might aggregate within families can be difficult.

4.3.1 Single Gene Defects and Myocarditis

"Mendelian" myocarditis is rare, and the available information is based on single case reports and small clinical series. Disease genes are either *immunity* genes or *non-immunity genes whose defects cause heritable cardiomyopathies* [2] and may eventually predispose to myocarditis.

4.3.1.1 Immunity Genes

These are cases of apparently sporadic myocarditis in patients with "primary immunodeficiency diseases" (PID), mainly autosomal recessive, which predispose to infections including those that cause myocarditis [25]. PID phenotypes are heterogeneous overall [26–28], and the genetic cause is not the infection itself, but the condition of immunodeficiency that underlies the predisposition and the occurrence of myocarditis. PIDs are predominantly observed in the pediatric age as the case of a child with disseminated *Mycobacterium avium* infection carrier of IL-12Rβ1 deficiency due to compound heterozygosity and who ultimately died of acute heart failure due to a Coxsackie myocarditis and a poor nutritional status [29]. In the adult it is rarer but possible. A toll-like receptor 3 mutation has been identified in an adult patient diagnosed with enteroviral (EV) myocarditis [30].

4.3.1.2 Non-immunity Genes: Do Genetic Cardiomyopathies Display Susceptibility to Myocarditis?

The possibility of deep molecular and genetic exploration of heart diseases may contribute to unravel the molecular pathogenetic mechanisms of heart diseases, either predisposition of genetic cardiomyopathies to infections which may trigger the first manifestation of the disease or simply infectious complications in patients with an established diagnosis of genetic cardiomyopathy. The question is whether genetically affected hearts are more vulnerable to inflammatory triggers than non-affected hearts [2, 31]. A recent in vitro and clinical study explored the hypothesis that human genetic factors might underlie acute viral myocarditis in previously healthy children. Authors tested the role of TLR3-interferon (IFN) immunity using human-induced pluripotent stem cell-derived cardiomyocytes (iPSC-CM) and performed whole-exome sequencing in 42 unrelated children with acute myocarditis, some with proven viral etiologies. *TLR3*- and *STAT1*-deficient iPSC-CM did not show more susceptibility to coxsackievirus B3 (CVB3) infection than control cells. CVB3 did not induce IFN-α/β and IFN-α/β-stimulated genes in control cardiomyocytes and exogenous IFN-α did not substantially protect cardiomyocytes against CVB3. Exome sequencing did not show mutations in *TLR3*- or *IFN-α/β*-related genes. Unexpectedly, seven of 42 patients (16.7%) were carriers of rare bi-allelic, nonsynonymous, or splice-site variations in six cardiomyopathy-associated genes (*BAG3*, *DSP*, *PKP2*, *RYR2*, *SCN5A*, or *TNNI3*). The authors concluded that "previously silent recessive defects of the myocardium may predispose to acute heart failure presenting as acute myocarditis, notably after common viral infections" [32]. The hypothesis that acute myocarditis reflects an active phase of ARVD that leads to changes in phenotype and abrupt progression of the disease has been investigated by Lopez-Ayala and colleagues [33]. They suggest that an active phase should be suspected in a patient with myocarditis associated with a family history of ARVD and that certain mutations may increase the susceptibility to superimposed myocarditis in ARVD [33]. Patients with dilated cardiomyopathy caused by defects of *dystrophin* and *dysferlin* demonstrate increased susceptibility to myocardial CVB3 infection by enhancing viral propagation to adjacent cardiomyocytes and disrupting the function that repairs the myocyte membrane [34–36]. The history of a recent flu episode in patients with XL-DCM caused by defects of dystrophin may confound the true clinical diagnosis, but the possibility that a viral flu triggers or unmasks the manifestation of preexisting asymptomatic disease cannot be excluded. Although myocarditis and the viral genome may not be found in the EMB from patients with XL-DCM [37], the myocardium with dystrophin defects could sustain greater damage from coxsackievirus proteases that are known to affect host cell proteins such as dystrophin [34–37]. As confirmation of the role or effect of myocarditis on the expression of dystrophin, there is evidence of focal disruption of the dystrophin–glycoprotein complex (DGC) in human coxsackievirus B myocarditis. DGC disruption can contribute to the pathogenesis of human enterovirus (EV)-induced dilated cardiomyopathy [38], and the disintegration of the sarcoglycan complex may, in addition to dystrophin cleavage, play an important role in the pathogenesis of enterovirus-induced cardiomyopathy [39].

4.3.2 Genetic Susceptibility and Enteroviral Myocarditis

The clinical presentation of EV infection may be relatively mild (fever, herpangina, conjunctivitis, hand-foot-mouth disease, tonsillitis, pharyngitis, lower respiratory tract infection, acute gastroenteritis) or, less commonly, very severe (pneumonia, meningitis, encephalitis, myocarditis, pericarditis, hepatic necrosis, and coagulopathy) [40]. EV myocarditis is often described in outbreaks of EV infections [41–46] (Table 4.2). The cardiotropic coxsackievirus B3 (CV-B3) is one of the most common causes of myocarditis [40]. The myocardial infection is initiated by the transmembrane coxsackievirus-adenovirus receptor (CAR) encoded by the *CXADR* gene (MIM∗602621); in experimental models, the ablation of CAR blocks viral infection of myocardial cells as well as inflammation in the myocardium [47]. Similarly,

Table 4.2 Enterovirus, outbreaks, and reports of EV myocarditis

Species	Types	Outbreaks with reports of myocarditis	Ref
A	• Coxsackievirus 1–8, 10, 12, 14, 16; • Enterovirus A71, A76, A89, A90, A114, A119, A120, A121	Severe hand-foot and mouth disease due to CVA6, CVA16, and A71	[41, 42]
B	• Coxsackie B 1–6, A9, • Echovirus 1–7, 9,11–21, 24–27, 29–33 • Enterovirus B 69, 73–75, 77–88, 93, 97, 98, 100, 101, 106 and 107	Neonatal sepsis due to CVB1	[43, 44]
C	• Coxsackie virus A1, 11, 13, 17, 19, 20, 21, 22, 24; • Enterovirus C 95, 96, 99, 102, 104, 105, 109, 113, 116–118; • Poliovirus 1–3	Small outbreaks of cVDPV and paralytic disease due to newer EV-C viruses	[45]
D	• EV D68 D70, D94, D111	Reports of EVD68 respiratory diseases, including myocarditis. Association with acute flaccid myelitis	[46]

increased cardiac expression of CAR may partially explain increased susceptibility to myocarditis [48]. However, to date, mutations in the *CXADR* gene have not been reported/identified. In CVB3-infected myocytes, the cell damage is induced by direct cytotoxicity and mediated by viral proteinases [49]. CVB3 replicates on the surface of autophagosomes [50, 51] and enhances replication by employing miRNA [52, 53]. CVB3-induced differential expression of miRNA modulates the expression of both host and viral genes.

Individual genetic make-up may favor EV infection. A recent investigation focuses on PI4KB/ACBD3 (phosphatidylinositol kinase 4, type 3 beta/acyl-CoA-binding domain-containing protein 3) interaction as facilitating mechanisms for efficient viral replication. Enteroviruses, as well as other positive-strand RNA viruses, reorganize host cellular membranes through recruiting phosphatidylinositol (PI) 4-kinase (*PI4KB*), whose defects cause the monogenic autosomal recessive perisylvian polymicrogyria, with cerebellar hypoplasia and arthrogryposis [54]. Acute inhibition of the enzyme PI4KA by kinase inhibitors causes sudden death [55]. The Golgi-residing protein, ACBD3 (Golgi phosphoprotein 1; GOLPH1), which is involved in the maintenance of Golgi structure and function, is responsible for proper localization of enteroviral 3A proteins in host cells. Mutants abrogating the ACBD3–PI4KB interaction showed that this interaction is crucial for enterovirus replication and allowed the identification of the minimal ACBD3 domains that are essential for enterovirus replication. Therefore, acyl-coenzyme A binding (ACB) and charged-amino-acid region (CAR) domains are dispensable for 3A-mediated PI4KB recruitment and efficient enterovirus replication [56]. The myocardial expression of *NOD2* (nucleotide-binding oligomerization domain protein 2) gene has also been found to be higher in CVB3-positive patients compared with patients with myocarditis but without evidence of persistent CVB3 infection; no genetic variants in the gene have been reported to date [57].

4.3.3 Parvovirus B19 and Myocarditis: Genetic Studies Unravel Molecular Mechanisms But Do Not Demonstrate Heritable Predisposition

Human parvovirus B19 (B19V) belongs to genus Erythroparvovirus of the Parvoviridae family, which is composed of a group of DNA viruses with a linear single-stranded DNA genome [58]. B19V infects human erythroid progenitor cells (EPCs) and causes mild to severe hematological disorders [59]. It may also infect non-erythroid lineage cells such as myocardial endothelial cells [60]. The tropism of B19V for EPCs depends on the expression of viral receptors and co-receptors on the cell surface and by the viral use of host factors such as RNA binding motif protein 38 (RBM38) for the processing of its pre-mRNA during viral replication [61]. Variants in *RBM38* gene have not been reported so far. The RBM38 protein (coded by the RBM38 gene, 20q13.31, MIM*612428) interacts with the intronic splicing enhancer 2 (ISE2) element of B19V pre-mRNA and promotes 11-kDa protein expression that regulates the 11-kDa protein-mediated augmentation of B19V replication [62]. The B19V–antibody complex enters the cells through an endocytosis process mediated by the direct interaction of antibody-bound complement factor C1q with its receptor CD93 on the cell surface [63].

Infection by PVB19 causes fifth disease, arthropathy, anemia in immunocompromised patients and sickle cell disease patients, myocarditis, and hydrops fetalis in pregnant women [64–66]. The cardiac manifestations vary, from mild and nonspecific symptoms (e.g., fatigue, arrhythmias) to severe, including cardiogenic shock requiring mechanical support. PCR-based studies have reported B19V genome in myocardial tissue of patients with myocarditis and dilated cardiomyopathy, however also in control cases, disproving the hypothesis that persistent myocardial viral infection might be a frequent cause of DCM or myocarditis [67–69]. Similar findings have been reported in skin samples from patients with dermatological diseases in which the role of viral infection is debated [70]. It should be considered that no biopsy tissue sample is blood-free. In addition, remnant B19V DNA strands can be released from tissues without active viral replication; therefore, the PCR-based detection of B19V DNA in blood does not prove the presence of infectious virions and viral replication [71]. This finding suggests caution in the interpretation of the role of B19V infection when based on B19V DNA detection in blood, not only in myocarditis but also in other diseases that have been hypothesized to be causally linked with B19V. Finally, the viral load of PVB19 genomes in the myocardium is not related to the long-term outcome [72]. A possible hypothesis that could explain the role of B19V in myocarditis and cardiomyopathy is the potential trigger effect of the viral genome for innate immunity, inducing pro-inflammatory cytokine secretion [72] and myocardial inflammation. Although the hypothesis that individual susceptibility and modifier genes may influence the predisposition to myocarditis, there is no current proven evidence of gene variants potentially exerting this role.

4.3.4 Herpes Virus Infections: Heritability of Chromosomally Integrated HHV-6 (ciHHV-6)

A recently described case of myocarditis in a patient with chromosomally integrated HHV-6 (ciHHV-6) [73] links the herpes virus infection with an inherited risk of myocarditis. ciHHV-6 is a rare heritable condition in which the complete genome of the virus is integrated into the host germline genome (OMIM 604474) [74]. ciHHV-6 is characterized by high viral copy numbers in blood or sera (>6 log (10) copies/mL) with a prevalence of 0.8% of UK blood donors. Therefore, the finding of high HHV-6 viral loads in healthy normal individuals highlights the need to correctly interpret ciHHV-6, with its possible confounding effect in laboratory diagnosis of HHV-6 infection [75, 76] or its role in patients with DCM/heart failure [77]. The integrated viral genome eventually secreting viral chemokines can confer human genes with links to inflammatory pathology and supports ciHHV-6A reactivation as a source for emergent infection [77, 78].

4.3.5 Chagas Disease and Genetic Predisposition

Chagas disease (CD) is caused by the protozoan parasite *Trypanosoma cruzi* [79] through direct oral contact, contaminated blood transfusion, or bone marrow transplantation. There may also be vertical transmission from the mother to infant. CD is endemic in the southern USA, Mexico, Central America, and South America [10, 79, 80]. Contamination of food and drink has been reported in northern South America, where transmission cycles may involve wild vector populations and mammalian reservoir hosts [10, 79–82]. In the acute phase, the disease can manifest with myocarditis, conduction system abnormalities, and pericarditis. In untreated patients, the disease progresses to the chronic phase with development of chronic Chagas cardiomyopathy (CCC) [79]. Genetic susceptibility to the development of CCC is a matter of ongoing investigation of immunity genes to identify possible individual and population-based predisposition. Table 4.3 [83–91] lists the genes and related variants investigated to date in CD. Although some association studies tested positive, no genetic test is currently performed in the diagnostic work-up of CD.

4.3.6 Rheumatic Fever, Carditis, and Genetics

Rheumatic fever (RF) is an immune-mediated disease that affects predominantly children and adolescents in low-income and developing countries, in which the disease burden is still relevant [92, 93]. RF occurs in "genetically susceptible individuals", as sequelae of Group A Streptococcus (GAS) pyogenes infection. The clinical manifestations depend upon the tissues involved, including synovium (arthritis), heart valves (endocarditis), myocardium (pancarditis), brain

Table 4.3 Genetic association studies for susceptibility to Chagas Disease (CD) and pathophysiology of Chronic Chagas Cardiomyopathy (CCC)

Gene	Peptide	Monogenic disease and susceptibility in OMIM: MIM Phenotype	Monogenic disease and susceptibility in OMIM: Inheritance	Genetic variants variably associated with Chagas Disease	Ref
COLEC11	Collectin 11	3MC syndrome 2	AR	Association with the pathophysiology of Chagas disease	[83]
MASP2	Lectin complement activation pathway, defect, 2	MASP2 deficiency	AR		
Promoter region, IL18	Interleukin 18	–	–	Susceptibility to CD	[84]
VDR gene (rs731236, rs7975232, rs1544410 and rs2228570)	Vitamin D receptor	Rickets, vitamin D-resistant, type IIA	AR	rs2228570*A allele: Association with CD	[85]
IL17A G197A (rs2275913)	Interleukin 17A	–	–	Association with Chagas disease	[86]
IL17F T7488C (rs763780)	Interleukin 17F	Familial candidiasis, 6	AD		
CCR5 ➔ Δ32 (rs333) 59029 A/G (pm rs1799987)	Chemochine, CR motif, 5	– Susceptibility/resistance to HIV infection – West Nile virus, susceptibility to	–	CCR5 Δ32 no CCR5 59,029 A/G yes Association with CCC	[87]
CCR2-CCR5 genes and their haplotypes	Chemochine, CR motif, 2 Chemochine, CR motif, 5		–	Association with CCC	[88]
• TGFB1: rs8179181, rs8105161, rs1800469;	• Transforming growth factor B 1	• Camurati–Engelmann disease[a]	• AD	No association with clinical outcome in CCC	[89]
• IL10: rs1800890, rs1800871, rs1800896;	• Interleukin 10	• HIV susceptibility; RA progression	• –		
• IFNG: rs2430561;	• Interferon gamma	• TSC2 angiomyolipomas, renal, Mod.	• AD		
• TNF: rs1800629;	• Tumor necrosis factor	• Asthma and Sepsis susceptibility	• –		
• BAT1 (DDX39B): rs3853601;	• HLA-B-associated transcript 1	• –	• –		
• LTA: rs909253, rs2239704;	• Lymphotoxin alpha	• Leprosy and Psoriatic ar. susceptibility	• –		
• TNFR1 (TNFRSF1A): rs767455;	• Tumor necrosis factor receptor 1	• Periodic familial fever	• AR		
• TNFR2 (TNFRSF1B): rs1061624.	• Tumor necrosis factor receptor 2	• –	• –		

Table 4.3 (continued)

Gene	Peptide	Monogenic disease and susceptibility in OMIM: MIM Phenotype	Inheritance	Genetic variants variably associated with Chagas Disease	Ref
NLRP1 rs11651270,	NLR family, pyrin domain containing 1	Auto-inflammation with arthritis and dyskeratosis	AD, AR	NLRP1 rs11651270 & CARD rs6953573: Association with CCC	[90]
CARD (NOD2) rs6953573	Caspase recruitment domain containing protein 15	Blau syndrome	AD		
CASP1P2	Caspase 1 apoptosis-related cysteine protease	–	–		
TYK2 gene variants	Tyrosine kinase	Immunodeficiency 35	AR	Negative susceptibility study	[91]

[a]Inflammatory bowel disease, immunodeficiency, and encephalopathy

(Sydenham's chorea), kidney (glomerulonephritis), skin (erythema marginatum), and subcutaneous tissue (rheumatic nodules). Rheumatic heart disease (RHD) is the most common acquired cardiovascular disease in youths [2] and is associated with high morbidity and mortality [94].

4.3.6.1 Familial Susceptibility

Genetic susceptibility has repeatedly been claimed as a contributor to the pathogenesis of RHD, but, to date, no significant result has been identified or reproduced with GWAS study [95]. Rheumatic fever is an example of familial "non-genetic aggregation" and of difficulties in distinguishing familial genetic susceptibility from transient or persistent environmental factors to which members of the same families may be exposed. Historical research focused attention on family aggregation [96], exploring the field of immunogenetics. An early study published in *Nature* in 1979 [97] identified the B-cell alloantigen marker, 883, in patients previously diagnosed with RF with or without subsequent RHD. The 883 antigen on B cells was found in 71% of patients typed in New York and 74% of patients typed in Bogota as compared with 17% in the two disease-free control groups. The marker was not associated with any of the known major histocompatibility complex (MHC) antigens. A later study showed that two antibodies produced against this antigen were present in 92% of patients as compared with 21% of disease-free controls [98]. Another monoclonal antibody, labeled D8/17, which identified a B-cell antigen present in 100% of RF patients, was found in 14.6 and 13% of unaffected sibs and parents, respectively. The segregation of phenotypes (percentage D8/17-positive cells within HLA-typed rheumatic fever families) was consistent with autosomal recessive inheritance, which was not associated with the MHC gene system [99]. The D8/17 antibody was later considered a disease-specific marker with worldwide distribution: it may serve as a diagnostic tool in patients with suspected rheumatic fever [100]. Therefore, the hypothesis of an autosomal familial recessive predisposition/susceptibility that was not related to HLA genes remains doubtful. Nonetheless, more recent twin pairs' studies demonstrated a concordant risk for acute rheumatic fever of 44% in monozygotic twins and 12% in dizygotic twins. The estimated heritability across six meta-analyzed studies was 60% [101].

Genetic variants associated with increased risk of RHD have been investigated on the basis of the hypothesis that cytokine gene polymorphisms could play a role in the susceptibility of RHD in patients: TNF-α (-308G>A) and IL-1β (-511C>T) were significantly associated with increased risk of RHD, while IL-10 (-1082G>A) and IL-6 (-174G>C) were not associated with modified RHD risk [102]. Thereafter, research focused on the role of functional variants in genes encoding molecules of the complement activation pathways. The rationale is that tissue damage in RHD is mediated by autoantibodies resulting from molecular mimicry between GAS and cardiac tissue proteins. The GAS molecule N-acetyl-β-D-glucosamine (GlcNAc) and the M protein cross-react with valve and myocyte proteins of the host [103]. GlcNAc is the immunodominant cell wall antigenic epitope of GAS and is recognized by ficolins [104] that comprise pattern-recognition receptors (PRRs) of the complement [103, 105]. Of the three human ficolins [ficolin-1 (M-ficolin), ficolin-2 (L-ficolin), and ficolin-3 (H-ficolin also known as Hakata antigen)] [106], ficolin-1 is found both in soluble form and on the cell membrane [107–109] and binds sialic acid to capsular polysaccharides of pathogens including *Streptococcus agalactiae* [110, 111]. The levels of expression of ficolin-1 are influenced by promoter gene variants, all associated with increased FCN1 gene expression in whole blood or adipose subcutaneous tissue, but are also associated with increased protection against the disease [112, 113]. FCN1 polymorphisms may play a dual role in the physiopathology of RF. On the one hand, they increase the GAS infection and predispose the patient to RHD symptoms, once the infection is established [113]. Polymorphisms associated with low levels of L-ficolin level may predispose carriers to recurrent and/or more severe streptococcal infection [112]. The low levels of ficolin-1 levels reported in RHD have been interpreted as an effect of the considerable ficolin-1 consumption in RF (Table 4.4). In any case, ficolin-1 is a promising therapeutic target for autoimmune diseases [114].

FLC3 gene defects are associated with immunodeficiency due to ficolin-3 deficiency (MIM # 613860), an autosomal recessive disease characterized by increased susceptibility to infections and autoimmune diseases, and by defect in the lectin

Table 4.4 Ficolin levels in autoimmune diseases [115]

Disease	Ficolin-1 levels High	Low	Unmodified	CRP correlations ($mg\ dL^{-1}$)	REF
Rheumatic fever		+		–	[112]
Vasculitis	+			0.98 [0.19, 6.71]	[113]
Rheumatoid arthritis	+			0.81 [0.06, 2.52]	
Myositis			+	0.20 [0.04, 0.63]	
Systemic lupus erythematosus			+	0.15 [0.10, 0.48]	
Behcet's disease			+	0.05 [0.04, 0.80]	

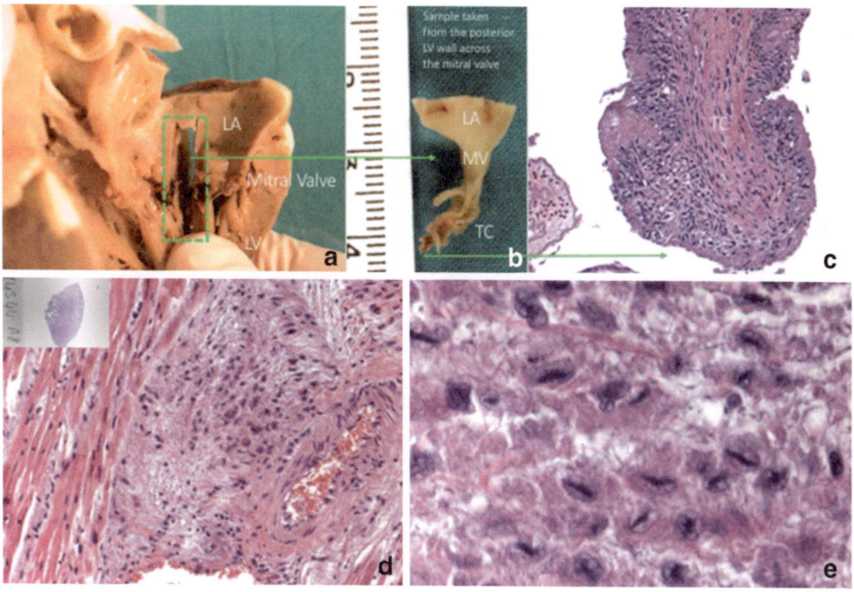

Fig. 4.2 Fatal rheumatic pancarditis with mitral chordal rupture in a boy with autosomal dominant osteogenesis imperfecta. The figure shows (**a**) the macroscopic view of the posterior atrioventricular wall. The sample in the (**b**) corresponds to the squared area in panel (**a**) and the histological panel (**c**) shows a ruptured chorda surrounded by inflammatory cells. The myocardial wall was extensively involved (**d**, **e**) and demonstrated the typical Anitschkow cells

activation pathway of the complement system. The specific biomarker is the decreased serum levels of ficolin-3. FLC3 deficiency is a rare disease of major scientific and clinical interest because heterozygous carriers have 50% reduction in circulating ficolin-3 levels. To date, only one case of cardiac disease has been described in an 11-month-old male infant who was operated on to repair a congenital heart defect [115]. Finally, the possibility exists that patients with genetic disease are more susceptible to RF [116]. This is a new area of clinical observation that also deserves attention due to the increasing number of genetic diseases that can now be correctly diagnosed [2]. As an example, the figure shows the case of a fatal rheumatic pancarditis in a boy with osteogenesis imperfecta (Fig. 4.2).

4.4 Non-Infectious Myocarditis

4.4.1 Sarcoidosis

Sarcoidosis is a chronic multisystem inflammatory disease of unknown etiology whose pathologic hallmark includes non-caseating, epithelioid granulomas primarily in the lungs and lung-draining lymph nodes [117, 118]. Sarcoidosis is considered a T-cell driven inflammatory disease in which mononuclear phagocytes (macrophages, monocytes, and dendritic cells) initiate and maintain T-cell activation and release cytokines that contribute to granuloma formation and maintenance [118, 119]. The data on incidence range from 3–4 to 35–80 per 100,000, reflecting ethnicity, geographic distribution, and gender. The prevalence is 10–40/100,000 persons in the USA and Europe, higher in the Scandinavian population, and lower in those of Turkish descent; in addition, the ratio of prevalence between African Americans and Caucasians is 10–17 to 1. Young women (20–40 years) are preferentially affected [119–121]. Cardiac involvement is influenced by ethnicity, approaching up to 58%, and constitutes the cause of death in up to 85% of Japanese patients [120, 122]. The disease typically occurs in the adult age; in children with suspected sarcoidosis, the autosomal dominant Blau syndrome has to be considered [123, 124]. This early aggressive form is associated with heterozygous mutations in CARD15 gene (NOD1) (MIM*605956) that cause constitutive NF-kappa-B activation [125].

The clinical manifestations of sarcoidosis are heterogeneous due to the involvement of many organs/organ systems and consist of polyarthritis, iridocyclitis, skin rash, and arteritis, in addition to potential heart, kidney, and nervous system involvement [117, 118, 124]. The heart is affected in 2–7% of patients diagnosed with systemic sarcoidosis [117, 122] (Fig. 4.3). Cardiac involvement is clinically manifest in about 5% of patients with sarcoidosis (sarcoid granulomas can be clinically silent), while it is asymptomatic in about 25% of cases, as confirmed by pathology, i.e., autopsy studies [126, 127], and imaging series, either CMR or fluorodeoxyglucose positron emission tomography (PET) [128, 129]. Simultaneous PET/MR increases the diagnostic accuracy and offers complementary information on disease pathophysiology [129, 130]. Therefore, given that sarcoid granulomas can be clinically silent, the real proportion of cardiac sarcoidosis is likely higher than clinically apparent.

Sarcoidosis can manifest acutely (Löfgren's syndrome) or with gradual onset (non-Löfgren's syndrome). The acute Löfgren's syndrome is characterized by hilar lymphadenopathy, erythema nodosum, and fever [131]; it mainly affects women and is common in Scandinavian, Irish, African, and Puerto Rican populations. The prognosis is good, with>90% of patients experiencing disease resolution within 2 years. On the other hand, resolution is difficult when lupus pernio, cardiac, or neurologic involvement is present.

4.4.1.1 Familial Monogenic Sarcoidosis: The BLAU Syndrome and Early-Onset Sarcoidosis (EOS)

Blau syndrome is an early-onset, chronic, granulomatous auto-inflammatory disease that is inherited by an autosomal dominant pattern [124]. The original clinical manifestations were described as a triad constituted by granulomatous dermatitis, arthritis, and uveitis [124]. Additional manifestations include erythema nodosum, fever, sialadenitis, lymphadenopathy, leukocytoclastic vasculitis, transient neuropathies, granulomatous glomerular and interstitial nephritis, interstitial lung disease, arterial hypertension, pulmonary hypertension, pericarditis, pulmonary embolism, hepatic granulomas, splenic involvement, and chronic renal failure [132–138]. Cardiac involvement is rare [136–140]. The pathologic hallmark is the

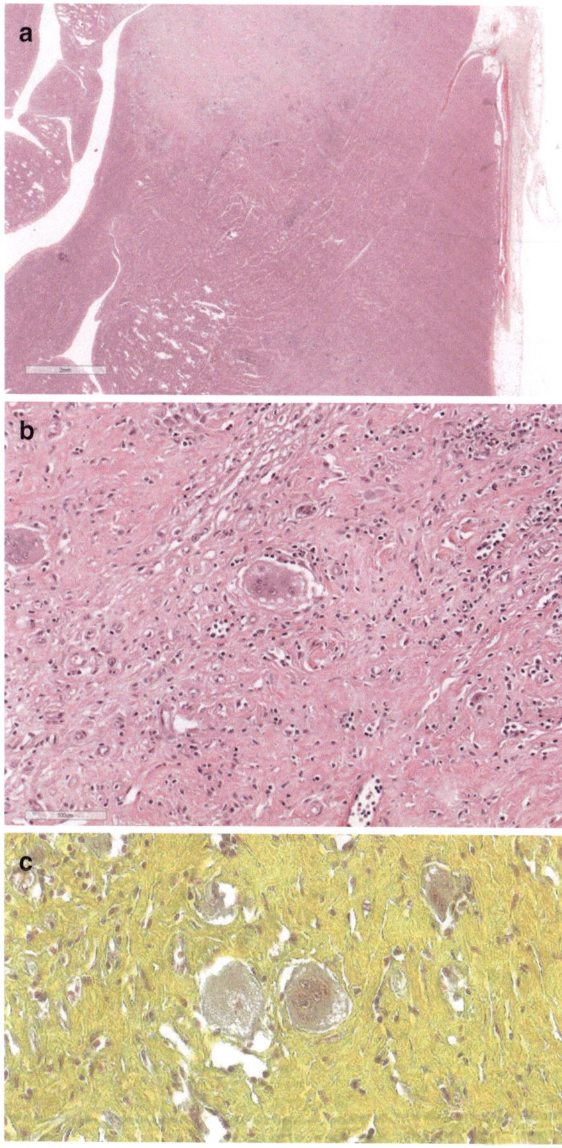

Fig. 4.3 End-stage fibrotic phase of adult-onset sarcoidosis. The patient underwent heart transplantation because of the extensive, multifocal scarring (**a**); residual giant cells are visible, with asteroid bodies, both H&E (**b**) and Movat Pentachrome stain (**c**)

non-caseating epithelioid cell Blau granuloma. Blau syndrome is caused by mutations in the Caspase Recruitment Domain Gene 15 (CARD15 or NOD1) (MIM∗605956) on chromosome 16q12.1 [125]. The mutations are systematically collected in the international Infevers Registry [fmf.igh.cnrs.fr/infevers] [139]. Blau syndrome is allelic to early-onset sarcoidosis (EOS) [140, 141]. The diagnosis is usually suspected in the clinical context of rheumatology or dermatology or ophthalmology issues. It is unusual for patients to manifest cardiac involvement at onset. Cardiologists are more likely to be involved in the clinical management of patients diagnosed with the disease [126]. Myocarditis is not specifically mentioned in the complex phenotype of the disease, but pericarditis is a known possible complication and myocardial involvement and cardiac infiltration have been reported in early-onset sarcoidosis associated with CARD15 mutations [140, 141].

4.4.1.2 Non-monogenic Sarcoidosis: Candidate Genes, Familial Aggregation, and Susceptibility

Outside of Blau syndrome and EOS, sarcoidosis is usually considered an autoimmune disease with possible family susceptibility in a way that does not conform to a classic Mendelian mode of inheritance [142, 143]. The susceptibility loci and the genes identified to date are summarized in Table 4.5. SNPs in major histocompatibility complex *HLA-DRA* and *BTNL2* genes have been associated with susceptibility to sarcoidosis. A recent multi-population study demonstrates that at least a part of these associations are *HLA-DRB1* independent (unrelated with linkage disequilibrium) and shared across ancestral origins. The variants that were independent of *HLA-DRB1* associations acted as e-quantitative trait loci for *HLA-DRB1* and/or *-DRB5*, suggesting a role in regulating gene expression [144]. The *BTNL2* gene variant G16071A seems to be a predisposing factor for sarcoidosis except in Caucasian postmenopausal women with sarcoid uveitis in whom the GG genotype prevails [145]. Other loci associated with genetic susceptibility of sarcoidosis are pending and many candidate genes are reported but not yet confirmed (*ACE, ADAM33, ANXA11, BTNL2, NOD2, CCDC88B, CCR2, GREM1, HLA-DRB1, IL23R, NOTCH4, C6ORF67, OS9, PRDX5, SLC11A1, TGFB1, TLR9*, and *TNFA*) [146–149]. Genes influencing clinical presentation of sarcoidosis are likely to be different from those that underlie disease susceptibility. To date, no genetic testing has entered the clinical diagnostic path of sarcoidosis. Whole-exome sequencing studies identified rare genetic variations in families with pulmonary sarcoidosis [150]. The family-based exome sequencing study identified 40 plausible functional rare genetic variants among German families. The findings highlighted the calcium ion-related biological activities and immune responsive genes with possible involvement in pathways of immune/inflammatory response regulation, leukocyte proliferation, and defense response to bacteria, among the major mechanisms. The KEGG pathway mapping analysis indicated inflammatory bowel disease as most relevant. The complexity of the phenotype (severity, chronicity, clinical course) and the overlapping of concurrent lung disease partly explain the difficulties encountered in the studies that investigate the genetic basis of sarcoidosis [150].

4.4.1.3 Familial Genetic Risk: Clinical Evaluation

On a clinical level, it is useful to be aware of the risk of recurrence of sarcoidosis in relatives of affected patients. The ACCESS study (A Case Controlled Etiologic Sarcoidosis Study) demonstrated that first-degree relatives of patients with sarcoidosis have a five times higher relative risk of developing sarcoidosis than control subjects [151–153]. A more recent study (Swedish National Patient Register using International Classification of Diseases codes, 1964–2013) confirmed that having at least one first-degree relative with sarcoidosis is associated with a 3.7-fold increase in the risk of sarcoidosis [154]. The relative risk increases in those with two or more relatives (relative risk 4.7) and in Löfgren's syndrome (relative risk 4.1). The percentage of heritability was 39% (95% CI 12–65%). Therefore, having a relative with sarcoidosis is a strong risk factor for the disease. In clinical practice, the family history (uveitis and lung diseases in particular) should be explored with the aim of verifying whether there are other family members diagnosed with sarcoidosis [155]. Instead, in the Japanese population in which sarcoidosis is particularly frequent, the occurrence of cardiac sarcoidosis in female patients is associated with the presence of *HLA-DQB1∗0601* and the allele *TNFA2* [156, 157]. Loci formally listed in the OMIM catalogue are described in Table 4.5 [155, 158–161] and genetic variants investigated in sarcoidosis are reported in Table 4.6.

4.4.2 Giant Cell Myocarditis and Genetics

Giant cell myocarditis (GCM) is a rare and potentially fatal illness of unknown etiology characterized by myocardial inflammation with multinucleated giant cells and myocyte necrosis [162, 163]. GCM is currently considered a "multifactorial disease triggered by different causes" [164–187]. Etiologic hypotheses include systemic autoimmune diseases [164–168], drug toxicity [169], infections [170–172], and complex combination of autoimmunity, infections and drug toxicity [173]. Infections reported in GCM include coxsackie B2 virus [170], parvovirus B19 [171], HCMV [172] and HIV1 infection [173–184]. In most cases, GCM is an isolated entity, while in about one-fifth of cases GCM occurs in association with autoimmune/immune-mediated diseases (Table 4.7), infections, drug toxicity, or syndromes such as immune reconstitution inflammatory syndrome (IRIS) in patients undergoing highly active antiretroviral therapy (HAART) against human immunodeficiency virus type 1 (HIV-1) [173, 184, 185] or even in patients taking common medications such as amoxicillin [183]. To date, the autoimmune/immune-mediated hypothesis is the most accredited pathogenic theory supported both by the aforementioned associations with systemic autoimmune diseases (Table 4.7) and by the partial remission of GCM in patients treated with immunosuppression as well as by the non-aggressive occurrence (10–50%) of the disease during immunosuppression treatment in transplanted patients [186, 187].

Table 4.5 Genetic susceptibility in sarcoidosis: loci formally included in OMIM catalogue

Susceptibility loci	Mapping	Association with variants in:	Ref
SS1	6p21.3	HLA-DRB1 (HLA-DRB1∗03)	[155, 157]
SS2	6p21.3	BTNL2 (butyrophilin-like protein, major histocompatibility complex class II-associated BTL II)	[159]
SS3	10q22–q23	ANXA11 (Annexin XI)	[160, 161]

Table 4.6 Systemic sarcoidosis: familial aggregation and genetic predisposition

Family studies		
Series	Relatives	Risk compared with the general population
210 twin pairs	Twins, monozygotic	80-fold
	Twins, dizygotic	7-fold
ACCESS (*A* *C*ase-*C*ontrol *E*tiologic *S*tudy in *S*arcoidosis)	First or second degree relative of a patient with sarcoidosis	4.7-fold
Genetic studies		
Genetic association	Chromosome 6, MHC genes	• Acute sarcoidosis: HLA-DRB1*0301 • Remitting disease: HLA-DQB1*0201-DRB1*0301 • Chronic active disease: DQB1*0602-DRB1*150101 • Extra-pulmonary manifestations: HLA-DRB1*11
Candidate genes	Case-control studies and family-based studies	• Variation of TNF production: TNFA1/TNFA2; rs1800629 • Chronic sarcoidosis: IL23R: rs11209026 (Arg381Gln) • Sarcoidosis and uveitis: IL23R: rs11209026 (Arg381Gln)
GWAS	Susceptibility loci and candidate genes	• *Butyrophilin-like 2 (BTNL2)* gene: rs2076530 A • Annexin A11 (ANXA11) gene: rs1049550 • Ras-related protein Rab-23 (RAB23): rs1040461 • Osteosarcoma amplified 9 (OS9): rs1050045 • Coiled-coil domain containing 88B (CCDC88B) • Peroxiredoxin 5 (PRDX5) gene • Neurogenic locus notch homolog protein 4 (NOTCH4) gene region: SNP rs715299
Gene–environment interactions	1101 patients with extrapulmonary sarcoidosis and exposed to insecticide, molds, and musty odors	HLADRB1*

Table 4.7 Giant cell myocarditis in inflammatory autoimmune diseases

Disease	References
Inflammatory bowel disease, both Crohn's disease (CD) and ulcerative colitis (UC); drug reaction is a possible trigger	[174–176]
Spondyloarthropathy	[177]
Thymoma, myasthenia gravis	[168, 178]
Vasculitis	[179]
Orbital myositis, vitiligo	[180]
Autoimmune hepatitis	[164]
Systemic lupus erythematosus	[181]
Sjogren's syndrome	[182]
Immune reconstitution inflammatory syndrome (IRIS) that may occur in patients undergoing highly active antiretroviral therapy (HAART) against human immunodeficiency virus type 1 (HIV-1)	[185]

Clinical manifestations of GCM are variable. Most patients present with cardiogenic shock or acute heart failure, requiring mechanical circulatory support. However, conduction disease such as atrio-ventricular nodal or infra-nodal heart block or atrial or ventricular arrhythmias can be the first manifestation. The rare "atrial variant" is characterized by atrial fibrillation and severe atrial dilation but preserved ventricular function [188, 189]. A precise diagnosis of GCM is established only when typical pathologic features are demonstrated on EMB or surgical samples [190] (Fig. 4.4). The inflammatory infiltrate is constituted by CD8-positive lymphocytes, eosinophils, and multinucleated giant cells; myocytes show damage and necrosis [162, 163]. The origin of giant cells, from myocytes and/or histiocytes, remains a matter of investigation. Differential diagnosis between GCM and cardiac sarcoidosis relies on pathologic features (non-caseating epithelioid granulomas with CD68-positive giant cells in sarcoidosis) and is supported by the different T-cell subsets, CD4+ in sarcoidosis and CD8+ in GCM. GCM carries a poor prognosis, with a median survival of 5.5 months from the onset of symptoms; up to 90% patients either die or require cardiac

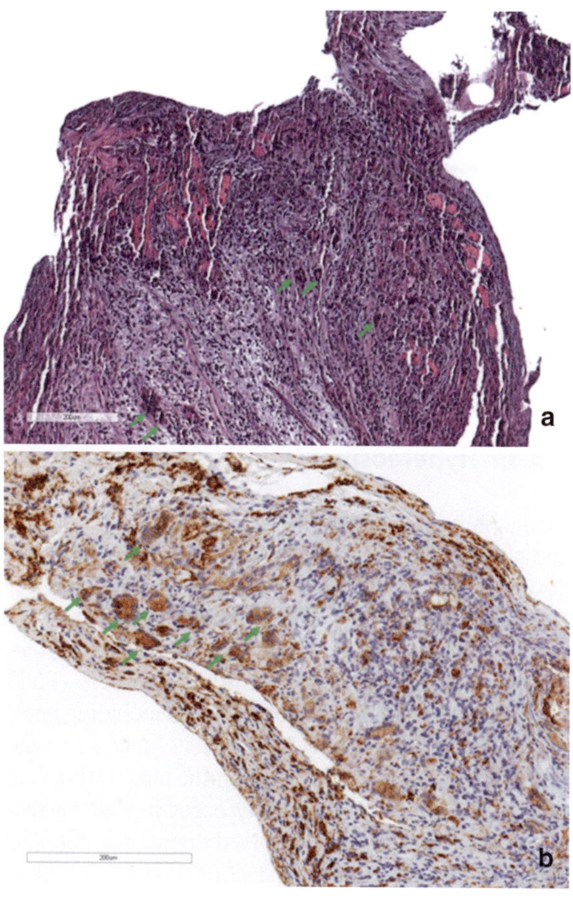

Fig. 4.4 The figure shows the EMB done in a 42-year-old patient with fulminant clinical manifestation of giant cell myocarditis. Death occurred 52 hours after admission to the emergency room, despite ventricular support, including medications and ECMO. (**a**) H&E; (**b**) Anti-CD68 immunostain showing specific immune-reaction of giant cells. Green arrows indicate the giant cells in both panels

transplantation. Data on management, including medications and mechanical circulatory support for bridge to recovery or to transplantation, are given in the dedicated chapter of this book.

The occurrence of GCM in Mendelian diseases is either underreported or unexplored or anecdotal and extremely rare. Myocarditis and giant cell hepatitis have been diagnosed in a patient with spinal muscular atrophy with respiratory distress (SMARD1) that was genetically caused by a nonsense mutation in the immunoglobulin-mu-binding protein 2, *IGHMBP2* disease gene. Mutations in this gene typically cause the autosomal recessive Charcot–Marie–Tooth disease, axonal, type 2S, and the distal hereditary motor neuronopathy type IV. This evidence does not causally link GCM with the genetic defect but rather represents a possible complication of the disease [191].

The association between GCM and myasthenia gravis (MG) and thymoma warrants special mention for two reasons: (1) the fair number of reports of GCM in patients with myasthenia gravis and (2) the association of giant cell polymyositis and myocarditis with myasthenia gravis and thymoma [168, 178, 192–195] and the possible responsiveness of myositis to novel biological drugs such as rituximab when steroids, acetylcholinesterase inhibitors, and immunosuppressive agents fail [193]. Cardiomyositis and subclinical cardiac dysfunction have been described in patients with thymoma and late-onset myasthenia gravis [192, 193].

To date, gene expression studies have not identified disease genes but rather have contributed to unraveling some pathophysiologic mechanisms of disease. Cardiac gene expression profiling has revealed upregulation of genes involved in the T-cell immune response, with the majority of upregulated genes involved in T-cell activation of the Th1 subset [196]. Plakoglobin expression was reduced in GCM and cardiac sarcoidosis as well as in ARVC, but not in lymphocytic myocarditis. A redistribution of plakoglobin from intercellular junctions to intracellular location was attributed to the mediation of IL-17 and TNF-alpha; both are considered to be mediators of granulomatous myocarditis [197].

4.4.3 Hypereosinophilic Syndromes (HES) and Myocarditis

Eosinophils are involved in host immune response to infection, cancer surveillance, and maintenance of other immune cells [198, 199]. The normal range of circulating eosinophils is 3–5%, which corresponds to an absolute count of 350–500/mm^3 [198]. Eosinophilia (hypereosinophilia) refers to an increased absolute eosinophilic count in peripheral blood and is graded as mild (from upper normal limit to 1500/mm^3), moderate (1500–5000/mm^3), and severe (>5000/mm^3) [200]. Eosinophilia encompasses a broad range of disorders including hematologic eosinophilia (clonal, **n**eoplastic, primary, HE_N), non-hematologic (secondary or **r**eactive HE_R), eosinophilic diseases of **u**nknown **s**ignificance (HE_{US}), and **f**amilial diseases (HE_F) (Table 4.8). Organ damage may occur in each of these forms [201]. The heart is either the major or solely involved organ or is potentially involved in systemic diseases. Diagnostic criteria of HES [201] were modified in 2006 when the definition

Table 4.8 Classification of HE eosinophilic syndromes

Class	Abbreviation	Pathogenesis/definition
Hereditary (familial, FA) HE	HE_{FA}	Pathogenesis unknown; familial clustering; absence of hereditary immunodeficiency; and absence of a reactive or neoplastic condition/disorder underlying HE
HE of undetermined significance (US)	HE_{US}	No underlying cause of HE, no family history, no evidence of a reactive or neoplastic condition/disorder underlying HE, and no end-organ damage attributable to HE
Primary (clonal/neoplastic) (N) HE[a]	HE_{N}	Underlying stem cell, myeloid, or eosinophilic neoplasm, as classified by WHO criteria; eosinophils considered neoplastic cells[b]
Secondary (reactive) HE[a]	HE_{R}	Underlying condition/disease in which eosinophils are considered nonclonal cells[b]; HE considered cytokine driven in most cases[c]

[a]HEN and HER should guide further diagnostic evaluations but cannot serve as final diagnoses
[b]Proven clonality: a myeloid or stem cell neoplasm typically manifesting with clonal HE; typical molecular defect is demonstrable (e.g., *PDGFR* or *FGFR* mutations or *BCR/ABL1*); eosinophilia should be considered clonal
[c]In a group of patients, HER might be caused/triggered by other as yet unknown processes because no increase in eosinophilopoietic cytokine levels can be documented

was expanded to include other previously distinct diseases associated with eosinophilia [eosinophilic granulomatosis with polyangiitis (EGPA), formerly known as Churg–Strauss syndrome, chronic eosinophilic pneumonia, and eosinophilic gastrointestinal disorders (EGID)] [200–202]. In 2010, the 6-month diagnostic period was substituted with the criterion of elevation of the absolute eosinophilic count >1500/mm^3 on at least two occasions [203]; it was recommended that the diagnosis had to be formulated in patients with "tissue eosinophilia and marked peripheral eosinophilia." The definition of HES was also expanded in order to include molecular evidence of end-organ damage [203]. HES has an age-adjusted prevalence of approximately 0.036 per 100,000 wherein the estimates are based on the ICDO (International Classification of Disease for Oncology Version 3), coding 9964/3 (HES including chronic eosinophilic leukemia), and the SEER database (Surveillance, Epidemiology, and End Results) [204].

4.4.3.1 Somatic Mutations

HES with somatic genetic mutation PDGFRA/B-FGFR1 fusion accounts for a minority of cases (median = 23%, range 3–56%) [205]. In developing countries, FIP1L1-PDGFRA fusion occurs in approximately 10–20% of patients with idiopathic hypereosinophilia [205, 206], usually young adults/adults and, less commonly, children and elderly [207–210]. Most patients with FIP1L1-PDGFRA fusion or myeloproliferative variants are male [205, 211, 212], while other eosinophilia subtypes do not show gender differences. Other rearrangements such as BCR/ABL1 are far less common than FIP1L1-PDGFRA.

4.4.3.2 HES: The Clinical Phenotype

The clinical presentation of HES is heterogeneous and nonspecific (weakness, fatigue, dyspnea, myalgias, angioedema, rash, fever, rhinitis, and diarrhea) [213]. Patients demonstrate leukocytosis (e.g., 20,000–30,000/mm^3 or higher) with eosinophilia in the range of 30–70%, neutrophilia, basophilia, myeloid immaturity, and both mature and immature eosinophils with varying degrees of dysplasia [214]. Anemia occurs in more than 50% of patients; thrombocytopenia, bone marrow eosinophilia with Charcot–Leyden crystals, and possible increased blasts and marrow fibrosis can also recur [198, 202]. Skin is the most commonly affected tissue (about 70% of patients), followed by lung and gastrointestinal manifestations in 40% and 30% of cases, respectively.

4.4.3.3 Eosinophilic Disease: The Cardiac Phenotype

Cardiac involvement occurs in 20% of patients [214, 215] and affects the myocardium, endocardium, and valves. The release of toxic mediators by interstitial eosinophils is associated with heart failure. Endocardial infiltration causes mural thrombi with increased embolic risk. Late phases are characterized by endocardial fibrosis manifesting with restrictive physiology. Valve regurgitation occurs when mural endocardial thrombosis and fibrosis involve mitral or tricuspid valve leaflets [214, 215]. Cardiac involvement is a major cause of morbidity and mortality in HES [216–219]. The disease course is divided into three stages: (1) an acute necrotic stage, (2) a thrombotic stage, and (3) a fibrotic stage. The *early, acute necrotic stage* is characterized by eosinophilic and lymphocytic infiltration; eosinophils undergo degranulation in the myocardial interstitium, releasing biologically active factors that cause myocyte injury (Fig. 4.5). In the *thrombotic stage*, mural thrombi stratify on the endocardium. Endocardial thrombophilia is likely promoted by the release of antifibrinolytic mediators such as PAI-2 and thrombomodulin-eosinophilic proteins that impair the anticoagulant property of the endocardial cells [209]. Thrombi most commonly involve the ventricular apex and further extend to subvalvular regions

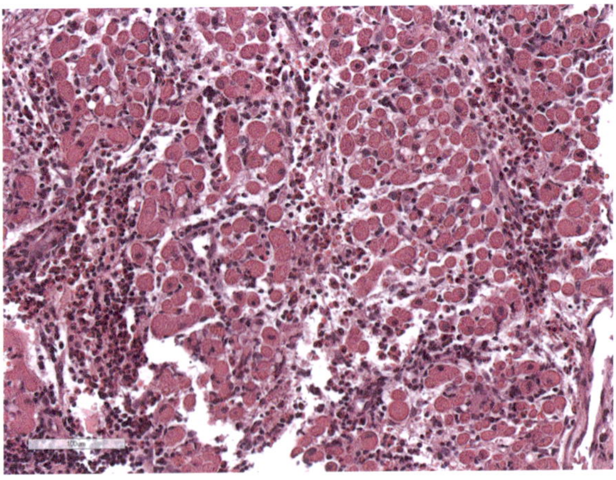

Fig. 4.5 Acute eosinophilic myocarditis in a patient with HE without known triggers/toxic substances. The FIP1L1-PDGFRA rearrangements tested negative. Full clinical recovery occurred in 4 weeks after steroid treatment

and, occasionally, to atria. In the *scarring (fibrotic) stage,* both ventricles and subvalvular structures of the atrio-ventricular valves are involved. The functional phenotype is typically restrictive, as in endomyocardial fibrosis [217, 218].

4.4.3.4 EGPA (formerly Churg–Strauss Syndrome): Familial Clustering and Genetics

EGPA is a systemic necrotizing vasculitis that affects small-to-medium-sized vessels [202]. EGPA belongs to the group of antineutrophil cytoplasm antibody (ANCA)-associated vasculitis (AAV) and is characterized by blood and tissue eosinophilia and asthma, thus distinct from granulomatosis with polyangiitis (Wegener's) and microscopic polyangiitis. ANCA positivity ranges from 30 to 70% in EGPA patients but is usually less frequently observed than in other AAV. Diagnostic and management algorithms for EGPA are reported in the corresponding chapter of this book. Although repeatedly mentioned in review articles, the contribution of germline mutations to EGPA remains elusive. A few reports describe familial clustering of EGPA: a sib pair, brother and sister [220], two sisters [221], and father and son [222]. The precise cause is unknown and genetic determinants or contributors remain unexplored. However, exceptional cases of organ transplantation in identical twins and different reactions to the same medication seem to exclude a genetic basis or predisposition to EGPA. One is a pair of twins in which one affected by EGPA received the identical twin graft with rejection-free excellent clinical results [223]. The second example is a pair of twins, both affected by asthma and treated with the same drug (leukotriene receptor antagonists, by instance, suspected to cause EGPA): one twin developed EGPA and the other did not [224]. Nevertheless, the search for risk factors or susceptibility continues to be an object of interest. Genetic studies that investigate the group of AAV [granulomatosis with polyangiitis (Wegener's) (GPA), microscopic polyangiitis (MPA), and Churg–Strauss syndrome (CSS)] showed that the genetic variants may vary in the three groups of AAV. As an example, the PTPN22 620 W allele confers susceptibility to the development of GPA but not to MPA or CSS [225]. The Lys656Asn SNP in the LEPR gene is positively associated with Wegener granulomatosis but not with CSS [226]. SNPs in the CCL26 gene (MIM*604697) that encode the chemokine Eotaxin-3 were initially described as associated with disease susceptibility and were later found not to predict the risk of disease, irrespective of the fact that serum eotaxin-3 is a sensitive and specific marker for the diagnosis of active CSS suitable for routine clinical practice [227]. Therefore, current evidence does not support a role for genetic variants in susceptibility to EGPA.

4.5 Inherited Primary Immunodeficiency Diseases (PID): Myocarditis and VARIABLE Cardiovascular Involvement

In PIDs, infections and inflammation are the complication and not the cause. The number of correctly diagnosed PID patients is progressively growing, with increased identification of previously unknown disease genes and availability of specific genetic tests. PIDs encompass a broad spectrum of inheritable disorders that are associated with increased susceptibility to infections, immune dysregulation, and malignancies [228]. PIDs are complex diseases with wide overlap (infection and/or malignancy) and immune dysregulation (auto-inflammation, auto-immunity, and/or allergy). The last classification guides the genetic and molecular diagnosis of patients with these rare diseases [228, 229]. However, the classification is complex (Table 4.9) and the extent and impact of these diseases on the cardiovascular system is far from being elucidated. Nonetheless, cardiologists are involved in the management of these patients, especially when myocarditis complicates the course of the disease. An example of PID with divergent cardiac

Table 4.9 Primary immunodeficiency syndromes (PID)

PID type	Inheritance and disease genes
Cellular and humoral immunity	• X-linked: *IL2RG* • Autosomal recessive *JAK3, IL7RA, PTPRC, CD3D, CD3E, CD3Z, CORO1A, RAG1, RAG2, ARTEMIS, PRKDC, VDj, LIG4, AK2, ADA, DOCK2, CD40LG, CD40, ICOS, CD3G, CD8A, ZAP70, TAP1, TAP2, TAPBP, B2M, CIITA, RFXANK, RFX5, RFXAP, ITK, MAGT1, DOCK8, RHOH, STK4, TRAC, B2M, IL21, MAP3K, CTPS1, LCK, MALT1, CARD11, BCL10, IL21, IL21R, OX40, IKBKB, LRBA, CD27, NIK, CTPS1, Omenn syndrome (hypomorphic mutations in RAG1, RAG2, Artemis, IL7RA, RMRP, ADA, DNA Ligase IV, IL2RG, AK2*) or associated with DiGeorge syndrome
Combined immunodeficiencies with associated or syndromic features	• X-linked: *Wiskott–Aldrich syndrome (WAS); WAS gene* • Autosomal recessive: *WIPF1, ATM, NBS1, BLM, DNMT3B, ZBTB24, PMS2, RNF168, MCM4,* *Contiguous gene deletion in chromosome 22q11.2 or mutation of a gene within this deletion region, TBX1 (DiGeorge Syndrome); CHARGE Syndrome (CHD7, SEMA3E, FOXN1, RMRP, SMARCAL1, STAT3, SPINK5, PGM3, DKC1, NOLA2, NOLA3, RTEL1, TERC, TERT, TINF2, TPP1, DCLRE1B, PARN, TCN2, SLC46A1, MTHFD, NEMO /IKBKG, IKBA (NFKIAB), ORAI1, STIM1, SP110, POLE1, TTC7A, EPG5, PNP, HOIL1/RBCK1, HOIP1 (/RNF31), CCBE1, STA5B*
Predominantly antibody deficiencies	1. ↓ of serum immunoglobulin isotypes with decreased or absent B cells • X-linked: *BKT,* • Autosomal recessive: *IGHM, IGLL1, CD79A, CD79B, BLNK, PIK3R1, TCF3,* 2. ↓ of at least two serum immunoglobulin isotypes with normal or low number of B cell • Autosomal recessive: *CD19, CD81, CD20, TNFRSF13B, TNFRSF13C, TWEAK (TNFSF12), NFKB2, TRNT1, TTC37,* 3. ↓ of serum IgG and IgA with normal/elevated IgM and normal numbers of B cells • Autosomal recessive: *AICDA, UNG, MSH6,* 4. Isotype or light chain deficiencies with generally normal numbers of B cells • Autosomal dominant: *PIK3CD, PIK3R1, CARD11* • Autosomal recessive: *deletion at 14q32, Kappa constant gene, CARD11*

Table 4.9 (continued)

PID type	Inheritance and disease genes
Diseases of immune dysregulation	1. Familial hemophagocytic lymphohistiocytosis (FHL) syndromes 1.1 FHL syndromes without hypopigmentation • X-linked: *SH2D1A, XIAP* • Autosomal recessive: *PRF1, UNC13D, STX11, STXBP2.* 1.2 FHL syndromes with hypopigmentation • Autosomal recessive: *LYST, RAB27A, AP3B1, PLDN,* 2. T-regulatory cells genetic defects • X-linked: *FOXP3,* • Autosomal recessive: *IL2RA* • Autosomal dominant: *CTLA4*
Congenital defects of phagocyte number, function, or both	1. Congenital neutropenias • Autosomal dominant: *ELANE, GFI1,* • Autosomal recessive: *HAX1, G6PC3, VPS45, G6PT1, ROBLD3/LAMTOR2, TAZ, CPH1, C16ORF57 (USB1), JAGN1, CLPB, CSF3R,* • X-linked: *WAS,* 2. Defects of motility • Autosomal recessive: *IRGB2, KINDLIN3, FPR1, CTSC, C/EBPE, SBDS,* • Autosomal dominant: *RAC2, ACTB* 3. Defects of respiratory burst • X-linked: *CYBB* • Autosomal recessive: *CYBA, NCF1, NCF2, NCF4,* 4. Other defects: • Autosomal dominant: *GATA4, CSF2RA*
Defects in intrinsic and innate immunity	1. Mendelian susceptibility to mycobacterial disease (MSMD) • X-linked: *CYBB* • Autosomal recessive: *IL12RB1, IL12B, IFNGR1* (also AD), *IFNGR2, STAT1, TYK2, ISG15, RORC, TMC6, TMC8, CXCR4,* • Autosomal dominant: *IRF8* 2. Epidermodysplasia verruciformis • Autosomal recessive: *TMC6, TMC8, CXCR4,* 3. Predisposition to severe viral infection • Autosomal recessive: STAT1, STAT2, IRF7, CD16, 4. Herpes simplex encephalitis (HSE) • Autosomal dominant and autosomal recessive: *TLR3, TRIF,* • Autosomal dominant: *TRAF3, TBK1,* • Autosomal recessive: *UNC93B1* 5. Predisposition to invasive fungal diseases • Autosomal recessive: *CARD9* 6. Chronic mucocutaneous candidiasis (CMC) • Autosomal dominant: *IL17F, STAT1,* • Autosomal recessive: *IL17RA, IL17RC, ACT1 (TRAF3IP2),* 7. TLR signaling pathway deficiency • Autosomal dominant: *RPSA, APOL-I (trypanosomiasis)* • Autosomal recessive: *IARK4, MYD88,*
Auto-inflammatory disorders	1. Defects effecting the inflammasome • Autosomal dominant and autosomal recessive: *MEFV,* • Autosomal dominant: *NLRP3, NLRP12, NLRP3, NLRC4, PLCG2, PLCG2, TNFRSF1A, PSTPIP1 (C2BP1), NOD2 (CARD15), CARD14, SH3BP2, COPA,* • Autosomal recessive: *MVK, ADAM17, LPIN2, IL1RN, IL36RN, SLC29A3, PSMB8,*

(continued)

Table 4.9 (continued)

PID type	Inheritance and disease genes
Complement deficiencies	1. Integral complement cascade component deficiencies • Autosomal dominant*: C3* • Autosomal recessive*: C1QA, C1QB, C1QC, C1R, C1S, C4A, C4B, C2, C3, C5, C6, C7, C8A, C8G, C9, MASP2, FCN3,* 2. Complement regulatory defect*s* • X-linked*:* CF • Autosomal dominant and autosomal recessive*: CFH, CFHR1-5,* • Autosomal dominant*: SERPING1, CFB, THBD, CD46,* • Autosomal recessive*: CFD, CFI, ITGAM, CD59*
Phenocopies of PID	Associated with somatic mutations • *TNFRSF6, KRAS, NRAS, NLRP3,* Associated with autoantibodies • *AIRE*

phenotypes (HCM and myocarditis) seems appropriate to give the perception of the complexity of the clinical manifestations.

4.5.1 The Omenn Syndrome (OMIM# 603554)

Children with Omenn Syndrome may have erythroderma, lymphadenopathy, eosinophilia, and profound immunodeficiency hepatosplenomegaly, failure to thrive, diarrhea, and alopecia; common laboratory abnormalities are eosinophilia and increased IgE, lymphocytosis, anemia, hypogammaglobulinemia, hypoproteinemia, and reduced lymphoproliferative responses to mitogens. Characteristic pathology includes thymic dysplasia, loss of B-cell-containing regions within the reticuloendothelial system, and extensive infiltrates of eosinophils and interdigitating reticular cells. The spectrum of cardiac involvement ranges from myocarditis to hypertrophic cardiomyopathy (HCM). In children with Omenn syndrome, cytomegalovirus (CMV) infections, which often run asymptomatic, can cause fatal CMV myocarditis [230]. Pathology may show pancarditis with eosinophil-rich inflammatory infiltrate in the myocardium [231]. Endomyocardial biopsy may show a mild T lymphocyte and histiocyte infiltrate and lack of myocyte hypertrophy [232]. Other manifestations include biventricular hypertrophy, impaired left ventricular systolic function, and severe sinus bradycardia, possibly secondary to endomyocardial disease caused by eosinophilia [233]. Successful bone marrow transplantation (BMT) has been reported in a patient with hypertrophic nonobstructive cardiomyopathy who developed BCG infection following neonatal vaccination [234].

4.5.2 Myocarditis in Immunocompromised Patients: Humoral Immunity

4.5.2.1 Agammaglobulinemia

Patients with X-linked agammaglobulinemia (XLA), a primary immunodeficiency caused by mutations in the gene that codes for Bruton tyrosine kinase (BTK), demonstrate deficient development of B lymphocytes and hypogammaglobulinemia. Infections are the most common clinical presentation (85%), followed by a positive family history (41%) and neutropenia (11%). Myocardial involvement is rare. Patients commonly manifest otitis (70%), pneumonia (62%), sinusitis (60%), chronic/recurrent diarrhea (23%), conjunctivitis (21%), pyoderma and/or cellulitis (18%), meningitis/encephalitis (11%), sepsis (10%), septic arthritis (8%), hepatitis (6%), and osteomyelitis (3%) [235]. BTK inhibitors are used for treatment of leukemia; these patients are exposed to high risk of pneumonia; the risk of myocarditis is unknown. However, polymorphisms in genes coding IL-6 and IL-10 and Fcg RIIa receptors (B lymphocyte growth and differentiation factors) increase susceptibility to pneumonia. In case of humoral immunodeficiency, antibody replacement therapy may be indicated [236].

4.5.2.2 Hypogammaglobulinemia

Patients with hypogammaglobulinemia, both inherited and acquired, are exposed to high risk of infections, in particular to those controlled through humoral immunity, such as picornaviridae infections. Bi-allelic mutations in *LRBA* (from *Lipopolysaccharide-responsive and beige-like anchor protein*) cause primary immunodeficiency with clinical features ranging from hypogammaglobulinemia and lymphoproliferative syndrome to inflammatory bowel disease and heterogeneous autoimmune manifestations [237]. A recent report describes the case of a 16-year-old female affected by systemic lupus erythematosus that was diagnosed 6 years before. She was admitted to hospital with chest pain and dyspnea. Her hypogammaglobulinemia was iatrogenic and secondary to rituximab treatment. The key clinical diagnosis was myocarditis caused by human parechovirus (HPeV) (*Picornaviridae* family of RNA viruses). The diagnosis of myocarditis was clinically suspected and confirmed with endomyocardial biopsy. IVIG therapy did not prevent encephalitis [238]. Patients, especially children, affected by hematologic-oncologic disorders and solid organ malignancies and appropriately treated for their disease, may develop neutropenia and decrease of their serum immunoglobulin levels. In these patients, the risk of myocarditis (bacterial and viral) is high; as such, when presenting with signs of heart failure, myocarditis should be considered and a precise diagnosis (presence of myocarditis and cause) should be obtained because of the associated mortality, even in patients with disease remission [239].

4.5.3 Congenital Neutropenia

The term "congenital neutropenia" encompasses a large group of permanent and intermittent neutropenic diseases defined by severely ($<0{\cdot}5 \times 10^9$/L) or mildly ($0{\cdot}5$ and $1{\cdot}5 \times 10^9$/L) reduced neutrophil count. The diseases are characterized by clinical and genetic heterogeneity and may affect the pancreas, central nervous system, heart, bone, muscle, and skin. The prevention and/or control of infections, the management of associated organ dysfunction, and the prevention of leukemic transformation constitute the main treatment targets [240]. Information on cardiac involvement in the numerous and complex types of congenital neutropenia is in its infancy and many of these diseases have recently been characterized on the genetic-molecular level. In addition, they are very rare, clinically heterogeneous, and often burdened by early extracardiac complications that may limit their complete phenotypic expression. However, future scientific developments can broaden horizons for expanding the knowledge of the pathogenic mechanisms of cardiac infections. The heart is involved in many of these diseases. For some of them, cardiac manifestations are being characterized and classified, with two possible major phenotypes: congenital heart disease (CHD) and myocarditis/cardiomyopathy. Two examples can underscore the importance of ongoing clinical research in this area.

4.5.3.1 Severe Congenital Neutropenia Type IV (SCN IV or SCN4) or G6PC3 Deficiency

SCN4 is an autosomal recessive disease characterized by severe congenital neutropenia, intermittent thrombocytopenia, prominent superficial venous circulation, congenital heart defects [atrial septal defect (ASD) being the most common], and urogenital malformations [241]. Although most cases are syndromic, non-syndromic forms are also reported [242]. The description of the spectrum of the phenotype is expanding and definitive SCN4 phenotype/genotype has not been established thus far. The recurrent p.Gly260Arg mutation has been identified in nine different patients with ASD type 2 [241, 243–245]. Treatment with granulocyte colony-stimulating factor restores the absolute neutrophil count and neutrophil functional competence. Myocarditis has not been described. However, this new field of knowledge, given the cardiovascular relevance and the possibility that SCN4 manifests with non-syndromic phenotype, must at least be known by cardiologists and reported to hematologists when these patients present with neutropenia and/or thrombocytopenia and/or associated CHD.

4.5.3.2 Shwachman–Diamond Syndrome (SDS)

SDS is an autosomal recessive disorder characterized by bone marrow failure and exocrine pancreatic dysfunction [246]. Two kinds of cardiac involvement have been described: "cardiomyopathies with heart failure (myocardial fibrosis and histopathological necrosis)" and CHD [247–249]. Recently, a case of dilated cardiomyopathy with refractory heart failure was reported in a 15-year-old girl with SDS [250]. Of 102 patients with genetically proven SDS, 12 had cardiac abnormalities: six had cardiomyopathy and six had CHD [251]. The pathologic substrates of systolic dysfunction are still unexplored, with few sporadic cases describing DCM with myocardial fibrosis. However, cardiac evaluation is also a major clinical need before and during cardiotoxic chemotherapy in case of hematopoietic stem cell transplantation (HSCT) [252]. The cardiac marker potentially predicting the progression to heart failure is circumferential strain ε(cc) that is abnormal in 33% of cases prior to HSCT and 33% of those who had undergone HSCT in those with normal left ventricular ejection fraction [253].

4.6 Auto-Inflammatory Syndromes (AIS) and Myocarditis

4.6.1 Introduction

Auto-inflammatory syndromes (AIS) encompass a large group of diseases clinically characterized by recurring inflammatory manifestation with variable organ involvement and febrile episodes [254]. The classification is complex and the number of diseases and related genetic causes is continuously expanding [255, 256]. The term auto-inflammation links the phenotypes with the defects of innate immune-mediated inflammation and distinguishes the related diseases from those caused by the dysfunction of adaptive immune function, i.e., those associated with autoimmune disorders. The number of myocarditis described in auto-inflammatory disease is low. The reasons may be that myocarditis is indeed very rare, or that, in the syndromic setting in which myocarditis may occur, the involvement of other organs and systems determines the phenotype and the course of the disease, or that our limited knowledge prevents precise phenotype description of AIS with myocardial involvement. Nevertheless, myocarditis deserves to be mentioned in the context of the AIS because it can occur and because its presence and evolution can seriously alter the clinical course of these patients.

4.6.2 Major Groups of AIS

IL-1-mediated auto-inflammatory syndromes include familial Mediterranean fever (FMF) that is the first systemic auto-inflammatory disorder to be genetically characterized. FMF is a rare autosomal recessive disease caused by homozygous or double heterozygous mutations in the *MEFV* gene encoding pyrin [257]. Another systemic auto-inflammatory disorder, the autosomal dominant receptor-associated periodic fever syndrome (TRAPS), was identified after the discovery of the *TNFR1* gene, which encodes the extracellular domains of the 55 kDa TNF receptor [258, 259]. Both FMF and TRAPS manifest with unexplained fevers, skin rashes, serositis, and arthralgias, in variable combinations. Myocarditis is uncommonly reported in both disorders and other IL-1-mediated auto-inflammatory syndromes [260], with pericarditis being much more common and potentially limiting the distinction of myocarditis from pericarditis.

In the IL-18-mediated auto-inflammation and susceptibility to macrophage-activation syndrome (MAS), myocarditis can be a complication of the underlying phenotype [261]. The disease gene is *NLRC4* and the diagnostic marker is the high level of IL18 that results from spontaneous and induced macrophage activation and pyroptosis. However, the levels of IL18 are not routinely measured in patients with suspected myocarditis; therefore, a diagnostic marker for a very rare disease is missing in clinical practice.

The A20 haplo-insufficiency-related syndromes are gaining attention for the new association with adult-onset Still's Disease (AOSD), a condition in which myocarditis is not uncommon. AOSD is a rare disease clinically characterized by fevers, arthritis, and skin rash. The etiology is unknown, but recent advances in the identification of the causes and characterization of the phenotypes of AIS are lending way to identifying the specific cause(s). As anticipated, A20 haplo-insufficiency (HA20) is one of the causes of AIS [262]. The A20 protein, which is encoded by the *TNFAIP3* gene, is a critical inhibitor of pro-inflammatory signaling pathways and is involved in negative regulation of auto-inflammation and autoimmunity [263]. The clinical phenotypes associated with HA20 are heterogeneous, including autoimmune diseases (Behçet's disease, hereditary fever-like condition, juvenile idiopathic arthritis, systemic lupus erythematosus, and rheumatoid arthritis) and, recently, AOSD: a splice site mutation on the *TNFAIP3* gene has been identified in a patient previously diagnosed with adult-onset Stills' disease (AOSD) [264]; once correctly diagnosed, the patient was successfully treated with anti-IL6 receptor biologic tocilizumab [265]. Myocarditis has been repeatedly reported in AOSD, presenting as myocarditis-pericarditis [265–274], with pericarditis occurring in more than 50% of cases [265]. Coronary arteritis has also been described [272]. In most cases, the diagnosis of myocarditis was formulated on the basis of clinical, biochemical, and imaging criteria. An appropriate endomyocardial biopsy study, however, should be performed to distinguish pericarditis from myocarditis, mostly because the chronic consequences can be different, irrespective of the cause.

The interferon-mediated auto-inflammatory diseases (or type I interferonopathies or IFN-mediated auto-inflammatory diseases (IMADs)) are defined by the chronic excessive type I interferon (IFN) production [275] and include the group of *Aicardi–Goutières Syndromes* (AGS), in which the "cardiomyopathy" phenotype is part of the spectrum of clinical manifestations of these diseases (Table 4.10).

Table 4.10 Aicardi-Goutieres syndromes

Phenotype	Phenotype MIM number	Inheritance	Chromosome	Gene/Locus	Gene/MIM number
Aicardi-Goutieres syndrome 1	225750	AD, AR	3p21.31	*TREX1*	606609
Aicardi-Goutieres syndrome 2	610181	AR	13q14.3	*RNASEH2B*	610326
Aicardi-Goutieres syndrome 3	610329	AR	11q13.1	*RNASEH2C*	610330
Aicardi-Goutieres syndrome 4	610333	AR	19p13.13	*RNASEH2A*	606034
Aicardi-Goutieres syndrome 5	612952	AR	20q11.23	*SAMHD1*	606754
Aicardi-Goutieres syndrome 6	615010	AR	1q21.3	*ADAR*	146920
Aicardi-Goutieres syndrome 7	615846	AD	2q24.2	*IFIH1*	606951

AGS are characterized by hypothyroidism, chilblains, glaucoma, cardiomyopathy, intracerebral vasculitis, peripheral neuropathy, bowel inflammation, and systemic lupus erythematosus [276]. AGSs (types 1–7) are auto-inflammatory diseases caused by mutations of genes involved in nucleic acid metabolism/signaling (*TREX1*, *RNASEH2A*, *RNASEH2B*, *RNASEH2C*, *SAMHD1*, *ADAR*, or *IFIH1)* and can manifest with in utero disease onset or with postnatal presentation, usually within the first year of life, with subacute encephalopathy (Table 4.10) [277]. The pathology of affected hearts is still largely unexplored. Cardiac involvement has been described as infantile-onset hypertrophic cardiomyopathy with hypothyroidism and demyelinating peripheral neuropathy. Whether the pathologic substrate of the cardiomyopathy has inflammatory origin is still unknown [278]. The absence of Trex1 (*TREX1* is one of the known disease genes causing AGS) in mice causes myocarditis [278]. The enzyme degrades endogenous retro-elements, thus linking them to autoimmune disease. In the Trex1-null mouse, an FDA-approved drug that inhibits reverse transcriptase can improve the myocarditis, indicating that retro-elements (RE) play a role in this hereditary form of autoimmunity and that administration of RE inhibitors might ameliorate AGS [279]. The possible association of mutations in other genes associated with *AGS* and myocarditis is still unexplored. However, mutations in *IFIH1* cause *Singleton-Merten syndrome 1* (SMS1), which is allelic at the same locus of *AGS7* and may manifest with cardiomegaly, heart failure, and conduction disease. The syndrome (aortic calcification, dental anomalies, osteopenia and acro-osteolysis, glaucoma, psoriasis, muscle weakness, joint laxity and abnormal facies traits with broad forehead, high anterior hairline, smooth philtrum, and thin upper vermilion border) is unlikely to escape clinical detection [280]. In addition, very recent experimental studies explored the involvement of adenosine deaminases acting on RNA 1 (*ADAR1*) (AGS6) in inflammatory diseases, cancer, and host defenses against viral infections. ADARs are enzymes that regulate RNA metabolism through post-transcriptional mechanisms. In particular, the complex ADAR1p150/DICER promotes the expression of miRNA-222 that is highly expressed in cardiac myocytes in viral myocarditis. In cultured cells, miR-222 suppresses PTEN expression. These preliminary experimental studies suggest that ADAR1p150 could play a role in gene expression in viral myocarditis [281]. The cardiovascular impact of type I interferonopathies such as AGS (TREX1 and IFIH1 in particular) could go beyond possible myocardial inflammation and expand to primary pulmonary hypertension [282] as well as to the risk of coronary artery disease [283].

4.7 Conclusions

Based on the current state of knowledge on myocarditis, we can say that infectious myocarditis is not in fact a genetic disease, as in the absence of an infectious pathogen, there is no myocarditis. However, a rigorous attempt is being made to establish who and why, with equal exposure to the same pathogen, develops myocarditis. Individual gene variants are candidates to play a role in both disease susceptibility/

predisposition and contribute to the severity of phenotypes and outcomes observed in different patients with myocardial infections caused by the same pathogens.

Non-infectious myocarditis, excluding exogenous toxic exposures, may have a hereditary basis or be strongly influenced by genetic factors. It is clinically difficult to distinguish acquired and inherited forms, further because the hereditary forms are often passed as recessive traits. Finally, inherited diseases in immunodeficiency syndromes and auto-inflammatory diseases can have overlapping causes and phenotypes in which myocarditis may occur. These are often syndromic disorders. Many of them have been identified only recently, and the number of reported and proven cases is limited to a few case reports or small clinical series. This clinical area is also continuously expanding, and in the short term, we expect radical changes in our knowledge and understanding of the mechanisms and causes of myocarditis. A critical point remains unsolved: true myocarditis is that diagnosed on tissue biopsy, at least until molecular imaging techniques are readily and routinely available, to demonstrate not the myocardial edema, but the inflammatory interstitial cells. Until then, we can accept a scientific literature that is based on non-biopsy diagnoses, but we retain the belief that, in the absence of pathological evidence, not all diagnoses are correct. The cardiologist should lead the diagnostic work-up of these diseases as well as the clinical management of these patients.

References

1. Arbustini E, Agozzino M, Favalli V, Pinney S, Narula J. Myocarditis. In: Fuster V, Harrington RA, Narula J, Eapen ZJ, editors. Hurst's the heart, Chapter 63. 14th ed. New York: McGraw-Hill; 2017.
2. Bondue A, Arbustini E, Bianco A, et al. Complex roads from genotype to phenotype in dilated cardiomyopathy: scientific update from the Working Group of Myocardial Function of the European Society of Cardiology. Cardiovasc Res. 2018;114(10):1287–303.
3. Heidt T, Courties G, Dutta P, et al. Differential contribution of monocytes to heart macrophages in steady-state and after myocardial infarction. Circ Res. 2014;115:284–95.
4. Pinto AR, Paolicelli R, Salimova E, et al. An abundant tissue macrophage population in the adult murine heart with a distinct alternatively-activated macrophage profile. PLoS One. 2012;7:e36814.
5. Epelman S, Lavine KJ, Beaudin AE, et al. Embryonic and adult-derived resident cardiac macrophages are maintained through distinct mechanisms at steady state and during inflammation. Immunity. 2014;40:91–104.
6. Molawi K, Wolf Y, Kandalla PK, et al. Progressive replacement of embryo-derived cardiac macrophages with age. J Exp Med. 2014;211:2151–8.
7. Gomez I, Duval V, Silvestre JS. Cardiomyocytes and macrophages discourse on the method to govern cardiac repair. Front Cardiovasc Med. 2018;5:134.
8. Monnerat G, Alarcón ML, Vasconcellos LR, et al. Macrophage-dependent IL-1β production induces cardiac arrhythmias in diabetic mice. Nat Commun. 2016;7:13344.
9. Fung G, Luo H, Qiu Y, Yang D, McManus B. Myocarditis. Circ Res. 2016;118:496–514.
10. Stanaway JD, Roth G. The burden of Chagas disease: estimates and challenges. Glob Heart. 2015;10:139–44.
11. Chomel B. Lyme disease. Rev Sci Tech. 2015;34:569–76.
12. Caforio ALP, Pankuweit S, Arbustini E, European Society of Cardiology Working Group on Myocardial and Pericardial Diseases, et al. Current state of knowledge on aetiology,

diagnosis, management, and therapy of myocarditis: a position statement of the European Society of Cardiology Working Group on Myocardial and Pericardial Diseases. Eur Heart J. 2013;34(33):2636–48.
13. Caforio ALP, Adler Y, Agostini C, et al. Diagnosis and management of myocardial involvement in systemic immune-mediated diseases: a position statement of the European Society of Cardiology Working Group on Myocardial and Pericardial Disease. Eur Heart J. 2017;38(35):2649–62.
14. Banoo S, Bell D, Bossuyt P, TDR Diagnostics Evaluation Expert Panel, et al. Evaluation of diagnostic tests for infectious diseases: general principles. Nat Rev Microbiol. 2010;8:S17–29.
15. Rostoff P, Nessler B, Pikul P, Golinska-Grzybala K, Miszalski-Jamka T, Nessler J. Fulminant adrenergic myocarditis complicated by pulmonary edema, cardiogenic shock and cardiac arrest. Am J Emerg Med. 2018;36(2):344.e1–4.
16. Bissel SJ, Winkler CC, DelTondo J, Wang G, Williams K, Wiley CA. Coxsackievirus B4 myocarditis and meningoencephalitis in newborn twins. Neuropathology. 2014;34(5):429–37.
17. Amdani SM, Kim HS, Orvedahl A, John AO, Said A, Simpson K. Successful treatment of fulminant neonatal enteroviral myocarditis in monochorionic diamniotic twins with cardiopulmonary support, intravenous immunoglobulin and pocapavir. BMJ Case Rep. 2018;2018:bcr-2017-224133.
18. Cho HJ, Ma JS. Left ventricular non-compaction progression to dilated cardiomyopathy following acute myocarditis in an early infant twin. Minerva Pediatr. 2015;67(2):199–202.
19. Bajanowski T, Rossi L, Biondo B, et al. Prolonged QT interval and sudden infant deathDOUBLEHYPHENreport of two cases. Forensic Sci Int. 2001;115(1–2):147–53.
20. Cognet T, Lairez O, Marchal P, Roncalli J, Galinier M. A family history of dilated cardiomyopathy induced by viral myocarditis. Case Rep Cardiol. 2012;2012:204371.
21. Sharma K, Orbai AM, Desai D, et al. Brief report: antisynthetase syndrome-associated myocarditis. J Card Fail. 2014;20(12):939–45.
22. Tsirpanlis G, Moustakas G, Sakka E, et al. Catastrophic antiphospholipid syndrome in a 14-year-old child. Pediatr Nephrol. 2005;20(4):519–21.
23. Roubille F, Cayla G, Gahide G, Mourad G, Macia JC. Acute myocarditis and tumor necrosis factor receptor-associated periodic (TRAP) syndrome: first case described and discussion. Eur J Intern Med. 2009;20(2):e25–6.
24. Cunha-Neto E, Chevillard C. Chagas disease cardiomyopathy: immunopathology and genetics. Mediat Inflamm. 2014;2014:683230.
25. Hintenberger R, Falkinger A, Danninger K, Pieringer H. Cardiovascular disease in patients with autoinflammatory syndromes. Rheumatol Int. 2018;38(1):37–50.
26. Bousfiha A, Jeddane L, Al-Herz W, et al. The 2015 IUIS phenotypic classification for primary immunodeficiencies. J Clin Immunol. 2015;35(8):727–38.
27. Casanova JL. Human genetic basis of interindividual variability in the course of infection. Proc Natl Acad Sci U S A. 2015;112(51):E7118–27.
28. Casanova JL. Severe infectious diseases of childhood as monogenic inborn errors of immunity. Proc Natl Acad Sci U S A. 2015;112(51):E7128–37.
29. Haerynck F, Holland SM, Rosenzweig SD, et al. Disseminated Mycobacterium avium infection in a patient with a novel mutation in the interleukin-12 receptor-beta1 chain. J Pediatr. 2008;153(5):721–2.
30. Gorbea C, Makar KA, Pauschinger M, et al. A role for toll-like receptor 3 variants in host susceptibility to enteroviral myocarditis and dilated cardiomyopathy. J Biol Chem. 2010;285(30):23208–23.
31. Cannatà A, Artico J, Gentile P, Merlo M, Sinagra G. Myocarditis evolving in cardiomyopathy: when genetics and offending causes work together. Eur Heart J Suppl. 2019;21(Suppl B):B90–5.
32. Belkaya S, Kontorovich AR, Byun M, et al. Autosomal recessive cardiomyopathy presenting as acute myocarditis. J Am Coll Cardiol. 2017;69(13):1653–65.
33. Lopez-Ayala JM, Pastor-Quirante F, Gonzalez-Carrillo J, et al. Genetics of myocarditis in arrhythmogenic right ventricular dysplasia. Heart Rhythm. 2015;12(4):766–73.

34. Wang C, Wong J, Fung G, et al. Dysferlin deficiency confers increased susceptibility to coxsackievirus-induced cardiomyopathy. Cell Microbiol. 2015;17:1423–30.
35. Badorff C, Lee GH, Lamphear BJ, et al. Enteroviral protease 2A cleaves dystrophin: evidence of cytoskeletal disruption in an acquired cardiomyopathy. Nat Med. 1999;5:320–6.
36. Xiong D, Lee GH, Badorff C, et al. Dystrophin deficiency markedly increases enterovirus-induced cardiomyopathy: a genetic predisposition to viral heart disease. Nat Med. 2002;8:872–7.
37. Diegoli M, Grasso M, Favalli V, et al. Diagnostic work-up and risk stratification in X-linked dilated cardiomyopathies caused by dystrophin defects. J Am Coll Cardiol. 2011;58:925–34.
38. Badorff C, Knowlton KU. Dystrophin disruption in enterovirus-induced myocarditis and dilated cardiomyopathy: from bench to bedside. Med Microbiol Immunol. 2004;193(2–3):121–6.
39. Lee GH, Badorff C, Knowlton KU. Dissociation of sarcoglycans and the dystrophin carboxyl terminus from the sarcolemma in enteroviral cardiomyopathy. Circ Res. 2000;87(6):489–95.
40. Garmaroudi FS, Marchant D, Hendry R, et al. Coxsackievirus B3 replication and pathogenesis. Future Microbiol. 2015;10:629–53.
41. Jiang M, Wei D, Ou WL, et al. Autopsy findings in children with hand, foot, and mouth disease. N Engl J Med. 2012;367(1):91–2.
42. Chang LY, Lin TY, Hsu KH, et al. Clinical features and risk factors of pulmonary oedema after enterovirus-71-related hand, foot, and mouth disease. Lancet. 1999;354:1682–6.
43. Verma NA, Zheng XT, Harris MU, et al. Outbreak of life-threatening coxsackievirus B1 myocarditis in neonates. Clin Infect Dis. 2009;49:759–63.
44. Wikswo ME, Khetsuriani N, Fowlkes AL, et al. Increased activity of Coxsackievirus B1 strains associated with severe disease among young infants in the United States, 2007–2008. Clin Infect Dis. 2009;49:e44–51.
45. Duintjer Tebbens RJ, Pallansch MA, et al. Oral poliovirus vaccine evolution and insights relevant to modeling the risks of circulating vaccine-derived polioviruses (cVDPVs). Risk Anal. 2013;33(4):680–702.
46. Antona D, Kossorotoff M, Schuffenecker I, et al. Severe paediatric conditions linked with EV-A71 and EV-D68, France, May to October 2016. Euro Surveill. 2016;21(46):30402.
47. Shi Y, Chen C, Lisewski U, Wrackmeyer U, et al. Cardiac deletion of the coxsackievirus-adenovirus receptor abolishes coxsackievirus B3 infection and prevents myocarditis in vivo. J Am Coll Cardiol. 2009;53:1219–26.
48. Noutsias M, Fechner H, de Jonge H, et al. Human coxsackie-adenovirus receptor is colocalized with integrins alpha(v)beta(3) and alpha(v)beta(5) on the cardiomyocyte sarcolemma and upregulated in dilated cardiomyopathy: implications for cardiotropic viral infections. Circulation. 2001;104:275–80.
49. Jagdeo JM, Dufour A, Fung G, et al. Heterogeneous nuclear ribonucleoprotein M facilitates enterovirus infection. J Virol. 2015;89:7064–78.
50. Alirezaei M, Flynn CT, Wood MR, Harkins S, Whitton JL. Coxsackievirus can exploit LC3 in both autophagy-dependent and-independent manners in vivo. Autophagy. 2015;11:1389–407.
51. Robinson SM, Tsueng G, Sin J, et al. Coxsackievirus B exits the host cell in shed microvesicles displaying autophagosomal markers. PLoS Pathog. 2014;10:e1004045.
52. Hemida MG, Ye X, Zhang HM, et al. MicroRNA-203 enhances coxsackievirus B3 replication through targeting zinc finger protein-148. Cell Mol Life Sci. 2013;70:277–91.
53. Corsten MF, Papageorgiou A, Verhesen W, et al. MicroRNA profiling identifies microRNA-155 as an adverse mediator of cardiac injury and dysfunction during acute viral myocarditis. Circ Res. 2012;111:415–25.
54. Pagnamenta AT, Howard MF, Wisniewski E, et al. Germline recessive mutations in PI4KA are associated with perisylvian polymicrogyria, cerebellar hypoplasia and arthrogryposis. Hum Mol Genet. 2015;24(13):3732–41.
55. Bojjireddy N, Botyanszki J, Hammond G, et al. Pharmacological and genetic targeting of the PI4KA enzyme reveals its important role in maintaining plasma membrane phosphatidylinositol 4-phosphate and phosphatidylinositol 4,5-bisphosphate levels. J Biol Chem. 2014;289(9):6120–32.

56. Lyoo H, van der Schaar HM, Dorobantu CM, et al. ACBD3 is an essential pan-enterovirus host factor that mediates the interaction between viral 3A protein and cellular protein PI4KB. MBio. 2019;10(1):e02742-18.
57. Tschöpe C, Müller I, Xia Y, et al. NOD2 (nucleotide-binding oligomerization domain 2) is a major pathogenic mediator of coxsackievirus B3-induced myocarditis. Circ Heart Fail. 2017;10(9):e003870.
58. Rogo LD, Mokhtari-Azad T, Kabir MH, Rezaei F. Human parvovirus B19: a review. Acta Virol. 2014;58:199–213.
59. Kerr JR. A review of blood diseases and cytopenias associated with human parvovirus B19 infection. Rev Med Virol. 2015;25:224–40.
60. Adamson-Small LA, Ignatovich IV, Laemmerhirt MG, et al. Persistent parvovirus B19 infection in non-erythroid tissues: possible role in the inflammatory and disease process. Virus Res. 2014;190:8–16.
61. Ganaie SS, Chen AY, Huang C, Xu P, Kleiboeker S, Du A, Qiu J. RNA binding protein RBM38 regulates expression of the 11-Kilodalton protein of parvovirus B19, which facilitates viral DNA replication. J Virol. 2018;92(8):e02050-17.
62. Xu P, Chen AY, Ganaie SS, Cheng F, Shen W, Wang X, Kleiboeker S, Li Y, Qiu J. The 11-kilodalton nonstructural protein of Human parvovirus B19 facilitates viral DNA replication by interacting with Grb2 through its Proline-rich motifs. J Virol. 2018;93(1):e01464-18.
63. Von Kietzell K, Pozzuto T, Heilbronn R, et al. Antibody-mediated enhancement of parvovirus B19 uptake into endothelial cells mediated by a receptor for complement factor C1q. J Virol. 2014;88:8102–15.
64. Kerr JR. The role of parvovirus B19 in the pathogenesis of autoimmunity and autoimmune disease. J Clin Pathol. 2016;69(4):279–91.
65. Koliou M, Karaoli E, Soteriades ES, et al. Acute hepatitis and myositis associated with erythema infectiosum by parvovirus B19 in an adolescent. BMC Pediatr. 2014;14:6.
66. Page C, Duverlie G, Sevestre H, et al. Erythrovirus B19 and autoimmune thyroid diseases. Review of the literature and pathophysiological hypotheses. J Med Virol. 2015;87:162–9.
67. Moimas S, Zacchigna S, Merlo M. Idiopathic dilated cardiomyopathy and persistent viral infection: lack of association in a controlled study using a quantitative assay. Heart Lung Circ. 2012;21:787–93.
68. Schenk T, Enders M, Pollak S, et al. High prevalence of human parvovirus B19 DNA in myocardial autopsy samples from subjects without myocarditis or dilative cardiomyopathy. J Clin Microbiol. 2009;47:106–10.
69. Linhartová K, Hubáček P, Zemánek D, Kodetová D, Zajac M, Setina M, Veselka J. Presence of the viral genome in the myocardial tissue of patients without clinical suspicion of myocarditis. Cardiovasc Pathol. 2013;22(1):113–4.
70. Santonja C, Santos-Briz A, Palmedo G, Kutzner H, Requena L. Detection of human parvovirus B19 DNA in 22% of 1815 cutaneous biopsies of a wide variety of dermatological conditions suggests viral persistence after primary infection and casts doubts on its pathogenic significance. Br J Dermatol. 2017;177(4):1060–5.
71. Molenaar-de Backer MW, Russcher A, Kroes AC, Koppelman MH, Lanfermeijer M, Zaaijer HL. Detection of parvovirus B19 DNA in blood: viruses or DNA remnants? J Clin Virol. 2016;84:19–23.
72. Greulich S, Kindermann I, Schumm J, et al. Predictors of outcome in patients with parvovirus B19 positive endomyocardial biopsy. Clin Res Cardiol. 2016;105(1):37–52.
73. Nguyen AB, Chung BB, Sayer G, Mullane K, Uriel N. Acute myocarditis secondary to reactivated chromosomally-integrated human herpesvirus 6. J Card Fail. 2017;23(7):576–7.
74. Pellett PE, Ablashi DV, Ambros PF, et al. Chromosomally-integrated HHV-6 (ciHHV-6) is a rarer condition in which the complete genome of the virus is integrated into the host germline genome chromosomally integrated human herpesvirus 6: questions and answers. Rev Med Virol. 2012;22(3):144–55.
75. Leong HN, Tuke PW, Tedder RS, et al. The prevalence of chromosomally integrated human herpesvirus 6 genomes in the blood of UK blood donors. J Med Virol. 2007;79:45–51.

76. Daibata M, Taguchi T, Nemoto Y, Taguchi H, Miyoshi I. Inheritance of chromosomally integrated human herpesvirus 6 DNA. Blood. 1999;94:1545–9.
77. Kühl U, Lassner D, Wallaschek N, et al. Chromosomally integrated human herpesvirus 6 in heart failure: prevalence and treatment. Eur J Heart Fail. 2015;17:9–19.
78. Tweedy J, Spyrou MA, Hubacek P, Kuhl U, Lassner D, Gompels UA. Analyses of germline, chromosomally integrated human herpesvirus 6A and B genomes indicate emergent infection and new inflammatory mediators. J Gen Virol. 2015;96(Pt 1.2):370–89.
79. Bern C. Chagas' disease. N Engl J Med. 2015;373(5):456–66.
80. Shikanai-Yasuda MA, Carvalho NB. Oral transmission of Chagas disease. Clin Infect Dis. 2012;54:845–52.
81. Garcia MN, Woc-Colburn L, Aguilar D, Hotez PJ, Murray KO. Historical perspectives on the epidemiology of human chagas disease in Texas and recommendations for enhanced understanding of clinical chagas disease in the Southern United States. PLoS Negl Trop Dis. 2015;9(11):e0003981.
82. World Health Organization. Chagas disease in Latin America: an epidemiological update based on 2010 estimates. Wkly Epidemiol Rec. 2015;90:33–43.
83. Sandri TL, Andrade FA, Lidani KCF, et al. Human collectin-11 (COLEC11) and its synergic genetic interaction with MASP2 are associated with the pathophysiology of Chagas disease. PLoS Negl Trop Dis. 2019;13(4):e0007324.
84. Leon Rodriguez DA, Carmona FD, Echeverría LE, González CI, Martin J. IL18 gene variants influence the susceptibility to Chagas disease. PLoS Negl Trop Dis. 2016;10(3):e0004583.
85. Leon Rodriguez DA, Carmona FD, González CI, Martin J. Evaluation of VDR gene polymorphisms in Trypanosoma cruzi infection and chronic Chagasic cardiomyopathy. Sci Rep. 2016;6:31263.
86. Reis PG, Ayo CM, de Mattos LC, et al. Genetic polymorphisms of IL17 and Chagas disease in the south and southeast of Brazil. J Immunol Res. 2017;2017:1017621.
87. Oliveira AP, Bernardo CR, Camargo AV, et al. Genetic susceptibility to cardiac and digestive clinical forms of chronic Chagas disease: involvement of the CCR5 59029 A/G polymorphism. PLoS One. 2015;10(11):e0141847.
88. Juiz NA, Estupiñán E, Hernández D, et al. Association study between CCR2-CCR5 genes polymorphisms and chronic Chagas heart disease in Wichi and in admixed populations from Argentina. PLoS Negl Trop Dis. 2019;13(1):e0007033.
89. Alvarado-Arnez LE, Batista AM, Alves SM, et al. Single nucleotide polymorphisms of cytokine-related genes and association with clinical outcome in a Chagas disease case-control study from Brazil. Mem Inst Oswaldo Cruz. 2018;113(6):e170489.
90. Clipman SJ, Henderson-Frost J, Fu KY, Bern C, Flores J, Gilman RH. Genetic association study of NLRP1, CARD, and CASP1 inflammasome genes with chronic Chagas cardiomyopathy among Trypanosoma cruzi seropositive patients in Bolivia. PLoS One. 2018;13(2):e0192378.
91. Leon Rodriguez DA, Acosta-Herrera M, Carmona FD, et al. Comprehensive analysis of three TYK2 gene variants in the susceptibility to Chagas disease infection and cardiomyopathy. PLoS One. 2018;13(1):e0190591.
92. Steer AC. Historical aspects of rheumatic fever. J Paediatr Child Health. 2015;51(1):21–7.
93. Bono-Neri F. Acute rheumatic fever: global persistence of a preventable disease. J Pediatr Health Care. 2017;31(3):275–84.
94. Zühlke LJ, Beaton A, Engel ME, et al. Group A streptococcus, acute rheumatic fever and rheumatic heart disease: epidemiology and clinical considerations. Curr Treat Options Cardiovasc Med. 2017;19(2):15.
95. Tian C, Hromatka BS, Kiefer AK, et al. Genome-wide association and HLA region finemapping studies identify susceptibility loci for multiple common infections. Nat Commun. 2017;8(1):599.
96. Wilson MG, Schweitzer MD, Lubschez R. The familial epidemiology of rheumatic fever: genetic and epidemiological studies. J Pediatr. 1943;97(2519):335–6.

97. Patarroyo ME, Winchester RJ, Vejerano A, et al. Association of a B-cell alloantigen with susceptibility of rheumatic fever. Nature. 1979;278:173–4.
98. Zabriskie JB, Lavency D, Williams RC, et al. Rheumatic fever associated B-cell alloantigen as identified by monoclonal antibodies. Arthritis Rheum. 1985;28:1047–51.
99. Khanna AK, Buskirk RD, Williamsa RC Jr, et al. Presence of a non-HLA B cell antigen in rheumatic fever patients and their families as defined by a monoclonal antibody. J Clin Invest. 1989;83:1710–6.
100. Harel L, Zeharia A, Kodman Y, Straussberg R, Zabriskie JB, Amir J. Presence of the d8/17 B-cell marker in children with rheumatic fever in Israel. Clin Genet. 2002;61:293–8.
101. Engel ME, Stander R, Vogel J, Adeyemo AA, Mayosi BM. Genetic susceptibility to acute rheumatic fever: a systematic review and meta-analysis of twin studies. PLoS One. 2011;6(9):e25326.
102. Bhatt M, Kumar S, Siddiqui MH, Garg N, Mittal B. Influence of cytokine gene polymorphism on the risk of rheumatic heart disease - a meta-analysis. Immunol Lett. 2018;194:69–78.
103. Guilherme L, Kalil J. Rheumatic heart disease: molecules involved in valve tissue inflammation leading to the autoimmune process and anti-S. pyogenes vaccine. Front Immunol. 2013;4:352.
104. Matsushita M. Ficolins in complement activation. Mol Immunol. 2013;55(1):22–6.
105. Garred P, Honoré C, Ma YJ, Rørvig S, Cowland J, Borregaard N, Hummelshøj T. The genetics of ficolins. J Innate Immun. 2010;2(1):3–16.
106. Garred P, Borregaard N. The ficolins. J Innate Immun. 2010;2(1):1–2.
107. Honoré C, Hummelshoj T, Hansen BE, Madsen HO, Eggleton P, Garred P. The innate immune component ficolin 3 (Hakata antigen) mediates the clearance of late apoptotic cells. Arthritis Rheum. 2007;56:1598–607.
108. Rørvig S, Honore C, Larsson L-I, et al. Ficolin-1 is present in a highly mobilizable subset of human neutrophil granules and associates with the cell surface after stimulation with fMLP. J Leukoc Biol. 2009;86:1439–49.
109. Zhang J, Yang L, Ang Z, et al. Secreted M-Ficolin anchors onto monocyte transmembrane G protein-coupled receptor 43 and cross talks with plasma C-reactive protein to mediate immune signaling and regulate host defense. J Immunol. 2010;185:6899–910.
110. Kjaer TR, Hansen AG, Sørensen UBS, et al. Investigations on the pattern recognition molecule M-ficolin: quantitative aspects of bacterial binding and leukocyte association. J Leukoc Biol. 2011;90:425–37.
111. Ren Y, Ding Q, Zhang X. Ficolins and infectious diseases. Virol Sin. 2014;29:25–32.
112. Messias-Reason IJ, Schafranski MD, Kremsner PG, Kun JF. Ficolin 2 (FCN2) functional polymorphisms and the risk of rheumatic fever and rheumatic heart disease. Clin Exp Immunol. 2009;157(3):395–9.
113. Catarino SJ, Andrade FA, Boldt ABW, Guilherme L, Messias-Reason IJ. Sickening or healing the heart? The association of ficolin-1 and rheumatic fever. Front Immunol. 2018;9:3009.
114. Katayama M, Ota K, Nagi-Miura N, et al. Ficolin-1 is a promising therapeutic target for autoimmune diseases. Int Immunol. 2019;31(1):23–32.
115. Michalski M, Świerzko AS, Pągowska-Klimek I, et al. Primary Ficolin-3 deficiencyDOUBLEHYPHENis it associated with increased susceptibility to infections? Immunobiology. 2015;220(6):711–3.
116. Kumar P, Gupta D, Sagar RK. A rare combination of Marfan's syndrome, rheumatic heart disease and muscular dystrophyDOUBLEHYPHENa case report. Indian Heart J. 1994;46(6):351–2.
117. Lee LS, Rose CS, Maier LA. Sarcoidosis. N Engl J Med. 1997;336:1224–34.
118. Iannuzzi MC, Rybicki BA, Teirstein AS. Sarcoidosis. N Engl J Med. 2007;357(21):2153–65.
119. Chen ES, Moller DR. Etiologies of Sarcoidosis. Clin Rev Allergy Immunol. 2015;49:6–18.
120. Rybicki BA, Major M, Popovich J Jr, et al. Racial differences in sarcoidosis incidence: a 5-year study in a health maintenance organization. Am J Epidemiol. 1997;145:234–41.

121. Burke RR, Stone CH, Havstad S, Rybicki BA. Racial differences in sarcoidosis granuloma density. Lung. 2009;187:1–7.
122. Lynch JP, Hwang J, Bradfield J, et al. Cardiac involvement in sarcoidosis: evolving concepts in diagnosis and treatment. Semin Respir Crit Care Med. 2014;35:372–90.
123. Liu D, Birnbaum AD. Update on sarcoidosis. Curr Opin Ophthalmol. 2015;26:512–6.
124. Blau EB. Familial granulomatous arthritis, iritis, and rash. J Pediatr. 1985;107(5):689–93.
125. Miceli-Richard C, Lesage S, Rybojad M, et al. CARD15 mutations in Blau syndrome. Nat Genet. 2001;29(1):19–20.
126. Tan JL, Fong HK, Birati EY, Han Y. Cardiac Sarcoidosis. Am J Cardiol. 2019;123(3):513–22.
127. Iwai K, Tachibana T, Takemura T, et al. Pathological studies on sarcoidosis autopsy. I. Epidemiological features of 320 cases in Japan. Acta Pathol Jpn. 1993;43:372–6.
128. Iwai K, Takemura T, Kitaichi M, et al. Pathological studies on sarcoidosis autopsy. II. Early change, mode of progression and death pattern. Acta Pathol Jpn. 1993;43:377–85.
129. Crouser ED, Ono C, Tran T, et al. Improved detection of cardiac sarcoidosis using magnetic resonance with myocardial T2 mapping. Am J Respir Crit Care Med. 2014;189:109–12.
130. Wicks EC, Menezes LJ, Barnes A, et al. Diagnostic accuracy and prognostic value of simultaneous hybrid 18F-fluorodeoxyglucose positron emission tomography/magnetic resonance imaging in cardiac sarcoidosis. Eur Heart J Cardiovasc Imaging. 2018;19(7):757–67.
131. Karakaya B, Kaiser Y, van Moorsel CHM, Grunewald J. Löfgren's syndrome: diagnosis, management, and disease pathogenesis. Semin Respir Crit Care Med. 2017;38(4):463–76.
132. Blau Wouters CH, Maes A, Foley KP, Bertin J, Rose CD. Blau syndrome, the prototypic auto-inflammatory granulomatous disease. Pediatr Rheumatol Online J. 2014;12:33. https://doi.org/10.1186/1546-0096-12-33.
133. Ebrahimiadib N, Samra KA, Domina AM, et al. A novel NOD2-associated mutation and variant blau syndrome: phenotype and molecular analysis. Ocul Immunol Inflamm. 2018;26(1):57–64.
134. Davoudi S, Navarro-Gomez D, Shen L, et al. NOD2 genetic variants and sarcoidosis-associated uveitis. Am J Ophthalmol Case Rep. 2016;3:39–42.
135. Whyte MP, Lim E, McAlister WH, et al. Unique variant of NOD2 pediatric granulomatous arthritis with severe 1,25-dihydroxyvitamin D-mediated hypercalcemia and generalized osteosclerosis. J Bone Miner Res. 2018;33(11):2071–80.
136. Milman N, Ursin K, Rødevand E, Nielsen FC, Hansen TV. A novel mutation in the NOD2 gene associated with Blau syndrome: a Norwegian family with four affected members. Scand J Rheumatol. 2009;38(3):190–7.
137. Li C, Zhang J, Li S, et al. Gene mutations and clinical phenotypes in Chinese children with Blau syndrome. Sci China Life Sci. 2017;60(7):758–62.
138. Mourad F, Tang A. Sinus of valsalva aneurysm in Blau's syndrome. J Cardiothorac Surg. 2010;5:16.
139. Touitou I, Lesage S, McDermott M, et al. Infevers: an evolving mutation database for auto-inflammatory syndromes. Hum Mutat. 2004;24(3):194–8.
140. Takeuchi Y, Shigemura T, Kobayashi N, et al. Early diagnosis of early-onset sarcoidosis: a case report with functional analysis and review of the literature. Clin Rheumatol. 2017;36(5):1189–96.
141. Okada S, Konishi N, Tsumura M, et al. Cardiac infiltration in early-onset sarcoidosis associated with a novel heterozygous mutation, G481D, in CARD15. Rheumatology. 2009;48:706–7.
142. Rybicki BA, Sinha R, Iyengar S, the SAGA Study Consortium, et al. Genetic linkage analysis of sarcoidosis phenotypes: the sarcoidosis genetic analysis (SAGA) study. Genes Immun. 2007;8:379–86.
143. Fischer A, Grunewald J, Spagnolo P, et al. Genetics of Sarcoidosis. Semin Respir Crit Care Med. 2014;35:296–306.
144. Wolin A, Lahtela EL, Anttila V, et al. SNP variants in major histocompatibility complex are associated with sarcoidosis susceptibility-a joint analysis in four European populations. Front Immunol. 2017;8:422.

145. Chaperon M, Pacheco Y, Maucort-Boulch D, Iwaz J, Perard L, Broussolle C, Jamilloux Y, Burillon C, Kodjikian L, Calender A, Seve P. BTNL2 gene polymorphism and sarcoid uveitis. Br J Ophthalmol. 2019;0:1–5. https://doi.org/10.1136/bjophthalmol-2018-312949.
146. Muller-Quernheim J, Schurmann M, Hofmann S, et al. Genetics of sarcoidosis. Clin Chest Med. 2008;29:391–414.
147. Kishore A, Petrek M. Immunogenetics of sarcoidosis. Int Trends Immun. 2013;1:43–53.
148. Fingerlin TE, Hamzeh N, Maier LA. Genetics of sarcoidosis. Clin Chest Med. 2015;36: 569–84.
149. Rivera NV, Ronninger M, Shchetynsky K, et al. High-density genetic mapping identifies new susceptibility variants in sarcoidosis phenotypes and shows genomic-driven phenotypic differences. Am J Respir Crit Care Med. 2016;193:1008–22.
150. Kishore A, Petersen BS, Nutsua M, et al. Whole-exome sequencing identifies rare genetic variations in German families with pulmonary sarcoidosis. Hum Genet. 2018;137(9): 705–16.
151. Rybicki BA, Iannuzzi MC, Frederick MM, et al. Familial aggregation of sarcoidosis. A case–control etiologic study of sarcoidosis (ACCESS). Am J Respir Crit Care Med. 2001;164:2085–91.
152. Baughman RP, Teirstein AS, Judson MA, Case Control Etiologic Study of Sarcoidosis (ACCESS) Research Group, et al. Clinical characteristics of patients in a case control study of sarcoidosis. Am J Respir Crit Care Med. 2001;164(10 Pt 1):1885–9.
153. Terwiel M, van Moorsel CHM. Clinical epidemiology of familial sarcoidosis: a systematic literature review. Respir Med. 2019;149:36–41.
154. Rossides M, Grunewald J, Eklund A, et al. Familial aggregation and heritability of sarcoidosis: a Swedish nested case control study. Eur Respir J. 2018;52(2):1800385.
155. Rossman MD, Thompson B, Frederick M, ACCESS Group, et al. HLA-DRB1∗1101: a significant risk factor for sarcoidosis in blacks and whites. Am. J Hum Genet. 2003;73:720–35.
156. Naruse TK, Matsuzawa Y, Ota M, et al. HLA-DQB1∗0601 is primarily associated with the susceptibility to cardiac sarcoidosis. Tissue Antigens. 2000;56(1):52–7.
157. Takashige N, Naruse TK, Matsumori A, Hara M, Nagai S, Morimoto S, Hiramitsu S, Sasayama S, Inoko H. Genetic polymorphisms at the tumour necrosis factor loci (TNFA and TNFB) in cardiac sarcoidosis. Tissue Antigens. 1999;54(2):191–3.
158. Grunewald J, Eklund A. Löfgren's syndrome: human leukocyte antigen strongly influences the disease course. Am J Respir Crit Care Med. 2009;179(4):307–12.
159. Rybicki BA, Walewski JL, Maliarik MJ, Kian H, Iannuzzi MC, ACCESS Research Group. The BTNL2 gene and sarcoidosis susceptibility in African Americans and whites. Am J Hum Genet. 2005;77:491–9.
160. Hofmann S, Franke A, Fischer A, et al. Genome-wide association study identifies ANXA11 as a new susceptibility locus for sarcoidosis. Nat Genet. 2008;40:1103–6.
161. Smith BN, Topp SD, Fallini C, et al. Mutations in the vesicular trafficking protein annexin A11 are associated with amyotrophic lateral sclerosis. Sci Transl Med. 2017;9:eaad9157.
162. Xu J, Brooks EG. Giant cell myocarditis: a brief review. Arch Pathol Lab Med. 2016;140(12):1429–34.
163. Vaideeswar P, Cooper L. Giant cell myocarditis: clinical and pathological disease characteristics in an Indian population. Cardiovasc Pathol. 2013;22:70–4.
164. Shariff S, Straatiamn L, Allard M, et al. Novel associations of giant cell myocarditis: two case reports and a review of the literature. Can J Cardiol. 2004;4:557–61.
165. Rosenstein ED, Zucker MJ, Kramer N. Giant cell myocarditis: most fatal of autoimmune diseases. Semin Arthritis Rheum. 2000;30(1):1–16.
166. Schumann C, Faust M, Gerharz M, et al. Autoimmune polyglandular syndrome associated with idiopathic giant cell myocarditis. Exp Clin Endocrinol Diabetes. 2005;113:302–7.
167. Varnavas VC, Reinsch N, Perrey M, et al. Recurrent lymphocytic myocarditis in a young male with ulcerative colitis. Eur J Med Res. 2014;19:11.
168. Joudinaud TM, Fadel E, Thomas-de-Montpreville V, et al. Fatal giant cell myocarditis after thymoma resection in myasthenia gravis. J Thorac Cardiovasc Surg. 2006;131:494–5.

169. Sasaki H, Yano M, Kawano O, et al. Thymoma associated with fatal myocarditis and polymyositis in a 58-year-old man following treatment with carboplatin and paclitaxel: a case report. Oncol Lett. 2012;3:300–2.
170. Lee M, Kwon GY, Kim JS, et al. Giant cell myocarditis associated with Coxsackievirus infection. J Am Coll Cardiol. 2010;56:e19.
171. Dennert R, Schalla S, Suylen RJ, et al. Giant cell myocarditis triggered by a parvovirus B19 infection. Int J Cardiol. 2009;134:115–6.
172. Gkouziouta A, Miliopoulos D, Karavolias G, et al. Acute cytomegalovirus infection triggering fatal giant cell myocarditis. Int J Cardiol. 2016;214:204–6.
173. Ikeda Y, Inomata T, Nishinarita R, et al. Giant cell myocarditis associated with multiple autoimmune disorders following highly active antiretroviral therapy for human immunodeficiency virus type 1 infection. Int J Cardiol. 2016;206:79–81.
174. Bunu DM, Timofte CE, Ciocoiu M, et al. Cardiovascular manifestations of inflammatory bowel disease: pathogenesis, diagnosis, and preventive strategies. Gastroenterol Res Pract. 2019;2019:3012509. https://doi.org/10.1155/2019/3012509.
175. Asadi J, Bhandari SS, Ahmed N. Mesalazine-induced myopericarditis in a patient with ulcerative colitis. Echo Res Pract. 2017;5(1):K1–5.
176. Okoro KU, Roby MD, Bankole AA. Myocarditis secondary to mesalamine-induced cardiotoxicity in a patient with ulcerative colitis. Case Rep Med. 2018;2018:9813893. https://doi.org/10.1155/2018/9813893.
177. Mitoff PR, Mesana TG, Mielniczuk LM, et al. Giant cell myocarditis in a patient with a spondyloarthropathy after a drug hypersensitivity reaction. Can J Cardiol. 2013;29(9):1138.e7–8.
178. Priemer DS, Davidson DD, Loehrer PJ, Badve SS. Giant cell polymyositis and myocarditis in a patient with thymoma and myasthenia gravis: a postviral autoimmune process? J Neuropathol Exp Neurol. 2018;77(8):661–4.
179. Bechman K, Gopalan D, Nihoyannopoulos P, Mason JC. A cohort study reveals myocarditis to be a rare and life-threatening presentation of large vessel vasculitis. Semin Arthritis Rheum. 2017;47(2):241–6.
180. Stevens AW, Grossman ME, Barr ML. Orbital myositis, vitiligo, and giant cell myocarditis. J Am Acad Dermatol. 1996;35(2 Pt 2):310–2.
181. Chung L, Berry GJ, Chakravarty EF. Giant cell myocarditis: a rare cardiovascular manifestation in a patient with systemic lupus erythematosus. Lupus. 2005;14(2):166–9.
182. Rasmussen TB, Dalager S, Andersen NH, Hansen TK, Nielsen-Kudsk JE. Fatal giant cell myocarditis in a patient with multiple autoimmune disorders. BMJ Case Rep. 2009;2009:bcr09.2008.0997. https://doi.org/10.1136/bcr.09.2008.0997.
183. Martinez S, Miranda E, Kim P, Pollanen MS. Giant cell myocarditis associated with amoxicillin hypersensitivity reaction. Forensic Sci Med Pathol. 2013;9(3):403–6.
184. Rogers JS, Zakaria S, Thom KA, Flammer KM, Kanno M, Mehra MR. Immune reconstitution inflammatory syndrome and human immunodeficiency virus-associated myocarditis. Mayo Clin Proc. 2008;83(11):1275–9.
185. Hill AM, Mitchell N, Hughes S, Pozniak AL. Risks of cardiovascular or central nervous system adverse events and immune reconstitution inflammatory syndrome, for dolutegravir versus other antiretrovirals: meta-analysis of randomized trials. Curr Opin HIV AIDS. 2018;13(2):102–11.
186. Kong G, Madden B, Spyrou N, et al. Response of recurrent giant cell myocarditis in a transplanted heart to intensive immunosuppression. Eur Heart J. 1991;12:554–7.
187. Maleszewski JJ, Orellana VM, Hodge DO, et al. Long-term risk of recurrence, morbidity and mortality in giant cell myocarditis. Am J Cardiol. 2015;115:1733–8.
188. Larsen BT, Maleszewski JJ, Edwards WD, et al. Atrial giant cell myocarditis: a distinctive clinicopathologic entity. Circulation. 2013;127(1):39–47.
189. Bose AK, Bhattacharjee M, Martin V, Kendall S. Giant cell myocarditis of the left atrium. Cardiovasc Pathol. 2010;19(2):e37–8.
190. Shih JA, Shih JA. Small steps for idiopathic giant cell myocarditis. Curr Heart Fail Rep. 2015;12:263–8.

191. Fanos V, Cuccu A, Nemolato S, Marinelli V, Faa G. A new nonsense mutation of the IGHMBP2 gene responsible for the first case of SMARD1 in a Sardinian patient with giant cell hepatitis. Neuropediatrics. 2010;41(3):132–4.
192. Kon T, Mori F, Tanji K, Miki Y, Kimura T, Wakabayashi K. Giant cell polymyositis and myocarditis associated with myasthenia gravis and thymoma. Neuropathology. 2013;33(3): 281–7.
193. Huang K, Shojania K, Chapman K, Amiri N, Dehghan N, Mezei M. Concurrent inflammatory myopathy and myasthenia gravis with or without thymic pathology: a case series and literature review. Semin Arthritis Rheum. 2019;48(4):745–51.
194. Gilhus NE, Nacu A, Andersen JB, Owe JF. Myasthenia gravis and risks for comorbidity. Eur J Neurol. 2015;22(1):17–23.
195. Saito N, Shimizu K, Kawaishi M, Araya J, Nakayama K, Kuwano K. A survival case of invasive thymoma accompanied by acute fulminant myocarditis. Respirol Case Rep. 2013;1(2):36–8.
196. Kittleson MM, Minhas KM, Irizarry RA, et al. Gene expression in giant cell myocarditis: altered expression of immune response genes. Int J Cardiol. 2005;102(2):333–40.
197. Asimaki A, Tandri H, Duffy E, et al. Altered desmosomal proteins in granulomatous myocarditis and potential pathogenic links to arrhythmogenic right ventricular cardiomyopathy. Circ Arrhythm Electrophysiol. 2011;4:743–52.
198. Wang SA. The diagnostic work-up of hypereosinophilia. Pathobiology. 2019;86(1):39–52.
199. Kita H. Eosinophils: multifaceted biological properties and roles in health and disease. Immunol Rev. 2011;242:161–77.
200. Valent P, Klion AD, Horny H-P, et al. Contemporary consensus proposal on criteria and classification of eosinophilic disorders and related syndromes. J Allergy Clin Immunol. 2012;130:607–612.e9.
201. Gotlib J. World Health Organization-defined eosinophilic disorders: 2011 update on diagnosis, risk stratification, and management. Am J Hematol. 2011;86:678–88.
202. Valent P, Gleich GJ, Reiter A, et al. Pathogenesis and classification of eosinophil disorders: a review of recent developments in the field. Expert Rev Hematol. 2012;5(2):157–76.
203. Simon H-U, Rothenburg ME, Bochner BS, et al. Refining the definition of hypereosinophilic syndrome. J Allergy Clin Immunol. 2010;126:45–9.
204. Crane MM, Chang CM, Kobayashi MG, et al. Incidence of myeloproliferative hypereosinophilic syndrome in the United States and an estimate of all hypereosinophilic syndrome incidence. J Allergy Clin Immunol. 2010;126:179–81.
205. Pardanani A, Ketterling RP, Li CY, et al. FIP1L1-PDGFRA in eosinophilic disorders: prevalence in routine clinical practice, long-term experience with imatinib therapy, and a critical review of the literature. Leuk Res. 2006;30:965–70.
206. Jovanovic JV, Score J, Waghorn K, et al. Low-dose imatinib mesylate leads to rapid induction of major molecular responses and achievement of complete molecular remission in FIP1L1-PDGFRA-positive chronic eosinophilic leukemia. Blood. 2007;109:4635–40.
207. Giovannini-Chami L, Hadchouel A, Nathan N, et al. Idiopathic eosinophilic pneumonia in children: the French experience. Orphanet J Rare Dis. 2014;9:28.
208. Tamse T, Rampersad A, Jordan-Villegas A, Ireland J. A case of idiopathic hypereosinophilic syndrome causing mitral valve papillary muscle rupture. Case Rep Pediatr. 2015;2015:538762.
209. Tai CP, Chung T, Avasarala K. Endomyocardial fibrosis and mural thrombus in a 4-year-old girl due to idiopathic hypereosinophilia syndrome described with serial cardiac magnetic resonance imaging. Cardiol Young. 2016;26:168–71.
210. Helbig G, Wiśniewska-Piąty K, Francuz T, Dziaczkowska-Suszek J, Kyrcz-Krzemień S. Diversity of clinical manifestations and response to corticosteroids for idiopathic hypereosinophilic syndrome: retrospective study in 33 patients. Leuk Lymphoma. 2013;54:807–11.
211. Cools J, DeAngelo DJ, Gotlib J, et al. A tyrosine kinase created by fusion of the PDGFRA and FIP1L1 genes as a therapeutic target of imatinib in idiopathic hypereosinophilic syndrome. N Engl J Med. 2003;348:1201–14.

212. Baccarani M, Cilloni D, Rondoni M, et al. The efficacy of imatinib mesylate in patients with FIP1L1-PDGFRalpha-positive hypereosinophilic syndrome. Results of a multicenter prospective study. Haematologica. 2007;92:1173–9.
213. Ogbogu PU, Bochner BS, Butterfield JH, et al. Hypereosinophilic syndromes: a multicenter, retrospective analysis of clinical characteristics and response to therapy. J Allergy Clin Immunol. 2009;124:1319–25.
214. Riley LK, Rupert J. Evaluation of patients with leukocytosis. Am Fam Physician. 2015;92(11):1004–11.
215. Mankad R, Bonnichsen C, Mankad S. Hypereosinophilic syndrome: cardiac diagnosis and management. Heart. 2016;102:100–6.
216. Séguéla PE, Iriart X, Acar P, Montaudon M, Roudaut R, Thambo JB. Eosinophilic cardiac disease: Molecular, clinical and imaging aspects. Arch Cardiovasc Dis. 2015;108(4):258–68.
217. Kleinfeldt T, Nienaber CA, Kische S, et al. Cardiac manifestation of the hypereosinophilic syndrome: new insights. Clin Res Cardiol. 2010;99:419–27.
218. Eicher JC, Bonnotte B, L'Huillier I, et al. Cardiovascular manifestations of eosinophilia: clinical and echocardiographic presentation. Rev Med Interne. 2009;30:1011–9.
219. Ginsberg F, Parrillo JE. Eosinophilic myocarditis. Heart Fail Clin. 2005;1(3):419–29.
220. Alyasin S, Khoshkhui M, Amin R. Familial Churg-Strauss syndrome in a sister and brother. Iran J Allergy Asthma Immunol. 2015;14(3):338–40.
221. Tsurikisawa N, Morita S, Tsuburai T, Oshikata C, Ono E, Taniguchi M, Saito H, Yanagihara Y, Akiyama K. Familial Churg-Strauss syndrome in two sisters. Chest. 2007;131(2):592–4.
222. Manganelli P, Giacosa R, Fietta P, Zanetti A, Neri TM. Familial vasculitides: Churg-Strauss syndrome and Wegener's granulomatosis in 2 first-degree relatives. J Rheumatol. 2003;30(3):618–21.
223. Schena S, Testa G, Setty S, Abcarian H, Benedetti E. Successful identical-twin living donor small bowel transplant for necrotizing enterovasculitis secondary to Churg-Strauss syndrome. Transpl Int. 2006;19(7):594–7.
224. Targońska-Stepniak B, Majdan M, Haberek G, Papuć E, Wnukowska K. Development of Churg-Strauss syndrome with severe multiple mononeuropathy after leukotriene receptor antagonist treatment in one of the monozygotic twins with asthma: case report. Pol Arch Med Wewn. 2009;119(11):761–4.
225. Martorana D, Maritati F, Malerba G, et al. PTPN22 R620W polymorphism in the ANCA-associated vasculitides. Rheumatology. 2012;51(5):805–12.
226. Wieczorek S, Holle JU, Bremer JP, et al. Contrasting association of a non-synonymous leptin receptor gene polymorphism with Wegener's granulomatosis and Churg-Strauss syndrome. Rheumatology. 2010;49(5):907–14.
227. Zwerina J, Bach C, Martorana D, et al. Eotaxin-3 in Churg-Strauss syndrome: a clinical and immunogenetic study. Rheumatology (Oxford). 2011;50(10):1823–7.
228. Human A, Murguia-Favela L, Benson L, Roifman I, Grunebaum E. Cardiovascular abnormalities in primary immunodeficiency diseases. Lympho Sign J. 2015;2(3):107–34.
229. Villa A, Notarangelo LD, Roifman CM. Omenn syndrome: inflammation in leaky severe combined immunodeficiency. J Allergy Clin Immunol. 2008;122(6):1082–6.
230. Chan Tack TA, Sandy S, Chan-Tack KM. Fatal cytomegalovirus myocarditis in an infant with Omenn's syndrome. Pediatr Infect Dis J. 2006;25(8):759–60.
231. Zago CA, Jacob CM, de Albuquerque Diniz EM, et al. Autoimmune manifestations in SCID due to IL7R mutations: Omenn syndrome and cytopenias. Hum Immunol. 2014;75(7):662–6.
232. Henderson LA, Frugoni F, Hopkins G, et al. First reported case of Omenn syndrome in a patient with reticular dysgenesis. J Allergy Clin Immunol. 2013;131(4):1227–9.
233. Brückmann C, Lindner W, Roos R, Permanetter W, Haas RJ, Haworth SG, Belohradsky BH. Severe pulmonary vascular occlusive disease following bone marrow transplantation in Omenn syndrome. Eur J Pediatr. 1991;150(4):242–5.
234. Heyderman RS, Morgan G, Levinsky RJ, Strobel S. Successful bone marrow transplantation and treatment of BCG infection in two patients with severe combined immunodeficiency. Eur J Pediatr. 1991;150(7):477–80.

235. Winkelstein JA, Marino MC, Lederman HM, et al. X-linked agammaglobulinemia: report on a United States registry of 201 patients. Medicine (Baltimore). 2006;85(4):193–202.
236. Rijkers GT, Holzer L, Dusselier T. Genetics in community-acquired pneumonia. Curr Opin Pulm Med. 2019;25(3):323–9.
237. Martínez Jaramillo C, Trujillo-Vargas CM. LRBA in the endomembrane system. Colomb Med (Cali). 2018;49(3):236–43.
238. Mardekian SK, Fortuna D, Nix A, et al. Severe human parechovirus type 3 myocarditis and encephalitis in an adolescent with hypogammaglobulinemia. Int J Infect Dis. 2015;36:6–8.
239. Scothorn DJ, Winick NJ, Timmons CF, Aquino VM. Rapidly fatal acute bacterial myocarditis in a nonneutropenic child with acute lymphoblastic leukemia in remission. J Pediatr Hematol Oncol. 2002;24(8):662–5.
240. Klein C. Genetic defects in severe congenital neutropenia: emerging insights into life and death of human neutrophil granulocytes. Annu Rev Immunol. 2011;29:399–413.
241. Boztug K, Appaswamy G, Ashikov A, et al. A syndrome with congenital neutropenia and mutations in G6PC3. N Engl J Med. 2009;360:32–43.
242. Banka S, Wynn R, Byers H, Arkwright PD, Newman WG. G6PC3 mutations cause non-syndromic severe congenital neutropenia. Mol Genet Metab. 2013;108(2):138–41.
243. Boztug K, Rosenberg PS, Dorda M, et al. Extended spectrum of human glucose-6-phosphatase catalytic subunit 3 deficiency: novel genotypes and phenotypic variability in severe congenital neutropenia. J Pediatr. 2012;160:679–83.
244. Xia J, Bolyard AA, Rodger E, et al. Prevalence of mutations in ELANE, GFI1, HAX1, SBDS, WAS and G6PC3 patients with severe congenital neutropenia. Br J Haematol. 2009;147:535–42.
245. McDermott DH, De Ravin SS, Jun HS, et al. Severe congenital neutropenia resulting from G6PC3 deficiency with increased neutrophil CXCR4 expression and myelokathexis. Blood. 2010;116:2793–802.
246. Dror Y, Donadieu J, Koglmeier J, et al. Draft consensus guidelines for diagnosis and treatment of Shwachman–Diamond syndrome. Ann N Y Acad Sci. 2011;1242:40–55.
247. Savilahti E, Rapola J. Frequent myocardial lesions in Shwachman's syndrome. Eight fatal cases among 16 Finnish patients. Acta Paediatr Scand. 1984;73:642–51.
248. Nivelon JL, Michiels R, Martres-Lassaunière MN, Passavy-Trouche AM, Petit A, Lorenzini JL. Myocardial fibrosis in Shwachman's syndrome: pathogenic discussion of cardiac complications. Pediatrie. 1978;33:461–9.
249. Graham AR, Walson PD, Paplanus SH, Payne CM. Testicular fibrosis and cardiomegaly in Shwachman's syndrome. Arch Pathol Lab Med. 1980;104:242–4.
250. Kopel L, Gutierrez PS, Lage SG. Dilated cardiomyopathy in a case of Shwachman–diamond syndrome. Cardiol Young. 2011;21:588–90.
251. Hauet Q, Beaupain B, Micheau M, et al. Cardiomyopathies and congenital heart diseases in Shwachman-Diamond syndrome: a national survey. Int J Cardiol. 2013;167(3):1048–50.
252. Toiviainen-Salo S, Pitkänen O, Holmström M, et al. Myocardial function in patients with Shwachman–Diamond syndrome: aspects to consider before stem cell transplantation. Pediatr Blood Cancer. 2008;51:461–7.
253. Ryan TD, Jefferies JL, Chin C, et al. Abnormal circumferential strain measured by echocardiography is present in patients with Shwachman-Diamond syndrome despite normal shortening fraction. Pediatr Blood Cancer. 2015;62(7):1228–31.
254. Pathak S, McDermott MF, Savic S. Autoinflammatory diseases: update on classification diagnosis and management. J Clin Pathol. 2017;70(1):1–8.
255. Comarmond C, Cacoub P. Myocarditis in auto-immune or auto-inflammatory diseases. Autoimmun Rev. 2017;16(8):811–6.
256. Broderick L. Hereditary autoinflammatory disorders: recognition and treatment. Immunol Allergy Clin N Am. 2019;39:13–29.
257. Consortium FF. A candidate gene for familial Mediterranean fever. Nat Genet. 1997;17:25–31.
258. McDermott MF, Aksentijevich I, Galon J, et al. Germline mutations in the extracellular domains of the 55 kDa TNF receptor, TNFR1, define a family of dominantly inherited autoinflammatory syndromes. Cell. 1999;97:133–44.

259. Masson V, Simon E, Hoppe P, et al. Tumor necrosis factor receptor-associated periodic syndrome (TRAPS): definition, semiology, prognosis, pathogenesis, treatment, and place relative to other periodic joint diseases. Joint Bone Spine. 2004;71:284–90.
260. Trost S, Rosé CD. Myocarditis and sacroiliitis: 2 previously unrecognized manifestations of tumor necrosis factor receptor associated periodic syndrome. J Rheumatol. 2005;32(1):175–7.
261. Parisi F, Paglionico A, Varriano V, Ferraccioli G, Gremese E. Refractory adult-onset still disease complicated by macrophage activation syndrome and acute myocarditis: a case report treated with high doses (8mg/kg/d) of anakinra. Medicine (Baltimore). 2017;96(24):e6656.
262. Zhou Q, Wang H, Schwartz DM, et al. Loss-of-function mutations in TNFAIP3 leading to A20 haploinsufficiency cause an early-onset autoinflammatory disease. Nat Genet. 2016;48(1):67–73.
263. Das T, Chen Z, Hendriks RW, Kool M. The A20/tumor necrosis factor α-induced protein 3 in immune cells controls development of autoinflammation and autoimmunity: lessons from mouse models. Front Immunol. 2018;9:104.
264. Lawless D, Pathak S, Scambler TE, Ouboussad L, Anwar R, Savic S. A case of adult-onset still's disease caused by a novel splicing mutation in TNFAIP3 successfully treated with tocilizumab. Front Immunol. 2018;9:1527.
265. Gerfaud-Valentin M, Sève P, Iwaz J, et al. Myocarditis in adult-onset Still disease. Medicine (Baltimore). 2014;93:280–9.
266. Bank I, Marboe CC, Redberg RF, Jacobs J. Myocarditis in adult Still's disease. Arthritis Rheum. 1985;28(4):452–4.
267. Sachs RN, Talvard O, Lanfranchi J. Myocarditis in adult Still's disease. Int J Cardiol. 1990;27:377–80.
268. Gonzalez FA, Beirao P, Adriao J, Coelho ML. Adult-onset Still's disease presenting as myopericarditis. BMJ Case Rep. 2014;2014:bcr2013202754.
269. Luconi N, Risse J, Busato T, et al. Myocarditis in a young man with adult onset Still's disease successfully treated with Il-1 blocker. Int J Cardiol. 2015;189:220–2.
270. Cavallasca JA, Vigliano CA, Perandones CE, Tate GA. Myocarditis as a form of relapse in two patients with adult Still's disease. Rheumatol Int. 2010;30:1095–7.
271. Jadhav P, Nanayakkara N. Myocarditis in adult onset Stills disease. Int J Rheum Dis. 2009;12:272–4.
272. Baratta L, Delfino M, Fiorentini A, et al. Alterations of the sympathovagal balance evaluated by heart rate variability in a rare case of adult Still's disease. Ann Ital Med Int. 2004;19:193–7.
273. Gupta D, Jagani R, Mendonca S, Rathi KR. Adult-onset Still's disease with myocarditis and hemophagocytic lymphohistiocytosis: rare manifestation with fatal outcome. Indian J Pathol Microbiol. 2016;59:84–6.
274. Meckenstock R, Therby A, Gibault-Genty G, Khau D, Monnier S, Greder-Belan A. Adult-onset Still's disease revealed by perimyocarditis and a concomitant reactivation of an EBV infection. BMJ Case Rep. 2012;2012:bcr0120113688.
275. Uggenti C, Lepelley A, Crow YJ. Self-awareness: nucleic acid-driven inflammation and the type I interferonopathies. Annu Rev Immunol. 2019;37:247–67.
276. Crow YJ. Aicardi-Goutières syndrome. 2005 Jun 29 [updated 2016 Nov 22]. In: Adam MP, Ardinger HH, Pagon RA, Wallace SE, Bean LJH, Stephens K, Amemiya A, editors. GeneReviews® [Internet]. Seattle: University of Washington, Seattle; 1993–2019. http://www.ncbi.nlm.nih.gov/books/NBK1475/.
277. Crow YJ, Chase DS, Lowenstein Schmidt J, et al. Characterization of human disease phenotypes associated with mutations in TREX1, RNASEH2A, RNASEH2B, RNASEH2C, SAMHD1, ADAR, and IFIH1. Am J Med Genet A. 2015;0(2):296–312.
278. Morita M, Stamp G, Robins P, et al. Gene-targeted mice lacking the Trex1 (DNase III) 3'-->5' DNA exonuclease develop inflammatory myocarditis. Mol Cell Biol. 2004;24(15):6719–27.
279. Beck-Engeser GB, Eilat D, Wabl M. An autoimmune disease prevented by anti-retroviral drugs. Retrovirology. 2011;8:91.
280. Feigenbaum A, Muller C, Yale C, et al. Singleton-Merten syndrome: an autosomal dominant disorder with variable expression. Am J Med Genet. 2013;161A:360–70.

281. Zhang X, Gao X, Hu J, et al. ADAR1p150 forms a complex with dicer to promote miRNA-222 activity and regulate PTEN expression in CVB3-induced viral myocarditis. Int J Mol Sci. 2019;20(2):E407.
282. Adang LA, Frank DB, Gilani A, et al. Aicardi goutières syndrome is associated with pulmonary hypertension. Mol Genet Metab. 2018;125(4):351–8.
283. Nelson CP, Schunkert H, Samani NJ, Erridge C. Genetic analysis of leukocyte type-I interferon production and risk of coronary artery disease. Arterioscler Thromb Vasc Biol. 2015;35(6):1456–62.

Viral Myocarditis: From Experimental Models to Diagnosis in Patients

5

Sabine Pankuweit and Karin Klingel

5.1 Introduction

In endomyocardial biopsies of patients with acute and chronic forms of myocarditis a variety of RNA and DNA viruses have been detected by molecular biological techniques such as in situ hybridization and nested or quantitative (RT)-PCR. Besides enteroviruses (EV), including coxsackieviruses of group B (CVB), parvovirus B19 (B19V), human herpesvirus-6 (HHV6), and Epstein–Barr virus (EBV) were found in a significant number of patients with myocarditis [1–5]. In addition, genomes of other virus infections including adenoviruses (ADV), influenza viruses, HIV, human herpesvirus type 1 (HSV1), and human cytomegalovirus (CMV) were amplified by (RT-) PCR in inflamed hearts [6, 7]. However, whereas the aetiopathogenetic role of enteroviruses and especially of CVB in the induction and progression of acute myocarditis to postviral cardiomyopathy was substantially confirmed by observations in CVB3-infected mice, it is rather unclear by which mechanisms herpesviruses, adenoviruses, or parvovirus B19 might contribute to cardiac damage and inflammation.

In order to improve the knowledge about the pathophysiology of viral myocarditis diverse animal models of DNA and RNA virus infections have been established. By investigation of infected immunocompetent as well as gene-targeted mice valuable new insights into virus pathogenicity and the host immune response were gained. It is important to note that considerable differences in the outcome and course of myocarditis in dependency of virus-induced pathogenicity and genetic factors of the host are present in these animal models (Fig. 5.1; for review see [8]).

S. Pankuweit (✉)
Department of Cardiology, University Hospital Gießen & Marburg, Marburg, Germany
e-mail: pankuwei@staff.uni-marburg.de

K. Klingel (✉)
Cardiopathology, Institute for Pathology and Neuropathology, University Hospital Tuebingen, Tuebingen, Germany
e-mail: karin.klingel@med.uni-tuebingen.de

A. L. P. Caforio (ed.), *Myocarditis*, https://doi.org/10.1007/978-3-030-35276-9_5

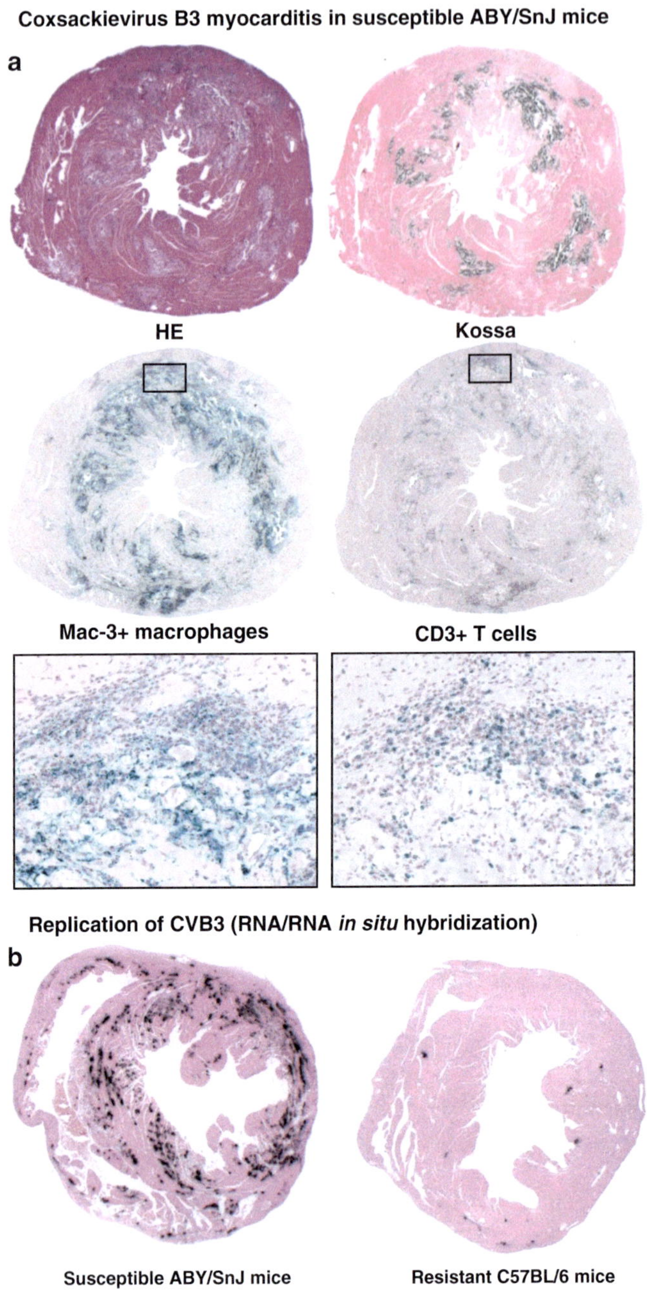

Fig. 5.1 Heart tissue sections of a susceptible ABY/SnJ obtained 2 weeks after infection with coxsackievirus B3 (CVB3) reveal massive calcification (Kossa staining) in areas of necrotic myocytes (HE) and ongoing inflammation as detected by MAC-3+ macrophages and CD3+ T lymphocytes (**a**). CVB3 replication in myocytes during acute infection as detected by radioactive in situ hybridization, cardiac damage, and inflammation is extensive in susceptible ABY/SnJ (H-2^b) mice compared to resistant C57BL/6 (H-2^b) mice which do not get a chronic myocarditis (**b**)

Thus, it is highly probable that also the different course of myocarditis in humans is determined by individual immune reactions on infection of specific cardiac cell types by the various RNA and DNA viruses. By means of light and electron microscopic in situ hybridization experiments it was possible to allocate specific virus infections to particular cardiac cell types in the human heart as well as in murine hearts [9, 10]. Coxsackieviruses belonging to the enteroviruses were found to infect primarily cardiomyocytes and due to extensive virus replication a rapid cytolysis of these cells occurs [11]. The consecutive antiviral immune response which involves NK cells, macrophages, and CD4+ and CD8+ T lymphocytes aims to eliminate CVB from the myocardium and is successful in most humans but some patients develop a chronic myocarditis on the basis of viral genome persistence [9]. At later stages of the disease, the virus-induced cytolysis may also trigger autoimmune reactions which are primed by the release of specific cellular antigens from necrotic myocytes such as to beta1-adrenergic receptors [12], myosin, or M2 muscarinic receptors which have also been observed in some animal models of myocarditis [13]. Further studies are needed to address the contribution of autoimmune reactions in comparison to those induced by persistent virus infections in the outcome of viral heart disease.

In contrast to enteroviruses, all other viruses often detected in the human heart cannot infect myocytes, e.g., due to absence of the correspondent viral receptors. Instead, some cardiotropic viruses infect exclusively endothelial cells as we have shown by radioactive in situ hybridization for B19V. This virus was exclusively found in endothelial cells of children and adult patients with myocarditis (Fig. 5.2). On the other hand herpesviruses including HHV6 and EBV which also do not infect cardiomyocytes were detected in cardiac inflammatory cells (macrophages, T or B lymphocytes) in patients with myocarditis (Fig. 5.2). Thus, numerous cardiotropic viruses do not damage the heart via cytolysis of cardiomyocytes but most likely via expression of cardiotoxic chemokines and cytokines from infected endothelial or immune cells, contributing to further attraction of potentially harmful immune cells into the heart. It is known that, e.g., HHV6 may induce the expression of the pro-inflammatory cytokine IL-6 which is decisive for the invasion of T cells into infected organs [14]. In order to delineate the differences of the cellular and molecular mechanisms in acute and chronic myocarditis induced by different viral triggers various animal models are discussed in the following chapters.

5.2 Murine Models of Coxsackievirus Myocarditis

The murine model of CVB3 myocarditis is by far the most thoroughly investigated animal model of viral myocarditis as genetically diverse mouse strains perfectly reflect the different course of enteroviral myocarditis in patients (Fig. 5.1) [15]. The induction of enteroviral myocarditis is mediated by the entry of the virus into the cardiomyocytes via internalization using the transmembrane receptor CAR (coxsackievirus and adenovirus receptor) (CAR) and the deflecting protein decay accelerating factor (DAF) as a coreceptor. CVB are able to lyse myocytes in vitro and

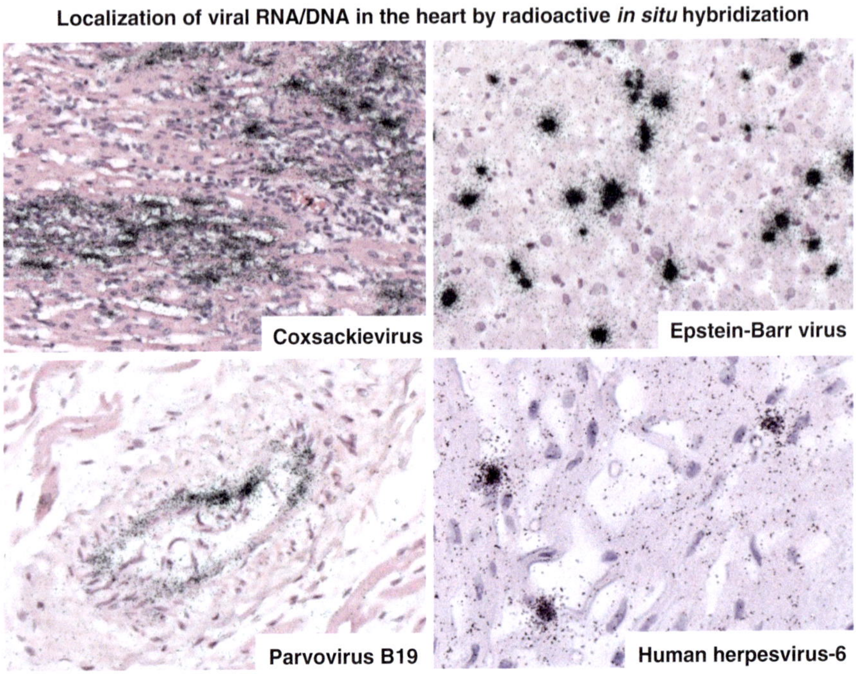

Fig. 5.2 Radioactive in situ hybridization demonstrates the localization of viral genomes in different cardiac cell types in patients with acute myocarditis (virus genomes are indicated by black silver grains). Coxsackieviruses infect mainly cardiomyocytes, whereas parvovirus B19 DNA is exclusively found in endothelial cells. Nucleic acids of Epstein–Barr virus and human herpesvirus-6 are present in interstitial immune cells (T cells, B cells, macrophages) but not in cardiomyocytes

in vivo very quickly due to pronounced viral replication as shown in Fig. 5.1 [10, 11]. In CVB3-infected mice myocytolysis due to virus replication was proven by electron microscopic in situ hybridization studies, demonstrating replicative RNA intermediates in close spatial association with vacuoles within myocytes [10]. Transgenic mice which express a replication-competent but not infectious full-length CVB3 cDNA reveal severe loss of myocytes and scarring, indicating that expression of viral proteins mediates cardiac dysfunction [16].

A decisive molecular mechanism by which enteroviruses contribute to the pathogenesis of myocarditis was described by Badorff et al. [17], demonstrating that CVB3 cleaves dystrophin via the viral proteinase 2A resulting in the disruption of cytoskeleton in myocytes. More recently, the intracellular protein degradation systems comprising the ubiquitin-proteasome and lysosome pathways have been identified as crucial factors of virus infectivity. Luo et al. [18] demonstrated that treatment of cells with proteasome inhibitors significantly decreased virus titers and prevented virus-induced cell death. Moreover, the virus-induced pro-inflammatory cytokine and chemokine production was found to be prevented by ONX 0914, an immunoproteasome-specific inhibitor [19].

As a consequence of viral replication in myocytes, the innate immune response is triggered. Pro-inflammatory cytokines such as interleukin-1 (IL-1), IL-6, tumor necrosis factor (TNFα), and interferons (type I and II) are released from resident cardiac cells, which consecutively activate macrophages. Also, the NLRP3 activity was enhanced during early stage of CVB3 infection, as evidenced by increased gene expression and/or secretion of IL-1β and caspase-1. NLRP3 and its upstream serine/threonine-protein kinase receptor-interacting protein 1/3 are degraded via the proteolytic activity of virus-encoded proteinases, thus counteracting the host defense response against CVB3 [20]. When IL-1ß in CVB3-infected mice is depleted, a reduction of cardiac inflammation and fibrosis is noted during the acute but also during the chronic phase of myocarditis in presence of persistent virus infection [21].

A major impact for the course of the disease emerged to be the type I interferon system. CVB3-infected type I-IFNR-deficient mice died within 2–4 days post infection [22]. In mice deficient for IFN-beta a downregulation of IFN-stimulated gene targets as well as increased cardiomyocyte injury was noted [23]. A disease-phase dependent role of interferon (IFN) regulatory factor 7 (IRF7) was suggested to robust IFN-beta induction in acute CVB3 myocarditis [24]. Various TLRs which are expressed on immune cells, comprising natural killer (NK) cells, dendritic cells (DCs), and macrophages have been implicated to be involved in the early immune response against enteroviruses. During acute CVB3-induced myocarditis *Tlr2*, *Tlr3*, *Tlr6*, *Tlr7*, and *Tlr9* displayed by far the highest increase of mRNA expression during acute disease [24]. CVB3-infected TLR3-knockout (ko) mice developed a severe ongoing myocarditis underlining the view that TLR3 plays a central role in the effective control of the infection [25]. TLR3 signaling in DCs and in other cells was found to be relevant for the activation and polarization of the CD4+ T lymphocyte response toward a Th1 profile and, consequently for a better outcome of CVB3 infection [26]. Monocytes, macrophages, dendritic cells express the colony-stimulating factor 1 receptor (CSF-1R). CSF-1R signaling screws mature monocytes into a pro-inflammatory state. Silencing the CSF-1 axis by siCSF-1 inverted virus-mediated immunopathology as reflected by lower troponin T levels, a reduction of accumulating myeloid cells in heart tissue and improved cardiac function [27].

Following the activation of the innate immunity, the adaptive immune response evolves around 6 days post infection (pi) (Fig. 5.1). As shown in CVB3-infected beta-2 microglobulin- [28] and CD8-deficient mice [29] the severity of disease was magnified, demonstrating protective effects of CD8+ T cells in the propagation of viral myocarditis. Dependent on the genetic background, susceptible animals such as A/J, ABY/SnJ, ASW/J, SWR/J, Balb/c develop a chronic myocarditis which may last for several months [15]. The failure to resolve viral RNA from the heart can be deleterious and results in ongoing myocarditis [15]. However, when the virus is completely cleared as observed in C57BL/6 mice 2 weeks pi, the downregulation of the inflammation in the heart occurs which is mediated by the production of anti-inflammatory cytokines such as transforming growth factor beta (TGFβ) and IL-10 by regulatory T cells and alternatively activated (M2) macrophages [30]. Adoptive

T_{reg} transfer in the inflammatory phase of CVB3 myocarditis was found to protect the heart against inflammatory damage and fibrosis via modulation of monocyte subsets [31]. Susceptible mice revealing chronic inflammation were found to have a delayed IFN-γ secretion and a highly diminished IL-10 production [32]. Findings in IL-10-deleted mice confirmed the regulatory role of IL-10 in the outcome of CVB3 myocarditis [32]. Recently, Li et al. [33] showed that the protection of female mice to excessive cardiac damage in the coxsackieviral mouse model is attributed to a larger presence of M2 macrophages in comparison to male mice. The consequences of chronic inflammation following CVB3 infection are cardiac fibrosis with remodeling of the extracellular matrix (EMC), which may finally result in dilated cardiomyopathy and heart failure. Important regulators of the ECM are matrix metalloproteinases (MMPs) which can degrade the different components in the interstitium. MMP-2, MMP-9, and MMP-12 transcription was increased during acute myocarditis, the tissue inhibitors of metalloproteinases-3 (TIMP-3) and TIMP-4 expression were found to be downregulated, indicating that cardiac remodeling is at least partially mediated via activation of MMPs [34]. Another protein that has been described to be involved in inflammatory responses and in the maintenance or reconfiguration of tissue integrity is osteopontin (OPN). In contrast to resistant C57BL/6 and OPN gene-deficient mice, transcription levels of matrix metalloproteinase-3, TIMP1, *urokinase-type plasminogen activator* (uPA), and transforming growth factor (TGF) beta1 were elevated in susceptible mice, and as a consequence, procollagen-1 mRNA expression and fibrosis were considerably enhanced but could be successfully treated with a vitamin D analog [35]. In addition to OPN [21] also connective tissue growth factor (CTGF), a member of the CCN protein family was found to be associated with the development of fibrosis in ongoing enteroviral myocarditis. CTGF which is known to be basically mediated by TGF-β was found to be extensively upregulated in CVB3-infected susceptible mice [36]. Interestingly, the matricellular protein Cyr61, another CCN protein was found not only to be linked with tissue repair but also to function as a modulator of immune cell migration as shown in a murine model of autoimmune myocarditis. The CCN1-driven modulation of immune cell migration is mimicked in part by cyclic RGD peptides which might offer a therapeutic option for the treatment of inflammatory heart diseases [37].

5.3 Murine Models of Encephalomyocarditis Virus Myocarditis

Encephalomyocarditis virus (EMCV) is another single-stranded picornavirus of the *Enterovirus* genus which has been studied to evaluate pathogenetic mechanisms in enteroviral myocarditis. Similar to CVB, EMCV was found to induce a necrotic myocarditis in mice but was also detected in the heart of young Rhesus macaques [38]. Whether transmission of EMCV to humans occurs is unclear. However, in 2009 EMCV was obviously isolated in two patients with fever, nausea, headache, and dyspnea supporting a role for EMCV in human infection and febrile illness [39].

In order to identify molecular mechanisms in EMCV myocarditis, mice lacking functional TLR3 were investigated. Correspondent to findings in CVB3-infected TLR3 ko mice [25], EMCV-infected TLR3 ko mice were found to be unable to control the proliferation of EMCV, subsequently resulting in increased cytopathogenic effects in cardiac myocytes and early death. The findings in this study implicate the importance of TLR3 signaling and antiviral effects of TNF-alpha and IL-6 in the very early stages of the heart disease [40]. On the other hand, it is well known that inflammatory cytokines including TNF-alpha may accelerate the pathology of EMCV-myocarditis and negatively influence the cardiac function [41]. Most recently, depletion of CD103+ conventional dendritic cell (cDC) was found to abrogate antigen-specific $CD8^+$ T cell proliferative expansion, transforming subclinical cardiac injury to overt heart failure [42].

5.4 Murine Models of Reovirus Myocarditis

Reoviruses which are enteric non-enveloped viruses with a double-stranded RNA genome have been widely used as model systems to study viral pathogenesis in the central nervous system, liver, and heart. The morphology of reovirus-induced myocarditis is generally characterized by mild inflammatory infiltrates but extensive myocardial necrosis. Comparable to findings in coxsackievirus infections, also, reovirus was found to induce a myocarditis in severe combined immunodeficient (SCID) mice, illustrating that reovirus myocarditis is primarily not an immune-mediated disease [43]. Correspondent to observations in CVB3 myocarditis [15) the extent of viral RNA synthesis during replication but not generation of infectious virus was found to be a determinant of reovirus-induced acute myocarditis [44].

Differences in the tropism and virulence have been linked to sensitivity of type I interferons [45]. The retinoic acid inducible gene I (RIG-I) and the RIG-I adaptor were found to be necessary for the activation of antiviral transcription factors including interferon regulatory factor 3 (IRF-3) and NF-κB [46]. The spontaneous activation of a mitochondrial antiviral signaling (MAVS) pathway in cardiac myocytes but not cardiac fibroblasts or skeletal muscle cells was found to determine high basal interferon-β expression in the heart [47].

5.5 Animal Models of Parvovirus Myocarditis

Human parvovirus B19 (B19V), the only human pathogenic parvovirus, is the causative agent of a wide spectrum of human diseases, including fifth disease (erythema infectiosum), hydrops fetalis in pregnant women, and transient aplastic crisis in patients. Numerous reports demonstrating the presence of B19V in the heart of patients with acute and chronic myocarditis further suggest that this virus may be associated with inflammatory heart disease. Our current understanding about the mechanisms by which B19V regulates disease progression is rather limited, also due to the lack of adequate animal models as infection of mice with B19V does not induce myocarditis. Interestingly, immunization of BALB/c mice with B19V VP1-unique region was found to result in dilated cardiomyopathy with cardiac fibrosis and progressive dilatation of left ventricle [48]. Recently, it was shown that parvovirus B19V non-structural protein-1 (NS-1) induced apoptotic bodies may elicit inflammation and degeneration in murine hearts [49]. Also, parvovirus B19-induced vascular damage in the heart was demonstrated to be associated with elevated circulating endothelial microparticles (EMPs) as detected in transgenic B19V-NS1-mice [50].

5.6 Murine Models of Herpesvirus Myocarditis

Epstein–Barr virus has been observed in the hearts of up to 8% of the patients with inflammatory heart disease [1]. The processes explaining cardiac inflammation and injury in EBV infection are uncertain mainly due to the absence of suitable animal models [51]. One animal model which might mimic in some aspects human EBV infection is infection of mice with the murine gamma herpesvirus MHV-68. Both viruses can induce a latent infection of B cells [52]. With regard to myocardial infection MHV-68 seems to replicate in the heart of immunocompetent mice showing a maximum replication between 5 and 10 days. Myocardial necrosis and focal inflammation, consisting mainly of T lymphocytes, occur after 10–12 days and 33–35 days, respectively. B- and T-cell deficient B6-(Rag1)™ mice revealed high myocardial viral loads but no myocardial necrosis, indicating that viral replication is not sufficient to explain myocardial damage. However, in this model it is still unclear which cells are infected in the heart and which molecular mechanisms lead to myocardial necrosis in BALB/c mice but not in C57BL/6 [52].

The evolvement of myocarditis has also been reported in mice infected with another herpesvirus, the murine cytomegalovirus (MCMV) [53]. The hearts of MCMV-infected BALB/c mice were found to be more susceptible than those of C57BL/6 for cardiac infiltration, which mainly consist of CD8+ and CD4+ T cells, macrophages, B cells, and neutrophils. In this model MCMV titres in the heart were low and replicative virus could not be isolated beyond the first week pi. Correspondent to human infection with cytomegalovirus (HCMV), also in cardiac MHV-68 and MCMV infection the direct lysis of myocytes due to virus replication in vivo was not proven [53]. In another study of MCMV-induced myocarditis in BALB/c mice it was shown that myocarditis-related pathological changes and increase in viral load were greatest at day 8 p.i., corresponding with peak cytokine transcription of TNF-alpha, IL-6, and IFN-γ, as well as of IL-10 mRNA transcripts [54]. Interestingly, treatment of MCMV-infected mice with IFNA6, A9, and B inhibited acute myocarditis, and IFNA6 was even found to reduce chronic cardiac inflammation, supporting the hypothesis that acute MCMV myocarditis does not reflect virus load but rather the immunomodulatory responses to this infection [55].

5.7 Molecular Diagnosis in Patients

Myocarditis in humans—a frequent cause of dilated cardiomyopathy and sudden cardiac death—typically results from cardiotropic viral infection followed by active inflammatory destruction of the myocardium. Advances in molecular detection of viruses by endomyocardial biopsy have improved our ability to diagnose and understand the pathophysiological mechanisms of this elusive disease, which have been summarized in 2013 by Klingel and Pankuweit [56]. Here, we present a condensed and updated summary of this review.

The diagnosis of virus-associated myocarditis was clearly facilitated by the introduction of endomyocardial biopsy techniques by Sakakibara and Konno in 1962 [57] in addition to the development of polymerase chain reaction (PCR) by Mullis et al. in 1982 [58]. The combination of both methods allowed for the first time the detection of viral genomes directly within the affected myocardial tissue in a patient with suspected myocarditis. A wide range of different PCR assays have been developed, which are suitable to identify different cardiac RNA and/or DNA viruses with a higher sensitivity in comparison to standard immunohistochemical methods used for the detection of viral proteins (for review [56, 59–62]).

By these molecular approaches enteroviruses have been identified as highly relevant pathogenic agents in myocarditis [63–71]. Moreover, the presence of genomes from adenoviruses (ADV), parvovirus B19 (B19V) [72], herpesviruses (human herpesvirus 6 (HHV6), cytomegalovirus (CMV), Epstein–Barr virus (EBV), herpes simplex virus type 1 (HSV1) [73], chlamydia pneumoniae [74], Borrelia burgdorferi [75, 76], as well as other infectious agents [77] was reported in patients with inflammatory heart disease.

One of the major problems associated with the analysis of cardiotropic agents by PCR is the fact that this technique only allows the detection of viral genomes without differentiating potentially infected cardiac cell types. In addition, active replication of the virus is generally not investigated by PCR [9]. Thus, in order to substantiate the etiopathogenetic role of an infectious agent, PCR must be carefully evaluated in the context of clinical, and histological and immunohistochemical findings of endomyocardial biopsies.

To overcome this diagnostic gap the in situ hybridization technique was established, which is capable to attribute viral sequences to specific cells types in the heart as illustrated in Fig. 5.2 and Table 5.1. Also, as shown for coxsackicviruses in

Table 5.1 Cardiotropic viruses infect different cell types in the heart

Coxsackieviruses	Cardiomyocytes, B cells, CD4+ T cells, macrophages, fibroblasts
Parvovirus B19	Endothelial cells
Epstein-Barr virus	B cells, T cells, macrophages
Human herpesvirus-6	T cells
Cytomegalovirus	Macrophages, fibroblasts, endothelial cells

situ hybridization allows the detection viral plus-strand RNA as well as the replicative minus-strand RNA intermediates, which are of particular interest for the diagnosis of active myocardial infections [9, 65–67, 78].

Starting from 2002, fluorescence-based real-time PCR assays were established for the evaluation of the viral load in the heart. Regarding the quantification of B19V genomes, real-time PCR assays have been developed for the use of the LightCycler system [79], fluorescence resonance energy transfer probes [80] as well as for the ABI Prism system [81, 82].

5.8 Prevalence of Cardiotropic Viruses in Endomyocardial Biopsies Assessed by Molecular Tools

Viral genomes were identified in a varying subset of patients with acute and chronic myocarditis and DCM, but the impact of these viral genomes on cardiac function and clinical outcome is still controversial [83]. The overall prevalence of cardiotropic viruses amplified by (RT-) PCR in endomyocardial biopsies of these patients differs widely: enteroviral genomes were detected in 3–53%, cytomegalovirus DNA in 3–40%, and adenoviruses in 3–23% in the myocardium of patients with inflammatory heart disease. In addition to the previous summaries [56, 59], the wide range of results that have been obtained by different molecular methods were summarized as follows with regard to the most prevalent cardiotropic viruses such as HHV6, EBV, and B19V.

5.9 Prevalence of Parvovirus B19 Genomes in Patients with Myocarditis and DCM

Investigations in adult patients with inflammatory heart diseases revealed a prevalence of B19V DNA in 19.5% of patients with myocarditis, 23% in patients with DCMi, and 16% in patients with DCM [84]. Prevalences for PVB19 genomes detected in patients with myocarditis or DCM ranged from 11–56% in patients with myocarditis and 10–51% in patients with DCM. As reported for enteroviruses also persistence of B19V in patients with LV dysfunction was found to be associated with a progressive impairment of LVEF [2]. In contrast to enteroviruses, spontaneous virus elimination of B19V was observed in only 22% of patients. These results suggest that persisting cardiac viral infections may constitute a major cause of progressive LV dysfunction in patients with past myocarditis or DCM. Interestingly, it was shown in 24 patients presented with acute onset of angina pectoris and ST-segment elevations or T-wave inversion mimicking acute myocardial infarction, that histological analysis excluded mostly active or borderline myocarditis, but B19V, EV, and ADV genomes were detected in the myocardium of 12, three, and two patients, respectively [85]. Here, virus genomes were found in 71% of patients with normal coronary anatomy, clinically mimicking acute myocardial infarction, an observation which was first published in a patient with lethal myocarditis by Bültmann et al. [86]. In this female patient with clinical signs of myocardial infarction and histopathological fulminant myocarditis in situ hybridization studies of the autopsy heart revealed the presence of B19V genomes exclusively in endothelial cells of the smaller intramyocardial vessels. Immunohistochemical stainings exhibited marked expression of E-selectin on endothelial cells, a finding indicative of endothelial dysfunction. These processes are likely to lead to disturbances in the coronary microcirculation and may explain the observation that many patients with B19V-associated myocarditis present with the clinical signs that are typical of ischemic heart disease.

However, the causal relationship of B19V infections to cardiac disease has been questioned, mainly because epidemiological data demonstrated a lifelong persistence of B19V genomes in various organs, apart from the heart [87, 88] and the fact, that B19V DNA was also detected in heart tissue from patients without clinical manifestations of inflammatory cardiomyopathy [89–91].

Nevertheless, parvovirus replication in myocardial endothelial cells was substantiated by the detection of B19V RNA replicative intermediates in the myocardium only in acutely inflamed hearts, whereas viral RNA was not detected in chronic dilated cardiomyopathy without inflammation or in control hearts [4]. On the basis of these data, it was suggested that viral loads of more than 500 genome equivalents per microgram isolated nucleic acid in endomyocardial biopsies are the clinically relevant threshold for the maintenance of myocardial inflammation.

In a recent publication with human samples, it was shown that endothelial derived microparticles were significantly different in B19V+ compared to B19V− patients and human controls, with an increase of apoptotic but not activated endothelial microparticles [50]. Other microparticles such as platelet-, leukocyte-, and monocyte-derived microparticles showed less specific patterns, indicating that differences in the subtypes of microparticles can be attributed to specific myocardial virus infections.

However, the molecular mechanisms responsible for a possible reactivation of B19V, the influence of the immune system triggering B19V replication and immune-independent viral pathogenesis in uninflamed hearts are the remaining gaps in our understanding of B19V pathogenicity in heart diseases [4].

5.10 Prevalence of Epstein–Barr Virus and Human Herpesvirus 6 and in Patients with Myocarditis and DCM

In immunocompetent patients, herpesviruses including EBV and HHV6 infections rarely induce cardiac symptoms. For example, EBV-linked acute pericarditis or myocarditis is only reported in some immunocompetent patients [92–94]. Also, HHV6-induced myocarditis has been published in a low number of patients, but sometimes with a fatal outcome [95, 96]. Investigation of autopsy material showed diffuse myocarditis with a granulocytic and monocytic infiltrate, necrotizing arteritis of the coronary arteries, and fulminant hepatitis with microvesicular steatosis and necrosis together with the detection of HHV6 genome in heart, liver, lung, and spleen [95]. In the larger series of patients with inflammatory heart diseases analyses for HHV6 and EBV were always included. Prevalences for HHV6 genomes detected in patients with myocarditis or DCM ranged from 8 to 20% and for EBV genomes from 0 to 8%. Nevertheless, the pathophysiological mechanisms of herpesviruses in acute myocarditis and especially the possible relevance of HHV-6 reactivation for the development of chronic cardiomyopathies remain to be assessed.

5.11 Prevalence of Influenza Virus RNA in Patients with Myocarditis and DCM

Last but not least several cases of acute myocarditis especially in juvenile patients have been reported in association with pandemic H1N1 influenza virus infections. Genomes of Influenza A/H1N1 virus were detected by RT-PCR analysis in blood as well as in myocardial tissue in patients with a lethal influenzavirus infection, however virus replication was not observed in heart muscle cells [6]. Nevertheless, fulminant myocarditis caused by H1N1 infection seems to be a rare but severe and often lethal complication not only in children [97, 98].

5.12 Prevalence of Double or Multiple Infections

In larger series of patients with myocarditis and dilated cardiomyopathy investigated by Kühl et al. [99] and Kandolf et al. [100] it has been shown that the detection of two or more cardiotropic viruses by PCR in the myocardium is rather common. In a series of 245 patients with DCM multiple infections were found in 27.3% of patients. Most often, HHV6 + B19V (10.6% of cases) and B19V + EV (3.7% of cases) genomes were amplified in parallel by PCR [99]. Comparably, in a published study of 3219 patients with cardiac dysfunction and suspected myocarditis, in 11.6% of the patients HHV6 and B19V genomes were concurrently detected in the heart [100]. However, there are no data available, whether clinical symptoms or cardiac histopathology differ in patients with multiple infections or whether prognosis in those patients is worse or different when compared to patients with only one virus type in the heart.

5.13 Diagnostic Implications

There is convincing evidence from animal models and investigations in humans that viral infections may induce a significant damage of the myocardium through direct virus-mediated injury of cardiomyocytes and secondary immune reactions, finally leading to chronic myocarditis and dilated cardiomyopathy. In addition, viral endomyocardial infections have also been reported as an independent predictor of graft loss in pediatric cardiac transplant recipients [101].

As a consequence from the investigations performed over more than 20 years the position statement of the European Society of Cardiology Working Group on

Myocardial and Pericardial Diseases with regard to "Current state of knowledge on aetiology, diagnosis, management, and therapy of myocarditis" was initiated [102]. There it is stated that the endomyocardial biopsy is the "gold standard" to diagnose myocarditis and should be performed early in the course of the disease to optimize diagnostic accuracy and reduce sampling error especially in focal myocarditis. Endomyocardial biopsy confirms the diagnosis of myocarditis and identifies the underlying etiology and the type of inflammation, which imply different treatments and prognosis [103–106]. Multiple specimens should be taken and immediately fixed in 10% buffered formalin at room temperature for light microscopy; additional 1–2 samples should be snap frozen in liquid nitrogen and stored at −80 °C or stored in RNA later tubes at room temperature for viral PCR [102, 103]. To increase the diagnostic sensitivity of myocarditis, immunohistochemistry is mandatory for the identification and characterization of the inflammatory infiltrate [102, 106, 107]. In addition to routine stainings (hematoxylin/eosin, Giemsa, Masson trichrome), immunohistochemistry is required to demonstrate infiltrating cells by applying antibodies specific for T and B lymphocytes, macrophages, major histocompatibility class 1 and class 2 antigens. Diagnosis of myocarditis in EMB requires ≥14 leucocytes/mm^2 in the interstitium [102].

The diagnostic contribution of EMB is significantly enhanced by molecular analysis with DNA/RNA extraction and (RT-) PCR amplification of viral genomes [102, 105, 107]. In this context it is worthy to note that patients with enterovirus myocarditis must not be treated by an immunosuppressive therapy comprising corticosteroids. In order to exclude systemic infection, peripheral blood should be investigated in parallel with EMB [102, 107]; quantification of virus load and determination of virus replication may add diagnostic value [4, 102]. For the detection of cardiotropic viruses total DNA and RNA should be extracted from the heart tissue samples. Primer pairs specific for enteroviruses, parvovirus B19 (B19V), cytomegalovirus (CMV), influenzaviruses (A, B), human herpesvirus-6 (HHV6) and Epstein–Barr virus (EBV) should be used to perform polymerase chain reaction (RT-) PCR, including quantitative real-time PCR in case of PVB19. These investigations are required to investigate, e.g., the success of an antiviral therapy.

Last but not least, as an innovative approach, next-generation sequencing was recently evaluated for detecting potential pathogens of acute myocarditis from sera [108]. In this small investigation virus-derived sequences were identified in seven of 17 cases, and the presence of viruses was confirmed by PCR or antigen testing in four patients. So far, the relationship between sequencing results and myocarditis remains to be clarified, but a NGS-based approach may have the potential to detect different viral pathogens and contribute to the clarification of the etiology of acute myocarditis.

References

1. Kindermann I, Kindermann M, Kandolf R, Klingel K, Bültmann B, Müller T, et al. Predictors of outcome in patients with suspected myocarditis. Circulation. 2008;118(6):639–48.
2. Kühl U, Pauschinger M, Seeberg B, Lassner D, Noutsias M, Poller W, Schultheiss HP. Viral persistence in the myocardium is associated with progressive cardiac dysfunction. Circulation. 2005;112(13):1965–70.

3. Trachtenberg BH, Hare JM. Inflammatory cardiomyopathic syndromes. Circ Res. 2017;121(7):803–18.
4. Bock CT, Klingel K, Kandolf R. Human parvovirus B19-associated myocarditis. N Engl J Med. 2010;362(13):1248–9.
5. Ruppert V, Meyer T, Balbach A, Richter A, Müller HH, Maisch B, Pankuweit S, German Heart Failure Network. Genotype-specific effects on left ventricular function in parvovirus B19-positive patients with dilated cardiomyopathy. J Med Virol. 2011;83(10):1818–25.
6. Gdynia G, Schnitzler P, Brunner E, Kandolf R, Bläker H, Daum E, Schnabel P, Schirmacher P, Roth W. Sudden death of an immunocompetent young adult caused by novel (swine origin) influenza A/H1N1-associated myocarditis. Virchows Arch. 2011;458(3):371–6.
7. Barbaro G. HIV-associated myocarditis. Heart Fail Clin. 2005;1(3):439–48. Review.
8. Esfandiarei M, McManus BM. Molecular biology and pathogenesis of viral myocarditis. Annu Rev Pathol. 2008;3:127–55. Review.
9. Klingel K, Sauter M, Bock CT, Szalay G, Schnorr JJ, Kandolf R. Molecular pathology of inflammatory cardiomyopathy. Med Microbiol Immunol. 2004;193(2–3):101–7.
10. Klingel K, Rieger P, Mall G, Selinka HC, Huber M, Kandolf R. Visualization of enteroviral replication in myocardial tissue by ultrastructural in situ hybridization: identification of target cells and cytopathic effects. Lab Investig. 1998;78(10):1227–37.
11. McManus BM, Chow LH, Wilson JE, Anderson DR, Gulizia JM, Gauntt CJ, Klingel KE, Beisel KW, Kandolf R. Direct myocardial injury by enterovirus: a central role in the evolution of murine myocarditis. Clin Immunol Immunopathol. 1993;68(2):159–69.
12. Jahns R, Boivin V, Hein L, Triebel S, Angermann CE, Ertl G, Lohse MJ. Direct evidence for a beta1-adrenergic receptor-directed autoimmune attack as a cause of idiopathic dilated cardiomyopathy. J Clin Invest. 2004;113(10):1419–29.
13. Caforio AL, Tona F, Bottaro S, Vinci A, Dequal G, Daliento L, Thiene G, Iliceto S. Clinical implications of anti-heart autoantibodies in myocarditis and dilated cardiomyopathy. Autoimmunity. 2008;41(1):35–45. Review.
14. Ogata M, Satou T, Kawano R, Takakura S, Goto K, Ikewaki J, Kohno K, Ikebe T, Ando T, Miyazaki Y, Ohtsuka E, Saburi Y, Saikawa T, Kadota J. Correlations of HHV-6 viral load and plasma IL-6 concentration with HHV-6 encephalitis in allogeneic stem cell transplant recipients. Bone Marrow Transplant. 2010;45(1):129–36.
15. Klingel K, Hohenadl C, Canu A, Albrecht M, Seemann M, Mall G, Kandolf R. Ongoing enterovirus-induced myocarditis is associated with persistent heart muscle infection: quantitative analysis of virus replication, tissue damage, and inflammation. Proc Natl Acad Sci U S A. 1992;89(1):314–8.
16. Wessely R, Klingel K, Santana LF, Dalton N, Hongo M, Jonathan Lederer W, Kandolf R, Knowlton KU. Transgenic expression of replication-restricted enteroviral genomes in heart muscle induces defective excitation-contraction coupling and dilated cardiomyopathy. J Clin Invest. 1998;102(7):1444–53.
17. Badorff C, Lee GH, Lamphear BJ, et al. Enteroviral protease 2A cleaves dystrophin: evidence of cytoskeletal disruption in an acquired cardiomyopathy. Nat Med. 1999;5(3):320–6.
18. Luo H, Zhang J, Cheung C, Suarez A, McManus BM, Yang D. Proteasome inhibition reduces coxsackievirus B3 replication in murine cardiomyocytes. Am J Pathol. 2003;163(2):381–5.
19. Althof N, Goetzke CC, Kespohl M, Voss K, Heuser A, Pinkert S, Kaya Z, Klingel K, Beling A. The immunoproteasome-specific inhibitor ONX 0914 reverses susceptibility to acute viral myocarditis. EMBO Mol Med. 2018;10(2):200–18.
20. Wang C, Fung G, Deng H, Jagdeo J, Mohamud Y, Xue YC, Jan E, Hirota JA, Luo H. NLRP3 deficiency exacerbates enterovirus infection in mice. FASEB J. 2019;33(1):942–52.
21. Kraft L, Erdenesuk T, Sauter M, Tschöpe C, Klingel K. Blocking the IL-1β signalling pathway prevents chronic viral myocarditis and cardiac remodeling. Basic Res Cardiol. 2019;114(2):11–27.
22. Wessely R, Klingel K, Knowlton KU, Kandolf R. Cardioselective infection with coxsackievirus B3 requires intact type I interferon signaling: implications for mortality and early viral replication. Circulation. 2001;103(5):756–61.

23. Deonarain R, Cerullo D, Fuse K, Liu PP, Fish EN. Protective role for interferon-beta in coxsackievirus B3 infection. Circulation. 2004;110(23):3540–3.
24. Becher PM, Hinrichs S, Fluschnik N, Hennigs JK, Klingel K, Blankenberg S, Westermann D, Lindner D. Role of toll-like receptors and interferon regulatory factors in different experimental heart failure models of diverse etiology: IRF7 as novel cardiovascular stress-inducible factor. PLoS One. 2018;13(3):e0193844.
25. Weinzierl AO, Szalay G, Wolburg H, Sauter M, Rammensee HG, Kandolf R, Stevanović S, Klingel K. Effective chemokine secretion by dendritic cells and expansion of cross-presenting CD4-/CD8+ dendritic cells define a protective phenotype in the mouse model of coxsackievirus myocarditis. J Virol. 2008;82(16):8149–60.
26. Sesti-Costa R, Françozo MCS, Silva GK, Proenca-Modena JL, Silva JS. TLR3 is required for survival following Coxsackievirus B3 infection by driving T lymphocyte activation and polarization: the role of dendritic cells. PLoS One. 2017;12(10):e0185819.
27. Meyer IS, Goetzke CC, Kespohl M, Sauter M, Heuser A, Eckstein V, Vornlocher HP, Anderson DG, Haas J, Meder B, Katus HA, Klingel K, Beling A, Leuschner F. Silencing the CSF-1 axis using nanoparticle encapsulated siRNA mitigates viral and autoimmune myocarditis. Front Immunol. 2018;9:2303.
28. Klingel K, Schnorr JJ, Sauter M, Szalay G, Kandolf R. Beta2-microglobulin-associated regulation of interferon-gamma and virus-specific immunoglobulin G confer resistance against the development of chronic coxsackievirus myocarditis. Am J Pathol. 2003;162(5):1709–20.
29. Opavsky MA, Penninger J, Aitken K, Wen WH, Dawood F, Mak T, Liu P. Susceptibility to myocarditis is dependent on the response of alphabeta T lymphocytes to coxsackieviral infection. Circ Res. 1999;85(6):551–8.
30. Frisancho-Kiss S, Coronado MJ, Frisancho JA, Lau VM, Rose NR, Klein SL, Fairweather D. Gonadectomy of male BALB/c mice increases Tim-3(+) alternatively activated M2 macrophages, Tim-3(+) T cells, Th2 cells and Treg in the heart during acute coxsackievirus-induced myocarditis. Brain Behav Immun. 2009;23(5):649–57.
31. Pappritz K, Savvatis K, Miteva K, Kerim B, Dong F, Fechner H, Müller I, Brandt C, Lopez B, González A, Ravassa S, Klingel K, Diez J, Reinke P, Volk HD, Van Linthout S, Tschöpe C. Immunomodulation by adoptive regulatory T-cell transfer improves Coxsackievirus B3-induced myocarditis. FASEB J. 2018;32(11):6066–78. https://doi.org/10.1096/fj.201701408R.
32. Szalay G, Sauter M, Hald J, Weinzierl A, Kandolf R, Klingel K. Sustained nitric oxide synthesis contributes to immunopathology in ongoing myocarditis attributable to interleukin-10 disorders. Am J Pathol. 2006;169(6):2085–93.
33. Li K, Xu W, Guo Q, Jiang Z, Wang P, Yue Y, Xiong S. Differential macrophage polarization in male and female BALB/c mice infected with coxsackievirus B3 defines susceptibility to viral myocarditis. Circ Res. 2009;105(4):353–64.
34. Cheung C, Luo H, Yanagawa B, Leong HS, Samarasekera D, Lai JC, Suarez A, Zhang J, McManus BM. Matrix metalloproteinases and tissue inhibitors of metalloproteinases in coxsackievirus-induced myocarditis. Cardiovasc Pathol. 2006;15(2):63–74.
35. Szalay G, Sauter M, Haberland M, Zuegel U, Steinmeyer A, Kandolf R, Klingel K. Osteopontin: a fibrosis-related marker molecule in cardiac remodeling of enterovirus myocarditis in the susceptible host. Circ Res. 2009;104(7):851–9.
36. Lang C, Sauter M, Szalay G, Racchi G, Grassi G, Rainaldi G, Mercatanti A, Lang F, Kandolf R, Klingel K. Connective tissue growth factor: a crucial cytokine-mediating cardiac fibrosis in ongoing enterovirus myocarditis. J Mol Med (Berl). 2008;86(1):49–60.
37. Rother M, Krohn S, Kania G, Vanhoutte D, Eisenreich A, Wang X, Westermann D, Savvatis K, Dannemann N, Skurk C, Hilfiker-Kleiner D, Cathomen T, Fechner H, Rauch U, Schultheiss HP, Heymans S, Eriksson U, Scheibenbogen C, Poller W. Matricellular signaling molecule CCN1 attenuates experimental autoimmune myocarditis by acting as a novel immune cell migration modulator. Circulation. 2010;122(25):2688–98.

38. Masek-Hammerman K, Miller AD, Lin KC, Mackey J, Weissenböck H, Gierbolini L, Burgos A, Perez H, Mansfield KG. Epizootic myocarditis associated with encephalomyocarditis virus in a group of rhesus macaques (Macacamulatta). Vet Pathol. 2012;49(2):386–92.
39. Oberste MS, Gotuzzo E, Blair P, Nix WA, Ksiazek TG, Comer JA, Rollin P, Goldsmith CS, Olson J, Kochel TJ. Human febrile illness caused by encephalomyocarditis virus infection, Peru. Emerg Infect Dis. 2009;15(4):640–6.
40. Hardarson HS, Baker JS, Yang Z, Purevjav E, Huang CH, Alexopoulou L, Li N, Flavell RA, Bowles NE, Vallejo JG. Toll-like receptor 3 is an essential component of the innate stress response in virus-induced cardiac injury. Am J Physiol Heart Circ Physiol. 2007;292(1):H251–8.
41. Yamada T, Matsumori A, Sasayama S. Therapeutic effect of anti-tumor necrosis factor-alpha antibody on the murine model of viral myocarditis induced by encephalomyocarditis virus. Circulation. 1994;89(2):846–51.
42. Clemente-Casares X, Hosseinzadeh S, Barbu I, Dick SA, Macklin JA, Wang Y, Momen A, Kantores C, Aronoff L, Farno M, Lucas TM, Avery J, Zarrin-Khat D, Elsaesser HJ, Razani B, Lavine KJ, Husain M, Brooks DG, Robbins CS, Cybulsky M, Epelman S. A CD103(+) Conventional Dendritic Cell Surveillance System Prevents Development of Overt Heart Failure during Subclinical Viral Myocarditis. Immunity. 2017;47(5):974–989.e8.
43. Sherry B, Li XY, Tyler KL, Cullen JM, Virgin HW 4th. Lymphocytes protect against and are not required for reovirus-induced myocarditis. J Virol. 1993;67(10):6119–24.
44. Sherry B, Baty CJ, Blum MA. Reovirus-induced acute myocarditis in mice correlates with viral RNA synthesis rather than generation of infectious virus in cardiac myocytes. J Virol. 1996;70(10):6709–15.
45. Sherry B, Torres J, Blum MA. Reovirus induction of and sensitivity to beta interferon in cardiac myocyte cultures correlate with induction of myocarditis and are determined by viral core proteins. J Virol. 1998;72(2):1314–23.
46. Holm GH, Zurney J, Tumilasci V, Leveille S, Danthi P, Hiscott J, Sherry B, Dermody TS. Retinoic acid-inducible gene-I and interferon-beta promoter stimulator-1 augment proapoptotic responses following mammalian reovirus infection via interferon regulatory factor-3. J Biol Chem. 2007;282(30):21953–61.
47. Rivera-Serrano EE, DeAngelis N, Sherry B. Spontaneous activation of a MAVS-dependent antiviral signaling pathway determines high basal interferon-β expression in cardiac myocytes. J Mol Cell Cardiol. 2017;111:102–13.
48. Bogomolovas J, Šimoliūnas E, Rinkūnaitė I, Smalinskaitė L, Podkopajev A, Bironaitė D, Weis CA, Marx A, Bukelskienė V, Gretz N, Grabauskienė V, Labeit D, Labeit S. A novel murine model of parvovirus associated dilated cardiomyopathy induced by immunization with VP1-unique region of parvovirus B19. Biomed Res Int. 2016;2016:1627184.
49. Puttaraksa K, Pirttinen H, Karvonen K, Nykky J, Naides SJ, Gilbert L. Parvovirus B19V non-structural protein NS1 induces dsDNA autoantibodies and end organ damage in non-autoimmune mice. J Infect Dis. 2019;219(9):1418–29.
50. Bachelier K, Biehl S, Schwarz V, Kindermann I, Kandolf R, Sauter M, Ukena C, Yilmaz A, Sliwa K, Bock CT, Klingel K, Böhm M. Parvovirus B19-induced vascular damage in the heart is associated with elevated circulating endothelial microparticles. PLoS One. 2017;12(5):e0176311.
51. Kawai C. From myocarditis to cardiomyopathy: mechanisms of inflammation and cell death: learning from the past for the future. Circulation. 1999;99(8):1091–100. Review.
52. Häusler M, Sellhaus B, Scheithauer S, Gaida B, Kuropka S, Siepmann K, Panek A, Berg W, Teubner A, Ritter K, Kleines M. Myocarditis in newborn wild-type BALB/c mice infected with the murine gamma herpesvirus MHV-68. Cardiovasc Res. 2007;76(2):323–30.
53. Lenzo JC, Fairweather D, Cull V, Shellam GR, James Lawson CM. Characterisation of murine cytomegalovirus myocarditis: cellular infiltration of the heart and virus persistence. J Mol Cell Cardiol. 2002;34(6):629–40.
54. Ritter JT, Tang-Feldman YJ, Lochhead GR, Estrada M, Lochhead S, Yu C, Ashton-Sager A, Tuteja D, Leutenegger C, Pomeroy C. In vivo characterization of cytokine profiles and

viral load during murine cytomegalovirus-induced acute myocarditis. Cardiovasc Pathol. 2010;19(2):83–93.

55. Cull VS, Bartlett EJ, James CM. Type I interferon gene therapy protects against cytomegalovirus-induced myocarditis. Immunology. 2002;106(3):428–37.
56. Pankuweit S, Klingel K. Viral myocarditis: from experimental models to molecular diagnosis in patients. Heart Fail Rev. 2013;18(6):683–702.
57. Sakakibara S, Konno S. Endomyocardial biopsy. Jpn Heart J. 1962;3:537–43.
58. Saiki RK, Scharf S, Faloona F, Mullis KB, Horn GT, Ehrlich HA, Arnheim N. Enzymatic amplification of β3-globin genomic sequences and restriction site analysis for diagnosis of sickle cell anemia. Science. 1985;230:1350–13541.
59. Pankuweit S, Portig I, Eckhardt H, Crombach M, Hufnagel G, Maisch B. Prevalence of viral genome in endomyocardial biopsies from patients with inflammatory heart muscle disease. Herz. 2000;25(3):221–6.
60. Jackson DP, Lewis FA, Taylor GR, Boylston AW, Quirke P. Tissue extraction of DNA and RNA and analysis by polymerase chain reaction. J Clin Pathol. 1990;43:499–504.
61. Chomczynski P, Sacchi N. Single-step method of RNA isolation by acid guanidinium thiocyanate-phenol-chloroform extraction. Anal Biochem. 1987;162:156–9.
62. Maniatis T, Fritsch EF, Sambrook J. Molecular cloning: a laboratory manual. New York: Cold Spring Harbor Laboratory; 1992.
63. Rotbart HA. Enzymatic RNA amplification of enteroviruses. J Clin Microbiol. 1990;28:438–42.
64. Martin AB, Webber S, Fricker J, Jaffe R, Demmler G, Kearney D, Zhang YH, Bodurtha J, Gelb B, Ni J. Acute myocarditis: rapid diagnosis in children. Circulation. 1994;90:330–9.
65. Kandolf R, Ameis D, Kirschner P, Canu A, Hofschneider PH. In situ detection of enteroviral genomes in myocardial cells by nucleic acid hybridization: an approach to the diagnosis of viral heart disease. Proc Natl Acad Sci U S A. 1987;84:6272–6.
66. Klingel K, Stephan S, Sauter M, Zell R, McManus BM, Bültmann B, Kandolf R. Pathogenesis of murine enterovirus myocarditis: virus dissemination and immune target cells. J Virol. 1996;70:8888–95.
67. Klump WM, Bergmann I, Müller BC, Ameis D, Kandolf R. Complete nucleotide sequence of infectious coxsackievirus B3 cDNA: two initial 5' uridine residues are regained during plus-strand RNA synthesis. J Virol. 1990;64:1573–83.
68. Archard L, Khan M, Soteriou BA, Zhang H, Why HJ, Robinson NM, Richardson PJ. Characterisation of coxsackie B virus RNA in myocardium from patients with dilated cardiomyopathy by nucleotide sequencing of reverse transcription-nested polymerase chain reaction products. Hum Pathol. 1998;29:578–84.
69. Chapman NM, Tracy S, Gauntt CJ, Fortmüller U. Molecular detection and identification of enteroviruses using enzymatic amplification and nucleic acid hybridisation. J Clin Microbiol. 1990;28:843–50.
70. Grasso M, Arbustini E, Silini E, Diegoli M, Percivalle E, Ratti G, Bramerio M, Gavazzi A, Vigano M, Milanesi G. Search for Coxsackievirus B3 RNA in idiopathic dilated cardiomyopathy using gene amplification by polymerase chain reaction. Am J Cardiol. 1992;69:658–64.
71. Tracy S, Chapman NM, McManus BM, Pallansch MA, Beck MA, Carstens J. A molecular and serologic evaluation of enteroviral involvement in human myocarditis. J Mol Cell Cardiol. 1990;22:403–14.
72. Schowengerdt K, Ni J, Denfield S, Gajarski RJ, Bowles NE, Rosenthal G, Kearney DL, Price JK, Rogers BB, Schauer GM, Chinnock RE, Towbin JA. Association of parvovirus B19 genome in children with myocarditis and cardiac allograft rejection. Diagnosis using the polymerase chain reaction. Circulation. 1997;96:3549–54.
73. Piiparinen H, Vaheri A. Genotyping of herpes simplex viruses by polymerase chain reaction. Arch Virol. 1991;119:541–8.
74. Weiss SM, Roblin PM, Gaydos CA, Cummings P, Patton DL, Schulhoff N, Shani J, Frankel R, Penney K, Quinn TC, Hammerschlag MR, Schachter J. Failure to detect chlamydia pneumoniae in coronary atheromas of patients undergoing atherectomy. J Infect Dis. 1996;173:957–62.

75. Goodman JL, Jurkovic P, Kramber JM, Johnson RC. Molecular detection of persistent Borrelia burgdorferi in the urine of patients with active Lyme disease. Infect Immunol. 1991;59:269–78.
76. Stanek G, Klein J, Bitnner R, Glogar D. Isolation of Borrelia burgdorferi from the myocardium of a patient with longstanding cardiomyopathy. N Engl J Med. 1990;322:249–52.
77. Nakhleh RE, Copenhaver CM, Werdin K. Lack of evidence for involvement of Epstein-Barr virus in the development of 'Quilty' lesion of transplanted hearts: an in situ hybridization study. J Heart Lung Transplant. 1991;10:504–7.
78. Kandolf R, Hofschneider PH. Molecular cloning of the genome of a cardiotropic coxsackie B3 virus: full-length reverse-transcribed recombinant cDNA generates infectious virus in mammalian cells. Proc Natl Acad Sci U S A. 1985;82:4818–22.
79. Manaresi E, Gallinella G, Zuffi E, Bonvicini F, Zerbini M, Musiani M. Diagnosis and quantitative evaluation of parvovirus B19 infections by real-time PCR in the clinical laboratory. J Med Virol. 2002;67:275–81.
80. Harder TC, Hufnagel M, Zahn K, Beutel K, Schmitt H-J, Ullmann U, Rautenberg P. New LightCycler PCR for rapid and sensitive quantification of parvovirus B19 DNA guides therapeutic decision-making in relapsing infections. J Clin Microbiol. 2001;39:4413–9.
81. Aberham C, Pendl C, Gross P, Zerlauth G, Gessner M. A quantitative, internally controlled real-time PCR assay for the detection of parvovirus B19 DNA. J Virol Methods. 2001;92:183–91.
82. Gruber F, Falkner FG, Dorner F, Hammerle T. Quantitation of viral DNA by real-time PCR applying duplex amplification, internal standardization, and two-color fluorescence detection. Appl Environ Microbiol. 2001;67:2837–9.
83. Yajima T, Knowlton KU. Viral myocarditis: from the perspective of the virus. Circulation. 2009;119:2615–24.
84. Pankuweit S, Moll R, Baantrup U, Portig I, Hufnagel G, Maisch B. Prevalence of the parvovirus B19 genome in endomyocardial biopsy specimens. Hum Pathol. 2003;34:497–500.
85. Kühl U, Pauschinger M, Bock T, Klingel K, Schwimmbeck CP, Seeberg B, Krautwurm L, Poller W, Schultheiss HP, Kandolf R. Parvovirus B19 infection mimicking acute myocardial infarction. Circulation. 2003;108(8):945–50.
86. Bültmann BD, Klingel K, Sotlar K, Bock CT, Baba HA, Sauter M, Kandolf R. Fatal parvovirus B19-associated myocarditis clinically mimicking ischemic heart disease: an endothelial cell-mediated disease. Hum Pathol. 2003;34:92–5.
87. Kuethe F, Lindner J, Matschke K, Wenzel JJ, Norja P, Ploetze K, Schaal S, Kamvissi V, Bornstein SR, Schwanebeck U, Modrow S. Prevalence of parvovirus B19 and human bocavirus DNA in the heart of patients with no evidence of dilated cardiomyopathy or myocarditis. Clin Infect Dis. 2009;49:1660–6.
88. Lotze U, Egerer R, Glück B, Zell R, Sigusch H, Erhardt C, Heim A, Kandolf R, Bock T, Wutzler P, Figulla HR. Low level myocardial parvovirus B19 persistence is a frequent finding in patients with heart disease but unrelated to ongoing myocardial injury. J Med Virol. 2010;82:1449–57.
89. Corcioli F, Zakrzewska K, Rinieri A, Fanci R, Innocenti M, Civinini R, De Giorgi V, Di Lollo S, Azzi A. Tissue persistence of parvovirus B19 genotypes in asymptomatic persons. J Med Virol. 2008;80:2005–11.
90. Schenk T, Enders M, Pollak S, Hahn R, Huzly D. High prevalence of human parvovirus B19 DNA in myocardial autopsy samples from subjects without myocarditis or dilative cardiomyopathy. J Clin Microbiol. 2009;47:106–10.
91. Stewart GC, Lopez-Molina J, Gottumukkala RV, Rosner GF, Anello MS, Hecht JL, Winters GL, Padera RF, Baughman KL, Lipes MA. Myocardial parvovirus B19 persistence: lack of association with clinicopathologic phenotype in adults with heart failure. Circ Heart Fail. 2011;4(1):71–8.
92. Richter J, Quintanilla-Martinez L, Bienemann K, Zeus T, Germing U, Sander O, Kandolf R, Häussinger D, Klingel K. An unusual presentation of a common infection. Infection. 2013;41(2):565–9.

93. Zafrir B, Aviv A, Reichman N, Flatau E. Epstein-Barr virus associated pericarditis and pericardial effusion: case report and diagnostic aspects. Eur J Intern Med. 2005;16:528–30.
94. Roubille F, Gahide G, Moore-Morris T, Granier M, Davy JM, Vernhet H, Piot C. Epstein Barr virus (EBV) and acute myopericarditis in an immunocompetent patient: first demonstrated case and discussion. Intern Med. 2008;47(7):627–9.
95. Chang YL, Parker ME, Nuovo G, Miller JB. Human herpesvirus 6–related fulminant myocarditis and hepatitis in an immunocompetent adult with fatal outcome. Hum Pathol. 2009;40(5):740–5.
96. Leveque N, Boulagnon C, Brasselet C, Lesaffre F, Boutolleau D, Metz D, Fornes P, Andreoletti L. A fatal case of human herpesvirus 6 chronic myocarditis in an immunocompetent adult. J Clin Virol. 2011;52(2):142–5.
97. Bratincsák A, El-Said HG, Bradley JS, Shayan K, Grossfeld PD, Cannavino CR. Fulminant myocarditis associated with pandemic H1N1 influenza A virus in children. J Am Coll Cardiol. 2010;55:928–9.
98. Liao YC, Hsieh YC, Chang WC, Huang JL, Ting CT, Wu TJ. Fulminant myocarditis in an adult with 2009 pandemic influenza A (H1N1 influenza) infection. J Chin Med Assoc. 2011;74(3):130–3.
99. Kuhl U, Pauschinger M, Noutsias M, Seeberg B, Bock T, Lassner D, Poller W, Kandolf R, Schultheiss HP. High prevalence of viral genomes and multiple viral infections in the myocardium of adults with idiopathic left ventricular dysfunction. Circulation. 2005;111:887–93.
100. Kandolf R, Bültmann B, Klingel K, Bock CT. Molecular mechanisms and consequences of cardiac viral infections. Pathologe. 2008;29(Suppl 2):112–7.
101. Moulik M, Breinholt JP, Dreyer WJ, Kearney DL, Price JF, Clunie SK, Moffett BS, Kim JJ, Rossano JW, Jefferies JL, Bowles KR, O'Brian Smith E, Bowles NE, Denfield SW, Towbin JA. Viral endomyocardial infection is an independent predictor and potentially treatable risk factor for graft loss and coronary vasculopathy in pediatric cardiac transplant recipients. J Am Coll Cardiol. 2010;56(7):582–92.
102. Caforio A, Pankuweit S, Charron P, Cooper L, Basso C, Felix S, Fu M, Gimeno R, Helio T, Heymans S, Jahns R, McKenna WJ, Klingel K, Linhart A, Maisch B, Mogensen J, Monserrat L, Pinto Y, Ristic A, Schultheiss HP, Seggewiss H, Tavazzi L, Yilmaz A, Elliott P. Current state of knowledge on aetiology, diagnosis, management and therapy of myocarditis: a position statement of the European Society of Cardiology Working Group on Myocardial and Pericardial Diseases. Eur Heart J. 2013;34(33):2636–48.
103. Richardson P, McKenna W, Bristow M, Maisch B, Mautner B, O'Connell J, Olsen E, Thiene G, Goodwin J, Gyarfas I, Martin I, Nordet P. Report of the 1995 World Health Organization/International Society and Federation of Cardiology Task Force on the definition and classification of cardiomyopathies. Circulation. 1996;93:841–2.
104. Leone O, Veinot JP, Angelini A, Baandrup UT, Basso C, Berry G, Bruneval P, Burke M, Butany J, Calabrese F, d'Amati G, Edwards WD, Fallon JT, Fishbein MC, Gallagher PJ, Halushka MK, McManus B, Pucci A, Rodriguez ER, Saffitz JE, Sheppard MN, Steenbergen C, Stone JR, Tan C, Thiene G, van der Wal AC, Winters GL. 2011 consensus statement on endomyocardial biopsy from the Association for European Cardiovascular Pathology and the Society for Cardiovascular Pathology. Cardiovasc Pathol. 2012;21:245–74.
105. Kindermann I, Barth C, Mahfoud F, Ukena C, Lenski M, Yilmaz A, Klingel K, Kandolf R, Sechtem U, Cooper LT, Bohm M. Update on myocarditis. J Am Coll Cardiol. 2012;59:779–92.
106. Sagar S, Liu PP, Cooper LT. Myocarditis. Lancet. 2012;379:738–47.
107. Dennert R, Crijns HJ, Heymans S. Acute viral myocarditis. Eur Heart J. 2008;29:2073–82.
108. Takeuchi S, Kawada JI, Okuno Y, Horiba K, Suzuki T, Torii Y, Yasuda K, Numaguchi A, Kato T, Takahashi Y, Ito Y. Identification of potential pathogenic viruses in patients with acute myocarditis using next-generation sequencing. J Med Virol. 2018;90(12):1814–21.

Autoimmune Myocarditis: Animal Models

6

Valeria Poli, Katelyn A. Bruno, and DeLisa Fairweather

Abbreviations

BL	C57BL
CFA	Complete Freund's adjuvant
CR	Complement receptor
CVB3	Coxsackievirus B3
DCM	Dilated cardiomyopathy
DCs	Dendritic cells
EAM	Experimental autoimmune myocarditis
IFN	Interferon
Ig	Immunoglobulin
IL	Interleukin
IL-12R	IL-12 receptor
IL-1R	IL-1 receptor
ILC	Innate lymphoid cell
ip	Intraperitoneally
LPS	Lipopolysaccharide

V. Poli
Department of Molecular Biotechnology and Health Sciences, University of Turin, Turin, Italy
e-mail: valeria.poli@unito.it

K. A. Bruno
Department of Cardiovascular Medicine, Mayo Clinic, Jacksonville, FL, USA
e-mail: Bruno.Katelyn@mayo.edu

D. Fairweather (✉)
Department of Cardiovascular Medicine, Mayo Clinic, Jacksonville, FL, USA

Department of Environmental Health Sciences, Johns Hopkins Bloomberg School of Public Health, Baltimore, MD, USA
e-mail: Fairweather.DeLisa@mayo.edu

A. L. P. Caforio (ed.), *Myocarditis*, https://doi.org/10.1007/978-3-030-35276-9_6

MCMV	Murine cytomegalovirus
MHC	Major histocompatibility complex
NK	Natural killer
pi	Post infection
sc	Subcutaneously
sST2	Soluble ST2
TGF	Transforming growth factor
Th	T helper
Tim3	T cell immunoglobulin mucin
TLR	Toll-like receptor
TNF	Tumor necrosis factor
Treg	Regulatory T cells
TSPO	Translocator protein 18 kDa

6.1 Introduction

Autoimmune models of myocarditis were developed in the late 1980s to 1990s by several laboratories [1–4]. Two main approaches were used to induce disease: either complete Freund's adjuvant (CFA) supplemented with *Mycobacterium tuberculosis* or a mildly infectious virus injected with cardiac myosin or other self-peptides [5, 6]. Characterization of the models revealed that both experimental autoimmune myocarditis (EAM) and the viral + self-peptide models involve two phases: acute myocarditis around day 7–14 after inoculation or infection and a second, much less severe phase of myocarditis associated with fibrosis and dilated cardiomyopathy (DCM) starting around day 35–42 (Fig. 6.1) [4, 7]. Originally, murine cytomegalovirus (MCMV) infection and coxsackievirus B3 (CVB3) infection were thought to be viral models of myocarditis that induced autoimmune myocarditis (i.e., the DCM phase) as a secondary feature of the pathogenesis of disease [4, 7–9]. Later it was realized that the viral infection acts like an "adjuvant" to activate the innate immune response and promote autoimmune disease in the presence of self-peptides, similar to the role of CFA in EAM [10–13]. The viral autoimmune myocarditis models produce a disease remarkably similar to EAM and to human disease. Autoantibodies against cardiac myosin are detected early after injection of self-peptide in all three models and persist throughout the time-course of disease [3, 4, 14]. Microarray analysis of hearts with myocarditis compared to undiseased controls revealed that the genes/proteins that lead to remodeling and fibrosis are upregulated during the first phase of disease during acute myocarditis, and that it takes around 3 weeks before fibrosis appears in the heart resulting in dilatation that can be detected using echocardiography (Fig. 6.1) [15–19].

The virus + self-peptide models of myocarditis differ from virus-only (without self-peptide) models in a number of important ways that are reviewed in [10–12]. Briefly, CVB3, for example, replicates in the heart in virus-only models at a much higher level than in the virus + self-peptide models (10^9 vs. 10^4 plaque forming units/PFU, respectively) causing widespread apoptosis and cardiomyocyte necrosis.

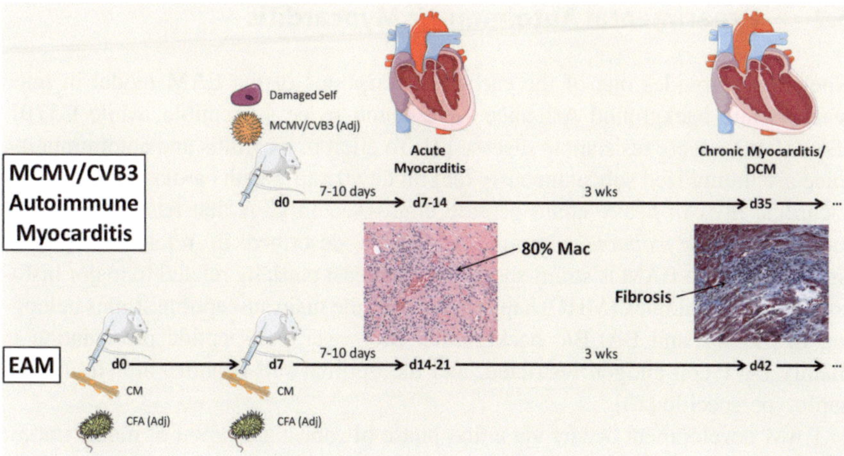

Fig. 6.1 Induction of biphasic myocarditis and DCM in susceptible strains of mice using viruses or CFA as the adjuvant (Adj). Viruses, including murine cytomegalovirus (MCMV) or coxsackievirus B3 (CVB3), are injected intraperitoneally at day 0 (d0) and acute myocarditis develops 7–10 days later followed by chronic myocarditis and DCM around 3 weeks after acute myocarditis in susceptible strains of mice. Similarly, experimental autoimmune myocarditis (EAM) is induced using self-peptide (i.e., purified cardiac myosin (CM)) subcutaneously on day 0 and 7 (d7). Acute myocarditis in the EAM model occurs around day 14–21 and about 3 weeks later disease progresses to DCM. The predominant immune infiltrate during acute myocarditis includes macrophages (Mac), while the chronic myocarditis stage is characterized by fibrosis and dilated cardiomyopathy (DCM). Cartoons licensed for use by https://creativecommons.org/licenses/by/3.0 from the following site https://smart.server.com. The liscencsee does not endorse the authors or their use of the cartoons. Photographs by D. Fairweather

In contrast, no apparent necrosis is observed histologically in the virus + self-peptide models. Another important difference in the two viral models is that acute myocardial inflammation occurs at a very low level (i.e., 5–10% of heart section) in virus-only models in wild type mice but at a high level in virus + self-peptide models (i.e., 30–60% of the heart section). Additionally, most of the mice (60–80%) die during acute myocarditis (day 7–14 after infection) in the virus-only models compared to no mortality in the virus + self-peptide models using wild type mice. As a consequence of the high mortality during acute myocarditis, few mice survive to allow researchers to study the second, chronic myocarditis/DCM stage of disease in the virus-only models.

Several other animal models of autoimmune myocarditis exist like porcine cardiac myosin-induced EAM in mice [20, 21], EAM in the Lewis rat [22, 23], and troponin-induced autoimmune myocarditis [24, 25]. However, this chapter does not present the findings of these models. Additionally, because sex differences in autoimmune myocarditis have predominantly been studied in the CVB3 model but not in other models, the chapter does not summarize findings according to sex for all of the models. The purpose of this chapter is to summarize and compare the key immunological characteristics of the EAM, MCMV, and CVB3 autoimmune myocarditis mouse models in order to assess their usefulness for the clinical setting.

6.2 Experimental Autoimmune Myocarditis

Noel Rose provides one of the earliest descriptions of the EAM model in mice where white background A/J mice were found to be susceptible, while C57BL (BL)/10 mice were resistant to disease [3]. To elicit myocarditis and autoimmunity, mice are immunized subcutaneously (sc) on day 0 and 7 with cardiac myosin or an α-cardiac myosin heavy chain peptide emulsified in CFA that has been supplemented with *Mycobacterium tuberculosis* as described in references [5, 6]. Susceptibility to EAM is strain-specific and at least partially related to major histocompatibility complex (MHC) haplotypes, with the main susceptible strains belonging to the A/J and BALB/c background. Moreover, self-peptide presentation is mainly IA-T cell antigen restricted, and the optimal self-peptides are strain- and haplotype-specific [26].

EAM development occurs via a first phase of robust activation of innate immunity, with strong leukocyte infiltration in the myocardium, required for the ensuing adaptive myocardium-specific immune response mainly driven by antigen-specific T cells and producing significant self-reactive antibody production and immunoglobulin (Ig) deposition on cardiac cells [26]. Interleukin (IL)-1β/IL-1 receptor (IL-1R)/MyD88 signaling are necessary in the EAM model for the development of acute myocarditis as well as remodeling and fibrosis leading to chronic myocarditis and DCM [27, 28]. Additionally, IL-1R signaling on dendritic cells (DCs) leads to the generation of autoreactive $CD4^+$ T cells during EAM [29]. Lipopolysaccharide (LPS) activates TLR4 signaling on antigen presenting cells like mast cells, macrophages, and DCs leading to IL-1β production. Importantly, EAM was found to require innate activation by Toll-like receptor (TLR)3 via dsRNA/poly (I:C), TLR4 via LPS and/or TLR9 via CpG to prime DCs to generate a $CD4^+$ T cell adaptive autoimmune response [30].

In keeping with the knowledge that infection with *M. tuberculosis* induces a protective T helper (Th)17-type immune response in animal models and humans [31, 32], CFA supplemented with *M. tuberculosis* is known to work at least partially by increasing IL-6 levels during EAM [13]. In turn, IL-6 together with IL-1β and IL-23 are known drivers of Th17-type immune responses that play an important role in promoting the progression from myocarditis to DCM during EAM [28, 33, 34]. Indeed, a Th17-type immune response is a key feature of the adaptive immune response in EAM. The biphasic disease course produced by this inoculation regimen results in acute myocarditis (i.e., peak inflammation) developing about 2 weeks after the second injection (i.e., day 7 CFA) from day 14 to 21, followed 3 weeks later by the second phase of chronic inflammation appearing around day 42 associated with fibrosis and the development of DCM (Fig. 6.1). IgG autoantibodies against cardiac myosin are produced in both strains of mice although only white background mice like BALB/c and A/J develop myocarditis/DCM using the EAM model [3]. However, while the central function of autoreactive $CD4^+$ T lymphocytes are well established in the pathogenesis of EAM, the role of autoreactive antibodies against the heart in promoting disease has not been clearly demonstrated even though the production of autoantibodies against cardiac myosin are present during EAM [35–37].

The key role of IL-6 was clearly demonstrated by experiments with IL-6 null mice, which were protected from EAM development correlating with impaired induction of complement C3 expression and heart deposition [38]. Indeed C3 has been shown to be important in promoting EAM by activating mast cells and macrophages that in turn activate autoreactive T and B cells. Depletion of C3 using cobra venom factor reduced EAM by globally decreasing tumor necrosis factor (TNF)α and IL-1β as well as Th1- and Th2-type immune responses and autoantibodies against cardiac myosin [4, 39], and a similar effect was achieved by inhibiting CR1/2 by either blocking monoclonal antibodies or gene deletion [4, 39]. Moreover, IL-6 was shown to increase the number of $CD4^+$ T cells that were autoreactive to cardiac myosin [26]. Inhibition of the transcription factor STAT3, the main mediator of IL-6 signaling and Th17 differentiation, was also found to impair EAM development when administered at the peak of heart inflammation and at the onset of DCM, improving heart function as shown by echocardiography [28, 40]. Moreover, the expression of constitutively active STAT3 was sufficient to elicit the spontaneous development of an immune-mediated form of myocarditis very similar to EAM, increasing Th17 cell responses and IL-6 signaling partially rescued by depletion of CD4+ T cells, recombinant antibody-mediated IL-6 neutralization and complement depletion by cobra venom factor [40].

IL-23 was also shown to promote myocarditis in EAM via the induction of an IL-17A/Th17A-type immune response, and to be particularly relevant for the development of chronic myocarditis/DCM by increasing remodeling and fibrosis [41, 42]. Sustained IL-23 was necessary to maintain a Th17 response during EAM [42] and IL-17A was shown to increase $CD11b^+$ myeloid immune infiltrate in the heart, which represents the main population of heart immune cells during acute myocarditis in EAM [16, 43]. However, $CD11b^+$ immune cells were also found to reduce acute inflammation in EAM by inhibiting Th17 T cell function [43]. IL-17A was also shown to increase IL-1β, IL-6, and TNFα levels in the heart leading to remodeling, fibrosis, and DCM, but not to alter the overall level of inflammation during acute myocarditis in the EAM model [15].

Susceptibility to EAM in A/J and BALB/c mice depends on the production of an IL-4/Th2-type immune response, which in mice is associated with eosinophils, elevated IgG1 autoantibodies against cardiac myosin, and elevated IgE [19, 37]. Inhibiting interferon (IFN)γ using monoclonal antibody or gene inactivation promotes a Th2-type immune response that increases acute myocarditis, pericarditis, and DCM in the EAM model [37, 39, 40, 44]. After inactivation of IFNγ and IL-17A genes, severe Th2-associated eosinophilic myocarditis and heart failure ensued [45]. Inhibiting Th1-driven natural killer (NK) cells also led to the development of eosinophilic myocarditis, fibrosis, DCM, and heart failure [46]. IL-12/STAT4 was found to promote EAM but, paradoxically, IFNγ reduces EAM by preventing progression to the chronic second phase of myocarditis, DCM, and heart failure [39, 40, 44, 47–49].

6.3 Virally-Induced Autoimmune Myocarditis

6.3.1 MCMV-Induced Autoimmune Myocarditis

The first reports of the development of MCMV-induced myocarditis came from two different laboratories in 1986 [1, 2]. Soon thereafter came the description of the production of autoantibodies against cardiac tissue following MCMV infection of mice with myocarditis [14, 50–52]. IgM and IgG autoantibodies against cardiac myosin were detected in the sera of BALB/c and BL mice from day 7 to 100 post infection (pi), with significantly higher autoantibody levels in BALB/c compared to BL mice [4, 50]. The presence of a strong autoantibody response to cardiac myosin after MCMV infection and the presence of autoreactive T cells provide evidence that MCMV-induced myocarditis is an autoimmune disease [4, 53].

Interestingly, purified MCMV is not used to induce the model; but rather MCMV is propagated through salivary glands which are the tissue with the greatest tropism for MCMV [54], homogenized during peak viral replication in the salivary gland, and the supernatant containing damaged salivary gland self-tissue and infectious virus (10^4 PFU) injected intraperitoneally (ip) on day 0 with myocarditis peaking around day 10 pi [4, 10]. Molecular mimicry, or cross-reactivity of a small sequence of viral peptides with those of cardiac myosin or other autoantigens, has been postulated as a mechanism for how MCMV could lead to autoimmune diseases like myocarditis [12, 51, 55, 56]. However, little evidence aside from cross-reactivity has been provided for the theory and a number of inconsistencies exist, which are discussed in references [11, 12]. Although un-researched, it is interesting to speculate whether one reason for how a salivary gland homogenate of MCMV could promote myocarditis could be due to injection of innate proinflammatory cytokines like IL-1β, IL-6, TNFα and/or IL-33 present in the supernatant that become upregulated during MCMV infection of the salivary gland and released by homogenizing the tissue and are able to promote activation of the innate immune response. LPS, which leads directly to IL-1β production by activating TLR4, or TNFα injected ip were shown to increase the severity of MCMV myocarditis and autoantibody levels in BALB/c and BL mice [57]. LPS, TNFα, IL-1β, and IL-33 have been demonstrated to increase CVB3-induced myocarditis [17, 58–60]. IL-33 increases CVB3 myocarditis at least in part by increasing IL-1β [60].

Autoimmune myocarditis induced by MCMV is biphasic in BALB/c mice, with BL mice developing only very low levels of acute myocarditis and being resistant (i.e., not progressing) to chronic myocarditis/DCM [4, 61]. Although BL mice do not develop the chronic phase of myocarditis/DCM, virus can be detected in the heart by PCR indicating that viral persistence is not the driving factor leading to chronic inflammation and dilatation in this model [61]. In contrast, IFN therapy has been found to prevent the progression from myocarditis to DCM in MCMV myocarditis [62]. Treatment of mice with several subtypes of IFNα or IFNβ decreased acute and chronic MCMV-induced myocarditis/DCM and reduced autoantibody levels in BALB/c mice [63–66]. Antiviral drugs used clinically to reduce MCMV infections, ganciclovir and cidofovir, were found to decrease acute and chronic

MCMV-induced myocarditis/DCM provided they were administered during the innate immune response or during acute myocarditis, but had no effect on the chronic stage of disease if administered after the acute myocarditis stage [67]. NK cells and $CD8^+$ T cells are associated with type I (IFNα subtypes, IFNβ) and type II IFN (IFNγ) cytokines that are effective at clearing MCMV infection. $NK1.1^+$ immune cells (i.e., NK cells and/or innate lymphoid cells (ILC)1) were found to reduce MCMV levels in the heart and decrease MCMV-induced autoimmune myocarditis [4, 62, 63, 66, 68]. BALB/c mice with MCMV autoimmune myocarditis develop a dominant IL-4 cytokine response indicative of a Th2-type immune response, while BL mice developed a dominant IFNγ response indicative of a Th1-type immune response [65]. The cardiac inflammatory infiltrate during MCMV myocarditis consists primarily of macrophages and T cells with lower numbers of neutrophils, NK and B cells [61, 66, 69]. Reduction of NK cells or T cells (CD4 or CD8) significantly reduced MCMV-induced myocarditis [4]. Studies examining the role of macrophages in MCMV-induced myocarditis have not been reported in the literature. Additionally, published studies of MCMV-induced autoimmune myocarditis did not report the sex of the mice used in the experiments and no reports describe whether sex differences exist in the pathogenesis of disease.

6.3.2 CVB3-Induced Autoimmune Myocarditis

The first description of the CVB3-induced autoimmune myocarditis model was a comparison of the MCMV and the CVB3 model in a review article in 2001 [4]. The first data paper to describe the model showed that IL-12 receptor (IL-12R)β1 and TLR4 signaling increase myocardial inflammation and cardiac viral replication via IL-1β and IL-18 [70]. Similar to the MCMV-induced autoimmune model, CVB3 from tissue culture is passaged through the heart of mice and supernatant from the tissue homogenate containing self-antigenic heart proteins such as cardiac myosin and a low titer infectious virus (10^3 PFU) are used to induce myocarditis [5, 6, 71]. The heart-passaged CVB3 supernatant induces biphasic myocarditis in susceptible strains of mice like BALB/c and A/J mice with the peak of acute myocarditis around day 10 pi and chronic myocarditis/DCM beginning at day 35 pi, which is similar to the time-course observed for MCMV-induced myocarditis and EAM but shifted by 1 week (Fig. 6.1) [4, 9, 71]. Also similar to the MCMV model, BL mice develop acute myocarditis, but do not progress to chronic inflammation or DCM. IgM and IgG autoantibodies against cardiac myosin are present, similar to the MCMV-myocarditis autoimmune model, from day 7 until day 56 pi following CVB3 infection, and autoantibody levels are higher in BALB/c compared to BL mice [4]. Historically, autoimmune disease was thought to be induced in this model by viral damage that occurs to the heart during acute myocarditis releasing self-antigen (i.e., cardiac myosin) with the second, chronic phase of myocarditis/DCM being considered to be the "autoimmune phase" [4, 8, 9, 12, 71]. However, it is now clear that the second phase of the disease is caused by remodeling genes that are "turned on" during acute myocarditis (day 7–10 pi) and so the biphasic disease process parallels the biphasic autoimmune disease observed in the EAM model. Peak acute myocarditis (day 21) and chronic myocarditis (day 42) are shifted 1 week in the EAM model most likely because of the requirement for a second injection at day 7 in order to induce EAM (Fig. 6.1) [5, 17]. Thus, autoantibodies and autoimmune T cells are present in CVB3 autoimmune myocarditis due to the injection of heart tissue at day 0 that contains cardiac myosin and other self-antigens providing the self-antigen component while injection of the low replicating virus acts as the "adjuvant" similar to CFA in the EAM model (Fig. 6.1) [12].

During the innate immune response to CVB3 infection in this autoimmune model BALB/c mice develop higher TLR4 expression and elevated levels of TNFα, IL-4, IL-1β, and IL-10 in the heart than BL mice [72, 73]. Similar to EAM and as found in the MCMV autoimmune myocarditis model, susceptible mice develop a dominant IL-4/Th2-type immune response during the acute phase of myocarditis [60, 72, 74–76]. A Th2-type immune response is also needed for progression from CVB3 autoimmune myocarditis to DCM [60, 72, 74–76]. A stronger IL-4, Th2-type immune response in BALB/c mice is likely due to the presence of high numbers of mast cells in the spleen of BALB/c mice that are not present in BL mice following CVB3 infection [72]. The innate immune response to CVB3 in the spleen is also characterized by increased expression of genes associated with cholesterol metabolism and steroidogenesis in male BALB/c mice [77]. The androgen receptor and translocator protein 18kDa (TSPO), the rate limiting step with STAR for steroid synthesis, were decreased in CVB3 infected BALB/c male mice compared to females consistent with activation of the receptors. These data suggest that cholesterol metabolism in the spleen may drive the testosterone-mediated increase in inflammation observed following CVB3 infection in male BALB/c mice.

One of the early observations in the CVB3 autoimmune myocarditis model was that myocardial inflammation was far more severe in male BALB/c mice than females [73]. Males had increased expression of TLR4 on mast cells and macrophages and higher levels of CD11b, which is also known as complement receptor (CR)3 or Itgam and is expressed on activated neutrophils, macrophages, granulocytes, mast cells, and some subsets of dendritic cells [73, 78]. During the innate immune response in the spleen 12 h pi and in the heart during acute myocarditis at day 10 pi, mast cells and macrophages from male mice displayed greater expression of TLR4 and reduced expression of the inhibitory receptor T cell immunoglobulin mucin (Tim)3 compared to females [73, 78]. Antibody-mediated inhibition of Tim3 in male mice led to increased myocarditis by enhancing the number of $CR3^+$/$CD11b^+$ immune cells in the heart, increased TLR4 expression on mast cells and macrophages, upregulating the activating receptor CD28 on T cells and globally elevating cardiac cytokines such as TNFα, IL-1β, IL-4, IFNγ, and IL-10 [78]. In contrast, male mice deficient in TLR4 signaling displayed decreased myocarditis, decreased numbers of heart-infiltrating $CR3^+$/$CD11b^+$ macrophages, and enhanced expression of Tim3 on cardiac mast cells and macrophages during acute myocarditis [70, 73]. Complement component C3b binds CR3/CD11b activating mast cells and macrophages [79]. CR1 inhibits C3b levels resulting in reduced mast cell and macrophage activation [80]. Male A/J mice deficient in CR1 developed more severe myocarditis, increased numbers of macrophages in the heart, increased cardiac IL-1β levels, increased fibrosis, DCM, and increased levels of autoantibodies that bind C3 to form immune complexes followed by deposition on the pericardium, leading to severe pericarditis, DCM, and heart failure [81].

The primary infiltrate in the heart of male BALB/c mice with CVB3 myocarditis are cells that express CD11b including macrophages, neutrophils, MCs, and CD11c$^+$ dendritic cells [73]. In contrast, female BALB/c mice have higher levels of T cells, B cells, and regulatory T cells (Treg) than males. Increased cardiac inflammation in males is not due to increased viral replication in the heart, which does not differ between the sexes and is cleared at the same rate in males and females [73, 82]. The dominant cytokine response in the heart of BALB/c males with acute CVB3 myocarditis is elevated IL-1β, IL-18, IL-33, and IFNγ, while females have increased IL-4 [17, 73, 82]. IL-12-induced STAT4 was found to increase TNFα and IFNγ levels in the heart of male BALB/c mice during acute myocarditis and reduce viral replication, but not to alter the overall level of inflammation in the heart [83]. IFNγ was found to contribute to the sex difference in myocarditis—increasing cardiac inflammation in males compared to females; however, not via IL-12/STAT4 suggesting that increased inflammation associated with IFNγ in males could be mediated by TLR4-induced IL-18, which strongly induces IFNγ [9, 82]. TLR4-induced IL-1β, released from mast cells and macrophages, and serpin A3n or α1-antichymotrypsin, which is released from MCs, were also found to be increased by testosterone during acute myocarditis in BALB/c males and to promote remodeling and fibrosis in the heart [17]. Gonadectomy of male BALB/c mice decreased circulating testosterone levels, CVB3 myocarditis, and CD11b$^+$ cells while shifting the immune response to an IL-4, Th2-type immune response with elevated Treg and T cells that express Tim3 and CTLA4 [84]. Macrophages in gonadectomized males expressed more GR1 and Tim3 and less IL-1β than sham operated controls indicating a shift to a more inhibitory or Th2-associated macrophage phenotype [84]. Importantly, all of the genes that promote remodeling in the heart such as IL-1, IL-33, serpin A3n, matrix metalloproteinases, and collagens, for example, were upregulated during acute myocarditis in male but not female mice [17], indicating that the proinflammatory and profibrotic factors that are elevated in the heart of males during acute myocarditis lead to the remodeling that results in chronic myocarditis and DCM several weeks later.

Male BALB/c mice progress from acute CVB3 myocarditis to chronic myocarditis and DCM (for example, ten out of ten male BALB/c mice develop DCM by echocardiography that is normally distributed) while most females do not (for example, two out of ten female BALB/c mice develop mild DCM) [17]. Development of DCM requires a Th2-type immune response which is why white background mice develop DCM while BL do not. If the Th response is skewed to a Th2 response in IFNγ deficient mice, then myocarditis is worse and DCM and pericarditis develop [74]. As stated previously, DCM only occurs in BALB/c mice while BL background mouse strains do not develop DCM regardless of sex. Resistance to DCM can be overcome, however, if BL background mice are forced from a dominant Th1-type to a Th2-type immune response by removal of a key Th1-inducing pathway like TLR3 or TRIF by gene deletion [75, 76]. Male BL mice that are deficient in TLR3 or TRIF (TRIF is a transcription factor downstream of TLR3 and TLR4 signaling) develop significantly more acute CVB3 myocarditis, have increased viral replication in the heart, worse cardiac function, and rapidly progress to DCM [75, 76]. TLR3 deficiency in BL males causes a shift from a dominant IFNγ/Th1-type immune response to an IL-4, IL-13, transforming growth factor (TGF)β1/Th2-type immune response and skewing of macrophages to a more alternatively activated phenotype with higher expression of arginase-1, Ym1, IL-4R, and Tim3 [76]. IL-4 was found to promote the progression to DCM following CVB3 myocarditis in males [76]. BALB/c males deficient in IFNγ also develop more severe acute CVB3 myocarditis and DCM characterized by a shift from an IFNγ/Th1-type immune response to an IL-4/Th2-type immune response with increased IL-4, IL-1β, TGFβ1 and histamine levels in the heart and cardiac MC activation associated with increased remodeling and fibrosis [74]. In contrast, IFNβ rather than IFNγ was reduced in BL mice deficient in TRIF with an increase in the Th2-associated cytokine IL-33 rather than IL-4 and macrophages expressed more Mrc1 [75]. DCM, remodeling/fibrosis, and heart failure were far more severe in male BL mice deficient in TRIF that expressed more IL-33 in the heart and in BL males given recombinant IL-33 compared to BL males deficient in TLR3 [75]. Thus, IL-33 promotes progression to DCM following CVB3 myocarditis in BL mice. IL-33 similarly increases progression to DCM in male BALB/c mice with CVB3 myocarditis by increasing IL-4, IL-1β, and IL-6 levels in the heart and soluble ST2 (sST2) levels in the sera [60]. ST2 is the receptor for IL-33 which can be cleaved to become sST2 or it can be secreted from cells [85]. DCM only occurs in BALB/c mice with CVB3 autoimmune myocarditis from day 35pi onwards, but in mice treated with recombinant IL-33 disease progresses more rapidly so that mice develop heart failure during acute myocarditis [60]. This form of disease is characterized by elevated eosinophils that resemble eosinophilic or giant cell myocarditis. Recently, male BALB/c mice were found to produce higher levels of sST2 in the sera that correlate to elevated cardiac IL-1β levels and inflammation as well as worse cardiac function [86]. Administration of recombinant IL-1β to male BALB/c mice was found to increase CVB3 myocarditis and sST2 levels in the sera [86]. Testosterone increased IL-1β levels in the heart and sST2 levels in the sera [17, 86].

6.4 Translation to Clinical Disease

The test of an experimental animal model is how similar its representation is to human disease. Experimental autoimmune models of myocarditis closely match their human counterparts. For example, autoantibodies against cardiac myosin are associated with myocarditis in autoimmune animal models [3, 4, 50] and in patients with myocarditis and DCM [87–89]. TLRs are important in driving the autoimmune response in T and B cells in animal models and patients [29, 30, 90]. Myocarditis is more severe in male than female mice and clinically more men develop myocarditis than women (sex ratio of 3.5:1 men to women) [82, 86]. Myocarditis occurs primarily in young adults and we recently reported that sera sST2 levels associate with New York Heart Association class III–IV heart failure in men that are 50 years or younger and not in women and in mice with CVB3 autoimmune myocarditis [86]. In mice, sera sST2 levels correlate to cardiac inflammation and cardiac IL-1β levels in male mice with CVB3 myocarditis [86]. Remodeling and fibrosis occur more often in men with myocarditis than women and lead to DCM and heart failure, which has been found also in mouse models [17, 75, 91]. More men develop DCM and heart failure than women requiring a heart transplant, and more male mice progress to DCM than female mice [17, 92]. The presence and severity of cardiac inflammation predicts progression to DCM in patients with myocarditis and in autoimmune animal models of myocarditis [83, 86, 93]. TLR4 was found to be expressed more often in patients with myocarditis and DCM than controls and to correlate to expression of CVB3 capsid protein VP1 in the heart [94, 95]. These clinical studies did not report whether sex differences in TLR4 were present. Similarly, in the CVB3 autoimmune myocarditis model TLR4 increases myocarditis and CVB3 replication in the heart of male BALB/c mice [70]. TLR2 has been found to bind cardiac myosin leading to elevated circulating IL-1β, IL-6, IL-23, and IL-17A levels in men with myocarditis and DCM, but not women [90]. Similarly, IL-1β, IL-6, IL-23, and IL-17A have been demonstrated to promote cardiac remodeling and fibrosis in EAM that leads to DCM [13, 15, 38, 42, 74]. Additionally, IL-17A has been found to promote progression from myocarditis to DCM in patients with myocarditis [90]. Treating mice or patients with type I IFNs have been found to reduce viral load in the heart, reduce acute and chronic myocarditis/DCM and prevent heart failure [62–66, 96]. Likewise, the three complement pathways were found to be expressed at higher levels in the sera of patients with myocarditis that progressed to DCM compared to controls [97]. And elevated complement C3 or reduced CR1/2 was found to promote myocarditis and DCM in EAM and CVB3 autoimmune myocarditis models [35, 38, 81].

Although the study of myocarditis and DCM using animal models has revealed many important aspects of the innate and autoimmune adaptive immune response to self-peptide, many gaps in our understanding still remain. A few of those gaps include the need for a better understanding of sex differences in the pathogenesis of disease, identification of biomarkers to better identify patients at greatest risk of heart failure, and immunological tools that could improve diagnosis of disease which is often missed resulting in unnecessary deaths. Continued research using animal models of autoimmune myocarditis/DCM should be able to provide clinically relevant answers for all of these gaps and many others.

6.5 Summary

Two primary animal models have been developed to study the pathogenesis of autoimmune myocarditis and DCM. The most commonly used model, EAM, involves sc injection of purified cardiac myosin emulsified in CFA on day 0 and 7. Disease progresses from acute myocarditis to chronic myocarditis. The second phase of disease is associated with remodeling, fibrosis, DCM, and heart failure. A similar biphasic disease is induced using mild viral infections plus damaged self-peptide from the salivary gland or heart with either MCMV or CVB3 infection, respectively. The cytokine and immune cell response to either of these models of autoimmune myocarditis are remarkably similar. IL-4/IL-33/Th2-type immune responses have been demonstrated to promote progression from myocarditis to DCM in susceptible white background mice. In contrast, a black background either does not develop disease at all (in EAM) or develops only acute myocarditis but not DCM (viral + self-peptide models). An IL-12/STAT4/IFNγ/Th1-type immune response increases acute myocarditis but prevents progression to DCM in both mouse strains. In contrast, an IL-23/IL-17A/Th17-type immune response has been demonstrated to not alter acute myocarditis but to promote the remodeling and fibrosis that is needed to develop DCM and heart failure. Complement, TLR4/IL-1β and IL-6/STAT3 increase acute myocarditis promote the development of chronic myocarditis/DCM. Future studies are needed to define sex differences in the immune response during myocarditis and DCM for all three autoimmune models of myocarditis and DCM. A better understanding of the pathogenesis of autoimmune disease using animal models is needed in order to develop better diagnostic tools and therapies for a disease with few disease-specific therapeutic options.

References

1. Gang DL, Barrett LV, Wilson EJ, Rubin RH, Medearis DN. Myopericarditis and enhanced dystrophic cardiac calcification in murine cytomegalovirus infection. Am J Pathol. 1986;124(2):207–15.
2. Leung WC, Hata J, Hashimoto K. Murine cytomegalovirus infection model in Balb/c mice--2. Pericarditis with myocardial involvement during virus infection. Tokai J Exp Clin Med. 1986;11(4):303–11.
3. Neumann DA, Lane JR, Wulff SM, Allen GS, LaFond-Walker A, Herskowitz A, et al. In vivo deposition of myosin-specific autoantibodies in the hearts of mice with experimental autoimmune myocarditis. J Immunol. 1992;148(12):3806–13.
4. Fairweather D, Kaya Z, Shellam GR, Lawson CM, Rose NR. From infection to autoimmunity. J Autoimmun. 2001;16(3):175–86.
5. Cihakova D, Sharma RB, Fairweather D, Afanasyeva M, Rose NR. Animal models for autoimmune myocarditis and autoimmune thyroiditis. Methods Mol Med. 2004;102:175–93.
6. Myers JM, Fairweather D, Huber SA, Cunningham MW. Autoimmune myocarditis, valvulitis, and cardiomyopathy. Curr Protoc Immunol. 2013;Chapter 15:Unit 15.4.1–51.
7. Cihakova D, Rose NR. Pathogenesis of myocarditis and dilated cardiomyopathy. Adv Immunol. 2008;99:95–114.
8. Fairweather D, Rose NR. Type 1 diabetes: virus infection or autoimmune disease? Nat Immunol. 2002;3(4):338–40.
9. Fairweather D, Frisancho-Kiss S, Rose NR. Viruses as adjuvants for autoimmunity: evidence from Coxsackievirus-induced myocarditis. Rev Med Virol. 2005;15(1):17–27.
10. Fairweather D, Stafford KA, Sung YK. Update on coxsackievirus B3 myocarditis. Curr Opin Rheumatol. 2012;24(4):401–7.
11. Root-Bernstein R, Fairweather D. Complexities in the relationship between infection and autoimmunity. Curr Allergy Asthma Rep. 2014;14(1):407.

12. Root-Bernstein R, Fairweather D. Unresolved issues in theories of autoimmune disease using myocarditis as a framework. J Theor Biol. 2015;375:101–23.
13. Fontes JA, Barin JG, Talor MV, Stickel N, Schaub J, Rose NR, et al. Complete Freund's adjuvant induces experimental autoimmune myocarditis by enhancing IL-6 production during initiation of the immune response. Immun Inflamm Dis. 2017;5(2):163–76.
14. Bartholomaeus WN, O'Donoghue H, Foti D, Lawson CM, Shellam GR, Reed WD. Multiple autoantibodies following cytomegalovirus infection: virus distribution and specificity of autoantibodies. Immunology. 1988;64(3):397–405.
15. Baldeviano GC, Barin JG, Talor MV, Srinivasan S, Bedja D, Zheng D, et al. Interleukin-17A is dispensable for myocarditis but essential for the progression to dilated cardiomyopathy. Circ Res. 2010;106(10):1646–55.
16. Barin JG, Baldeviano GC, Talor MV, Wu L, Ong S, Quader F, et al. Macrophages participate in IL-17-mediated inflammation. Eur J Immunol. 2012;42(3):726–36.
17. Coronado MJ, Brandt JE, Kim E, Bucek A, Bedja D, Abston ED, et al. Testosterone and interleukin-1beta increase cardiac remodeling during coxsackievirus B3 myocarditis via serpin A 3n. Am J Physiol Heart Circ Physiol. 2012;302(8):H1726–36.
18. Diny NL, Hou X, Barin JG, Chen G, Talor MV, Schaub J, et al. Macrophages and cardiac fibroblasts are the main producers of eotaxins and regulate eosinophil trafficking to the heart. Eur J Immunol. 2016;46(12):2749–60.
19. Diny NL, Baldeviano GC, Talor MV, Barin JG, Ong S, Bedja D, et al. Eosinophil-derived IL-4 drives progression of myocarditis to inflammatory dilated cardiomyopathy. J Exp Med. 2017;214(4):943–57.
20. Wang Y, Afanasyeva M, Hill SL, Rose NR. Characterization of murine autoimmune myocarditis induced by self and foreign cardiac myosin. Autoimmunity. 1999;31(3):151–62.
21. Wang Y, Afanasyeva M, Hill SL, Kaya Z, Rose NR. Nasal administration of cardiac myosin suppresses autoimmune myocarditis in mice. J Am Coll Cardiol. 2000;36(6):1992–9.
22. Galvin JE, Hemric ME, Kosanke SD, Factor SM, Quinn A, Cunningham MW. Induction of myocarditis and valvulitis in Lewis rats by different epitopes of cardiac myosin and its implications in rheumatic carditis. Am J Pathol. 2002;160(1):297–306.
23. Li Y, Heuser JS, Kosanke SD, Hemric M, Cunningham MW. Cryptic epitope identified in rat and human cardiac myosin S2 region induces myocarditis in the Lewis rat. J Immunol. 2004;172(5):3225–34.
24. Goser S, Andrassy M, Buss SJ, Leuschner F, Volz CH, Ottl R, et al. Cardiac troponin I but not cardiac troponin T induces severe autoimmune inflammation in the myocardium. Circulation. 2006;114(16):1693–702.
25. Muller AM, Fischer A, Katus HA, Kaya Z. Mouse models of autoimmune diseases - autoimmune myocarditis. Curr Pharm Des. 2015;21(18):2498–512.
26. Barin JG, Cihakova D. Control of inflammatory heart disease by CD4+ T cells. Ann N Y Acad Sci. 2013;1285:80–96.
27. Marty RR, Dirnhofer S, Mauermann N, Schweikert S, Akira S, Hunziker L, et al. MyD88 signaling controls autoimmune myocarditis induction. Circulation. 2006;113(2):258–65.
28. Blyszczuk P, Kania G, Dieterle T, Marty RR, Valaperti A, Berthonneche C, et al. Myeloid differentiation factor-88/interleukin-1 signaling controls cardiac fibrosis and heart failure progression in inflammatory dilated cardiomyopathy. Circ Res. 2009;105(9):912–20.
29. Eriksson U, Kurrer MO, Sonderegger I, Iezzi G, Tafuri A, Hunziker L, et al. Activation of dendritic cells through the interleukin 1 receptor 1 is critical for the induction of autoimmune myocarditis. J Exp Med. 2003;197(3):323–31.
30. Eriksson U, Ricci R, Hunziker L, Kurrer MO, Oudit GY, Watts TH, et al. Dendritic cell-induced autoimmune heart failure requires cooperation between adaptive and innate immunity. Nat Med. 2003;9(12):1484–90.
31. Li Q, Li J, Tian J, Zhu B, Zhang Y, Yang K, et al. IL-17 and IFN-gamma production in peripheral blood following BCG vaccination and Mycobacterium tuberculosis infection in human. Eur Rev Med Pharmacol Sci. 2012;16(14):2029–36.

32. Shen H, Chen ZW. The crucial roles of Th17-related cytokines/signal pathways in M. tuberculosis infection. Cell Mol Immunol. 2018;15(3):216–25.
33. Eriksson U, Kurrer MO, Schmitz N, Marsch SC, Fontana A, Eugster HP, et al. Interleukin-6-deficient mice resist development of autoimmune myocarditis associated with impaired upregulation of complement C3. Circulation. 2003;107(2):320–5.
34. Camporeale A, Poli V. IL-6, IL-17 and STAT3: a holy trinity in auto-immunity? Front Biosci (Landmark Ed). 2012;17:2306–26.
35. Kaya Z, Afanasyeva M, Wang Y, Dohmen KM, Schlichting J, Tretter T, et al. Contribution of the innate immune system to autoimmune myocarditis: a role for complement. Nat Immunol. 2001;2(8):739–45.
36. Cihakova D, Barin JG, Afanasyeva M, Kimura M, Fairweather D, Berg M, et al. Interleukin-13 protects against experimental autoimmune myocarditis by regulating macrophage differentiation. Am J Pathol. 2008;172(5):1195–208.
37. Afanasyeva M, Wang Y, Kaya Z, Park S, Zilliox MJ, Schofield BH, et al. Experimental autoimmune myocarditis in A/J mice is an interleukin-4-dependent disease with a Th2 phenotype. Am J Pathol. 2001;159(1):193–203.
38. Camporeale A, Marino F, Papageorgiou A, Carai P, Fornero S, Fletcher S, et al. STAT3 activity is necessary and sufficient for the development of immune-mediated myocarditis in mice and promotes progression to dilated cardiomyopathy. EMBO Mol Med. 2013;5(4):572–90.
39. Afanasyeva M, Georgakopoulos D, Fairweather D, Caturegli P, Kass DA, Rose NR. Novel model of constrictive pericarditis associated with autoimmune heart disease in interferon-gamma-knockout mice. Circulation. 2004;110(18):2910–7.
40. Afanasyeva M, Georgakopoulos D, Belardi DF, Bedja D, Fairweather D, Wang Y, et al. Impaired up-regulation of CD25 on CD4+ T cells in IFN-gamma knockout mice is associated with progression of myocarditis to heart failure. Proc Natl Acad Sci U S A. 2005;102(1):180–5.
41. Rangachari M, Mauermann N, Marty RR, Dirnhofer S, Kurrer MO, Komnenovic V, et al. T-bet negatively regulates autoimmune myocarditis by suppressing local production of interleukin 17. J Exp Med. 2006;203(8):2009–19.
42. Wu L, Diny NL, Ong S, Barin JG, Hou X, Rose NR, et al. Pathogenic IL-23 signaling is required to initiate GM-CSF-driven autoimmune myocarditis in mice. Eur J Immunol. 2016;46(3):582–92.
43. Valaperti A, Marty RR, Kania G, Germano D, Mauermann N, Dirnhofer S, et al. CD11b+ monocytes abrogate Th17 CD4+ T cell-mediated experimental autoimmune myocarditis. J Immunol. 2008;180(4):2686–95.
44. Afanasyeva M, Wang Y, Kaya Z, Stafford EA, Dohmen KM, Sadighi Akha AA, et al. Interleukin-12 receptor/STAT4 signaling is required for the development of autoimmune myocarditis in mice by an interferon-gamma-independent pathway. Circulation. 2001;104(25):3145–51.
45. Barin JG, Baldeviano GC, Talor MV, Wu L, Ong S, Fairweather D, et al. Fatal eosinophilic myocarditis develops in the absence of IFN-gamma and IL-17A. J Immunol. 2013;191(8):4038–47.
46. Ong S, Ligons DL, Barin JG, Wu L, Talor MV, Diny N, et al. Natural killer cells limit cardiac inflammation and fibrosis by halting eosinophil infiltration. Am J Pathol. 2015;185(3):847–61.
47. Eriksson U, Kurrer MO, Sebald W, Brombacher F, Kopf M. Dual role of the IL-12/IFN-gamma axis in the development of autoimmune myocarditis: induction by IL-12 and protection by IFN-gamma. J Immunol. 2001;167(9):5464–9.
48. Eriksson U, Kurrer MO, Bingisser R, Eugster HP, Saremaslani P, Follath F, et al. Lethal autoimmune myocarditis in interferon-gamma receptor-deficient mice: enhanced disease severity by impaired inducible nitric oxide synthase induction. Circulation. 2001;103(1):18–21.
49. Barin JG, Talor MV, Baldeviano GC, Kimura M, Rose NR, Cihakova D. Mechanisms of IFNgamma regulation of autoimmune myocarditis. Exp Mol Pathol. 2010;89(2):83–91.
50. O'Donoghue HL, Lawson CM, Reed WD. Autoantibodies to cardiac myosin in mouse cytomegalovirus myocarditis. Immunology. 1990;71(1):20–8.

51. Lawson CM, O'Donoghue HL, Reed WD. Mouse cytomegalovirus infection induces antibodies which cross-react with virus and cardiac myosin: a model for the study of molecular mimicry in the pathogenesis of viral myocarditis. Immunology. 1992;75(3):513–9.
52. Fairweather D, Lawson CM, Chapman AJ, Brown CM, Booth TW, Papadimitriou JM, et al. Wild isolates of murine cytomegalovirus induce myocarditis and antibodies that cross-react with virus and cardiac myosin. Immunology. 1998;94(2):263–70.
53. Lawson CM, O'Donoghue H, Reed WD. The role of T cells in mouse cytomegalovirus myocarditis. Immunology. 1989;67(1):132–4.
54. Gupta M, Shorman M. Cytomegalovirus. Treasure Island: StatPearls; 2019.
55. Root-Bernstein R, Fairweather D. Autoimmune disease: mechanisms. Encyclopedia of life sciences. Chichester: Wiley; 2015. p. 1–7.
56. Hussein HM, Rahal EA. The role of viral infections in the development of autoimmune diseases. Crit Rev Microbiol. 2019;45(4):394–412.
57. Lenzo JC, Fairweather D, Shellam GR, Lawson CM. Immunomodulation of murine cytomegalovirus-induced myocarditis in mice treated with lipopolysaccharide and tumor necrosis factor. Cell Immunol. 2001;213(1):52–61.
58. Lane JR, Neumann DA, Lafond-Walker A, Herskowitz A, Rose NR. LPS promotes CB3-induced myocarditis in resistant B10.A mice. Cell Immunol. 1991;136(1):219–33.
59. Lane JR, Neumann DA, Lafond-Walker A, Herskowitz A, Rose NR. Interleukin 1 or tumor necrosis factor can promote Coxsackie B3-induced myocarditis in resistant B10.A mice. J Exp Med. 1992;175(4):1123–9.
60. Abston ED, Barin JG, Cihakova D, Bucek A, Coronado MJ, Brandt JE, et al. IL-33 independently induces eosinophilic pericarditis and cardiac dilation: ST2 improves cardiac function. Circ Heart Fail. 2012;5(3):366–75.
61. Lenzo JC, Fairweather D, Cull V, Shellam GR, James Lawson CM. Characterisation of murine cytomegalovirus myocarditis: cellular infiltration of the heart and virus persistence. J Mol Cell Cardiol. 2002;34(6):629–40.
62. Cull VS, Bartlett EJ, James CM. Type I interferon gene therapy protects against cytomegalovirus-induced myocarditis. Immunology. 2002;106(3):428–37.
63. Bartlett EJ, Cull VS, Brekalo NL, Lenzo JC, James CM. Synergy of type I interferon-A6 and interferon-B naked DNA immunotherapy for cytomegalovirus infection. Immunol Cell Biol. 2002;80(5):425–35.
64. Cull VS, Broomfield S, Bartlett EJ, Brekalo NL, James CM. Coimmunisation with type I IFN genes enhances protective immunity against cytomegalovirus and myocarditis in gB DNA-vaccinated mice. Gene Ther. 2002;9(20):1369–78.
65. Lenzo JC, Mansfield JP, Sivamoorthy S, Cull VS, James CM. Cytokine expression in murine cytomegalovirus-induced myocarditis: modulation with interferon-alpha therapy. Cell Immunol. 2003;223(1):77–86.
66. Bartlett EJ, Lenzo JC, Sivamoorthy S, Mansfield JP, Cull VS, James CM. Type I IFN-beta gene therapy suppresses cardiac CD8+ T-cell infiltration during autoimmune myocarditis. Immunol Cell Biol. 2004;82(2):119–26.
67. Lenzo JC, Shellam GR, Lawson CM. Ganciclovir and cidofovir treatment of cytomegalovirus-induced myocarditis in mice. Antimicrob Agents Chemother. 2001;45(5):1444–9.
68. Ivanova DL, Denton SL, Fettel KD, Sondgeroth KS, Munoz Gutierrez J, Bangoura B, et al. Innate lymphoid cells in protection, pathology, and adaptive immunity during apicomplexan infection. Front Immunol. 2019;10:196.
69. Ritter JT, Tang-Feldman YJ, Lochhead GR, Estrada M, Lochhead S, Yu C, et al. In vivo characterization of cytokine profiles and viral load during murine cytomegalovirus-induced acute myocarditis. Cardiovasc Pathol. 2010;19(2):83–93.
70. Fairweather D, Yusung S, Frisancho S, Barrett M, Gatewood S, Steele R, et al. IL-12 receptor beta 1 and Toll-like receptor 4 increase IL-1 beta- and IL-18-associated myocarditis and coxsackievirus replication. J Immunol. 2003;170(9):4731–7.
71. Fairweather D, Rose NR. Coxsackievirus-induced myocarditis in mice: a model of autoimmune disease for studying immunotoxicity. Methods. 2007;41(1):118–22.

72. Fairweather D, Frisancho-Kiss S, Gatewood S, Njoku D, Steele R, Barrett M, et al. Mast cells and innate cytokines are associated with susceptibility to autoimmune heart disease following coxsackievirus B3 infection. Autoimmunity. 2004;37(2):131–45.
73. Frisancho-Kiss S, Davis SE, Nyland JF, Frisancho JA, Cihakova D, Barrett MA, et al. Cutting Edge: Cross-regulation by TLR4 and T cell Ig mucin-3 determines sex differences in inflammatory heart disease. J Immunol. 2007;178(11):6710–4.
74. Fairweather D, Frisancho-Kiss S, Yusung SA, Barrett MA, Davis SE, Gatewood SJ, et al. Interferon-gamma protects against chronic viral myocarditis by reducing mast cell degranulation, fibrosis, and the profibrotic cytokines transforming growth factor-beta 1, interleukin-1 beta, and interleukin-4 in the heart. Am J Pathol. 2004;165(6):1883–94.
75. Abston ED, Coronado MJ, Bucek A, Bedja D, Shin J, Kim JB, et al. Th2 regulation of viral myocarditis in mice: different roles for TLR3 versus TRIF in progression to chronic disease. Clin Dev Immunol. 2012;2012:129486.
76. Abston ED, Coronado MJ, Bucek A, Onyimba JA, Brandt JE, Frisancho JA, et al. TLR3 deficiency induces chronic inflammatory cardiomyopathy in resistant mice following coxsackievirus B3 infection: role for IL-4. Am J Physiol Regul Integr Comp Physiol. 2013;304(4):R267–77.
77. Onyimba JA, Coronado MJ, Garton AE, Kim JB, Bucek A, Bedja D, et al. The innate immune response to coxsackievirus B3 predicts progression to cardiovascular disease and heart failure in male mice. Biol Sex Differ. 2011;2:2.
78. Frisancho-Kiss S, Nyland JF, Davis SE, Barrett MA, Gatewood SJ, Njoku DB, et al. Cutting Edge: T cell Ig mucin-3 reduces inflammatory heart disease by increasing CTLA-4 during innate immunity. J Immunol. 2006;176(11):6411–5.
79. Hillion S, Arleevskaya MI, Blanco P, Bordron A, Brooks WH, Cesbron JY, et al. The innate part of the adaptive immune system. Clin Rev Allergy Immunol. 2019. https://doi.org/10.1007/s12016-019-08740-1.
80. Holers VM. Complement receptors and the shaping of the natural antibody repertoire. Springer Semin Immunopathol. 2005;26(4):405–23.
81. Fairweather D, Frisancho-Kiss S, Njoku DB, Nyland JF, Kaya Z, Yusung SA, et al. Complement receptor 1 and 2 deficiency increases coxsackievirus B3-induced myocarditis, dilated cardiomyopathy, and heart failure by increasing macrophages, IL-1beta, and immune complex deposition in the heart. J Immunol. 2006;176(6):3516–24.
82. Frisancho-Kiss S, Nyland JF, Davis SE, Frisancho JA, Barrett MA, Rose NR, et al. Sex differences in coxsackievirus B3-induced myocarditis: IL-12Rbeta1 signaling and IFN-gamma increase inflammation in males independent from STAT4. Brain Res. 2006;1126(1):139–47.
83. Fairweather D, Frisancho-Kiss S, Yusung SA, Barrett MA, Davis SE, Steele RA, et al. IL-12 protects against coxsackievirus B3-induced myocarditis by increasing IFN-gamma and macrophage and neutrophil populations in the heart. J Immunol. 2005;174(1):261–9.
84. Frisancho-Kiss S, Coronado MJ, Frisancho JA, Lau VM, Rose NR, Klein SL, et al. Gonadectomy of male BALB/c mice increases Tim-3(+) alternatively activated M2 macrophages, Tim-3(+) T cells, Th2 cells and Treg in the heart during acute coxsackievirus-induced myocarditis. Brain Behav Immun. 2009;23(5):649–57.
85. Griesenauer B, Paczesny S. The ST2/IL-33 Axis in immune cells during inflammatory diseases. Front Immunol. 2017;8:475.
86. Coronado MJ, Bruno KA, Blauwet LA, Tschope C, Cunningham MW, Pankuweit S, et al. Elevated sera sST2 is associated with heart failure in men ≤50 years old with myocarditis. J Am Heart Assoc. 2019;8(2):e008968.
87. Lauer B, Schannwell M, Kuhl U, Strauer BE, Schultheiss HP. Antimyosin autoantibodies are associated with deterioration of systolic and diastolic left ventricular function in patients with chronic myocarditis. J Am Coll Cardiol. 2000;35(1):11–8.
88. Jahns R, Boivin V, Hein L, Triebel S, Angermann CE, Ertl G, et al. Direct evidence for a beta 1-adrenergic receptor-directed autoimmune attack as a cause of idiopathic dilated cardiomyopathy. J Clin Invest. 2004;113(10):1419–29.
89. Simpson KE, Cunningham MW, Lee CK, Ward K, Tong A, Danon S, et al. Autoimmunity against the heart and cardiac myosin in children with myocarditis. J Card Fail. 2016;22(7):520–8.

90. Myers JM, Cooper LT, Kem DC, Stavrakis S, Kosanke SD, Shevach EM, et al. Cardiac myosin-Th17 responses promote heart failure in human myocarditis. JCI Insight. 2016;1(9):e85851.
91. Cocker MS, Abdel-Aty H, Strohm O, Friedrich MG. Age and gender effects on the extent of myocardial involvement in acute myocarditis: a cardiovascular magnetic resonance study. Heart. 2009;95(23):1925–30.
92. McNamara DM, Starling RC, Cooper LT, Boehmer JP, Mather PJ, Janosko KM, et al. Clinical and demographic predictors of outcomes in recent onset dilated cardiomyopathy: results of the IMAC (intervention in myocarditis and acute cardiomyopathy)-2 study. J Am Coll Cardiol. 2011;58(11):1112–8.
93. Kindermann I, Kindermann M, Kandolf R, Klingel K, Bultmann B, Muller T, et al. Predictors of outcome in patients with suspected myocarditis. Circulation. 2008;118(6):639–48.
94. Satoh M, Nakamura M, Akatsu T, Iwasaka J, Shimoda Y, Segawa I, et al. Expression of Toll-like receptor 4 is associated with enteroviral replication in human myocarditis. Clin Sci (Lond). 2003;104(6):577–84.
95. Satoh M, Nakamura M, Akatsu T, Shimoda Y, Segawa I, Hiramori K. Toll-like receptor 4 is expressed with enteroviral replication in myocardium from patients with dilated cardiomyopathy. Lab Investig. 2004;84(2):173–81.
96. Schultheiss HP, Piper C, Sowade O, Waagstein F, Kapp JF, Wegscheider K, et al. Betaferon in chronic viral cardiomyopathy (BICC) trial: effects of interferon-beta treatment in patients with chronic viral cardiomyopathy. Clin Res Cardiol. 2016;105(9):763–73.
97. Cooper LT Jr, Onuma OK, Sagar S, Oberg AL, Mahoney DW, Asmann YW, et al. Genomic and proteomic analysis of myocarditis and dilated cardiomyopathy. Heart Fail Clin. 2010;6(1):75–85.

Electrocardiography

7

Claudio Rapezzi, Alberto Foà, and Raffaello Ditaranto

7.1 Introduction

Standard ECG is one of the essential diagnostic tools when approaching a patient with suspected myocarditis. Most of the knowledge on ECG correlates was mainly collected in the 1970s when myocarditis was diagnosed on the basis of endomyocardial biopsy (EMB) findings.

Over the last two decades, the introduction and the widespread use of cardiac magnetic resonance (CMR) has broadened the number of myocarditis diagnoses, especially among patients with mild forms who might have not received an EMB according to current indications.

Myocarditis is no longer considered a single entity, but rather a spectrum of clinical conditions, so that diagnostic work-up, risk stratification, and therapeutic management are nowadays challenging. Namely, the 2013 ESC myocarditis Task Force position statement [1] identified four main clinical scenarios of myocarditis presentation: acute coronary syndrome (ACS) like, new onset or worsening heart failure, chronic heart failure, life threatening condition (i.e. life threatening arrhythmias/aborted sudden death, cardiogenic shock, and severely impaired left ventricle [LV] function).

This chapter summarizes the available data on ECG characteristics of acute, subacute, and chronic myocarditis according to clinical presentation as well as the underlying etiology, trying to identify the most relevant findings that may be useful for differential diagnosis and prognostic stratification.

C. Rapezzi (✉) · A. Foà · R. Ditaranto
Cardiology, Department of Experimental Diagnostic and Specialty Medicine, Alma Mater Studiorum-University of Bologna, Bologna, Italy
e-mail: claudio.rapezzi@unibo.it; alberto.foa@gmail.com, alberto.foa2@unibo.it; raffaello.ditaranto@studio.unibo.it

A. L. P. Caforio (ed.), *Myocarditis*, https://doi.org/10.1007/978-3-030-35276-9_7

7.2 The Spectrum of ECG Findings in Different Clinical Presentations of Myocarditis: Prevalence, Electrogenesis, Diagnostic Implications, and Differential Diagnosis

A wide spectrum of ECG findings can be found in acute myocarditis [2] including ST elevation and depression, atrioventricular blocks of different degrees, PR segment depression/elevation, QRS enlargement and bundle branch blocks, abnormal Q waves, reduced QRS voltage, T wave inversion, and QT interval prolongation. Furthermore, atrial and ventricular arrhythmias frequently coexist. Nevertheless, it should be noted that patients affected by acute myocarditis might have a normal ECG [3] at first medical contact and develop only mild abnormalities throughout the disease.

The correct ECG interpretation cannot be detached from clinical background. In this regard the current myocarditis classification [1], differentiated according to clinical presentation, meets this requirement.

7.2.1 Acute Coronary Syndrome (ACS)

Acute myocarditis can mimic an ACS, with chest pain (frequently starting within 1–4 weeks from a respiratory or gastrointestinal infection), ST/T wave changes, increased serum troponin levels (more commonly with prolonged and sustained release over several weeks or months). Global or regional LV or right ventricular (RV) dysfunction can be observed at imaging. Viral lymphocytic myocarditis is presumed to be the most frequent cause, although other infectious/inflammatory causes might be responsible of the scenario. These ECG findings are thought to be the result of a combination of inflammation, necrosis and, in some circumstances, coronary vasospasm as shown in parvovirus B19 (PVB19) endothelial cells infection [4], causing vascular dysfunction.

The presence of ST elevation (STE) in patients with acute myocarditis might lead to a wrong ST-segment elevation myocardial infarction (STEMI) diagnosis. Typically, in these cases, myocarditis causes isolated saddle-shaped (concave) STE without specular repolarization changes, or a widespread STE with diffuse distribution (except for aVR). However, STE topography may be localized and associated with specular ST depression, perfectly mimicking a coronary pattern, and ST may have a convex aspect (Fig. 7.1). A long-lasting STE (paralleling troponin kinetics) with a slow regression of ECG abnormalities is in favor of acute myocarditis. On the other hand, in anterior STEMI due to distal or mid-level left descendent anterior coronary occlusion (after the first diagonal branch), reciprocal ST depression in the inferior leads is absent and ST segment can even be elevated in both anterior and inferior leads [5, 6] (Fig. 7.2). The electrocardiographic ambiguity of myocarditis and ACS contributes to a relevant risk of diagnostic mistakes, even in specialized and ultra-specialized settings [7–12]. This is clearly evident in data coming from different PCI networks [7–13], showing a high frequency (up to 39%) of inappropriate cardiac catheterization laboratories' activation for primary PCI. Within these false positives, a relevant percentage of patients received a diagnosis of acute myocarditis at the end of work-up. Awareness of this phenomenon and of the possible role of acute myocarditis is fundamental to avoid the simplistic

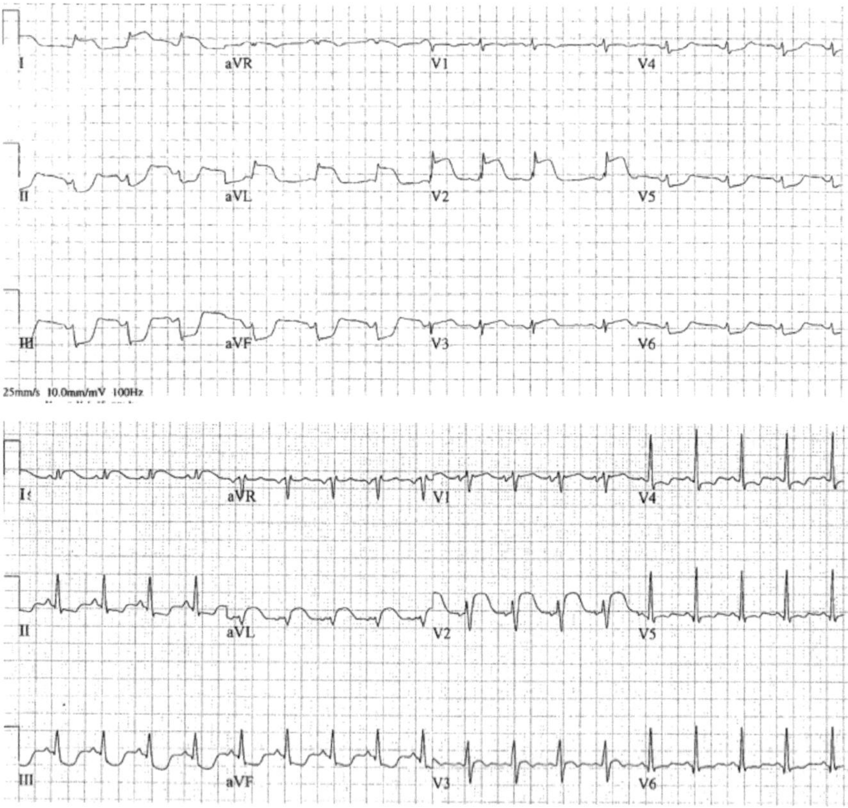

Fig. 7.1 Two cases of acute myocarditis presenting with ST segment elevation in the lateral leads and marked ST depression in the inferior leads. In both cases precordial leads show an "inconsistent" isolated ST elevation in V2

label of ACS with normal coronary arteries or myocardial infarction with nonobstructive coronary arteries (MINOCA) and to address patients towards a tailored diagnostic evaluation and appropriate management.

While in STEMI the value of ECG in localizing the affected regions is unquestionable, ECG is an unreliable tool to localize involved heart muscle sites in acute myocarditis. Different studies [3, 14, 15] tried to assess the ability of ECG to predict inflammatory process localization, using cardiac magnetic resonance as reference for in vivo tissue characterization. All available data showed poor correlation. Particularly, Meléndez-Ramírez et al. [14] found only a moderate agreement for the inferolateral localization of late gadolinium enhancement (LGE) and STE, but not in the other regions. Nucifora et al. [15] reported a topographic agreement between LGE and STE site in 59% of patients presenting with anterolateral STE, in 46% of those with inferolateral STE, with an overall agreement between the LGE and STE site reaching 68%. These data might reflect a limited resolution of CMR, unable to detect small areas of myocardial damage that are, however, large enough to modify the ECG. Conversely, the magnitude of STE and a late ST normalization were found to be significantly and independently related to the extent of LGE, identifying the

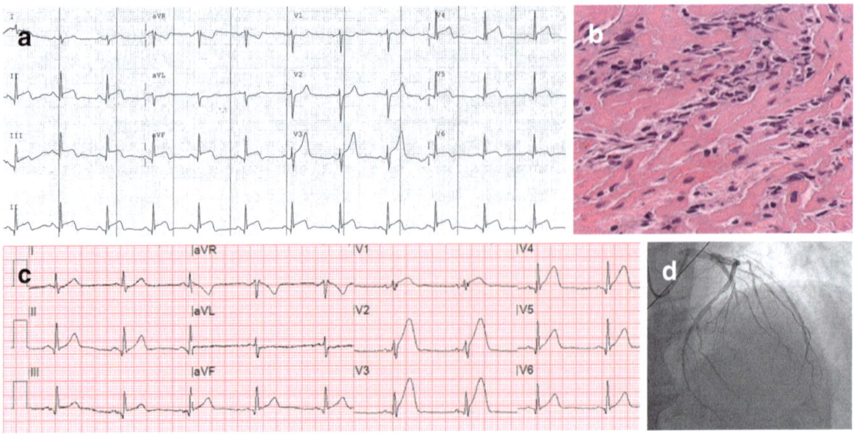

Fig. 7.2 Two examples of anterolateral ST segment elevation without reciprocal changes (**a**) and (**c**). In both cases ST elevation involves both anterior and inferior leads. (**b**) shows the underlying acute myocarditis with lymphocytic infiltrates while in (**d**) a mid-level occlusion of the left anterior descending artery is evident resulting in the same electrocardiographic pattern. *Courtesy of Dr. Ornella Leone and Dr. Nevio Taglieri*

ECG as an easy bedside tool for predicting the extent of myocardial damage, irrespective of its localization.

Another ECG feature that may be helpful in differential diagnosis is the Q wave. More specifically, although Q waves can be present in the acute phase of myocarditis, they may be overlooked due to their brief appearance. In myocardial infarction Q waves persist indefinitely, due to irreversible myocardial injury, whereas Q waves in myocarditis might disappear along with the inflammatory process resolution. Supposedly, Q waves in myocarditis reflect the transiently decreased electrical and mechanical activity in the inflamed regions, not necessarily implying cellular death. This view is in keeping with the clinical observation that LV function improvement usually occurs when Q waves disappear. Myocarditis patients with Q waves generally have more thickened myocardium, more depressed LV function (with an inverse correlation between the number of leads showing Q waves and reduced LV ejection fraction) and a higher incidence of severe complications, e.g. hemodynamic instability and conduction disturbances.

The ECG in acute myocarditis can also simulate acute myocardial infarction without ST segment elevation (NSTEMI). Inverted symmetric T waves, typically short lasting, may be documented, resembling those seen in coronary artery disease. These findings can be isolated or associated with ST depression (or sometimes following ST elevation), localized at two or more contiguous leads or present in all standard leads except for aVR, the so-called diffuse inversion (Fig. 7.3). The reported prevalence of T-waves inversion (TWI) varies from 9% to 48% and likely reflects the underlying myocardial edema and dyshomogeneity of cardiomyocyte repolarization between spared endocardial and diseased epicardial layers. Similarly to STE, concordance between TWI location at ECG leads and affected LV segments at cardiac imaging is poor. Considering any pattern of myocardial edema, De Lazzari et al. [16] reported an overall topographic agreement not exceeding 57%. However, focusing only on areas affected by transmural myocardial edema, the

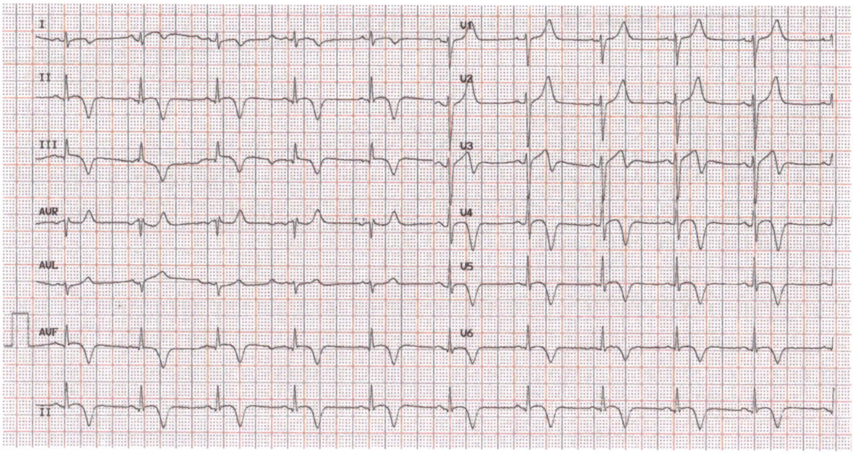

Fig. 7.3 Diffuse (giant) T wave inversion in a young adult with lymphocytic myocarditis presenting with chest pain

overall agreement raised to 88%, supporting the hypothesis that the occurrence of TWI mostly depends on the extent of transmural myocardial edema. Furthermore, the development of TWI was significantly and independently associated with the extent of myocardial LGE. This study underlines the ability of the ECG, once again, to estimate the amount rather than the topography of myocardial damage.

A peculiar form of acute myocarditis often characterized by a pseudo-ACS presentation is represented by *myocarditis associated with pericarditis*, a still widely debated clinical entity. The term indicates a condition in which a typical acute pericarditis is accompanied by echocardiographic or CMR evidence of new onset global/regional wall motion abnormalities or by an abnormal troponin release.

Notably, since the pericardium is electrically silent, the classical ECG changes detected in pericarditis are actually generated in response to myocardial inflammation of subepicardial layers. In this context, the diffuse STE without reciprocal ST segment depression, the PR segment depression and the evolution towards transient negative T waves, reflect an existing "epicarditis." Accordingly, the magnitude of ST-T abnormalities usually correlates with the extent of myocardial inflammation.

Although various and often non-specific ECG patterns may accompany myocarditis associated with pericarditis, ECG may provide useful clues to identify myocardial involvement among patients with pericarditis. Imazio et al. in a series of 234 cases of isolated acute pericarditis compared with 40 cases of myocarditis associated with pericarditis described in the latter a higher prevalence of ST segment elevation (90 vs 70%) and an "atypical" ECG evolution, not necessarily following the classic 4 stages of pericarditis [17]. In fact, among patients with myocarditis associated with pericarditis, negative T waves may be detected before ST segment normalization. Furthermore, patients with myocarditis associated with pericarditis show a much greater arrhythmogenic burden, mainly characterized by ventricular arrhythmias [17]. Lastly, a prolonged QT interval may be detected as an expression of acute myocardial damage.

7.2.2 New Onset or Worsening Heart Failure

The clinical scenario of acute heart failure associated with imaging evidence of a dilated/hypokinetic cardiomyopathy phenotype underlies two possible conditions: sudden onset symptoms in the context of a pre-existing cardiomyopathy or, alternatively, a new onset ventricular dysfunction. In this setting, ECG findings integrated with clinical characteristics, echocardiography, and eventually CMR imaging may address a differential diagnosis.

Acute Phase Indicators The most typical ECG findings in this setting are ST elevation or depression, low QRS voltages, impaired atrioventricular conduction, prolonged QT interval, and transient Q waves. Notably, reduced QRS voltages, frequently associated with sinus tachycardia, suggest extensive myocardial edema (Fig. 7.4) or pericardial effusion. Differently from what observed in an ischemic setting or in chronic cardiomyopathies, this ECG presentation in the acute phase is not necessarily associated with irreversible muscle loss: in fact, as myocardial inflammation resolves, QRS voltages increase paralleling the improvement in ventricular ejection fraction.

Chronic Phase Indicators Conversely, the absence of relevant repolarization abnormalities, an abnormal QRS duration, left bundle brunch block, left ventricular hypertrophy, left atrial enlargement, and atrial fibrillation/flutter suggest a pre-existing condition.

7.2.3 Chronic Heart Failure

ECG findings in patients with inflammatory cardiomyopathy showing a dilated/hypokinetic phenotype are usually indistinguishable from those seen in non-inflammatory dilated cardiomyopathies. In fact, baseline ECG shows signs of chambers' remodeling due to hemodynamic overload, secondary to diastolic and systolic ventricular dysfunction as well as chronic wall inflammation. Specifically, variable degrees of intraventricular delay, left ventricular hypertrophy, left atrial enlargement, and atrial flutter or fibrillation are often detected. Cardiac sarcoidosis and Chagas disease represent two exceptions and are further described in detail.

7.2.4 Life Threatening Conditions

Sudden cardiac death (SCD) occurs in patients with myocarditis and can be the first disease presentation. Ventricular arrhythmias (VA, Fig. 7.5) and bradyarrhythmia (namely, high-degree/complete atrioventricular blocks, Fig. 7.6) can be documented both in acute and chronic myocarditis, with a wide spectrum of clinical presentations, ranging from palpitations to acute heart failure or cardiac arrest. Although they might be present in virtually all forms of myocarditis, the arrhythmogenic burden is generally greater in cases of giant cell myocarditis (GCM) and cardiac sarcoidosis.

The risk of VA is associated with the degree of tissue damage and inflammation. On the other hand, bradyarrhythmias are infrequently encountered, except for some

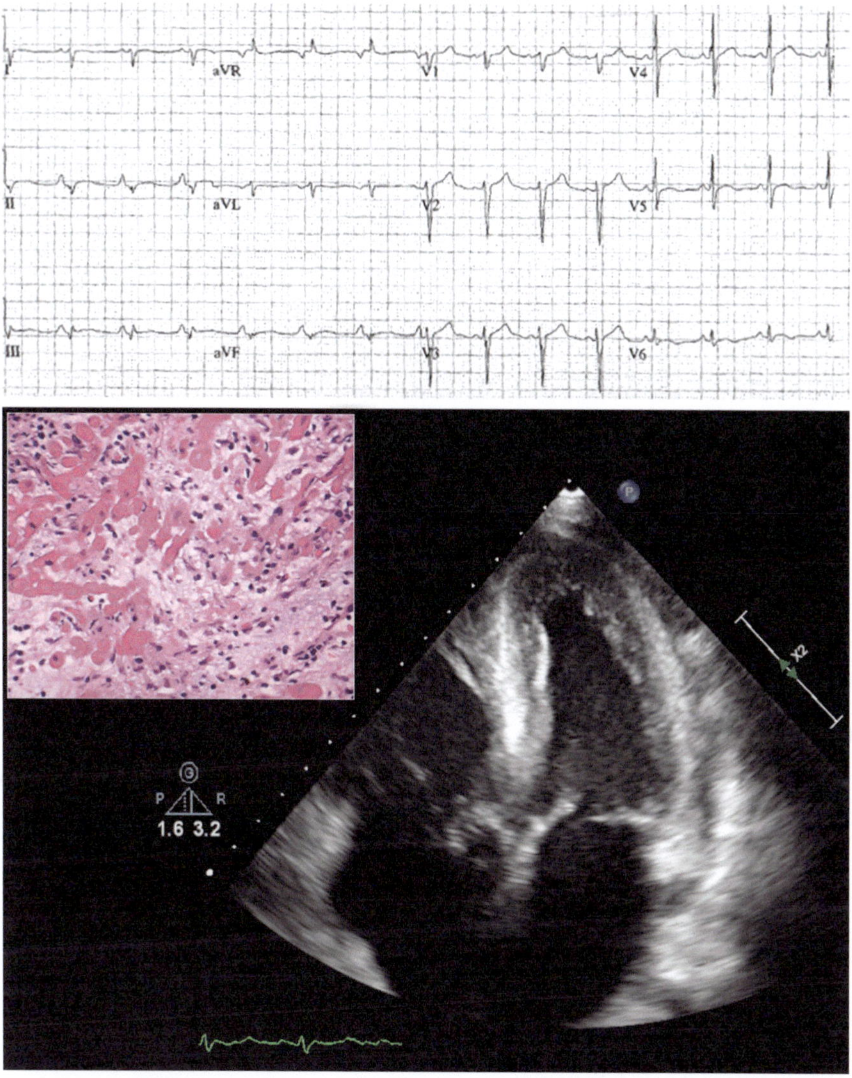

Fig. 7.4 Low QRS voltages in a patient with acute myocarditis admitted for acute heart failure. Echocardiogram showed a thickened and sparkling myocardium. At histology diffuse lymphocytic infiltrates are evident with extensive intramyocardial edema. *Courtesy of Dr. Ornella Leone*

peculiar forms (GCM, Lyme disease, Chagas heart disease, cardiac sarcoidosis). Various pathophysiologic mechanisms have been proposed to explain electrogenesis of VA in the acute setting [18]: electrical instability due to myocyte membrane lysis as a consequence of viral infection or other causes, ischemia from coronary macro/microvascular disease, abnormal calcium handling and ion channel function, and gap junction dysfunction related to abnormal myocardial expression of connexins. In the chronic stage, two kinds of mechanisms can trigger VA: reentry and enhanced

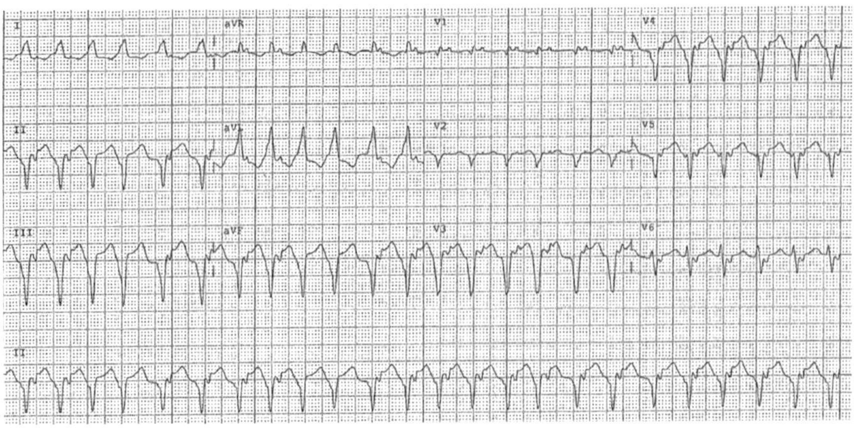

Fig. 7.5 Sustained ventricular tachycardia in a case of acute lymphocytic myocarditis admitted for heart failure

automaticity. Reentry scar-related ventricular tachyarrhythmias, after inflammation resolution, are due to re-entrant circuits secondary to myocardial fibrosis. Indeed, the presence of LGE has been described as a predictor of VA in viral myocarditis. Baseline ECG, in patients with reentry VA, may show signs of the underlying dilated cardiomyopathy, including reduced R wave amplitude, left bundle branch block or intraventricular conduction delay, abnormal Q waves, low voltages and repolarization abnormalities. However, reentry VA can also develop in the setting of normal ECG and/or echocardiogram, especially among young people. Secondly, VA in the chronic setting [18] can be the expression of infection and/or (auto) inflammatory persistence or reactivation: new onset electrical abnormalities may indicate underlying disease activity. Arrhythmic instability with iterative VA, associated with new onset monster ST-T abnormalities, is highly suggestive of acute myocarditis.

7.3 Specific Etiologies

Within the wide spectrum of abnormalities some electrocardiographic patterns may suggest specific etiologies of myocarditis.

Conduction system abnormalities may complicate all forms of myocarditis, as a reflection of inflammatory changes (edema/fibrosis) of the conduction fibers. *Lyme carditis* represents a typical example of intermittent and variable AV block, usually followed by a favorable outcome. A recent review analyzing 45 cases of Lyme carditis showed that 80% of patients presented complete AV block at admission. Atrioventricular blocks may vary in degree and most cases tend to show a benign course with complete regression after adequate antibiotic therapy [19, 20]. However, autoptic cases of sudden cardiac death have been described [21, 22] as well as the possible development of ventricular arrhythmias [23]. Additionally,

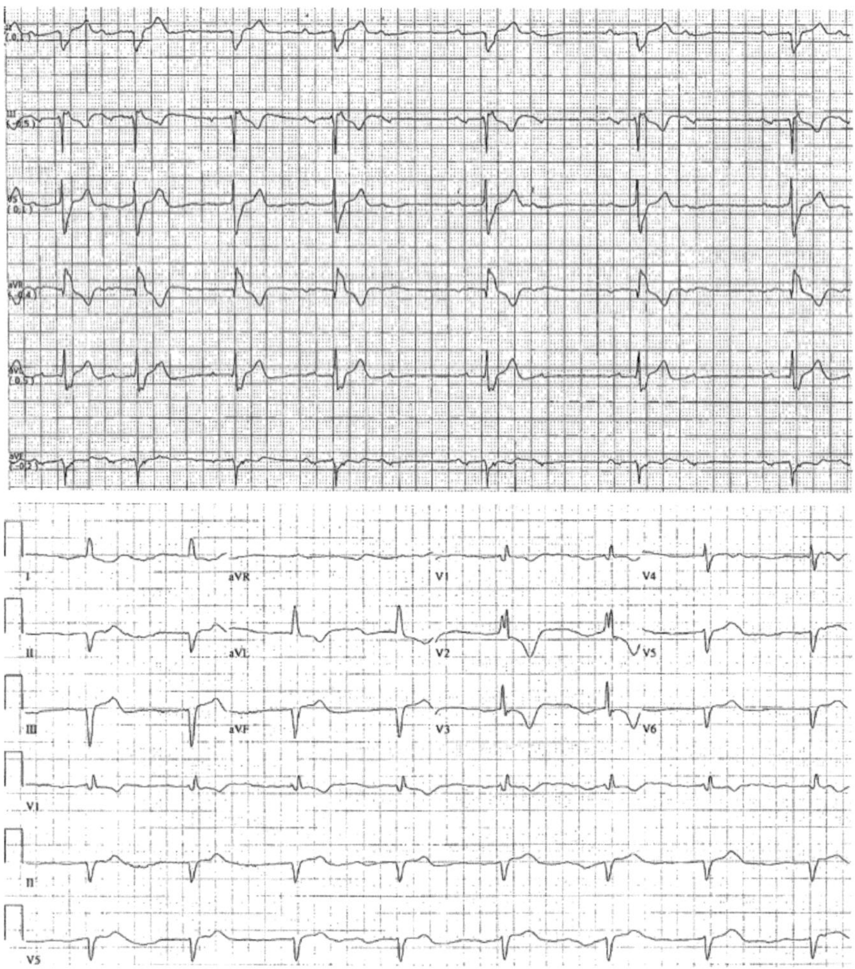

Fig. 7.6 Advanced atrioventricular block in two patients with acute myocarditis. On top a case of 2:1 atrioventricular block; on bottom a case of atrial fibrillation, complete heart block, and escape junctional rhythm

supraventricular arrhythmias may occur; sporadic cases of atrial fibrillation have been described [24, 25].

Although western world countries have established a routine vaccination regimen against diphtheria, this condition is still common in developing countries. Myocardial involvement may be present, often manifesting with conduction disturbances. In fact, a small Indian series of 6 patients with diphtheritic myocarditis revealed the presence of complete heart block, persistent or intermittent, in all cases [26].

ECG is often abnormal in patients with *cardiac sarcoidosis*. In fact, epithelioid granulomas together with the surrounding myocardial fibrosis represent the ideal histopathologic substrate for conduction disturbances. Moreover, the preferential involvement of the basal region of the interventricular septum, spreading to the atrioventricular junction and His-Purkinje system, often results in varying degrees of AV block as well as bundle brunch blocks. Notably, several series have shown that complete heart block is the most common ECG presentation among symptomatic patients, accounting for up to 30% of cases. An interesting observational study on young and middle-aged adults with unexplained II- and III-degree AV block found that in almost 20% the underlying disease was isolated cardiac sarcoidosis and in 4 cases giant cell myocarditis [27]. Moreover, these patients showed a worse outcome (a composite end-point of cardiac death, heart transplantation, ventricular fibrillation, and treated ventricular tachycardia) as compared to idiopathic AV blocks [27]. The typical inflammatory process of sarcoidosis may also trigger tachyarrhythmias. As a result of scar-mediated reentry, ventricular tachycardia, monomorphic rather than polymorphic, is quite common in this scenario. The arrhythmic burden may vary depending on disease activity: an insightful study on 15 patients with cardiac sarcoidosis showed that complete heart block occurred more often during the active phases of the disease, while sustained VT prevailed in the quiescent phase, mostly in patients with a lower ejection fraction [28].

Clinical presentation of *giant cell myocarditis* is mainly characterized by acute heart failure, which may require mechanical circulatory support. In addition, these patients often show electrical instability with a high frequency of ventricular tachycardia both at presentation and during follow-up (Fig. 7.7), with a reported incidence of life-threatening VA reaching 55% at 5 years from symptom onset [29]. Clinical manifestations may also include bradyarrhythmia as shown in a series of 32 patients where high-degree AV block exceeded 30% of cases at presentation [30].

Chagas disease [31], caused by the protozoan parasite Trypanosoma cruzi and endemic in Southern America, is characterized by frequent cardiac involvement, with a predilection for the conduction system and the myocardium. The description of ECG and arrhythmias in Chagas cardiomyopathy by Rosenbaum and his school represents a milestone of history of electrocardiography. The most common initial ECG signs are left anterior fascicular block, left posterior fascicular block, and right bundle branch block. Sinus tachycardia is often present and the heart rate is usually higher than attributable to fever alone. Later findings include sinus node dysfunction, leading to severe bradycardia, high-degree atrioventricular blocks,

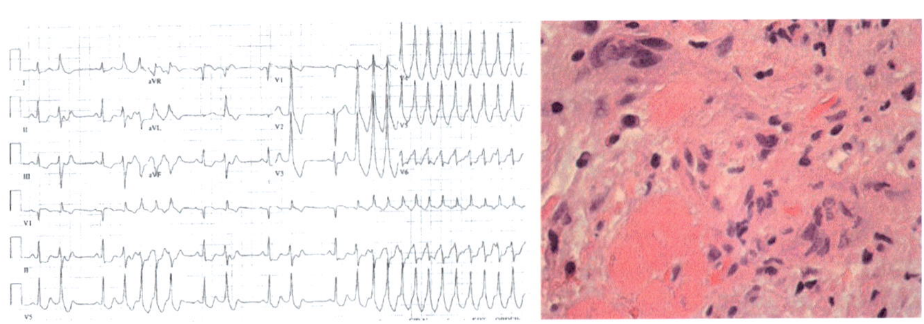

Fig. 7.7 Nonsustained monomorphic ventricular tachycardia in a 33-year-old man with giant cell myocarditis. *Courtesy of Dr. Ornella Leone*

nonsustained or sustained ventricular tachycardia, and low QRS voltages associated with the progression towards a dilated cardiomyopathy with congestive heart failure and apical aneurysms. Rassi et al. [32] developed a score system to predict mortality in Chagas' heart disease and identified, among different ECG variables, nonsustained VT on 24-H Holter monitoring and low QRS voltages as reliable risk factors for long-term mortality.

7.4 Prognostic Implications

Clinical and instrumental presentation of myocarditis is typically extremely heterogeneous. In this setting, the identification of prognostic factors may provide a substantial contribution towards an adequate therapeutic management. The availability and inexpensiveness of ECG have stimulated investigators to look for potential prognostic ECG indicators (Table 7.1).

Ischemic like ST-T abnormalities are common in patients with acute myocarditis, often mimicking acute coronary syndromes. The prognostic role of such ECG findings has been investigated with reassuring results; in fact subjects with this ECG pattern seem to fully recover [33].

Some studies have focused on the clinical and prognostic significance of Q waves. This finding has been detected in more advanced forms of myocarditis with a tendency towards hemodynamic instability and conduction systems

Table 7.1 ECG findings associated with poor outcome

Study	Sample	Follow-up	End point	Identified risk factor
Ukena, Eur Heart J (2011)	186	55 ± 105.1 months	Cardiac death or heart transplantation	QRS ≥ 120 ms QTc ≥ 440 ms (only at univariate analysis)
Morgera, Am Heart J (1992)	42	44 ± 26 months	Mortality	Abnormal QRS complex and LBBB
Lee, Int J Cardiol (2006)	35	In-hospital	Fulminant course	Prolonged QRS duration
Chen, J Card Fail (2018)	193	5.7 years	Death or heart failure	QRS-T angle ≥100°
Ogunbayo, Heart Lung Circ (2019)	31,760	In-hospital	In-hospital mortality and morbidity (cardiogenic shock, cardiac arrest, respiratory and renal failure)	High-degree AV block (Mobitz II second-degree AV block and complete heart block)
Hung, Acta Cardiol Sin (2016)	40	In-hospital	Fulminant course	Prolonged QRS duration Prolonged QTc interval

LBBB left bundle branch block, *AV* atrioventricular

abnormalities; authors have reported a non-significantly higher in-hospital mortality among these patients, with a favorable long-term follow-up [34].

Several series have investigated the prognostic relevance of QRS duration and of QT interval in patients admitted for acute myocarditis. Some studies have shown that both prolonged QRS duration and corrected QT interval are markers of a fulminant course [36, 37]. Ukena and colleagues [35] have partially reinforced this evidence. In a series of 186 cases they identified a prolonged QRS duration (>120 ms) as a risk factor for cardiac death or heart transplantation. Additionally, regression analysis revealed that QTc > 440 ms was associated with a poor outcome but the result was not confirmed at multivariate analysis.

Abnormal QRS complexes, with a particular focus on LBBB, tended to be associated with progression to dilated cardiomyopathy and were shown to be predictors of mortality and sudden cardiac death; in fact, histopathological findings underlying an abnormal QRS complex include left ventricular hypertrophy and myocardial fibrosis, both ideal arrhythmia substrates [38].

Chen et al. proposed the angle between ventricular depolarization and repolarization vectors as a possible outcome indicator [39]. A QRS-T angle ≥100° was found to be a predictor of poor prognosis both in terms of mortality and morbidity, possibly reflecting impaired systolic function [39].

A recent review [40] has investigated the prognostic role of AV conduction disturbances in over 30,000 patients with a diagnosis of myocarditis. The presence of first degree AV block or Mobitz type I second-degree AV block did not affect inpatient outcome. Conversely, patients with high-degree AV block—Mobitz type II or complete heart block—showed a worse outcome with a higher incidence of in-hospital mortality, cardiogenic shock, cardiac arrest, and acute renal failure. After adjustment for patients' baseline characteristics and comorbidities, high-degree AV was found to be independently associated with mortality.

References

1. Caforio AL, et al. Current state of knowledge on aetiology, diagnosis, management, and therapy of myocarditis: a position statement of the European Society of Cardiology Working Group on Myocardial and Pericardial Diseases. Eur Heart J. 2013;34:2636–2648, 2648a-2648d.
2. Jhamnani S, Fuisz A, Lindsay J. The spectrum of electrocardiographic manifestations of acute myocarditis: an expanded understanding. J Electrocardiol. 2014;47:941–7.
3. Di Bella G, et al. Electrocardiographic findings and myocardial damage in acute myocarditis detected by cardiac magnetic resonance. Clin Res Cardiol. 2012;101:617–24.
4. Yilmaz A, et al. Coronary vasospasm as the underlying cause for chest pain in patients with PVB19 myocarditis. Heart. 2008;94:1456–63.
5. Oreto G. Elettrocardiogramma: un mosaico a 12 tessere. Torino: Centro Scientifico Editore; 2009.
6. Taglieri N, et al. Diagnostic performance of standard electrocardiogram for prediction of infarct related artery and site of coronary occlusion in unselected STEMI patients undergoing primary percutaneous coronary intervention. Eur Heart J Acute Cardiovasc Care. 2014;3:326–39.
7. Gu YL, Svilaas T, van der Horst IC, Zijlstra F. Conditions mimicking acute ST-segment elevation myocardial infarction in patients referred for primary percutaneous coronary intervention. Neth Hear J. 2008;16:325–31.

8. Larson DM, et al. "False-positive" cardiac catheterization laboratory activation among patients with suspected ST-segment elevation myocardial infarction. JAMA. 2007;298:2754–60.
9. Perugini E, et al. What is the acceptable rate of false positives for STEMI within a primary PCI network? Insights from a metropolitan system with direct ambulance-based access. Int J Cardiol. 2012;154:356–8.
10. Prasad SB, Richards DA, Sadick N, Ong AT, Kovoor P. Clinical and electrocardiographic correlates of normal coronary angiography in patients referred for primary percutaneous coronary intervention. Am J Cardiol. 2008;102:155–9.
11. Widimsky P, et al. The incidence, treatment strategies and outcomes of acute coronary syndromes in the "reperfusion network" of different hospital types in the Czech Republic: results of the Czech evaluation of acute coronary syndromes in hospitalized patients (CZECH) registry. Int J Cardiol. 2007;119:212–9.
12. Youngquist ST, Shah AP, Niemann JT, Kaji AH, French WJ. A comparison of door-to-balloon times and false-positive activations between emergency department and out-of-hospital activation of the coronary catheterization team. Acad Emerg Med. 2008;15:784–7.
13. McCabe JM, et al. Prevalence and factors associated with false-positive ST-segment elevation myocardial infarction diagnoses at primary percutaneous coronary intervention-capable centers: a report from the Activate-SF registry. Arch Intern Med. 2012;172:864–71.
14. Meléndez-Ramírez G, de Micheli A, Soto ME, Meave-González A, Kimura-Hayama E, Alcántara M, González-Pacheco H. Agreement between ST elevation and late enhancement evaluated by MRI in patients with acute myocarditis. J Electrocardiol. 2014;47:212–8.
15. Nucifora G, et al. Infarct-like acute myocarditis: relation between electrocardiographic findings and myocardial damage as assessed by cardiac magnetic resonance imaging. Clin Cardiol. 2013;36:146–52.
16. De Lazzari M, et al. Relationship between T-wave inversion and transmural myocardial edema as evidenced by cardiac magnetic resonance in patients with clinically suspected acute myocarditis: clinical and prognostic implications. J Electrocardiol. 2016;49:587–95.
17. Imazio M, et al. Myopericarditis versus viral or idiopathic acute pericarditis. Heart. 2008;94:498–501.
18. Peretto G, et al. Arrhythmias in myocarditis: state of the art. Heart Rhythm. 2019;16:793.
19. Fish AE, Pride YB, Pinto DS. Lyme carditis. Infect Dis Clin North Am. 2008;2:275–88, vi.
20. Forrester JD, Mead P. Third-degree heart block associated with lyme carditis: review of published cases. Clin Infect Dis. 2014;59:996–1000.
21. Centers for Disease, Control and Prevention. Three sudden cardiac deaths associated with lyme carditis - United States, November 2012-July 2013. MMWR Morb Mortal Wkly Rep. 2013;62:993–6.
22. Muehlenbachs A, et al. Cardiac tropism of Borrelia burgdorferi: an autopsy study of sudden cardiac death associated with lyme carditis. Am J Pathol. 2016;186:1195–205.
23. Yoon EC, et al. Lyme disease: a case report of a 17-year-old male with fatal lyme carditis. Cardiovasc Pathol. 2015;24:317–21.
24. Kennel PJ, et al. A case of lyme carditis presenting with atrial fibrillation. Case Rep Cardiol. 2018;2018:5265298.
25. Wenger N, Pellaton C, Bruchez P, Schlapfer J. Atrial fibrillation, complete atrioventricular block and escape rhythm with bundle-branch block morphologies: an exceptional presentation of lyme carditis. Int J Cardiol. 2012;160:e12–4.
26. Varghese MJ, et al. Complete heart block due to diphtheritic myocarditis in the present era. Ann Pediatr Cardiol. 2013;6:34–8.
27. Kandolin R, Lehtonen J, Kupari M. Cardiac sarcoidosis and giant cell myocarditis as causes of atrioventricular block in young and middle-aged adults. Circ Arrhythm Electrophysiol. 2011;4:303–9.
28. Banba K, et al. Relationship between arrhythmogenesis and disease activity in cardiac sarcoidosis. Heart Rhythm. 2007;4:1292–9.

29. Ekstrom K, et al. Incidence, risk factors, and outcome of life-threatening ventricular arrhythmias in giant cell myocarditis. Circ Arrhythm Electrophysiol. 2016;9(12):e004559.
30. Kandolin R, et al. Diagnosis, treatment, and outcome of giant-cell myocarditis in the era of combined immunosuppression. Circ Heart Fail. 2013;6:15–22.
31. Perez-Molina JA, Molina I. Chagas disease cardiomyopathy treatment remains a challenge – Authors' reply. Lancet. 2018;391:2209–10.
32. Rassi A Jr, et al. Development and validation of a risk score for predicting death in Chagas' heart disease. N Engl J Med. 2006;355:799–808.
33. Gerzen P, Granath A, Holmgren B, Zetterquist S. Acute myocarditis. A follow-up study. Br Heart J. 1972;34:575–83.
34. Nakashima H, et al. Q wave and non-Q wave myocarditis with special reference to clinical significance. Jpn Heart J. 1998;39:763–74.
35. Ukena C, et al. Prognostic electrocardiographic parameters in patients with suspected myocarditis. Eur J Heart Fail. 2011;13:398–405.
36. Hung Y, et al. The prognostic role of QTc interval in acute myocarditis. Acta Cardiol Sin. 2016;32:223–30.
37. Lee CH, et al. Predictive factors of a fulminant course in acute myocarditis. Int J Cardiol. 2006;109:142–5.
38. Morgera T, et al. Electrocardiography of myocarditis revisited: clinical and prognostic significance of electrocardiographic changes. Am Heart J. 1992;124:455–67.
39. Chen S, et al. Electrocardiographic predictors of morbidity and mortality in patients with acute myocarditis: the importance of QRS-T angle. J Card Fail. 2018;24:3–8.
40. Ogunbayo GO, et al. Outcomes of heart block in myocarditis: a review of 31,760 patients. Heart Lung Circ. 2019;28:272–6.

Standard and Advanced Echocardiography

8

Silvia Gianstefani, Anna Baritussio, Chun-Yan Cheng, Luigi P. Badano, Alida L. P. Caforio, and Sabino Iliceto

8.1 Introduction

The diagnosis of myocarditis is challenging, mainly due to its heterogeneous clinical presentation, and usually requires a high level of suspicion. Clinical scenarios range from mild and atypical cardiac complaints to infarct like chest pain, unexplained heart failure, or signs and symptoms of arrhytmia. Myocarditis' onset can be abrupt and life threatening with cardiogenic shock, or even sudden cardiac death (SCD) or chronic and insidious leading to non-ischemic dilated cardiomyopathy (DCM). It affects patients of all ages, but predominantly young individuals, representing a main cause of SCD in the young and a well-known DCM precursor [1]. Due to the insidious nature of myocarditis, the use of appropriate diagnostic tools at presentation is mandatory, aiming at achieving a correct and early diagnosis and possibly identifying the cause.

The standard clinical approach, including clinical history, patient's examination, ECG, blood test is often non-specific. Therefore, an appropriate use of basic and advanced cardiac imaging modalities becomes fundamental in the diagnostic process. The European Working Group on Myocardial and Pericardial Diseases recommends that all patients with clinically suspected myocarditis should undergo a standard transthoracic echocardiography (TTE) at presentation [1]. TTE should be repeated during hospitalization if there is any worsening of hemodynamics and during follow-up [1].

S. Gianstefani (✉) · A. Baritussio · C.-Y. Cheng · A. L. P. Caforio
Cardiology, Department of Cardiological, Thoracic and Vascular Sciences and Public Health, Padua University, Padova, Italy

Cardioimmunology Outpatient Clinic, Padua University, Padova, Italy
e-mail: silviagians@yahoo.it; anna.baritussio@gmail.com; 073047chengchunyan@163.com; alida.caforio@unipd.it

L. P. Badano · S. Iliceto
Cardiology, Department of Cardiological, Thoracic and Vascular Sciences and Public Health, Padua University, Padova, Italy
e-mail: lpbadano@gmail.com; sabino.iliceto@unipd.it

A. L. P. Caforio (ed.), *Myocarditis*, https://doi.org/10.1007/978-3-030-35276-9_8

8.2 Trans-Thoracic Echocardiography (TTE)

Due to its accessibility, reliability, cost-effectiveness, and unique ability to provide real-time images of the beating heart, TTE represents the first-line imaging technique. It is invaluable in the diagnostic workup, in monitoring the efficacy of treatment, in prognostic stratification, and follow-up.

TTE delivers an excellent assessment of regional wall motion abnormalities, chamber size, wall thickness, left and right ventricular systolic function, diastolic function, valvular function, intracardiac and pulmonary artery pressure estimations, stroke volume, and cardiac output.

It also provides an important contribution to the differential diagnosis as well as to the exclusion of some specific non-inflammatory etiologies such as:

- Ischemic cardiomyopathy,
- Restrictive or hypertrophic cardiomyopathy,
- Valvular heart disease,
- Amyloidosis,
- Congenital heart disease.

TTE findings may range from a completely normal heart (Fig. 8.1a) to severe biventricular dysfunction (Fig. 8.1b). In a patient with clinically suspected myocarditis, it is recommended to investigate the following features:

1. Size and geometry (spherical vs. elliptical) of the ventricles
2. Pattern of contractility (regional or global); left ventricular (LV)/right ventricular (RV) function
3. Associated valvular regurgitation
4. Cardiac output and loading conditions (assessment of filling pressures and pulmonary hypertension)

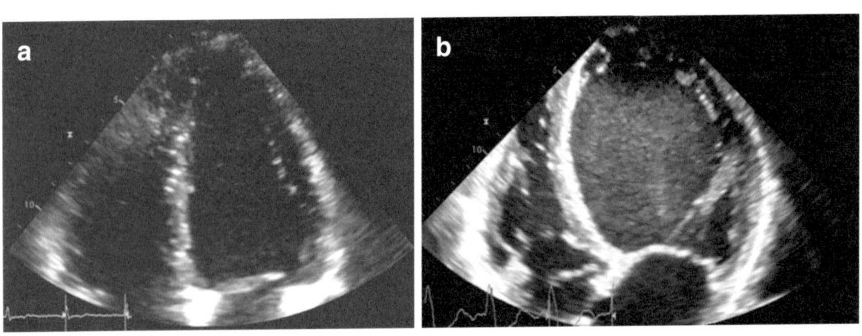

Fig. 8.1 Left ventricular shape in myocarditis. (**a**) magnified four chamber (4ch) view of a normally shaped left ventricle in a patient with active lymphocytic myocarditis and pseudo-infarct presentation. (**b**) magnified 4ch view of a spherically shaped LV in a patient with active lymphocytic myocarditis and heart failure presentation

5. LV wall thickness and changes in image texture
6. Pericardial effusion
7. Presence of intracavity thrombus

8.2.1 Size and Geometry (Spherical Vs. Elliptical) of the Ventricles

Increased sphericity has been described by Mendes et al. [2]. In patients with active myocarditis, they observed that chamber dilatation occurred primarily along the mid-cavity diameter (Fig. 8.1b). Increased left ventricular volume was associated with a more spherical chamber and left ventricular ejection fraction was lower compared to controls. The spherically shaped ventricle may remodel to a more elliptical shape over few months [2].

8.2.2 Pattern of Contractility (Regional or Global); LV/RV Function

In the acute setting, the presence of regional wall motion abnormalities (mainly with a non-coronary distribution) might suggest an inflammatory background. However, wall motion abnormalities may also be indistinguishable from those observed during an acute coronary syndrome [1, 3]. In biopsy-proven myocarditis, it is not uncommon to find LV dilatation and systolic dysfunction (Fig. 8.1b). These features are predictors of poor prognosis as demonstrated by Caforio et al. [3]. The authors showed in a prospective cohort of 174 patients with biopsy-proven myocarditis that biventricular dysfunction at diagnosis was the main predictor of death/transplantation [3].

Right ventricular dysfunction, if present, is in fact a powerful independent predictor of death or cardiac transplantation in myocarditis [3, 4]. It may be related to the inflammatory myocardial disease per se or to pulmonary hypertension due to hemodynamic impairment and LV dysfunction (Figs. 8.2 and 8.3).

8.2.3 Associated Valvular Regurgitation

The most common mechanism of atrio-ventricular valve regurgitation is the lack of leaflets' coaptation mainly due to tethering from dilated ventricles, annular dilatation, and consequent displacement of the papillary muscles (Fig. 8.2). This usually results in a central or posteriorly directed jet (Fig. 8.2 middle panel). The structure and function of both valves should be carefully assessed, in order to identify the mechanism of regurgitation and rule out ventricular dysfunction related to significant valvular disease. It is always useful to record a continuous wave (CW) Doppler of the regurgitant jet, even in the presence of minimal/mild mitral regurgitation (MR), as it provides information about LV systolic function. DP/dT and jet peak

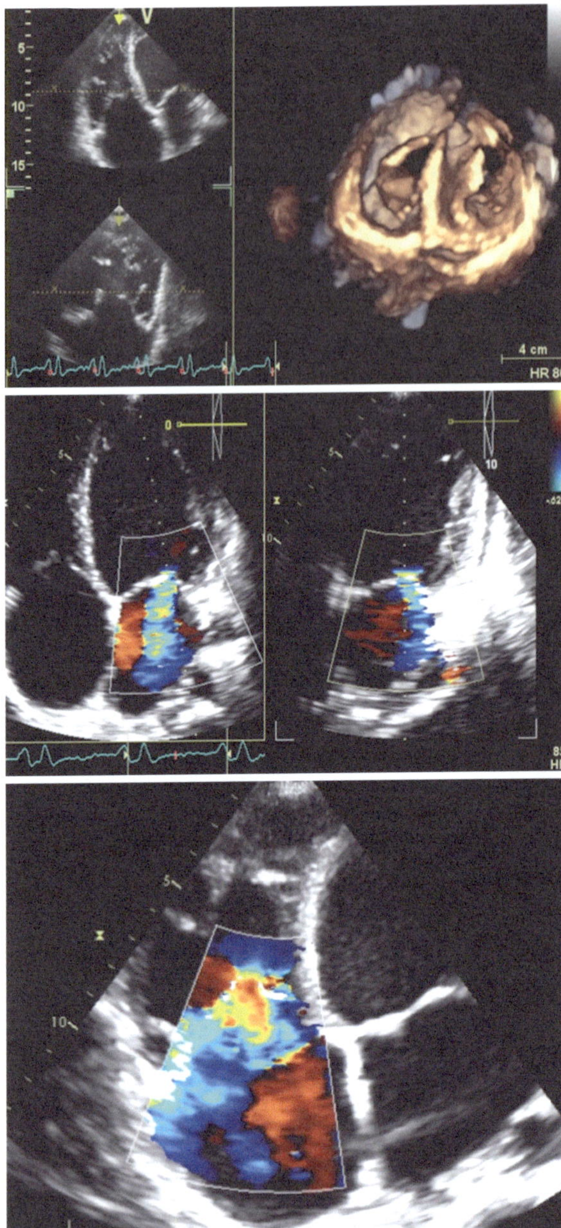

Fig. 8.2 Echo findings in a patient with severe biventricular dysfunction, active lymphocytic myocarditis with heart failure presentation and atrio-ventricular valve regurgitation. Top panel: Right side: 3D rendering of the tricuspid (on the left) and mitral (on the right) valves, seen from the LV apex. Left side: two perpendicular planes cutting across the tricuspid valve annulus at its maximum and minimum diameters, pointing the level (dotted line) and the direction (yellow arrow) of the 3D cropping. Mid panel: Secondary mitral regurgitation (MR), due to lack of leaflets' coaptation by tethering from a dilated left ventricle, dilated mitral valve annulus, and displacement of the papillary muscles. The MR is visualized in two perpendicular planes by the muliplane 3D reconstruction. Bottom panel: 2D color Doppler of torrential secondary tricuspid regurgitation

velocity, as well as indexes of LV contractility are particularly useful in this setting, since the increased preload can lead to an overestimation of LV systolic function. Color flow imaging is used to evaluate direction and area of the regurgitant jet. In order to fully assess the severity of valvular disease, it is important to include in the evaluation CW Doppler spectral intensity, pulmonary vein systolic flow reversal or

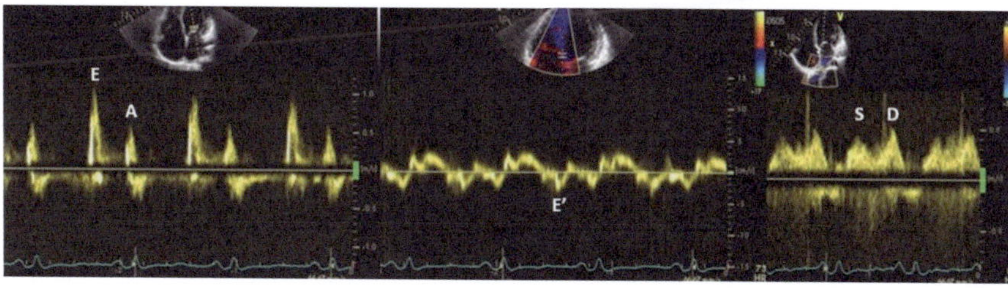

Fig. 8.3 Diastolic dysfunction grade III in same patient from Fig. 8.2 with active lymphocytic myocarditis and heart failure presentation. Left panel: Mitral valve inflow spectral Doppler shows an E/A > 2. Mid panel: left ventricular septal tissue Doppler shows reduction in relaxation (septal e′ < 7 cm/s) and increase in left ventricular end-diastolic pressure (E/e′ = 17). Right panel: Reduced (<1) S/D ratio in pulmonary venous flow is shown (indirect sign of elevated left ventricular filling pressure)

blunting (in the case of MR), presence and size of vena contracta and proximal isovelocity surface area (PISA) for quantifying the regurgitant volume and the effective regurgitant orifice area. MR is an important determinant of progressive ventricular remodelling, symptoms, and outcome [5].

8.2.4 Cardiac Output and Loading Conditions

TTE is a unique tool to assess loading conditions, pulmonary and LV filling pressures. Diastolic dysfunction (frequently related to LV dysfunction) and pulmonary hypertension suggest hemodynamic impairment and increased severity of the disease. Diastolic dysfunction should be assessed with pulsed-wave (PW) Doppler of the mitral valve and tissue Doppler imaging (TDI). If in doubt between a normal or pseudonormal pattern, it is also useful to perform a Valsalva maneuver as the presence of a pseudonormal or restrictive filling pattern has functional and prognostic implications [6] (Fig. 8.3).

Spectral Doppler echocardiography, CW and PW Doppler provide an accurate, non-invasive assessment of cardiovascular hemodynamics. This is obtained by translating changes in wavelengths from red blood cells into velocities displayed against time.

TDI detects lower-velocity, higher-amplitude signals arising from myocardial motion. PW TDI assesses peak myocardial velocities, reflecting the shortening of myocardial fibers in the longitudinal plane and providing a relatively load-independent value. Peak systolic myocardial velocity (positive waveform) is used to measure LV systolic function. The negative waveforms include mitral annular early diastolic velocity (e′), corresponding to early filling, and atrial contraction (a′) measuring the diastolic function. In the most recent guidelines [7] diastolic dysfunction is identified by four variables (with abnormal cut-off values): annular e′ velocity (septal e′ < 7 cm/s, lateral e′ < 10 cm/s), average E/e′ ratio > 14, LA maximum volume index >34 mL/m^2, and peak TR velocity >2.8 m/s (Fig. 8.3).

In a few cases of biopsy-proven myocarditis in which no abnormalities were shown using two-dimensional echocardiography, TDI showed a reduction of myocardial velocities [8, 9] and myocardial velocity gradient in systole and diastole. One of the main TDI limitations is that it reflects only a single point of interest on the myocardium, thus, for example, an akinetic segment of the myocardium may have a near-normal tissue velocity if dragged by a normally contracting segment. This issue is overcome by strain imaging.

8.2.5 LV Wall Thickness and Changes in Image Texture

The presence of thickened and bright myocardial walls in an inflammatory setting should immediately suggest myocardial edema (Fig. 8.4a, b). Myocardial interstitial edema from increased inflammatory cell infiltration and vascular permeability can cause transient LV hypertrophy, increasing hydrostatic pressure within the interstitial space as well as causing ischemic necrosis due to capillary compression. The presence of edema contributes to systolic and diastolic dysfunction, reducing

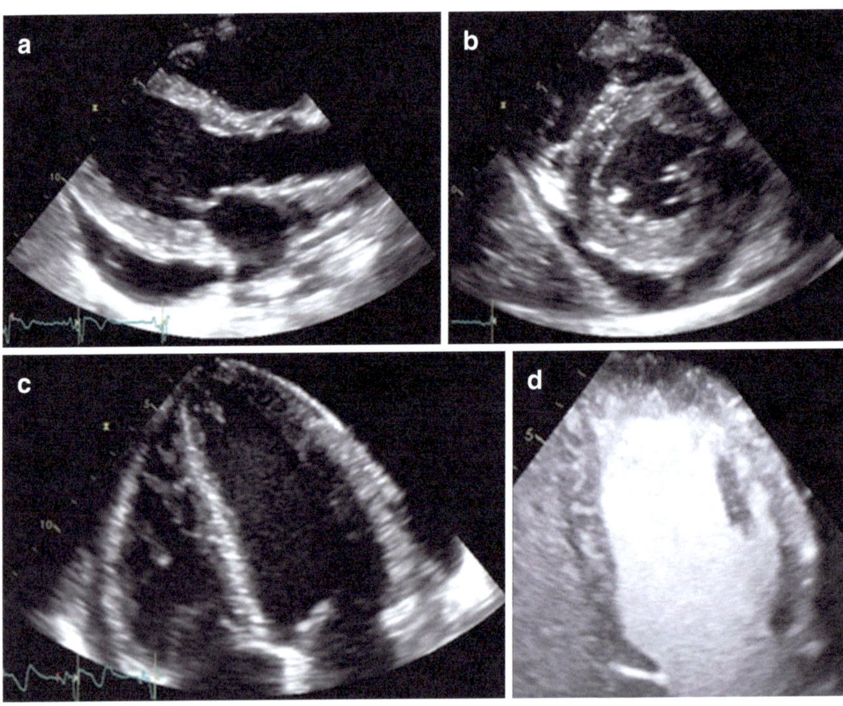

Fig. 8.4 Echo findings in a patient with fulminant lymphocytic myocarditis. (**a**) Parasternal long axis (PLAX), the inferolateral wall is bright and thickened due to edema. There is a moderate pericardial effusion. (**b**) Short axis (SAX) shows thickened inferior and inferolateral walls and mild–moderate pericardial effusion. (**c**) Trabeculated apex, suspicious for an apical thrombus is shown. (**d**) After contrast injection (Sonovue Bracco) no thrombus is confirmed in the left ventricular apex

ventricular compliance and increasing wall stiffness, and, if persistent, can lead to interstitial fibrosis. Moreover, it has an impact on electrical stability and intramyocardial conduction, triggering arrhythmias [10]. Edema and inflammatory changes in the myocardium modify myocardial texture and influence myocardial density and backscatter properties.

Lieback et al. [11] analyzed myocardial texture in 106 patients with biopsy-proven myocarditis and highlighted that the average brightness was appreciably higher in cases of myocarditis than in controls. Some case reports also suggest that increase in brightness, heterogeneity, and contrast may be useful to suspect acute myocarditis [12, 13]. In patients with biopsy-proven myocarditis, it was shown that interventricular septal and left ventricular wall thickness significantly decreased from the acute phase to follow-up and that edema was present in most patients in the acute phase and only in a minority of patients in the convalescent phase [13].

8.2.6 Pericardial Effusion

The extension of myocardial inflammation to the pericardium can lead to pericardial effusion (Fig. 8.4a, b) due to pericarditis. Pericardial effusion, if present, should be described in its location and maximum thickness and quantified as mild (<10 mm), moderate (between 10 and 20 mm), or severe (>20 mm), as recommended for isolated pericarditis. In addition, echocardiographic and Doppler findings suggestive of cardiac tamponade, such as abnormal collapse of the right atrium and ventricle at end-diastole, increased respiratory variation of the Doppler inflow across the atrio-ventricular valves, should be carefully evaluated if pericardial effusion is present. However, most patients with myocarditis have none or minimal pericardial effusion.

8.2.7 Presence of Intracavitary Thrombus

In acute myocarditis, there is an increased risk of thrombus formation because of inflammation, associated hypercoagulable states, and stasis due to LV systolic dysfunction [14]. Viral infections trigger hyperactivity of the immune system increasing tissue factor expression with a procoagulant and thrombogenic action [15]. Characteristic trabeculations may be found if inflammation is substantial. Contrast echocardiography is useful in this setting to confirm or exclude the suspicion of apical or intracavitary thrombus (Fig. 8.4c, d). Contrast agents are composed of microbubbles, containing a high molecular weight gas, which enhances the scattering of the incident ultrasound waves and increase the intensity of the returning signal. Contrast alleviates near-field artifacts and significantly improves the assessment of LV apical anatomy. It is also used to enhance and better delineate LV endocardial borders for an accurate assessment of systolic function in the presence of suboptimal images (when ≥2 consecutive segments cannot be clearly visualized) [16] and to assess LV structural abnormalities.

Advanced applications of echo contrast include the assessment of myocardial perfusion in real time. This has been used in clinically suspected myocarditis revealing, in the affected myocardial segments, attenuated perfusion with delayed contrast replenishment (in comparison with non-affected segments). These findings were attributed to compromised myocardial blood flow and compromised microvascular integrity of the capillary bed in areas of necrosis and inflammation which may result in myocardial perfusion defects, as previously demonstrated by nuclear perfusion imaging [17].

8.3 Specific Settings

Echocardiography may provide additional findings suggestive of specific clinical settings, in particular in fulminant myocarditis, and in endomyocardial fibrosis or eosinophilic myocarditis.

8.3.1 Fulminant Myocarditis

Fulminant myocarditis (FM) is an acute illness, defined by profound and sudden hemodynamic compromise, usually in young previously healthy subjects, characterized by the need of inotropes, vasopressor, and/or mechanical circulatory support (MCS) to maintain the circle. Echocardiography in this acute setting is the first-line, bedside tool for a prompt diagnosis.

The initial presentation could be misleading and difficult to distinguish from ischemic or infiltrative cardiomyopathy. The main echo findings of FM include regional wall motion abnormalities, significant wall thickening with normal LV volume, systolic dysfunction, or severe diastolic dysfunction (restrictive pattern) (Fig. 8.4). Less frequently, it could be characterized by intracardiac thrombus, pericardial effusion, and significant mitral regurgitation [18, 19]. RV dysfunction when present is the strongest predictor of poor outcome [20].

A pathognomonic characteristic of FM is progressive wall thickening, due to edema, in particular of the inferior/inferolateral walls, the septum, and occasionally the papillary muscles, often resulting in a complete normalization at follow-up scans. For its accurate evaluation, it was suggested to measure both end-diastolic septal and inferolateral LV walls thickness at mid-short axis views [19]. Severe edema may sometimes mimic concentric hypertrophy.

Patients with FM often need intra-aortic balloon pump, extracorporeal membrane oxygenator (ECMO), or a ventricular-assist device. Echocardiography has a paramount role in the evaluation of adequacy of circulatory support. It also provides aid with cannula placement, assessment of ventricular filling, and detection of intracardiac thrombus.

Peripheral ECMO is the first-choice device in patients with low cardiac output (CO), non-dilated LV, and absence of MR or pulmonary stasis [21]. During ECMO placement transesophageal echocardiography (TEE) is used to confirm the correct position of the cannulas and should be repeated daily to exclude their displacement, or other complications such as cardiac tamponade or LV distention.

Impella is usually utilized when adequate ventricular unloading is necessary, because of severe LV dilatation, MR, or tricuspid regurgitation (TR). Impella is an axial pump placed across the aortic valve, aspirating blood from the LV to the ascending aorta. Left ventricular ejection fraction (LVEF) >20% and CO >1.5 L/min are required before inserting the device, as it supplies only submaximal flow. In a dilated LV (e.g., end-diastolic volume >120 mL) Impella can work at its highest performance without a risk of malfunction due to wall contact. If the walls are too thickened due to edema, this can interfere with the cannula and lead to arrhythmia, with difficult management and poor device performance. In the post insertion period, TTE helps in optimizing ventricular preload, excluding device displacement, malfunction, or cardiac tamponade.

The use of paracorporeal devices is mandatory in the presence of a very poor CO, LVEF <10%, severe MR, and pulmonary edema, or if biventricular support is needed.

Before apical cannulation, echocardiography is necessary to exclude LV thrombus, atrial septal defects/patent foramen ovale, as they can create a right-to-left shunt, systemic desaturation or paradoxic embolus, as well as aortic regurgitation, as it worsens left ventricular emptying.

In the perioperative assessment, TTE identifies patients who need LV support alone or patients at risk of RV failure. After left ventricular-assist device (LVAD) insertion, an increased flow in the systemic circulation will increase the venous return to the RV which must be capable of increasing its output. RV failure can be unmasked early after LVAD implantation and it may be associated with unfavorable clinical course. In this event the use of a right ventricular-assist device (RVAD) decreases right-sided pressures, reduces liver congestion, and increases LVAD flow. Echocardiographic predictors of RV failure after LVAD implant include: RV wall akinesia, severe RV dilatation, RV fractional area change (FAC) <25%, tricuspid annular plane systolic excursion (TAPSE) <10 mm, RV outflow tract fractional shortening (FS) <20%, and RV–RA pressure drop <30 mmHg [21].

TTE/TEE is also required in the post-operative setting to monitor the device's performance. This is considered effective in the presence of:

- Adequate LV filling and RV function (neutral septum position while a rightward septal shift indicates poor LV offloading)
- Correct orientation of inflow cannula
- Mild or absent MR
- Closed aortic valve
- Detection of unidirectional flow through inflow and outflow cannulae (with color Doppler and PW Doppler)
- No evidence of spontaneous contrast echo into the left atrium (LA) and the LV

In the weaning phase from mechanical devices the role of echocardiography is paramount in assessing LVEF, recommended to be ≥35%, with RV FAC ≥40% and wall thickness reduction to <1.0 cm [19]. Right and left ventricular distention, cardiac tamponade, or intracavity thrombus should also be ruled out.

Felker et al. [20] demonstrated that FM can be distinguished from acute myocarditis (AM) by echo criteria. Typical of AM is a marked left ventricular dilation, normal septal thickness, and reduced ventricular function. Surprisingly in the FM group, there was a high likelihood of ventricular recovery at 6 months compared with those with AM. This was considered related to the fact that in patients with established inflammatory cardiomyopathy and evidence of diffuse fibrosis, even if the presentation is less severe, the degree of recovery may be minor. However, a recent larger series [22] demonstrated that patients with FM have a worse outcome compared with those with non-fulminant presentation (NFM). LVEF in patients with FM was significantly impaired, most of them survived the acute phase with mechanical support; LVEF, despite improvements during hospitalization, remained lower at long-term follow-up. This was supposed to be due to extensive myocardial damage, precluding a complete recovery. In the whole population ($n = 187$), the rate of in-hospital death or heart transplantation was 25.5% versus 0% in FM versus NFM, respectively ($P < 0.0001$). However, in this study only a minority of patients with FM (39 of 55) and of NFM (11/132) had biopsy-proven myocarditis and none had confirmation of infectious etiology by polymerase chain reaction (PCR) on endomyocardial biopsy [22]; this study limitation may account for the discrepancy on outcome in FM compared to the results by Felker et al. [20].

8.3.2 Eosinophilic Myocarditis

Eosinophilic myocarditis (EM) is a rare disease characterized by eosinophilic infiltration of the myocardium caused by several etiologies. These include parasitic infection, chronic eosinophilia as a component of the hypereosinophilic syndrome or of Eosinophilic granulomatosis with polyangiitis (EGPA), formerly Churg–Strauss syndrome, hypersensitivity to drugs and allergens [1]. Loeffler, in 1936, during a postmortem examination first described EM which is also known as Loeffler endocarditis.

The knowledge of typical echocardiographic characteristics of EM is of paramount importance as, if not promptly diagnosed, it often has unfavorable clinical course [23].

EM is characterized by three pathologic stages. In the first *early acute necrotic stage*, usually clinically asymptomatic, the damage occurs on endomyocardial tissue, and the echocardiogram is generally normal.

In a subsequent *thrombotic stage*, intramural thrombi develop on the damaged endocardial tissue, typically obliterating apically one or both ventricles (Fig. 8.5a, b). Accessory findings include regional wall motion abnormalities, hyperdynamic contraction of the spared ventricular walls, pericardial effusion, and increased myocardial wall thickening due to edema. The *fibrotic stage* is characterized by significant intramural fibrosis (Fig. 8.5c). Fibrosis leads to impaired cardiac function and output, progressive scarring of the valvular and subvalvular apparatus, resulting in

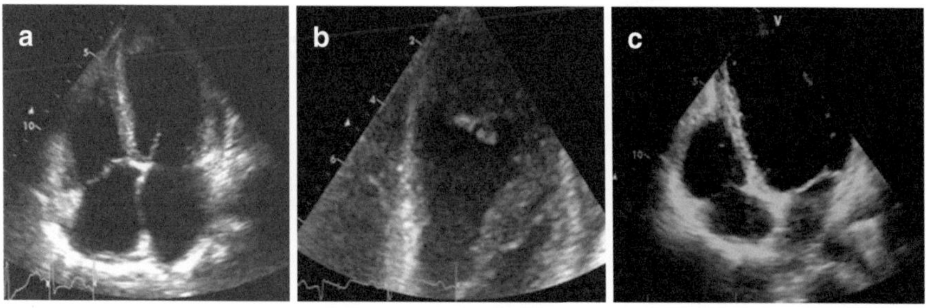

Fig. 8.5 Echo findings in eosinophilic myocarditis. (**a**) Four-chamber view showing apical thrombotic obliteration of the left ventricle. (**b**) Magnified view of the large apical left ventricular thrombus in the same patient. (**c**) Different case of eosinophilic myocarditis in the fibrotic stage. Four-chamber view showing scarring and obliteration of the right ventricular apex

valve damage and regurgitation. Ultimately, these patients may develop restrictive cardiomyopathy characterized by bilateral atrial enlargement with small ventricles and a restrictive pattern on echo-Doppler.

Echocardiography is an invaluable diagnostic tool to assess cardiac damage during the thrombotic and fibrotic stages [24]. In the differential diagnostic process, it is important to differentiate the apical deposition of thrombus from an apical hypertrophic cardiomyopathy, where the apical cavity is obliterated by hypertrophied myocardium. In this setting, the use of echo contrast can help in the diagnosis. After infusion, the contrast fills the LV cavity and it is possible to easily differentiate an intracardiac thrombus (dark filling defect) from a hypertrophied apex.

8.4 Advanced Techniques

8.4.1 3D Echocardiography

Three-dimensional echocardiography (3DE) has dramatically increased the clinical impact of echocardiography in diagnosis, management, and follow-up of heart disease. 3DE allows real-time acquisition of structures that can be seen from any spatial point of view and can be cut across infinite planes in space.

In myocarditis, 3DE has the greatest impact in accurately and reproducibly assessing cardiac chambers' volume and function. It is free from geometrical assumptions, prevents apical foreshortening and errors in imaging positioning. After the acquisition of a 3D full volume, a semi-automated border tracking software is used to create a mathematical cast of the LV throughout the cardiac cycle from which volumes and ejection fraction are extracted, discarding the need for geometric assumptions (Fig. 8.6). These measurements are easy to perform and have been proven to be more accurate than 2D or M-mode calculations when compared to cardiac magnetic resonance imaging (CMR), the current gold standard for mass and volumes. Correlation has been very good despite a tendency for 3DE to

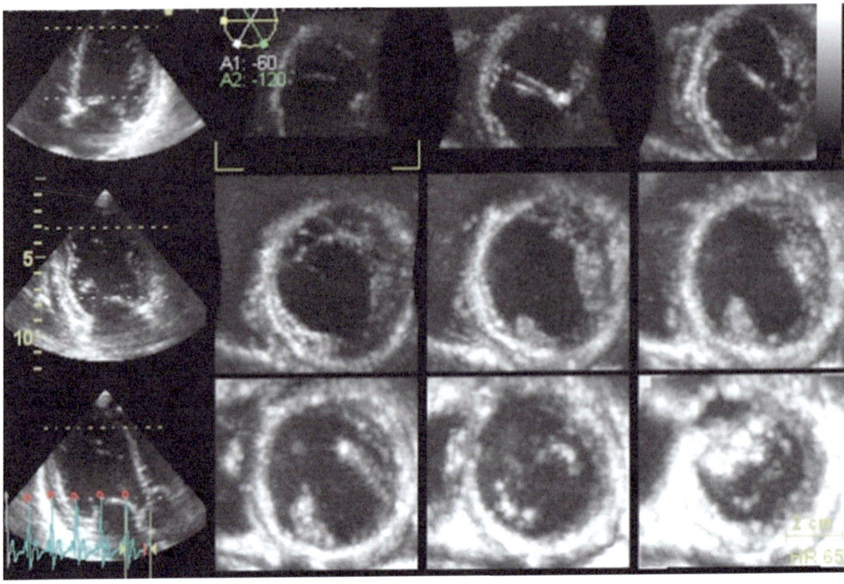

Fig. 8.6 3D echocardiography (3DE) in myocarditis. 3DE tomographic representation of a dilated, remodelled, and trabeculated LV in a patient with active lymphocytic myocarditis, troponin release, and heart failure presentation. The different slices are obtained cutting the left ventricle across multiple parallel short axis planes from apex to base. This specific view is particularly useful to assess regional wall motion abnormalities

slightly underestimate volumes, mainly due to the difference in endocardial border visualization [25].

Due to a better inter-observer, intra-observer, and test–retest variability [26] compared to 2D, 3DE is paramount in the decision-making and follow-up of patients undergoing sequential LVEF and volumes quantification as it provides an accurate and reproducible quantification with the lowest variability [27]. It is also very valuable in risk stratification and in guiding patients' selection for implantable defibrillators or biventricular pacemakers, which requires an accurate and reproducible LVEF [28, 29].

Three-dimensional echocardiography also provides an accurate estimation of RV volumes and RVEF. Three-dimensional echocardiography assessment of RV volumes has less variability than 2D estimation [30, 31]: in 2DE the complicated geometrical structure and asymmetry of the RV significantly limits an accurate quantification of RV size and function. Moreover, this chamber is often not explored enough with the standard RV projections and is subject to misinterpretation with the modified ones. Three-dimensional echocardiography analysis has been shown to be more accurate, compared to CMR, as it does not rely on geometrical assumptions that may be improperly applied to the right ventricle [32, 33]. Normal ranges of RV volumes and RVEF have been established [34] and new and more user-friendly software packages are available to perform quantitative analysis of 3DE data sets of the RV.

Three-dimensional echocardiography has also demonstrated an improved accuracy and reliability compared with 2D techniques in assessment of the left atrium (LA), with excellent correlation with CMR imaging [35, 36]. LA volumes by 3DE have shown an incremental prognostic value for detection of major adverse cardiovascular events and arrhythmias [37, 38].

Three-dimensional echocardiography is also extremely useful for an accurate assessment of mitral and tricuspid structure and function (Fig. 8.2 top and mid panels). The mitral and tricuspid valve and their subvalvular apparatus are optimally imaged by 3DE with an "en face" view of the valves from both LV and LA perspectives. In addition, 3DE provides the most accurate evaluation of the extent of annular dilation and leaflet tenting.

8.4.2 Speckle Tracking

The sensitivity of echocardiography to detect subtle regional wall motion abnormalities and areas of impaired contraction has been expanded by the advent of 2D speckle tracking (ST). This is particularly useful in myocarditis where, often, myocardial dysfunction derived from edema remains undiagnosed with standard TTE. Two-dimensional ST provides a non-invasive, objective, load-independent measurement of cardiac deformation and regional contractility and quantitatively measures myocardial mechanics (strain and strain rate). Strain and strain rate may be calculated by color TDI from Doppler velocity data; however, more recently, these data are obtained by ST strain analysis, directly measuring myocardial strain from tracking natural acoustic markers within the myocardium.

ST analysis is based on the physical principle that ultrasound interaction with the heart muscle generates acoustic markers equally distributed within the myocardium (speckles) that can be tracked in their displacement during the cardiac cycle using dedicated software. The regional deformation of the myocardium can be estimated with the geometric shift of the speckles in all directions within the image plane. Myocardial strain and strain rate can be estimated in longitudinal, radial, and circumferential directions [39] (Fig. 8.7).

LV myocardial fibers are oriented in different directions in space: circumferential fibers in the mid-wall; longitudinal fibers, responsible for most of the longitudinal deformation, forming a right-handed helix in the subendocardium; the subepicardium is instead characterized by a left-handed helix. During systole, the LV walls thicken (radial direction) and the LV shortens in its longitudinal and circumferential dimensions. Myocardial layers are not independent and myocardial fibers work in a complex way. Understanding the complex anatomic distribution of myocardial fibers is key to recognize the potential of ST analysis in imaging mechanical deformation accurately.

Systolic strain describes the regional relative change (deformation) in thickness or length of a myocardial segment in its longitudinal, circumferential, and radial components, in relation to its original dimension. A negative strain refers to a decrease in length, a positive strain to an increase in length, and it is measured in

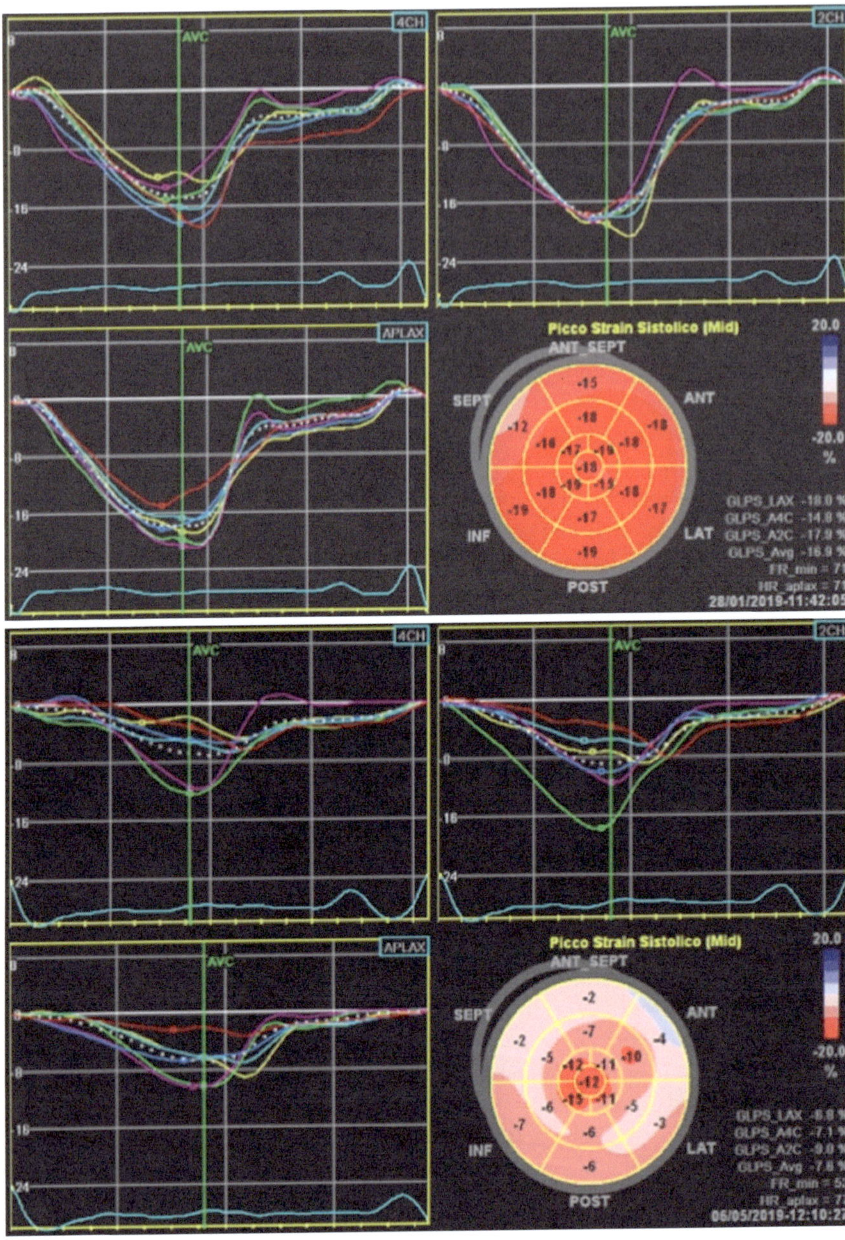

Fig. 8.7 Measurement of global longitudinal strain (GLS) in myocarditis. Longitudinal strain curves from the four chamber, two chamber, and two chamber views generating a bull's eye map of all the analyzed segments. Top panel: nearly normal GLS in a patient with infarct like myocarditis. Bottom panel: severely reduced GLS in the patient with myocarditis and heart failure

percentage. Strain rate is a measure of the velocity (rate) at which the deformation occurs, and it is measured in seconds. Using the 17-segment model of the American Heart Association, systolic segmental strain captures the 3D nature of cardiac contraction and relaxation, providing valuable information on global and segmental myocardial mechanics (Fig. 8.7). Strain imaging is considered a sensitive and reproducible tool to measure alterations in myocardial mechanics and adds value, accuracy, and prognostic information to standard TTE [40–42]. In different clinical settings (cardiomyopathy, coronary artery disease), a decreased systolic strain has been shown to detect subclinical LV dysfunction before changes in LVEF [43].

During myocarditis, the inflammatory infiltration is mainly located in the epicardial layer and often does not result in significant impairment of regional wall motion or LVEF. This happens because the whole myocardial thickening is mainly driven by the endocardium. However, a patchy edema distribution can be detected by global longitudinal strain (GLS) which has the capability to point out subtle changes or mild myocardial damage. There is a growing body of evidence that strain and strain rate measurements in patients with myocarditis are helpful in diagnosis. GLS (obtained with echocardiography) is reduced in areas of edema or fibrosis detected by CMR and decreased strain and strain rate might have prognostic implications, in particular as predictors of LV heart failure development [44–47].

Hsiao et al. [44] showed in clinically suspected myocarditis patients with decreased or normal LVEF that GLS, circumferential strain and strain rate predict major clinical events. Patients with clinically suspected acute myocarditis had decreased longitudinal and circumferential strain and strain rate values compared with healthy controls. The possibility of deterioration or event-free survival was consistently related to strain measures. Escher et al. [45] demonstrated, in a cohort of biopsy-proven myocarditis, that affected patients had a reduction in GLS and strain rate. At follow-up, these parameters were significantly lower in patients with inflammation than in patients without and correlated with the severity of lymphocytic infiltrates, predictors of poor outcome. The study suggests that strain echocardiography may be useful to identify longitudinal myocardial dysfunction derived from infiltration. Di Bella et al. [46] analyzed a group of patients with clinically suspected myocarditis who underwent echocardiography and CMR. They observed a significant GLS reduction in the myocarditis group, compared to controls, whereas no difference was found concerning circumferential and radial strain. Moreover, segments with late gadolinium enhancement (LGE) on CMR showed a significantly lower GLS in comparison with segments without LGE. In patients with acute myocarditis and preserved LVEF, there was a diffuse impairment of LV longitudinal strain whereas circumferential strain (CS) was only impaired in areas of subepicardial damage. They suggested that impaired GLS and CS, in the absence of wall motion abnormalities, may represent a useful diagnostic finding to support the diagnosis of acute myocarditis. Løgstrup et al. [47] evaluated the usefulness of 2D ST echocardiography (STE) in the diagnostic process of acute myocarditis. A significant correlation was found between GLS and presence of edema on CMR, suggesting that GLS could detect myocardial injury better than standard

2DE, especially in patients with preserved LVEF. They demonstrated that edema was mainly located in the infero-posterolateral segments of the left ventricle (on CMR) and this was also visualized by the predominance of an infero-posterolateral segmental strain decrease by 2D STE. They also observed alterations in GLS reflecting the patchy distribution of myocardial edema and LGE on CMR.

Three-dimensional speckle tracking (3DST) has the capability to further improve these promising results. Due to LV fibers' complex orientation and simultaneous contraction in different directions, the LV mechanics is a 3D phenomenon; therefore, its accurate assessment requires a 3D method. This new tool has been implemented for measuring 3D strain, overcoming the limitations of 2DSTE including its time-consuming acquisition and post-processing. The speckles can be followed in the three dimensions and the entire LV data set can be acquired in full-volume mode from only one apical window with a reduction of processing time. However, at present 3D ST is still a research tool, not yet validated for clinical use: normal values are not standardized and it is not interchangeable with 2D ST [48]. As 2D ST, 3D ST is dependent on good echo windows for accurate measurements.

In conclusion, TTE is an invaluable tool in diagnosis, follow-up, and prognostic assessment in patients with myocarditis. Advanced echocardiography enhances its capabilities and represents a promising research field.

References

1. Caforio AL, Pankuweit S, Arbustini E, Basso C, Gimeno-Blanes J, Felix SB, Fu M, Heliö T, Heymans S, Jahns R, Klingel K, Linhart A, Maisch B, McKenna W, Mogensen J, Pinto YM, Ristic A, Schultheiss HP, Seggewiss H, Tavazzi L, Thiene G, Yilmaz A, Charron P, Elliott PM, European Society of Cardiology Working Group on Myocardial and Pericardial Diseases. Current state of knowledge on aetiology, diagnosis, management, and therapy of myocarditis: a position statement of the European Society of Cardiology Working Group on Myocardial and Pericardial Diseases. Eur Heart J. 2013;34(33):2636–48, 2648a–d.
2. Mendes LA, Picard MH, Dec GW, Hartz VL, Palacios IF, Davidoff R. Ventricular remodelling in active myocarditis. Myocarditis treatment trial. Am Heart J. 1999;138:303–8.
3. Caforio AL, Calabrese F, Angelini A, Tona F, Vinci A, Bottaro S, Ramondo A, Carturan E, Iliceto S, Thiene G, Daliento L. A prospective study of biopsy-proven myocarditis: prognostic relevance of clinical and aetiopathogenetic features at diagnosis. Eur Heart J. 2007;28(11):1326–33.
4. Mendes LA, Dec GW, Picard MH, Palacios IF, Newell J, Davidoff R. Right ventricular dysfunction: an independent predictor of adverse outcome in patients with myocarditis. Am Heart J. 1994;128:301–7.
5. Rossi A, Dini FL, Faggiano P, Agricola E, Cicoira M, Frattini S, Simioniuc A, Gullace M, Ghio S, Enriquez-Sarano M, Temporelli PL. Independent prognostic value of functional mitral regurgitation in patients with heart failure. A quantitative analysis of 1256 patients with ischaemic and non-ischaemic dilated cardiomyopathy. Heart. 2011;97:1675–80.
6. Xie GY, Berk MR, Smith MD, Gurley JC, DeMaria AN. Prognostic value of Doppler transmitral flow patterns in patients with congestive heart failure. J Am Coll Cardiol. 1994;24:132–9.
7. Nagueh SF, Smiseth OA, Appleton CP, Byrd BF 3rd, Dokainish H, Edvardsen T, Flachskampf FA, Gillebert TC, Klein AL, Lancellotti P, Marino P, Oh JK, Alexandru Popescu B, Waggoner AD. Recommendations for the evaluation of left ventricular diastolic function by echocardiography: an update from the American Society of Echocardiography

and the European Association of Cardiovascular Imaging. Eur Heart J Cardiovasc Imaging. 2016;17(12):1321–60. Review.
8. Adsett M, West MJ, Galbraith A, Duhig E, Lange A, Palka P. Eosinophilic heart: marked left ventricular wall thickening and myocardial dysfunction improving with corticosteroid therapy. Echocardiography. 2003;20:369–74.
9. Urhausen A, Kindermann M, Bohm M, Kindermann W. Images in cardiovascular medicine. Diagnosis of myocarditis by cardiac tissue velocity imaging in an Olympic athlete. Circulation. 2003;108:e21–2.
10. Friedrich MG. Myocardial edema--a new clinical entity? Nat Rev Cardiol. 2010;7(5):292–6. Review. https://doi.org/10.1038/nrcardio.2010.28.
11. Lieback E, Hardouin I, Meyer R, Bellach J, Hetzer R. Clinical value of echocardiographic tissue characterization in the diagnosis of myocarditis. Eur Heart J. 1996;17: 135–42.
12. Omi W, Nagai H, Takata S, Yuasa T, Sakagami S, Kobayashi K. Ultrasonic tissue characterization in acute myocarditis: a case report. Circ J. 2002;66:416–8.
13. Hiramitsu S, Morimoto S, Kato S, Uemura A, Kubo N, Kimura K, Sugiura A, Itoh T, Hishida H. Transient ventricular wall thickening in acute myocarditis: a serial echocardiographic and histopathologic study. Jpn Circ J. 2001;65(10):863–6. Review.
14. Thuny F, Avierinos JF, Jop B, Tafanelli L, Renard S, Riberi A, et al. Massive biventricular thrombosis as a consequence of myocarditis: findings from 2-dimensional and real-time 3-dimensional echocardiography. Circulation. 2006;113:e932–3.
15. Antoniak S, Boltzen U, Riad A, Kallwellis-Opara A, Rohde M, Dörner A, et al. Viral myocarditis and coagulopathy: increased tissue factor expression and plasma thrombogenicity. J Mol Cell Cardiol. 2008;45:118–26.
16. Senior R, Becher H, Monaghan M, Agati L, Zamorano J, Vanoverschelde JL, Nihoyannopoulos P, Edvardsen T, Lancellotti P, EACVI Scientific Documents Committee for 2014–16 and 2016–18, EACVI Scientific Documents Committee for 2014–16 and 2016–18. Clinical practice of contrast echocardiography: recommendation by the European Association of Cardiovascular Imaging (EACVI) 2017. Eur Heart J Cardiovasc Imaging. 2017;18(11):1205.
17. Afonso L, Hari P, Pidlaoan V, Kondur A, Jacob S, Khetarpal V. Acute myocarditis: can novel echocardiographic techniques assist with diagnosis? Eur J Echocardiogr. 2010;11(3):E5. https://doi.org/10.1093/ejechocard/jep183.
18. Skouri HN, Dec GW, Friedrich MG, Cooper LT. Non-invasive imaging in myocarditis. J Am Coll Cardiol. 2006;48:2085–93.
19. Shillcutt SK, Thomas WR, Sullivan JN, Duhachek-Stapelman A. Fulminant myocarditis: the role of perioperative echocardiography. Anesth Analg. 2015;120(2):296–9.
20. Felker GM, Boehmer JP, Hruban RH, Hutchins GM, Kasper EK, Baughman KL, Hare JM. Echocardiographic findings in fulminant and acute myocarditis. J Am Coll Cardiol. 2000;36:227–32.
21. Catena E, Paino R, Milazzo F, Colombo T, Marianeschi S, Lanfranconi M, Aresta F, Bruschi G, Russo C, Vitali E. Mechanical circulatory support for patients with fulminant myocarditis: the role of echocardiography to address diagnosis, choice of device, management, and recovery. J Cardiothorac Vasc Anesth. 2009;23(1):87–94.
22. Ammirati E, Cipriani M, Lilliu M, Sormani P, Varrenti M, Raineri C, et al. Survival and left ventricular function changes in fulminant versus nonfulminant acute myocarditis. Circulation. 2017;136:529–45.
23. Sohn IS, Park JC, Chung JH, Kim KH, Ahn Y, Jeong MH, et al. A case of acute eosinophilic myopericarditis presenting with cardiogenic shock and normal peripheral eosinophil count. Korean J Intern Med. 2006;21:136–40.
24. Shah R, Ananthasubramaniam K. Evaluation of cardiac involvement in hypereosinophilic syndrome: complementary roles of transthoracic, transesophageal, and contrast echocardiography. Echocardiography. 2006;23:689–91.
25. Mor-Avi V, Jenkins C, Kuhl HP, et al. Real-time 3-dimensional echocardiographic quantification of left ventricular volumes: multicentre study for validation with magnetic reso-

nance imaging and investigation of sources of error. J Am Coll Cardiol Img. 2008;1: 413–23.
26. Jenkins C, Bricknell K, Hanekom L, Marwick TH. Reproducibility and accuracy of echocardiographic measurements of left ventricular parameters using real-time three-dimensional echocardiography. J Am Coll Cardiol. 2004;44:878–86.
27. Zamorano JL, Lancellotti P, Rodriguez Muñoz D, Aboyans V, Asteggiano R, Galderisi M, Habib G, Lenihan DJ, Lip GYH, Lyon AR, Lopez Fernandez T, Mohty D, Piepoli MF, Tamargo J, Torbicki A, Suter TM, ESC Scientific Document Group. 2016 ESC position paper on cancer treatments and cardiovascular toxicity developed under the auspices of the ESC Committee for Practice Guidelines: the task force for cancer treatments and cardiovascular toxicity of the European Society of Cardiology (ESC). Eur Heart J. 2016;37(36):2768–801.
28. Gopal AS, Chukwu EO, Mihalatos DG, Katz AS, Mathew ST, Lachmann JS, et al. Left ventricular structure and function for postmyocardial infarction and heart failure risk stratification by three-dimensional echocardiography. J Am Soc Echocardiogr. 2007;20(8):949–58.
29. Hare JL, Jenkins C, Nakatani S, Ogawa A, Yu CM, Marwick TH. Feasibility and clinical decision-making with 3D echocardiography in routine practice. Heart. 2007;94(4):440–5.
30. Prakasa KR, Dalal D, Wang J, Bomma C, Tandri H, Dong J, James C, Tichnell C, Russell SD, Spevak P, Corretti M, Bluemke DA, Calkins H, Abraham TP. Feasibility and variability of three dimensional echocardiography in arrhythmogenic right ventricular cardiomyopathy. Am J Cardiol. 2006;97:703–9.
31. Jiang L, Siu SC, Handschumacher MD, Luis Guererro J, Vazquez de Prada JA, King ME, Picard MH, Weyman AE, Levine RA. Three-dimensional echocardiography. In vivo validation for right ventricular volume and function. Circulation. 1994;89:2342–50.
32. Niemann PS, Pinho L, Balbach T, et al. Anatomically oriented right ventricular volume measurements with dynamic three-dimensional echocardiography validated by 3-tesla magnetic resonance imaging. J Am Coll Cardiol. 2007;50:1668–76.
33. Khoo NS, Young A, Occleshaw C, Cowan B, Zeng IS, Gentles TL. Assessments of right ventricular volume and function using three-dimensional echocardiography in older children and adults with congenital heart disease: comparison with cardiac magnetic resonance imaging. J Am Soc Echocardiogr. 2009;22:1279–88.
34. Maffessanti F, Muraru D, Esposito R, et al. Age-, body size-, and sex-specific reference values for right ventricular volumes and ejection fraction by three-dimensional echocardiography: a multicentre echocardiographic study in 507 healthy volunteers. Circ Cardiovasc Imaging. 2013;6:700–10.
35. Buechel RR, Stephan FP, Sommer G, Bremerich J, Zellweger MJ, Kaufmann BA. Head-to-head comparison of two-dimensional and threedimensional echocardiographic methods for left atrial chamber quantification with magnetic resonance imaging. J Am Soc Echocardiogr. 2013;26:428–35. https://doi.org/10.1016/j.echo.2013.01.001.
36. Mor-Avi V, Yodwut C, Jenkins C, Kühl H, Nesser HJ, Marwick TH, Franke A, Weinert L, Niel J, Steringer-Mascherbauer R, Freed BH, Sugeng L, Lang RM. Real-time 3D echocardiographic quantification of left atrial volume: multicenter study for validation with CMR. JACC Cardiovasc Imaging. 2012;5:769–77.
37. Wu VC, Takeuchi M, Kuwaki H, Iwataki M, Nagata Y, Otani K, Haruki N, Yoshitani H, Tamura M, Abe H, Negishi K, Lin FC, Otsuji Y. Prognostic value of LA volumes assessed by transthoracic 3D echocardiography: comparison with 2D echocardiography. JACC Cardiovasc Imaging. 2013;6:1025–35. https://doi.org/10.1016/j.jcmg.2013.08.002.
38. Montserrat S, Gabrielli L, Borras R, Poyatos S, Berruezo A, Bijnens B, Brugada J, Mont L, Sitges M. Left atrial size and function by threedimensional echocardiography to predict arrhythmia recurrence after first and repeated ablation of atrial fibrillation. Eur Heart J Cardiovasc Imaging. 2014;15:515–22. https://doi.org/10.1093/ehjci/jet194.
39. Gianstefani S, Voigt JU, Monaghan MJ. New developments in echocardiography/advanced echocardiography. The ESC textbook of cardiovascular imaging (2nd). JL. Zamorano, J. Bax, J. Knuuti, U. Sechtem, P. Lancellotti, L. Badano 2015. Oxford University Press, Oxford

40. Stanton T, Leano R, Marwick TH. Prediction of all-cause mortality from global longitudinal speckle strain: comparison with ejection fraction and wall motion scoring. Circ Cardiovasc Imaging. 2009;2:356–64. https://doi.org/10.1161/CIRCIMAGING.109.862334.
41. Thavendiranathan P, Poulin F, Lim KD, Plana JC, Woo A, Marwick TH. Use of myocardial strain imaging by echocardiography for the early detection of cardiotoxicity in patients during and after cancer chemotherapy: a systematic review. J Am Coll Cardiol. 2014;63:2751–68.
42. Nahum J, Bensaid A, Dussault C, Macron L, Clémence D, Bouhemad B, Monin JL, Rande JL, Gueret P, Lim P. Impact of longitudinal myocardial deformation on the prognosis of chronic heart failure patients. Circ Cardiovasc Imaging. 2010;3:249–56.
43. Hare JL, Brown JK, Leano R, Jenkins C, Woodward N, Marwick TH. Use of myocardial deformation imaging to detect preclinical myocardial dysfunction before conventional measures in patients undergoing breast cancer treatment with trastuzumab. Am Heart J. 2009;158:294–301. https://doi.org/10.1016/j.ahj.2009.05.031.
44. Hsiao JF, Koshino Y, Bonnichsen CR, et al. Speckle tracking echocardiography in acute myocarditis. Int J Cardiovasc Imaging. 2013;29:275–84.
45. Escher F, Kasner M, Kuhl U, et al. New echocardiographic findings correlate with intramyocardial inflammation in endomyocardial biopsies of patients with acute myocarditis and inflammatory cardiomyopathy. Mediators Inflamm. 2013;2013:875420–9.
46. Di Bella G, Gaeta M, Pingitore A, et al. Myocardial deformation in acute myocarditis with normal left ventricular wall motion-a cardiac magnetic resonance and 2-dimensional strain echocardiographic study. Circ J. 2010;74:1205–13.
47. Løgstrup BB, Nielsen JM, Kim WY, et al. Myocardial oedema in acute myocarditis detected by echocardiographic 2D myocardial deformation analysis. Eur Heart J Cardiovasc Imaging. 2015;17:1018–26.
48. Muraru D, Niero A, Rodriguez-Zanella H, Cherata D, Badano L. Three-dimensional speckle-tracking echocardiography: benefits and limitations of integrating myocardial mechanics with three-dimensional imaging. Cardiovasc Diagn Ther. 2018;8(1):101–17.

Cardiac Magnetic Resonance Imaging in Myocarditis

9

Martina Perazzolo Marra and Alberto Cipriani

9.1 Introduction

Cardiac magnetic resonance (CMR) has emerged as a reliable and accurate diagnostic tool for the evaluation of patients with cardiac disease in several clinical settings and with proven additional diagnostic and prognostic value compared with other imaging modalities [1].

Non-invasive diagnosis of myocarditis and all spectrum of inflammatory cardiomyopathies can be very difficult in clinical practice due to the high heterogeneity of the clinical presentations in the absence of specific ECG and echocardiographic signs. In this setting CMR is a valuable diagnostic tool to non-invasively support the clinical diagnosis of myocarditis, representing an in vivo tissue characterization imaging modality. CMR represents not only the gold-standard for volume quantification and contractility assessment, but also provides myocardial tissue characterization, combining different sequences able to focus on all physiopathological aspects involved in myocardium inflammation, ranging from edema, to myocardial necrosis and subsequent scar.

The first CMR studies in myocarditis date back to the early 1990s [2]. More recently, multicenter studies and consensus documents [3] aimed at a global standardization of CMR acquisition protocols in inflammatory cardiomyopathies, as documented by both the American Heart Association (AHA) [4] and European Society of Cardiology (ESC) position statements. Data from different registries suggest that the early use of CMR may reduce hospitalization time and costs, mostly in patients with clinically suspected myocarditis presenting with troponin release and unobstructed coronary arteries [5].

M. P. Marra (✉) · A. Cipriani
Department of Cardiac Thoracic Vascular Sciences and Public Health, University of Padua Medical School, Padova, Italy
e-mail: martina.perazzolomarra@unipd.it; alberto.cipriani@unipd.it

A. L. P. Caforio (ed.), *Myocarditis*, https://doi.org/10.1007/978-3-030-35276-9_9

CMR indications in the setting of myocarditis include the whole spectrum of presentations, ranging from "infarct-like" with normal coronary arteries, to unexplained heart failure and arrhythmias. The systematic application of novel parametric CMR techniques has been recommended to increase the diagnostic accuracy of CMR in cases with concealed disease. Outcome data on prognosis are available, suggesting a role of late gadolinium enhancement (LGE) as predictor of poor prognosis in this heterogeneous group of diseases.

9.2 Technical Issues

CMR imaging sequences are sensitive to the tissue changes that occur during myocardial inflammation, regardless of its etiology. These pathophysiological changes include: hyperemia due to dilatation of the myocardial vascular bed; increased capillary leak; edema (both intracellular and interstitial); myocyte injury with loss of cell membrane integrity; myocyte necrosis; increase of the extracellular space due to infiltration of inflammatory cells or macrophages; and, ultimately, collagen deposition, interstitial fibrosis, and scar formation. The magnitude and spatial extent of these changes depend on the severity of inflammation, leading to varying ability of CMR visualization and detection, due to spatial resolution and different physical properties of the inflamed heart muscle.

The standard acquisition protocol includes cine images for volume quantification and evaluation of wall motion abnormalities. Biventricular volumes and *functional parameters* can be obtained by the acquisition of a set of ventricular short-axis views from the atrio-ventricular plane to the apex (with 6–8 mm slice thickness, possibly no gap between the slices, although the use of a 1–3 mm gap between slices is accepted). A balanced steady-state free precession (bSSFP) cine images with a temporal resolution of 45 ms or less and in-plane spatial resolution of less than 2 mm has to be used. Those bSSFP sequences are the method of choice for cine imaging because they provide high signal-to-noise ratio (SNR) and excellent contrast between myocardium and blood pool. In the setting of myocarditis, the ventricular dysfunction is neither a very sensitive nor a specific finding, since the inflammatory process may be focal, and the surrounding myocardium may compensate with an increase in contractility. Moreover, there is a predominant sub-epicardial involvement in myocarditis, and a relative sparing of the endocardium that provides up to 75% of the contractile force.

Besides providing anatomic and morphological information, the CMR provides tissue characterization by measuring T1 and T2 relaxation times and spin densities.

Active myocarditis is typically associated with myocyte injury, edema, and cellular swelling; assessment of relaxation times provides a sensitive measure for edema detection. Different CMR approaches can be used. *Myocardial edema* can be identified as an hyperintense area on images obtained with a T2-weighted short tau inversion recovery (STIR) FSE pulse sequence, generally acquired with a triple-inversion recovery protocol (double-inversion recovery and the third-inversion recovery pulse, with inversion time of 150 ms for a 1.5 T system); this type of sequence has the advantage to abolish signal from fat tissue, allowing edema detection [6]. In T2-weighted (T2W) images, that are no-contrast sequences, edema appears as regionally or globally increased signal hyperintensity. T2 mapping allows for the direct measurement of the water-induced prolongation of myocardial T2 relaxation time [7]. Edema also leads to an increase of myocardial T1 relaxation time [8], although the increase of T1 is less specific for active inflammation because it can also be seen in fibrotic areas where free water may accumulate [9].

Inflammatory changes include *hyperemia,* due to increased vascular permeability, and a net expansion of the extracellular space. The CMR techniques to target these changes include T1-weighted spin-echo images, acquired pre-administration and early post-administration of an extracellular gadolinium-based contrast agent [6]. Because gadolinium in its ligated form is an extracellular contrast agent, it is believed that the increased volume of distribution available for the gadolinium agent leads to greater contrast enhancement inflamed compared to not inflamed myocardium, although it ultimately remains unclear whether these methods can specifically reflect hyperemia or are just markers of an expansion of the extracellular space.

Following inflammatory-induced myocyte injury, the post-inflammatory repair phenomenon leads to replacement-type *fibrosis and scarring*. These changes substantially increase the volume of distribution available for gadolinium, as the contrast agent gains access to the intracellular space of myocytes that are injured or no longer viable. The no longer-viable scarred myocardium is notable as bright signal, i.e., late gadolinium enhancement (LGE) on post-contrast sequences. LGE images are obtained using two-dimensional or three-dimensional segmented inversion recovery GRE or SSFP pulse sequence. The acquisition of an inversion-time scout sequence is recommended before the acquisition of an LGE image to establish the appropriate inversion time.

The typical regional LGE patterns of post-inflammatory non-coronary related injury in the myocardium include a patchy, focal distribution, a sub-epicardial stria (in contrast to ischemic lesions that involve the sub-endocardium), and a midwall stria (Fig. 9.1). These patterns do not identify a specific myocarditis etiology (e.g., viral vs. autoimmune) and may also be found in non-inflammatory cardiomyopathies, i.e., the presence of LGE in the infero-lateral left ventricular wall in Fabry's or Becker's disease. Finally, myocardial inflammation secondary to hypereosinophilia syndromes typically shows a circumferential subendocardial LGE pattern that does not localize to any specific coronary territory.

More advanced tissue characterization can be obtained with parametric techniques, based on quantification of T1, T2 relaxation time, including the evaluation of extracellular volume (ECV) mapping.

T1 mapping is a newer technique for tissue characterization, based on the quantification of T1 value in each voxel or in the myocardial region of interest. T1 is the longitudinal relaxation time of a tissue; T1 values can be estimated acquiring multiple T1-weighted images and fitting the resulting signals to an appropriate exponential recovery curve: each tissue type exhibits a specific range of normal T1

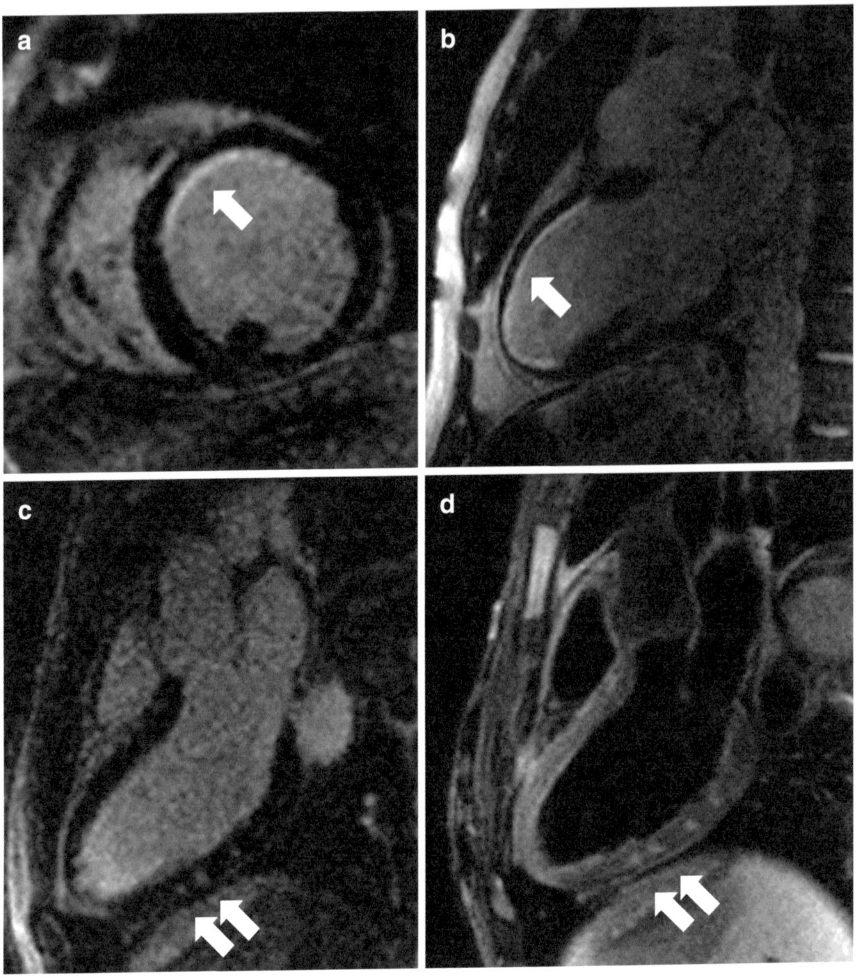

Fig. 9.1 Different CMR patterns in ischemic heart disease and myocarditis. A typical case of subendocardial post-infarction scar (late gadolinium enhancement, LGE) is shown in (**a**) (post-contrast short-axis view) and (**b**) (post-contrast long axis view) at the left ventricular anterior and antero-septal walls (white arrow). On the contrary in myocarditis LGE is detectable with a patchy, non-coronary related pattern, in this case at the infero-lateral wall (white arrow on **c**, post-contrast long axis view); acute inflammation is confirmed by the presence of edema on T2-weighted sequences at the same areas of LGE detection (white arrow on **d**)

values, deviation from which indicates a pathologic condition. After acquisition, T1 maps can be displayed using color scale to aid visual interpretation. T2 represents the transverse relaxation time, similar to T1 values; T2 values represent global signals from both intracellular and extracellular compartments. Myocardial T2 correlates with myocardial water content and edema.

The T1 signal can be measured 15 min after contrast and used to calculate the extracellular volume (ECV). ECV is increased in most cardiac diseases, due to expansion of the extracellular space as a result of interstitial non-cellular edema, infiltration, fibrosis, expansion of the intravascular compartment because of coronary vasodilation and ischemia.

The final CMR diagnosis is reached combining the results obtained with different tissue characterization techniques and parametric mapping.

9.3 The History of CMR in Myocarditis Detection

T2-weighted sequences were first applied for CMR diagnosis of myocarditis, since edema was considered the hallmark feature of myocardial inflammation. In the 1991, Gagliardi et al. [2] studied a pediatric population and described a significant difference in signal intensity between children with and without acute myocarditis on T2-weighted spin-echo sequences. Over the following years, additional steps were made towards a better understanding of the mechanisms and causes of inflammatory myocardial damage and its CMR depiction. In 2005, Abdel-Aty et al. [10] assessed the diagnostic accuracy of the available proposed CMR diagnostic approaches. They suggested that a combined application of T2-weighted and post-contrast imaging with early and LGE allowed to obtain a high diagnostic accuracy in suspected acute myocarditis. The following year, a cornerstone paper published by Mahrholdt et al. [11] elegantly observed and described the association of different clinical presentations and patterns of myocardial damage by analyzing 128 patients with a clinical suspicion of acute myocarditis. Forty-nine patients presented as a causative agent a PVB19 infection and 16 patients an HHV6 infection. Clinical presentation was different between groups, since PVB19 infections predominantly presented with severe acute chest pain mimicking myocardial infarction, whereas most patients infected by HHV6 showed symptoms of subacute new-onset heart failure, arrhythmias, and bundle branch block. LGE in these two subgroups also differed, since the PVB19 group had LGE in the infero-lateral segments, whereas the HHV6 group in the interventricular septum. This paper remains fundamental for CMR application since the correlation of biopsy findings with LGE is proof of concept for the use of this contrast agent in acute myocarditis. However, the reported association of specific LGE sites with specific viral infections was subsequently disproven; similarly it is nowadays established that LGE does not distinguish viral from other non-infectious causes of myocarditis.

In 2009, after the publication of many articles reporting different scan protocols, an expert consensus document was published; the study aim was to increase CMR diagnostic accuracy in suspected myocarditis by the identification of homogeneous diagnostic criteria and protocols. The document identified the so-called Lake Louise criteria (LLC) [3]: in keeping with LLC when myocardial edema, hyperemia, and LGE are studied, the presence of at least 2 out of these 3 tissue markers leads to a diagnostic accuracy of 78%. Therefore, in order to formulate a plausible myocarditis diagnosis by LLC at least 2 out of these 3 features are needed. These authors suggested that the detection of edema, hyperemia, and LGE over time could also have been useful to monitor the course of myocardial inflammation, providing information on possible reversible and irreversible cardiac damage, as well as differential CMR features of acute and healed myocarditis. The LLC provided a uniform diagnostic protocol, but the accuracy of CMR remained limited (i.e., accuracy estimated at 78%, with a sensitivity of 67% and a specificity of 91%) since it was calculated on a small number of patients in whom CMR was compared to histology.

Technical advances, specifically the development of pixel-wise mapping of T1 and T2 relaxation times, have led to multiple studies, suggesting that these newer techniques may have clinical potential in the diagnosis of suspected myocardial inflammation. To increase diagnostic accuracy recently the LLC have been revised [1], including new mapping techniques. The old LLC criteria were based on "any 2 out of 3" criteria (T2-weighted sequences, early enhancement, LGE). The new revised criteria suggest a different approach, defined "2 out of 2," i.e., with one positive T2-based criterion and one T1-based criterion to increase the specificity in the detection of acute myocardial inflammation. The tissue characterization target remains the same (edema, hyperemia, fibrosis) and the proposed *main criteria* include: *T2-based imaging* (regional high T2 signal intensity *or* global T2 signal intensity ratio ≥ 2.0 in T2W *or* regional or global increase of myocardial T2 relaxation time images) *and T1-based imaging* (regional or global increase of native myocardial T1 relaxation time *or* ECV or areas with high signal intensity in a non-ischemic distribution pattern in LGE images). *Supportive criteria* include: pericardial effusion in cine CMR images, high signal intensity of the pericardium in LGE images, T1-mapping or T2-mapping, T1 mapping or T2 mapping, systolic LV wall motion abnormality in cine images.

9.4 Indication and Differential Diagnosis

The indication to perform CMR in patients with troponin release, no coronary lesions, and suspected myocarditis has been extensively recommended in different consensus documents, since the first application of CMR. In particular, in this setting, CMR is indicated first of all to refine the clinical suspicion, to support invasive procedures (i.e., endomyocardial biopsy), to guide the site of endomyocardial biopsy, to suggest additional tests, such as positron emission tomography (PET) in suspected sarcoidosis. In the setting of myocarditis with "infarct-like" presentation, CMR findings are typically impressive, with widespread edema and patchy, often infero-lateral, necrosis in LGE images (Fig. 9.2). Conversely, in the same clinical context, a subendocardial LGE pattern may be useful to review the coronary angiography or perform a computed tomography (CT) to detect small vessel disease, non-atherosclerotic myocardial infarction caused by embolization, or distal dissection of a coronary vessel. Thus, in this context CMR has important impact on medical management.

Another clinical scenario that requires CMR is unexplained systolic and/or diastolic heart failure with clinically suspected myocarditis: in these patients more extensive myocardial involvement would be expected [12]. Last but not least,

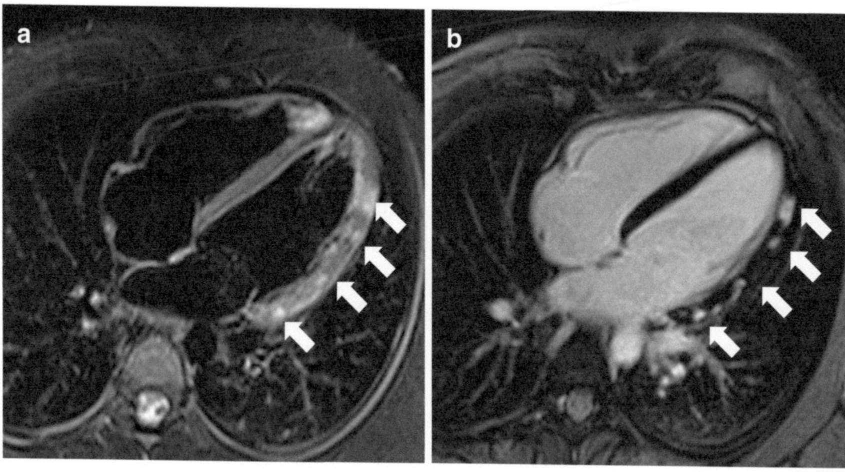

Fig. 9.2 Typical CMR feature of myocarditis. A typical case of acute myocarditis is shown on (**a**) (T2-weighted sequence, long axis view): the bright signal intensity with epicardial–midmural pattern on left ventricular wall (white arrows) represents areas of myocardial edema due to inflammation. On post-contrast sequence (**b**, long axis view) area of late gadolinium enhancement (white arrows on **b**), spatially corresponding to patchy edema on (**a**), represents area with more pronounced myocardial damage including necrosis

unexplained arrhythmias may also be an indication for CMR to detect the site and pattern of LGE, to relate it to the type of arrhythmia, and to strengthen the clinical suspicion of myocarditis [12].

Although CMR is appropriate in several clinical scenarios, and particularly to differentiate coronary-ischemic from inflammatory myocardial damage, no information regarding the etiology of myocarditis can be obtained from CMR images, both LGE and mapping. Some peculiar LGE findings may be found in specific myocarditis forms. In giant cell myocarditis large areas of high signal intensity at various, sometimes atypically subendocardial sites of the myocardium are detectable. Diffuse subendocardial areas of high signal intensity in LGE images, sometimes associated with small mural thrombosis may be found in eosinophilic myocarditis; such images look quite different from the more sub-epicardial or patchy intramyocardial LGE distribution patterns of viral myocarditis. Finally, sarcoidosis may be suspected when LGE involves the epicardial layer of the left ventricular inferior wall and the right side of the interventricular septum, associated with right ventricular involvement.

9.5 Prognostic Role

At CMR follow-up, edema disappears in the majority of patients, thus T2-based imaging becomes negative. At T1-based imaging LGE intensity of extent will also be reduced, persisting in a limited number of subjects; such persistent LGE is thought to represent, if T2-based imaging is negative, the final post-inflammatory scar. It should be considered to perform a CMR at follow-up to visualize the extent of persisting myocardial damage after the first episode. Definite consensus on the time interval to perform a follow-up CMR is lacking; it should be decided taking into consideration the clinical condition, the persistence of systolic dysfunction and/or arrhythmias, and the availability of the exam. If the clinical condition is stable, it seems reasonable to perform a second CMR at least within the first year.

The prognostic role of LGE persistence in myocarditis, independently from systolic dysfunction, remains to be proven, although initial observations suggested a worse prognosis (mainly in terms of arrhythmias) in patients with LGE persistence [13, 14].

9.6 Conclusion

The CMR is a non-invasive imaging tool to confirm the clinical suspicion of myocarditis, but does not provide information on myocarditis etiology. Recently the LLC diagnostic criteria have been updated to increase CMR accuracy, including T2-based and T1-based imaging. The application of CMR in the setting of myocardial inflammation is indicated first of all to confirm the clinical suspicion, to support subsequent more invasive procedures (i.e., endomyocardial biopsy), to guide the site of endomyocardial biopsy, and to suggest additional exams. The definite prognostic role of traditional LGE and of the novel techniques including T2 mapping, native T1, and ECV is under investigation.

References

1. Ferreira VM, Schulz-Menger J, Holmvang G, Kramer CM, Carbone I, Sechtem U, Kindermann I, Gutberlet M, Cooper LT, Liu P, Friedrich MG. Cardiovascular magnetic resonance in nonischemic myocardial inflammation: expert recommendations. J Am Coll Cardiol. 2018;72(24):3158–76.
2. Gagliardi MG, Bevilacqua M, Di Renzi P, Picardo S, Passariello R, Marcelletti C. Usefulness of magnetic resonance imaging for diagnosis of acute myocarditis in infants and children, and comparison with endomyocardial biopsy. Am J Cardiol. 1991;68(10):1089–91.
3. Friedrich MG, Sechtem U, Schulz-Menger J, Holmvang G, Alakija P, Cooper LT, White JA, Abdel-Aty H, Gutberlet M, Prasad S, Aletras A, Laissy JP, Paterson I, Filipchuk NG, Kumar A, Pauschinger M, Liu P, International Consensus Group on Cardiovascular Magnetic Resonance in Myocarditis. Cardiovascular magnetic resonance in myocarditis: a JACC White Paper. J Am Coll Cardiol. 2009;53(17):1475–87.
4. Bozkurt B, Colvin M, Cook J, et al. Current diagnostic and treatment strategies for specific dilated cardiomyopathies: a scientific statement from the American Heart Association. Circulation. 2016;134:e579–646.
5. Bruder O, Wagner A, Lombardi M, Schwitter J, van Rossum A, Pilz G, Nothnagel D, Steen H, Petersen S, Nagel E, Prasad S, Schumm J, Greulich S, Cagnolo A, Monney P, Deluigi CC, Dill T, Frank H, Sabin G, Schneider S, Mahrholdt H. European cardiovascular magnetic resonance (EuroCMR) registry – multi national results from 57 centers in 15 countries. J Cardiovasc Magn Reson. 2013;15:9.

6. Aquaro GD, Di Bella G, Castelletti S, Maestrini V, Festa P, Ait-Ali L, Masci PG, Monti L, di Giovine G, De Lazzari M, Cipriani A, Guaricci AI, Dellegrottaglie S, Pepe A, Marra MP, Pontone G. Clinical recommendations of cardiac magnetic resonance, part I: ischemic and valvular heart disease: a position paper of the working group 'Applicazioni della Risonanza Magnetica' of the Italian Society of Cardiology. J Cardiovasc Med (Hagerstown). 2017;18(4):197–208.
7. Fernández-Jiménez R, Sánchez-González J, Aguero J, Del Trigo M, Galán-Arriola C, Fuster V, Ibáñez B. Fast T2 gradient-spin-echo (T2- GraSE) mapping for myocardial edema quantification: first in vivo validation in a porcine model of ischemia/reperfusion. J Cardiovasc Magn Reson. 2015;17:92.
8. Ferreira VM, Piechnik SK, Dall'Armellina E, Karamitsos TD, Francis JM, Choudhury RP, Friedrich MG, Robson MD, Neubauer S. Non-contrast T1-mapping detects acute myocardial edema with high diagnostic accuracy: a comparison to T2-weighted cardiovascular magnetic resonance. J Cardiovasc Magn Reson. 2012;14:42.
9. Iles LM, Ellims AH, Llewellyn H, Hare JL, Kaye DM, McLean CA, Taylor AJ. Histological validation of cardiac magnetic resonance analysis of regional and diffuse interstitial myocardial fibrosis. Eur Heart J Cardiovasc Imaging. 2015;16:14–22.
10. Abdel-Aty H, Boyé P, Zagrosek A, Wassmuth R, Kumar A, Messroghli D, Bock P, Dietz R, Friedrich MG, Schulz-Menger J. Diagnostic performance of cardiovascular magnetic resonance in patients with suspected acute myocarditis: comparison of different approaches. J Am Coll Cardiol. 2005;45(11):1815–22.
11. Mahrholdt H, Wagner A, Deluigi CC, Kispert E, Hager S, Meinhardt G, Vogelsberg H, Fritz P, Dippon J, Bock CT, Klingel K, Kandolf R, Sechtem U. Presentation, patterns of myocardial damage, and clinical course of viral myocarditis. Circulation. 2006;114:1581–90.
12. Caforio AL, et al. Current state of knowledge on aetiology, diagnosis, management, and therapy of myocarditis: a position statement of the European Society of Cardiology Working Group on Myocardial and Pericardial Diseases. Eur Heart J. 2013;34:2636–48, 2648a-2648d.
13. Grün S, Schumm J, Greulich S, Wagner A, Schneider S, Bruder O, Kispert EM, Hill S, Ong P, Klingel K, Kandolf R, Sechtem U, Mahrholdt H. Long-term follow-up of biopsy-proven viral myocarditis: predictors of mortality and incomplete recovery. J Am Coll Cardiol. 2012;59(18):1604–15.
14. Aquaro GD, Negri F, De Luca A, Todiere G, Bianco F, Barison A, Camastra G, Monti L, Dellegrottaglie S, Moro C, Lanzillo C, Scatteia A, Di Roma M, Pontone G, Perazzolo Marra M, Di Bella G, Donato R, Grigoratos C, Emdin M, Sinagra G. Role of right ventricular involvement in acute myocarditis, assessed by cardiac magnetic resonance. Int J Cardiol. 2018;271:359–65.

Organ-Specific Autoimmune Myocarditis 10

Alida L. P. Caforio, Chun-Yan Cheng, Mara Seguso, Nicoletta Gallo, Renzo Marcolongo, and Sabino Iliceto

10.1 Introduction

Autoimmune disease results from the loss of tolerance to self-antigens, which is preserved in physiological conditions. An autoimmune disease must fulfill at least two major criteria proposed by Witebsky and later modified by Rose [1]. There are also minor criteria, some of which common to all autoimmune conditions, others found in a few of them [1]. Organ-specific autoimmune diseases develop as a result of both genetic predisposition and environmental factors. The genetic predisposition is responsible for both the fact that different autoimmune conditions may be associated in patients or in their family members, as well as for the well-known feature that single autoimmune diseases often occur in families. The inheritance of susceptibility is usually polygenic. Organ-specific autoimmune diseases are commonly associated with specific Human Leucocyte Antigens (HLA) class II

A. L. P. Caforio (✉) · C.-Y. Cheng
Cardiology, Department of Cardiological, Thoracic and Vascular Sciences and Public Health, University of Padua, Padua, Italy

Cardio Immunology outpatient clinic, University of Padua, Padua, Italy
e-mail: alida.caforio@unipd.it; 73047chengchunyan@163.com

M. Seguso · N. Gallo
Haematology and Clinical Immunology Unit, Department of Medicine, University of Padua, Padua, Italy
e-mail: mara.seguso@gmail.com; nicoletta.gallo@aopd.veneto.it

R. Marcolongo
Cardio Immunology outpatient clinic, University of Padua, Padua, Italy

Department of Laboratory Medicine, University of Padua, Padua, Italy
e-mail: renzo.marcolongo@tiscali.it

S. Iliceto
Cardiology, Department of Cardiological, Thoracic and Vascular Sciences and Public Health, University of Padua, Padua, Italy
e-mail: sabino.iliceto@unipd.it

A. L. P. Caforio (ed.), *Myocarditis*, https://doi.org/10.1007/978-3-030-35276-9_10

antigens, although the mechanisms by which multiple HLA and non-HLA genes, often involved in immune regulatory pathways [2–5] may determine disease predisposition are still undefined [1, 6].

Autoimmune disease is characterized by the presence of circulating autoantibodies, which are not always pathogenic but represent markers of on-going tissue damage. In non-organ specific autoimmune disease the autoantibodies are against ubiquitous autoantigens (e.g., nuclear antigens in systemic lupus erythematosus) and tissue damage is generalized. In organ-specific autoimmune disease, immunopathology is restricted to one organ or apparatus, and the autoimmune process, antibody and/or cell-mediated, is directed against autoantigens which are unique to the affected organ (e.g., thyroid peroxidase in Hashimoto's thyroiditis). The majority of organ-specific autoimmune diseases are chronic and apparently "idiopathic." The histological hallmark of organ-specific autoimmunity is an early mononuclear cell infiltrate in the affected organ, e.g., insulitis in Type 1 insulin-dependent diabetes mellitus (IDDM), with inappropriate expression of HLA Class II and of adhesion molecules. At a later stage inflammatory cells tend to disappear and the tissue undergoes fibrotic changes with end-stage atrophy and organ dysfunction (hypothyroidism in Hashimoto's thyroiditis). In other instances organ-specific autoimmunity may lead to enhanced target organ function (e.g., Basedow's disease).

Organ- and disease-specific antibodies are found in the affected patients. These antibodies are also detected in family members even years before the development of disease, and thus identify asymptomatic relatives at risk [1]. Involvement of organ-specific autoimmunity has been suspected in the postpericardiotomy and post-myocardial infarction (Dressler) syndromes, rheumatic carditis, Chagas' disease, idiopathic inflammatory cardiomyopathy, and brady or tachyarrhythmia [7]. The Rose--Witebski criteria for organ-specific autoimmunity are entirely fulfilled in infection-negative biopsy-proven myocarditis and in inflammatory cardiomyopathy (defined as myocarditis with myocardial dysfunction) that are covered in this chapter (Table 10.1).

10.2 The Clinical Continuum: Autoimmune Myocarditis and Inflammatory Cardiomyopathy/Dilated Cardiomyopathy (DCM)

The World Health Organization (WHO) classification of cardiomyopathies defines myocarditis as an inflammatory disease of the myocardium, which is diagnosed by endomyocardial biopsy (EMB) using established histological, immunological, and immunohistochemical criteria; in addition, myocarditis may be idiopathic, infectious, or autoimmune and may heal or evolve in dilated cardiomyopathy (DCM) [8–11]. The term "idiopathic" is nowadays only used in the absence of complete microbiological workup on endomyocardial biopsy (EMB).

DCM features include dilatation and impaired contraction of the left or both ventricles in the absence of known, specific causes of heart failure, including coronary artery disease; idiopathic, familial/genetic, viral, and/or immune DCM

Table 10.1 Fulfilled Rose–Witebsky autoimmune criteria in myocarditis/DCM: 2019 update

Major
* Mononuclear cell infiltration and abnormal HLA expression in the myocardium in the absence of infectious agents or other known causes: *yes*
* Circulating autoantibodies in patients and in unaffected family members: *yes*
* Autoantibody and/or autoreactive lymphocytes in situ within the myocardium: *yes*
* Identification and isolation of organ-specific autoantigen(s) involved: *yes*
* Disease induced in animals by immunization with relevant autoantigen, and/or passive transfer of serum, purified autoantibody and/or lymphocytes: *yes*
* Efficacy of immunosuppression in proven autoimmune myocarditis: *yes*
Minor
a) all autoimmune disorders
* Middle-aged women most frequently affected: *no*
* Familial aggregation: *yes*
* HLA association: *yes*
* Clinical course with hot phases and remissions: *yes*
* Autoimmune diseases associated in the same patient or in family members: *yes*
b) Organ-specific autoimmune disorders
* Autoantibodies against organ-specific autoantigens: *yes*
* Immunopathology mediated by type II, IV, V, VI reactions: *yes*
* Induction of antibodies induces an organ-specific disease/phenotype: *yes*
* Transfer of autoantibodies also transfers the disease/phenotype: *yes*

forms -are recognized [8, 9]. Histological EMB findings in DCM include myocyte loss, compensatory hypertrophy, fibrosis, and acute or chronic myocarditis in 30–40% of cases. Therefore, in a patient subset, myocarditis and DCM represent two sides of the same coin, e.g., an inflammatory disease of the myocardium, which can be infectious, post-infectious immune, or primarily organ-specific autoimmune [8–13].

10.3 Aetiopathogenesis of Myocarditis

Viral infections are presumed to be the most common cause in the Western world; frequency of viral genomes detected on EMB in patients with myocarditis and DCM by molecular techniques, mainly reverse transcriptase-(RT)-polymerase chain reaction (PCR), is variable [14–38]. Koch's postulates are used to establish whether an infectious agent causes disease. While many viruses are detected in the myocardium by PCR, fulfillment of Koch's postulates is limited to myocarditis caused by enterovirus and cytomegalovirus [14–38]. More studies are therefore needed to clarify whether a growing list of viruses really cause myocarditis or are detected coincidentally as remnants of past benign infections or as experimental contamination and artifact. At the state of current knowledge, myocarditis is defined as autoimmune if no infectious agents are identified on EMB and other known causes are excluded [6, 36]. Autoimmune myocarditis may develop with exclusive (organ-specific) cardiac involvement or in the context of autoimmune disorders with predominant extra-cardiac organ involvement [6, 19, 36]. Here we focus on organ-specific myocarditis/inflammatory cardiomyopathy.

10.4 Fulfilled Rose–Witebski Criteria for Organ-Specific Autoimmunity in Myocarditis/DCM

In several susceptible mouse strains viral genomic material and inflammation persist in the heart for weeks, triggering myocardial post-infectious autoimmune phenomena [6, 36–38]. However, the same genetically predisposed mouse strains, harboring specific major histocompatibility complex (MHC) and non-MHC genes, also develop autoimmune lymphocytic or giant cell myocarditis (and later on DCM) in the absence of a viral challenge, after immunization with specific cardiac autoantigens, e.g., cardiac myosin, or spontaneously [36, 37, 39–48]. Some MHC genes predisposing to organ-specific autoimmune myocarditis are also associated with Type 1 diabetes and other autoimmune diseases [37, 46, 48–50]. Both myocarditis and inflammatory DCM may be familial [51–56] and have been associated with HLA [57, 58]. A recent landmark large multicenter European genome-wide association study reported that, without a pre-specified hypothesis, HLA is a risk locus for DCM, in keeping with the autoimmune paradigm [58]. Biopsy-proven myocarditis has also been described in other cardiomyopathies, besides DCM [59, 60], and in some channelopathies [61]. It remains to be clarified whether this reflects involvement of autoimmunity as final common pathway of chronic cardiac damage in other genetically determined cardiomyopathies or an association of distinct diseases. More work should be focused on the identification of HLA and non-HLA immunogenetic basis of human myocarditis/DCM.

Fulfilled Rose–Witebski postulates in human myocarditis/DCM (Table 10.1) include myocardial mononuclear cell infiltrates, abnormal expression of HLA class II, and/or adhesion molecules on cardiac endothelium in the absence of viral genomes (as assessed by PCR on EMB) in index patients and family members [62–64]; increased serum levels of cytokines and cardiac autoantibodies (aabs) in patients and relatives [19, 36, 51–57, 65–136]; experimentally induced models of myocarditis/DCM after immunization with recognized autoantigen(s) [37, 39–50]; and response to immunosuppression or immunomodulation in patients with giant cell myocarditis and with autoimmune DCM [25, 35, 36, 67, 103, 104]. Many distinct cardiac aabs have been found in human myocarditis/DCM (Table 10.2). In keeping with the suggestion of a direct pathogenic role for some of these aabs, functional effects of cardiac aabs isolated from index patients have been shown in vitro [76, 99, 141]. In addition, the cardiac abnormalities seen in human post-myocarditic DCM have been reproduced in experimental animals following immunization with defined autoantigens, e.g., beta1-adrenergic or M2 muscarinic receptors, cardiac myosin, and cardiac troponin (cTNI) [41–43, 80–82, 86, 94, 95]. Myocardial pathology has also been produced by transfer of immune components from one experimental animal to another [82, 83, 86–89, 96]. Last but not least, improved cardiac morphology and function has been obtained by removal of beta1-adrenoceptor aabs (beta1-aabs) using immunoabsorption (IA) in rabbits, or by

Table 10.2 Circulating cardiac autoantibodies(Aab): frequency in myocarditis/DCM and in control groups (reprinted from reference 51 with permission)

Cardiac autoantibody (Ab)	% Aabs positive		% Antibody positive		References
	Myoc	DCM	OCD	Normal	
Muscle-specific ASA, (AFA,IFA,AMLA)	28–59[a]	9–41[a]	NT	0–25	[108–111]
Cardiac-specific AHA AIDA	41–56[a, b] 17[a, b]	26–30[a, b] 16[a, b]	1–4 2–4	3 0	[101] [19[a, b], 52[a, b], 53[a, b], 68[a, b], 69[a, b], 137[a, b]]
Anti-Beta1-AR	33 NT 73–96[a, b] NT	40–51[b] 35[a, b] 29–95[a, b] 27–28	13–55 16 8 10	0–13 7 0 0	[73, 75, 76, 89, 99, 100, 105, 112–120, 138]
Anti-Beta2-AR	NT NT NT	30–38[b] 13–14 30–75[a, b]	33 37	15 18	[74, 89, 121[b], 122]
Anti-muscarinic acetylcholine receptor-2	11 NT	30–77[c] 83[d]	23[e]–61	8–13	[93, 105, 115, 116, 118, 120, 123–127]
Cardiodepressant (Fγ-gamma-receptor 2a) Anti-Ky channel-interacting protein 2, KChIP2.6—ELISA)	NT NT	64 14	– 8	– 4	[104, 105, 128, 129, 139, 140]
Anti-alpha-MHC (cardiac-specific) Anti-Beta-MHC (muscle-cross reactive)	17–37[a, b]	20–46[a, b]	4–16	0–2.5	[66, 69–72[a, b], 106, 130[a, b]]
Anti-MLC 1v	NT	17[b]-35	25	0–15	[70[b], 132]
Anti-tropomyosin	NT	55[b]	21	NT	[132]
Anti-non-myofibrillar	NT	46[a, b]	17	0	[70[a, b]]
Anti-MHC	NT	67[b]	42	NT	[132]
Anti-actin	NT	71[b]	21	NT	[132]
Anti-troponin I,T	NT	1.7[b]–20[b]	0[b]–18	0–4	[105–107]
Anti-laminin	73	78	25–35	6	[133]
Anti-HSP60,70	NT	10–85[b]	1–42	3	[132, 134]
Anti-s.Na/K-ATPase	26[a]		NT	2	[90]
Anti- ANT Anti-M7 Anti-BCKD-E2	91[a, b] 13[a] 100	57[a, b] 31[a] 60	0 10 4	0 0 0	[84, 135, 136[a, b]] [91] [92]

[a]$P < 0.05$ vs normals
[b]$p < 0.05$ vs OCD
[c]77% (in Chagas-DCM)
[d]In selected ELISA-positive heart failure patients
[e]In atrial fibrillation patients
[a, b]Cardiac and disease-specific for myocarditis/DCM
AFA anti-fibrillary Ab, *AHA* organ-specific and partially organ-specific anti-heart aabs, *AIDA* anti-Intercalated disks-aabs, *ANT* adenine nucleotide translocator, *AMLA* anti-myolemmal aabs, *AR* adrenergic receptor, *ASA* anti-sarcolemmal aabs, *IFA* anti-interfibrillary aabs, *BCKD* branched chain alpha-ketoacid dehydrogenase dihydrolipoyl transacylase, *HSP* heat shock protein, *NT* not tested, *OCD* other cardiac disease, *MHC* myosin heavy chain, *MLC1v* myosin light chain 1 ventricular, *Myoc* myocarditis

specific scavenging of beta1-aabs by epitope-mimicking cyclic peptides in rats with autoimmune DCM [95, 96] . It has been reported that aabs-induced endoplasmic reticulum stress induces cardiomyocyte apoptosis [98]. It is worth noting that anti-cardiac myosin aabs, induced by immunization of rats against cardiac myosin, cross-react with cardiac membrane beta1-adrenergic receptors, and increase cAMP-dependent protein kinase A activity in myocytes [43]. Passive transfer of purified aabs from cardiac myosin-immunized rats leads to myocardial IgG deposits and increased myocyte apoptosis, leading to cardiomyopathy in recipients [43].

10.5 Serum Cardiac Autoantibodies (Aabs): Diagnostic and Clinical Relevance in Myocarditis/DCM

In patients with myocarditis/DCM and of their symptom-free relatives serum heart-reactive aabs recognize multiple antigens (Table 10.2), some of which are only expressed in the myocardium (e.g., organ-specific), others in heart and skeletal muscle (e.g., muscle-specific). Each of these aabs has different frequency in disease and normal control cohorts; the organ-specific and cross-reactive-1 types of anti-heart aabs (AHA) detected by standard indirect immunofluorescence (s-I IFL) shown in Fig. 10.1 are disease-specific for myocarditis/DCM (Table 10.2). Aabs of IgG class, if demonstrated to be cardiac and disease-specific for autoimme myocarditis/DCM, can be used as autoimmune markers for identifying patients in whom immunosuppression and/or immunomodulation therapy may be beneficial and their relatives at risk [19, 35, 51–53, 68, 69]. Some aabs may have a functional role and/or, being associated with hot phases of the disease, represent negative prognostic markers [71, 76, 78, 86, 87, 89–97, 100, 101, 104, 138, 141]. The ESC Task Force recommended to assess sera with clinically suspected or definite myocarditis for cardiac aabs, using one (or more) of the published tests, according to specific center expertise, preferably disease-specific aabs [36].

10.6 Specific Aabs Tests as Organ-Specific Autoimmune Markers in Myocarditis/DCM

10.6.1 Anti-Heart Aabs (AHA) and Anti-Intercalated Disk Aabs (AIDA) by Standard Indirect Immunofluorescence (s-I IFL)

Using indirect s-I IFL on 4 μm-thick unfixed fresh frozen cryostat sections of blood group O normal human heart and skeletal muscle, and absorption with human heart and skeletal muscle and rat liver, organ-specific IgG AHA giving a diffuse cytoplasmic staining pattern of myocytes and a negative pattern on skeletal muscle (Fig. 10.1, panels a, b) were found in about 30–56% of myocarditis/DCM patients and their symptom-free family members, in 1–4% of patients with other cardiac disease, in 3% of normal subjects, and in 17% of patients without cardiac disease, but with autoimmune polyendocrinopathy (Table 10.2) [53, 68, 69, 79]. AHA of the

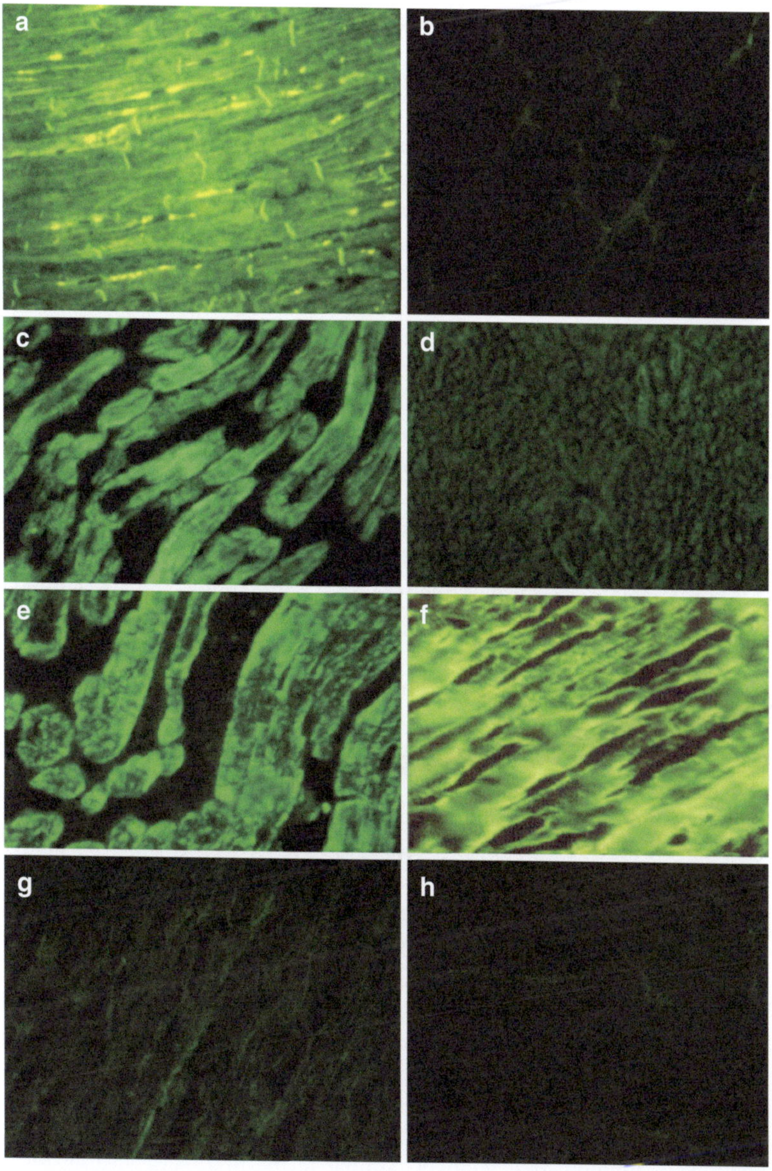

Fig. 10.1 Anti-heart aabs (AHA) patterns by indirect immunofluorescence test (reprint with permission from reference 51). *Organ-specific AHA and AIDA pattern:* panel (**a**) on human heart tissue: cytoplasmic diffuse staining of cardiac myocytes (organ-specific AHA pattern) and linear staining of the intercalated disks (AIDA pattern) (x400); panel (**b**) (x400) on human skeletal muscle tissue: negative. *Partially organ-specific (or cross-reactive 1) AHA pattern:* panel (**c**) on human heart tissue: strongly positive fine striational pattern (x400), and panel (**d**) on human skeletal muscle: weak positive fine striational pattern (x400). *Entirely cross-reactive (or cross-reactive 2) AHA pattern:* panel (**e**) on human heart tissue: strong positive broad striational (myasthenic) pattern (x400), and panel (**f**) on human skeletal muscle: broad striational (myasthenic) pattern (x400). *Negative AHA control serum pattern*: panel (**g**) on human heart tissue: negative (x400), and panel (**h**) on human skeletal muscle: negative (x400)

cross-reactive 1 type, partially cardiac-specific by absorption, gave a fine striational staining pattern on myocytes, but were negative or weakly stained skeletal muscle (Fig. 10.1, panels c, d), and were also more frequently detected in DCM/myocarditis than in controls. On the other hand, AHA of the cross-reactive 2 type, entirely skeletal muscle cross-reactive by absorption, gave a broad striational "myasthenic" pattern on heart and skeletal muscle (Fig. 10.1, panels e, f), and were found in similar proportions among groups [53, 68, 69, 79]. Anti-intercalated disk aabs (AIDA), giving a linear staining on cardiomyocytes (Fig. 10.1, panel a), are associated with myocarditis/DCM and with idiopathic recurrent acute pericarditis [137].

Clinical and Diagnostic Role of AHA in Symptom-Free DCM Relatives In autoimmune disorders, circulating aabs identify symptom-free subjects at risk years before clinical presentation. So far, the clinical and prognostic significance of cardiac aabs has been prospectively assessed only for AHA in symptom-free relatives of DCM index patients, not for the other published aabs shown in Table 10.2. In particular, healthy relatives of patients with DCM who have echocardiographic changes, including left ventricular enlargement (LVE) or depressed fractional shortening (dFS) at baseline, have increased medium-term risk for DCM development [142]. Approximately one-third of relatives from both familial and nonfamilial pedigrees have serum AHA at baseline [52]. AHA are independent predictors of DCM development in symptom-free relatives at 5 year follow-up [53] . In this study, baseline evaluation, including electrocardiography, echocardiography, and AHA, was performed in 592 asymptomatic relatives of 169 consecutive DCM patients (291 males, aged 36 ± 16 years) [53]. Relatives were classified in accordance with published echocardiographic criteria; those who did not have DCM were followed up (median of 58 months). DCM among relatives was diagnosed by echocardiography at follow-up. Of the 592 individuals evaluated, 77% were assessed as normal, 4.4% as having DCM, and 19% as possibly affected on the basis of dFS without ventricular dilatation in 17 and LVE without systolic dysfunction in 94. Five-year follow-up of 311 relatives revealed that 26 had progressed (13 to DCM, 11 to LVE, and 2 to dFS). Relatives who developed DCM were more frequently AHA-positive than those who did not (69% versus 37%, $P = 0.02$). Five-year probability of progression to DCM, among normal or possibly affected relatives, was higher in AHA-positive cases ($P = 0.03$). By Cox regression, positive AHA at baseline were independent predictors of progression (RR 2.26, CI 1 to 5.1, $P = 0.03$). Thus, it was suggested that LVE and dFS represent early, preclinical DCM or asymptomatic left ventricular dysfunction in symptom-free relatives, similar to the first-phase insulin response (FPIR) to intravenous glucose in prediabetes [53] AHA, similar to islet cell aabs in preclinical diabetes, preceded other diagnostic abnormalities of heart dysfunction. Positive AHA status alone had higher sensitivity (61%) than its combination with abnormal echocardiogram (sensitivity 27%) as a predictor of progression to DCM, LVE, or dFS. In other words, positive AHAs with a normal echocardiogram identified a proportion of relatives at risk of progression to DCM, or of progression from normal to preclinical DCM (e.g., LVE or dFS), that would not have been identified by echocardiography alone. Both techniques are necessary in DCM family screen-

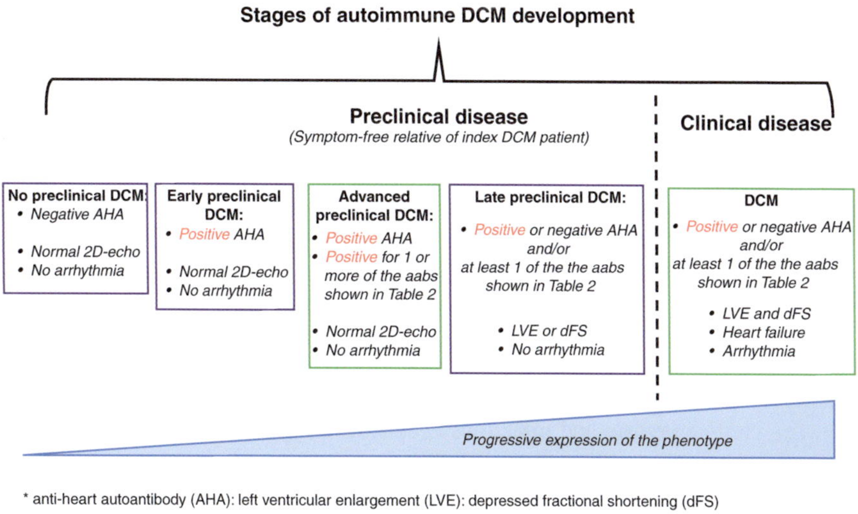

Fig. 10.2 Stages of autoimmune DCM development

ing and counseling. In fact, the positive predictive value (PPV) for progression to DCM was higher (18%) for both abnormal echocardiogram and positive AHA than for AHA alone (7%) or echocardiogram alone (10%). Similarly, the PPV for any progression (e.g., DCM, LVE, or dFS) was higher (18%) or both an abnormal echocardiogram and positive AHA than for AHA alone (13%) or echocardiogram alone (10%). The combination of abnormal echocardiography and positive AHA seemed to identify relatives at a more advanced stage of preclinical DCM, who need closer follow-up and could potentially benefit from therapeutic intervention to attenuate or prevent disease development. Negative AHAs alone or in combination with a normal echocardiogram had a good negative predictive value (98%) and allowed the identification of the majority of subjects at low risk of progression at least up to 5 years [53]. An important issue that needs further study is the long-term outcome of these AHA-negative relatives with normal echocardiograms. In type 1 diabetes mellitus, a staging of preclinical disease has been proposed for siblings of affected children based on a combination of the initial number of antibodies and FPIR to intravenous glucose, by analogy, if the same applies to DCM, the staging could be as shown in Fig. 10.2: no pre-DCM (negative AHAs, normal echocardiogram), early (positive AHAs, normal echocardiogram), advanced (AHA-positive and positivity for 1 or more of the other antibodies described in DCM), and late pre-DCM (at least 1 antibody marker and LVE or dFS). Although 98% of relatives with negative AHAs and normal echocardiograms did not progress up to 5 years, a long latency period and slow progression are features of organ-specific autoimmune disease, and therefore, a proportion of them may develop AHA in the future, thus becoming at risk [53]. Longer follow-up is needed to completely reassure these subjects, and it may be appropriate to provide echocardiographic and immunologic testing, although less frequently than for those with AHAs and/or abnormal echocardiography [53].

These recommendations have been incorporated in a recent expert consensus paper on DCM of the ESC working group on myocardial and pericardial diseases [12].

Autoantigens Recognized by AHA Although Aabs to α and β myosin heavy chain (MHC) have been detected by several groups and various techniques (Table 10.2), including enzyme-linked immunosorbent assay (ELISA) and immunoblotting, it has been shown that α and β MHC isoforms are two of the autoantigens recognized by the AHA detected by s-I IFL in DCM and in myocarditis [66, 69–72, 130]. The α isoform is exclusively expressed within the atrial myocardium, thus aabs to this molecule are organ-specific. In some studies the antimyosin aabs were associated with deterioration of cardiac function [72] or with negative inotropic effect in vitro [66]. Myosin is an intracellular protein. Major hypotheses to explain interruption of tolerance to myosin include molecular mimicry, since cross-reactive epitopes between cardiac myosin and infectious agents have been found, myocyte necrosis due to viral infection or other noxae [6], and cross-reactive mimicry between cardiac myosin and the β_1-adrenergic receptor, resulting in apoptosis of cardiac myocytes [43]. In some murine strains, e.g., Balb/c mice, Coxackie B3 virus-induced, or myosin-induced myocarditis is T cell-mediated [42], whereas in other strains, e.g., DBA/2 mice, it is an antibody-mediated [97] . These data have led to the hypothesis that the antimyosin aabs may be directly pathogenic in some, but not all patients with myocarditis/DCM according to different immunogenetic backgrounds, isotype [97], and/or subclass specificity of these aabs [72].

10.6.2 Aabs to β-Adrenergic and M_2: Muscarinic Receptors

Fu et al. showed anti-M2 aabs in 39% of DCM sera and 7% of the normal subjects by ELISA, using as antigen a synthetic peptide analogous to the 169–193 sequence of the second extra cellular loop of human M2 muscarinic receptors [93]. A significant inhibitory activity, attributed to anti-β_1-adrenoceptor IgG antibodies, was reported in 30–75% of DCM sera, 37% of disease controls, and 18% of sera from normal subjects by other groups, using a binding inhibition assay on rat cardiac membranes [73, 74]. Magnusson et al., using as antigens synthetic peptides analogous to the sequences of the second extra cellular loop of β_1- and β_2-adrenergic receptors by ELISA, found aabs in 31% of DCM patients, 12% of normal subjects and in none of the disease controls [75].

Antibody positive DCM sera [73] or the affinity purified β_1-receptor aabs [75] increased the beating frequency of isolated neonatal rat myocytes in vitro. β_1-blocking drugs inhibited the effect of the aabs. Stimulating anti β_1-receptor aabs were described in 96% of myocarditis, 26–95% of DCM sera, 8–10% of controls with ischemic heart disease, and 0–19% of normal individuals (Table 10.2). Functional fluorescence resonance energy transfer (FRET) assay using novel cAMP-sensors, a recent, sensitive screening technique for the detection of functional β_1-adrenoceptor aabs, is employed in the on-going prospective ETiCS-study in patients with biopsy-proven myocarditis [99, 101, 139, 143].

10.6.3 Cardiodepressant Aabs

Functional cardiodepressant aabs have been described in DCM sera using an in vitro bioassay system and isolated rat cardiomyocytes as antibody targets [78, 104]. The negative inotropic effect of these aabs, which may predict hemodynamic benefits from immunoadsorption (IA) therapy in DCM [139], could be mediated by binding of their FC fragments to cardiac FCgamma IIa receptors [140].

10.6.4 Aabs to Other Sarcolemmal Autoantigens and Heat Shock Proteins (HSP)

AAbs to heat shock proteins (HSP)-60 and HSP-70 [132, 134] and to troponin I and T have also been detected in DCM (Table 10.2) [105–107] . Cardiac troponin would be an organ-specific cardiac autoantigen, but the disease-specificity for myocarditis/DCM as compared to ischemic heart disease is not entirely clear [144]. Anti-Na-K-ATPase aabs were found by ELISA in 26% of DCM and in 2% of normal subjects, using porcine cerebral cortex sarcolemmal Na-K-ATPase as antigen, and were independently associated with cardiac sudden death [90]. On the basis of this association the authors hypothesized that the aabs might lead to electrical instability, because of abnormal Ca^{2+} handling by reduced Na-K-ATPase activity. Sarcolemmal Na-K-ATPase is not an organ-specific cardiac autoantigen [40].

10.6.5 Aabs to Mitochondrial Antigens

Aabs to several mitochondrial antigens were described, including the M7 [91], the adenine nucleotide translocator (ANT) [84, 135, 136] and the branched chain α-ketoacid dehydrogenase dihydrolipoyl transacylase (BCKD-E2) [92]. The M7 antibodies of IgG class, assessed by ELISA using beef heart mitochondria as antigenic substrate, were found in 31% of DCM patients, 13% of those with myocarditis, 33% of controls with hypertrophic cardiomyopathy, and were absent in controls with other cardiac disease, immune-mediated disorders, or in normal subjects [91]. ANT, a protein of the internal mitochondrial membrane, was purified from beef heart, liver, and kidney and used as antigen in a indirect micro solid-phase radioimmunoassay (SPRIA); anti-ANT antibodies were found in 57–91% of myocarditis/DCM sera, and in ischemic heart disease, or in normal subjects [91, 135, 136]. Although mitochondrial antigens have generally been classified as non-organ specific, the heart-specificity of the M7 aabs was shown by absorption studies. Experimentally induced affinity-purified anti-ANT antibodies cross-reacted with calcium channel complex proteins of rat cardiac myocytes, induced enhancement of transmembrane calcium current, and produced calcium-dependent cell lysis in the absence of complement [136]. Antibody-dependent cell lysis has not been reported using the aabs from patients' sera.

10.7 Immunosuppression to Treat Autoimmune Myocarditis/DCM

A major feature of autoimmune disease is its response to immunosuppressive therapy (Table 10.1). Current evidence shows benefit of immunosuppression in chronic virus-negative myocarditis/DCM [35, 103], in giant cell myocarditis [67], and in active autoimmune myocarditis (e.g., virus-negative and positive for cardiac aabs) [20], using a combination of azathioprine, steroids, and/or cyclosporine A. Conversely, immunosuppression had a neutral effect in the Myocarditis Treatment Trial, in myocarditis of unspecified etiology [34]. Immunosuppression is recommended by 2013 ESC Task Force experts [33] in proven autoimmune myocarditis forms, such as giant cell myocarditis [67], cardiac sarcoidosis [145], and virus-negative myocarditis associated with systemic immune-mediated disease [146] (Fig. 10.3). Steroids are indicated in cardiac sarcoidosis and in virus-negative eosinophilic or toxic myocarditis, with heart failure and arrhythmia [36, 147]. Immunosuppression may also be considered in virus-negative myocarditis refractory to standard therapy with no contraindications to immunosuppression [36, 103] (Fig. 10.3).

10.8 The Quest for New Treatments Targeting Functional Aabs

Potential new treatments targeting functional aabs in myocarditis/DCM [78, 139], as for other autoimmune disorders [148–152], include design of specific epitope-derived peptides to be used as antibody-scavengers, direct targeting/suppression of aab-producing B cells, and/or plasma-cells and immunoadsorption (IA) [77, 78, 97–100, 104, 139, 153–158]. IA is aimed at the removal of pathogenic aabs through the extracorporeal removal of patient immunoglobulin following plasmapheresis. IA is followed by supplemental administration of intravenous immunoglobulin to prevent infection or antibody production rebound [155–157]. A proportion of patients do not respond to IA which has limited its potential use; in addition, the therapy is expensive and requires an invasive procedure. It was reported that a subset of DCM patients with serum cardiodepressant aabs were responders to IA [104, 128]. The baseline presence of cardiodepressant antibodies in combination with myocardial gene expression profiles was found to improve prediction of treatment outcome [158].

10.9 Future Research Directions: Cell-Mediated Immunity and Cytokine Networks

Regulatory T cells (FOXP3, CD25, CD4+ cells) and Th17 cells are emerging as key players in development and fate of experimentally induced myocarditis [159]. Passive transfer of Treg induced disease remission in a mice with virus-induced

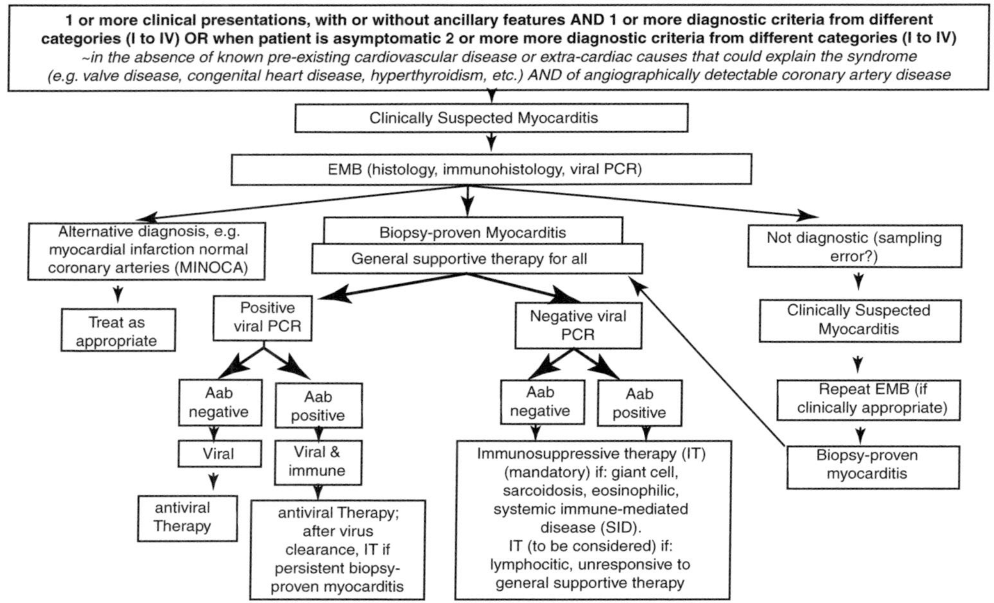

Fig. 10.3 Diagnostic workup and etiology-based management in myocarditis according to ESC 2013 Task Force criteria. Biopsy-proven myocarditis (acute or chronic, lymphocytic or other inflammatory infiltrate) = Dallas criteria positive (active or borderline myocarditis) and/or immunohistology positive, with positive or negative viral polymerase chain reaction (PCR) on endomyocardial biopsy (EMB), with or without a DCM clinical phenotype, with normal or depressed biventricular function. Specific myocarditis types would also be included in this definition according to standard histopathological diagnosis (e.g., giant cell, eosinophilic, polymorphic, granulomatous myocarditis). *Not diagnostic* Not diagnostic for myocarditis according to the Dallas histological criteria (or technically inadequate for histological diagnosis). A proportion of these cases may represent EMB false-negatives, thus clinical follow-up is recommended, and EMB may be repeated if clinically indicated. *No myocarditis* (*Alternative diagnosis*) Histological diagnosis alternative to myocarditis or DCM, e.g., cardiac amyloid, arrhythmogenic right ventricular cardiomyopathy, etc. This would reject the clinical suspicion of myocarditis and establish an alternative diagnosis. *EMB* endomyocardial biopsy, *PCR* polymerase chain reaction, *Aab* cardiac autoantibody

myocarditis [160]. Knockout models of Th17 cell-induced myocarditis hold promise for testing anti-IL17 monoclonal antibodies as therapeutic agents in experimental autoimmune myocarditis [161]. The role of these lymphocytic subtypes has not not yet explored in human biopsy-proven myocarditis. A role for T cells in humans is suggested by case reports of biopsy-proven or clinically suspected autoimmune myocarditis occurring in oncology patients treated with biologic agents, including anti-PD1, anti-CTLA-4, and anti-CD20 agents [162, 163]. A case of biopsy-proven rituximab-induced myocarditis has also been published [164]. However, in the this case, tissue PCR was positive for enteroviral genome, so it is possible that myocarditis was triggered by the immunosuppressive action of the anti-CD20 monoclonal antibody (MoAb) rather than by autoimmunity. Our group has reported a case of autoimmune giant cell myocarditis recurrence in a transplanted patient, refractory to standard immunosuppression, that was successfully treated with rituximab [165]. Therefore it seems mandatory that new treatments are tested in clinical trials recruiting patients with biopsy-proven autoimmune myocarditis.

In theory, immune-modulatory agents might influence systemic and organ-specific cytokine/lymphokine networks leading to cardiac dysfunction even in the absence of myocardial inflammatory infiltrates [166]. Future studies in patients should better clarify the cytokine and cellular networks fostering chronic myocarditis, as well as the final effector mechanisms of myocyte necrosis and/or dysfunction. Reversible severe ventricular dysfunction may be induced by cardio depressant factors in the absence or with minimal myocyte necrosis, in septic shock [167], Cushing's syndrome [168], pheocromocytoma, or Takotsubo cardiomyopathy [169, 170]. In addition, several groups have shown a pathogenic role for circulating cardiac Aabs in chronic DCM, in the absence of florid myocardial inflammation on EMB [43, 47, 65, 66, 71, 73–78, 81, 85, 86, 89, 94, 95, 100, 104, 105, 119, 128, 131, 136, 139–141, 156–158]. We may speculate that an "immune-mediated myocardial stunning/hibernation phenomenon" occurs in acute and/or chronic myocarditis/DCM, which, if reversed by tailored immune therapies before the occurrence of irreversible myocardial damage, could be clinically beneficial.

In conclusion, due to the complexity of the immune network in autoimmune myocarditis, future immunomodulatory trials will probably be designed for distinct patient subsets according to their specific cytokine and/or cellular immune biomarker profiles, e.g., personalized immune intervention.

References

1. Rose NR, et al. Defining criteria for autoimmune diseases (Witebsky's postulates revisited). Immunol Today. 1993;14:426–8.
2. The Wellcome Trust Case Control Consortium. Genome-wide association study of 14,000 cases of seven common diseases and shared controls. Nature. 2007;447:661–83.
3. The International Multiple Sclerosis Genetics Consortium. Risk alleles for multiple sclerosis identified by a genomewide study. N Engl J Med. 2007;357:1–12.

4. Todd JA, Genetics of type 1 diabetes in Finland, Simmonds MJ, Heward JM, Gough SC, Wellcome Trust case control consortium, Dunger DB, Wicker LS, Clayton DG, et al. Robust associations of four new chromosome regions from genome-wide analyses of type 1 diabetes. Nat Genet. 2007;39:857–64.
5. Lowe CE, et al. Large-scale genetic fine mapping and genotype-phenotype associations implicate a polymorphism in the IL2RA region in type 1 diabetes. Nat Genet. 2007;39:1074–82.
6. Rose NR. Myocarditis: infection versus autoimmunity. J Clin Immunol. 2009;29:730–7.
7. Caforio ALP, Marcolongo R, Malipiero G, Agostini C, Seguso M, Gallo N, Plebani M, Iliceto S. Organ-specific autoimmune myocardial diseases: from pathogenesis to diagnosis and management. In: Nussinovitch U, editor. The heart in rheumatologic, inflammatory and autoimmune diseases. Amsterdam: Elsevier; 2017. p. 25–43.
8. Richardson P, et al. Report of the 1995 World Health Organization/International Society and Federation of Cardiology Task Force on the definition and classification of cardiomyopathies. Circulation. 1996;93:841–2.
9. Jefferies JL, et al. Dilated cardiomyopathy. Lancet. 2010;375:752–62.
10. Aretz HT, et al. Myocarditis: a histopathologic definition and classification. Am J Cardiol Pathol. 1985;1:1–10.
11. Magnani JW, et al. Myocarditis. Current trends in diagnosis and treatment. Circulation. 2006;113:876–90.
12. Pinto Y, et al. Proposal for a revised definition of dilated diomyopathy, hypokinetic non-dilated cardiomyopathy, and its implications for clinical practice: a position statement of the ESC working group on myocardial and pericardial diseases. Eur Heart J. 2016;37:1850–8.
13. Schultheiss HP, Fairweather D, Caforio ALP, Escher F, Hershberger RE, Lipshultz SE, Liu PP, Matsumori A, Mazzanti A, McMurray J, Priori SG. Dilated cardiomyopathy. Nat Rev Dis Primers. 2019;5(1):32.
14. Angelini A, et al. Active versus borderline myocarditis: clinicopathological correlates and prognostic implications. Heart. 2002;87:210–5.
15. Angelini A, et al. Myocarditis mimicking acute myocardial infarction: role of endomyocardial biopsy in the differential diagnosis. Heart. 2000;84:245–50.
16. Maisch B, et al. Immunosuppressive and immunomodulatory treatment for myocarditis. Curr Opin Cardiol. 1996;11:310–24.
17. Yajima T, et al. Viral myocarditis:from the perspective of the virus. Circulation. 2009;119:2615–24.
18. Calabrese F, et al. Myocarditis and inflammatory cardiomyopathy: microbiological and molecular aspects. Cardiovasc Pathol. 2003;60:11–25.
19. Caforio ALP, et al. A prospective study of biopsy-proven myocarditis: prognostic relevance of clinical and etiopathogenetic features at diagnosis. Eur Heart J. 2007;28:1326–33.
20. Mahrholdt H, et al. Cardiovascular magnetic resonance assessment of human myocarditis: a comparison to histology and molecular pathology. Circulation. 2004;109:1250–8.
21. Bock CT, et al. Human parvovirus B19-associated myocarditis. N Engl J Med. 2010;362: 1248–9.
22. Liu P, et al. Viral myocarditis: balance between viral infection and immune response. Can J Cardiol. 1996;12:935–43.
23. Cambridge G, et al. Antibodies to Coxsackieviruses in congestive cardiomyopathy. Br Heart J. 1979;41:692–6.
24. Baboonian C, et al. Meta-analysis of the association of enteroviruses with human heart disease. Heart. 1997;78:539–43.
25. Schultheiss HP, et al. The management of myocarditis. Eur Heart J. 2011;32:2616–25.
26. Maisch B, et al. Cytomegalovirus associated inflammatory heart muscle disease. Scan J Infect Dis. 1993;88:135–48.
27. Martin AB, et al. Acute myocarditis, rapid diagnosis by PCR in children. Circulation. 1994;90:330–9.
28. Matsumori A, et al. Dilated cardiomyopathy associated with hepatitis C infection. Circulation. 1995;92:2519–225.

29. Pankuweit S, et al. Prevalence of parvovirus B 19 genome in endomyocardial biopsy specimen. Hum Pathol. 2003;34:80–6.
30. Kühl U, et al. High prevalence of viral genomes and multiple viral infections in the myocardium of adults with "idiopathic" left ventricular dysfunction. Circulation. 2005;111:887–93.
31. Kühl U, et al. Viral persistence in the myocardium is associated with progressive cardiac dysfunction. Circulation. 2005;112:1965–70.
32. Bowles NE, et al. Detection of viruses in myocardial tissues by polymerase chain reaction: evidence of adenovirus as a common cause of myocarditis in children and adults. J Am Coll Cardiol. 2003;42:466–72.
33. Magnani JW, et al. Survival in biopsy-proven myocarditis: a long-term retrospective analysis of the histopathological, clinical, and hemodynamic predictors. Am Heart J. 2006;151:463–70.
34. Mason JW, et al. A clinical trial of immunosuppressive therapy for myocarditis. N Engl J Med. 1995;333:269–75.
35. Frustaci A, et al. Immunosuppressive therapy for active lymphocytic myocarditis: virological and immunologic profile of responders versus nonresponders. Circulation. 2003;107:857–63.
36. Caforio ALP, et al. Current state of knowledge on aetiology, diagnosis, management and therapy of myocarditis. A position statement of the European Society of Cardiology Working Group on myocardial and pericardial diseases. Eur Heart J. 2013;34:2636–48.
37. Huber SA, et al. Enteroviruses and myocarditis: viral pathogenesis through replication, cytokine induction, and immunopathogenicity. Adv Virus Res. 1999;51:35–68.
38. Klingel K, et al. Ongoing enterovirus-induced myocarditis is associated with persistent heart muscle infection: quantitative analysis of virus replication, tissue damage, and inflammation. Proc Natl Acad Sci U S A. 1992;89(1):314–8.
39. MacLellan RW, et al. Dilated cardiomyopathy: learning to live with yourself. Nat Med. 2003;9:1455–6.
40. Rose NR. Viral damage or 'molecular mimicry'– placing the blame in myocarditis. Nat Med. 2000;6:631–2.
41. Neu N, et al. Cardiac myosin induces myocarditis in genetically predisposed mice. J Immunol. 1987;139:3630–6.
42. Smith SC, et al. Myosin-induced myocarditis is a T cell-mediated disease. J Immunol. 1991;147:2141–7.
43. Li Y, et al. Mimicry and antibody-mediated cell signaling in autoimmune myocarditis. J Immunol. 2006;177:8234–40.
44. Kodama M, et al. Rat dilated cardiomyopathy after autoimmune giant cell myocarditis. Circ Res. 1994;75:278–84.
45. Taneja V, et al. Spontaneous myocarditis mimicking human disease occurs in the presence of an appropriate MHC and non-MHC background in transgenic mice. J Mol Cell Cardiol. 2007;42:1054–64.
46. Elliott JF, et al. Autoimmune cardiomyopathy and heart block develop spontaneously in HLA-DQ8 transgenic IAbeta knockout NOD mice. Proc Natl Acad Sci U S A. 2003;100:13447–52.
47. Satoh M, et al. MyD88 signaling controls autoimmune myocarditis induction. Circulation. 2006; 113:258–265
48. Lv H, et al. Impaired thymic tolerance to α-myosin directs autoimmunity to the heartin mice and humans. J Clin Invest. 2011;121:1561–73.
49. Guler ML, et al. Two autoimmune diabetes loci influencing T cell apoptosis control susceptibility to experimental autoimmune myocarditis. J Immunol. 2005;174:2167–73.
50. Ono M, et al. Control of autoimmune myocarditis and multiorgan inflammation by glucocorticoid-induced TNF receptor family-related protein high, Foxp3-expressing $CD25^+$ and $CD25^-$ regulatory T cells. J Immunol. 2006;176:4748–56.
51. Caforio ALP, et al. Immune-mediated and autoimmune myocarditis: clinical presentation, diagnosis and management. Heart Fail Rev. 2013;18(6):715–32.
52. Caforio ALP, et al. Evidence from family studies for autoimmunity in dilated cardiomyopathy. Lancet. 1994;344:773–7.

53. Caforio ALP, et al. Prospective familial assessment in dilated cardiomyopathy. Cardiac autoantibodies predict disease development in asymptomatic relatives. Circulation. 2007;115:76–83.
54. Limas CJ, et al. Familial clustering of autoimmune diseases in patients with dilated cardiomyopathy. Am J Cardiol. 2004;93:1189–91.
55. Mestroni L, et al. Familial dilated cardiomyopathy:evidence for genetic and phenotypic heterogeneity. J Am Coll Cardiol. 1999;34:181–90.
56. Portig I, et al. Familial inflammatory dilated cardiomyopathy. Eur J Heart Fail. 2006;8:816–25.
57. Jin B, et al. HLA-DR4 antigen and idiopathic dilated cardiomyopathy susceptibility: a meta-analysis involving 11,761 subjects. Tissue Antigens. 2011;77:107–11.
58. Meder B, et al. A genome-wide association study identifies 6p21 as novel risk locus for dilated cardiomyopathy. Eur Heart J. 2014;35:1069–77.
59. Basso C, et al. Arrhythmogenic right ventricular cardiomyopathy: dysplasia, dystrophy or myocarditis? Circulation. 1996;94:983–91.
60. Frustaci A, et al. Myocarditis in hypertrophic cardiomyopathy patients presenting acute clinical deterioration. Eur Heart J. 2007;28:733–40.
61. Frustaci A, et al. Cardiac histological substrate in patients with clinical phenotype of Brugada syndrome. Circulation. 2005;112:3680–7.
62. Mahon NG, et al. Immunohistochemical evidence of myocardial disease in apparently healthy relatives of patients with dilated cardiomyopathy. J Am Coll Cardiol. 2002;39:455–62.
63. Wojnicz R, et al. Randomized, placebo controlled study for immunosuppressive treatment of inflammatory dilated cardiomyopathy. Two-year follow-up results. Circulation. 2001;104:39–45.
64. Kindermann I, et al. Predictors of outcome in patients with suspected myocarditis. Circulation. 2008;118:639–48.
65. Okazaki T, et al. Pathogenic roles of cardiac autoantibodies in dilated cardiomyopathy. Trends Mol Med. 2005;11:322–6.
66. Warraich RS, et al. Human cardiac myosin autoantibodies impair myocyte contractility: a cause-and-effect relationship. FASEB J. 2006;20:651–60.
67. Cooper LT Jr, Giant Cell Myocarditis Treatment Trial Investigators, et al. Usefulness of immunosuppression for giant cell myocarditis. Am J Cardiol. 2008;102(11):1535–9.
68. Caforio ALP, et al. Novel organ-specific circulating cardiac autoantibodies in dilated cardiomyopathy. J Am Coll Cardiol. 1990;15:1527–34.
69. Caforio ALP, et al. Circulating cardiac autoantibodies as markers of autoimmunity in clinical and biopsy-proven myocarditis. Eur Heart J. 1997;18:270–5.
70. Caforio ALP, et al. Identification of α- and β-cardiac myosin heavy chain isoforms as major autoantigens in dilated cardiomyopathy. Circulation. 1992;85:1734–42.
71. Lauer B, et al. Antimyosin autoantibodies are associated with deterioration of systolic and diastolic left ventricular function in patients with chronic myocarditis. J Am Coll Cardiol. 2000;35:11–8.
72. Warraich RS, et al. Subclass specificity of autoantibodies against myosin in patients with idiopathic dilated cardiomyopathy: proinflammatory antibodies in dilated cardiomyopathy patients. Biochem Biophys Res Commun. 1999;259:255–61.
73. Wallukat G, et al. Antibodies against the β-adrenergic receptor in human myocarditis and dilated cardiomyopathy: β-adrenergic agonism without desensitization. Eur Heart J. 1991;12(Suppl D):178–81.
74. Limas CJ, et al. β-receptor antibodies and genetics in dilated cardiomyopathy. Eur Heart J. 1991;12(Suppl D):175–7.
75. Magnusson Y, et al. Autoimmunity in idiopathic dilated cardiomyopathy: characterization of antibodies against the β_1-adrenoceptor with positive chronotropic effect. Circulation. 1994;89:2760–667.
76. Jahns R, et al. Modulation of β1-adrenoceptor activity by domain-specific antibodies and heart-failure associated autoantibodies. J Am Coll Cardiol. 2000;36:1280–7.
77. Muller J, et al. Immunoglobulin adsorption in patients with idiopathic dilated cardiomyopathy. Circulation. 2000;101:385–91.

78. Staudt A, et al. Potential role of autoantibodies belonging to the immunoglobulin G-3 subclass in cardiac dysfunction among patients with dilated cardiomyopathy. Circulation. 2002;106:2448–53.
79. Caforio ALP, et al. Organ-specific cardiac autoantibodies: new serological markers for systemic hypertension in autoimmune polyendocrinopathy. Lancet. 1991;337:1111–5.
80. Nishimura H, et al. Autoimmune dilated cardiomyopathy in PD-1 receptor-deficient mice. Science. 2001;291:319–22.
81. Okazaki T, et al. Autoantibodies against cardiac troponin I are responsible for dilated cardiomyopathy in PD-1-deficient mice. Nat Med. 2003;9:1477–83.
82. Göser S, et al. Cardiac troponin I but not cardiac troponin T induces severe autoimmune inflammation in the myocardium. Circulation. 2006;114:1693–702.
83. Kaya Z, et al. Identification of cardiac troponin I sequence motifs leading to heart failure by induction of myocardial inflammation and fibrosis. Circulation. 2008;118:2063–72.
84. Schultheiss HP, et al. Biomolecular changes in dilated cardiomyopathy. In: Baroldi G, Camerini F, Goodwin JF, editors. Advances in cardiomyopathies. Berlin: Springer; 1990. p. 221–34.
85. Schultheiss HP, et al. Antibody mediated enhancement of calcium permeability in cardiac myocytes. J Exp Med. 1988;168:2105–19.
86. Jahns R, et al. Direct evidence for a β1-adrenergic receptor directed autoimmune attack as a cause of idiopathic dilated cardiomyopathy. J Clin Invest. 2004;113:1419–29.
87. Liu J, et al. Adoptive passive transfer of rabbit beta1-adrenoceptor peptide immune cardiomyopathy into the Rag2−/− mouse: participation of the ER stress. J Mol Cell Cardiol. 2008;44:304–14.
88. Omerovic E, et al. Induction of cardiomyopathy in severe combined immunodeficiency mice by lymphocytes from patients with idiopathic dilated cardiomyopathy. Autoimmunity. 2000;32:271–80.
89. Jahns R, et al. Autoantibodies activating human beta1-adrenergic receptors are associated with reduced cardiac function in chronic heart failure. Circulation. 1999;99(5):649–54.
90. Baba A, et al. Autoantibodies against sarcolemmal Na-K-ATPase: possible upstream targets of arrhythmias and sudden death in patients with dilated cardiomyopathy. J Am Coll Cardiol. 2002;40:1153–9.
91. Klein R, et al. Demonstration of organ specific antibodies against heart mitochondria (anti-M7) in sera from patients with some forms of heart diseases. Clin Exp Immunol. 1984;58:283–92.
92. Ansari AA, et al. Epitope mapping of the branched chain α-ketoacid dehydrogenase dihydrolipoyl transacylase (BCKD-E2) protein that reacts with sera from patients with idiopathic dilated cardiomyopathy. J Immunol. 1994;153:4754–65.
93. Fu LX, et al. Localization of a functional autoimmune epitope on the muscarinic acetylcholine receptor-2 in patients with idiopathic dilated cardiomyopathy. J Clin Invest. 1993;91:1964–8.
94. Fu LXM, et al. A synthetic peptide corresponding to the second extracellular loop of the human M2 acetylcholine receptor induces pharmacological and morphological changes in cardiomyocytes by active immunization after 6 months in rabbits. Clin Immunol Immunopathol. 1996;78:203–7.
95. Jahns R, et al. Targeting receptor-antibodies in immune-cardiomyopathy. Semin Thromb Hemost. 2010;36:212–8.
96. Götz M, et al. Administration of the cyclic peptide COR-1 in humans (phase I study). Ex vivo measurements of anti-beta1-receptor antibody neutralisation and of immune parameters. Eur J Heart Fail. 2012;14(11):1230–9.
97. Kuan AP, et al. Immunoglobulin isotype determines pathogenicity in antibody-mediated myocarditis in naïve mice. Circ Res. 2000;86:281–5.
98. Mao W, et al. Cardiomyocyte apoptosis in autoimmune cardiomyopathy: mediated via endoplasmic reticulum stress and exaggerated by norepinephrine. Am J Physiol Heart Circ Physiol. 2007;293:H1636–45.
99. Nikolaev VO, et al. A novel fluorescent method for the rapid detection of functional beta1-adrenergic receptor autoantibodies in heart failure. J Am Coll Cardiol. 2007;50:423–31.

100. Mobini R, et al. Hemodynamic improvement and removal of autoantibodies against the β1-adrenergic receptor by immunoadsorption therapy in dilated cardiomyopathy. J Autoimmun. 2003;20:345–50.
101. Deubner N, et al. Cardiac beta1-adrenoceptor autoantibodies in human heart disease: rationale and design of the Etiology, Titre-Course, and Survival (ETiCS) Study—on behalf of the ETiCS-Study Group. Eur J Heart Fail. 2010;12:753–62.
102. Caforio ALP, et al. Cardiac autoantibodies in dilated cardiomyopathy become undetectable with disease progression. Heart. 1997;77:62–7.
103. Frustaci A, et al. Randomized study on the efficacy of immunosuppressive therapy in patients with virus-negative inflammatory cardiomyopathy: the TIMIC study. Eur Heart J. 2009;30:1995–2002.
104. Felix SB, et al. Removal of cardiodepressant antibodies in dilated cardiomyopathy by immunoadsorption. J Am Coll Cardiol. 2002;39:646–52.
105. Landsberger M, et al. Potential role of antibodies against cardiac Kv channel-interacting protein 2 in dilated cardiomyopathy. Am Heart J. 2008;156:92–9.
106. Leuschner F, et al. Absence of auto-antibodies against cardiac troponin I predicts improvement of left ventricular function after acute myocardial infarction. Eur Heart J. 2008;29:1949–55.
107. Shmilovich H, et al. Autoantibodies to cardiac troponin I in patients with idiopathic dilated and ischemic cardiomyopathy. Int J Cardiol. 2007;117:198–203.
108. Maisch B, et al. Diagnostic relevance of humoral and cytotoxic immune reactions in primary and secondary dilated cardiomyopathy. Am J Cardiol. 1983;52:1072–8.
109. Neumann DA, et al. Circulating heart-reactive antibodies in patients with myocarditis or cardiomyopathy. J Am Coll Cardiol. 1990;16:839–46.
110. Fletcher GF, et al. Autoimmune studies in patients with primary myocardial disease. Circulation. 1968;37:1032–5.
111. Kirsner AB, et al. Immunologic findings in idiopathic cardiomyopathy: a prospective serial study. Am Heart J. 1973;86:625–30.
112. Borda ES, et al. Antiadrenergic and muscarinic receptor antibodies in Chagas' cardiomyopathy. Int J Cardiol. 1996;54:149–56.
113. Christ T, et al. Autoantibodies against the beta1 adrenoceptor from patients with dilated cardiomyopathy prolong action potential duration and enhance contractility in isolated cardiomyocytes. J Mol Cell Cardiol. 2001;33:1515–25.
114. Iwata M, et al. Autoantibodies against the second extracellular loop of beta1-adrenergic receptors predict ventricular tachycardia and sudden death in patients with idiopathic dilated cardiomyopathy. J Am Coll Cardiol. 2001;37:418–24.
115. Matsui S, et al. Dilated cardiomyopathy defines serum autoantibodies against G-protein-coupled cardiovascular receptors. Autoimmunity. 1995;21:85–8.
116. Matsui S, et al. Characteristic distribution of circulating autoantibodies against G-protein coupled cardiovascular receptors in patients with idiopathic dilated and hypertrophic cardiomyopathy. Int J Cardiol. 1996;54:143–7.
117. Staudt Y, et al. Beta1-adrenoceptor antibodies induce apoptosis in adult isolated cardiomyocytes. Eur J Pharmacol. 2003;466:1–6.
118. Stavrakis S, et al. Opposing cardiac effects of autoantibody activation of beta-adrenergic and M2 muscarinic receptors in cardiac-related diseases. Int J Cardiol. 2011;148:331–6.
119. Wallukat G, et al. Anti-beta 1-adrenoceptor autoantibodies with chronotropic activity from the serum of patients with dilated cardiomyopathy: mapping of epitopes in the first and second extracellular loops. J Mol Cell Cardiol. 1995;27:397–406.
120. Zhang L, et al. Autoantibodies against the myocardial beta1-adrenergic and M2-muscarinic receptors in patients with congestive heart failure. Chin Med J. 2002;115:1127–31.
121. Chiale PA, et al. High prevalence of antibodies against beta 1- and beta 2-adrenoceptors in patients with primary electrical cardiac abnormalities. J Am Coll Cardiol. 1995;26:864–9.
122. Sterin-Borda L, et al. Antibodies to beta 1 and beta 2 adrenoreceptors in Chagas' disease. Clin Exp Immunol. 1988;74:349–54.

123. Baba A, et al. Autoantibodies against M2-muscarinic acetylcholine receptors: new upstream targets in atrial fibrillation in patients with dilated cardiomyopathy. Eur Heart J. 2004;25:1108–15.
124. Chiale PA, et al. Autoantibodies in Chagas' cardiomyopathy and arrhythmias. Autoimmunity. 2001;34:205–10.
125. Fu ML. Characterization of anti-heart M2 muscarinic receptor antibodies--a combined clinical and experimental study. Mol Cell Biochem. 1996;163-164:343–7.
126. Liu HR, et al. Screening of serum autoantibodies to cardiac beta1-adrenoceptors and M2-muscarinic acetylcholine receptors in 408 healthy subjects of varying ages. Autoimmunity. 1999;29:43–51.
127. Wallukat G, et al. Autoantibodies against the beta- and muscarinic receptors in cardiomyopathy. Herz. 2000;25:261–6.
128. Staudt A, et al. Fcgamma-receptor IIa polymorphism and the role of immunoadsorption in cardiac dysfunction in patients with dilated cardiomyopathy. Clin Pharmacol Ther. 2010;87:452–8.
129. Trimpert C, et al. Immunoadsorption in dilated cardiomyopathy: long-term reduction of cardiodepressant antibodies. Eur J Clin Investig. 2010;40:685–91.
130. Goldman JH, et al. Autoimmunity to alpha myosin in a subset of patients with idiopathic dilated cardiomyopathy. Br Heart J. 1995;74:598–603.
131. Warraich RS, et al. Immunoglobulin G3 cardiac myosin autoantibodies correlate with left ventricular dysfunction in patients with dilated cardiomyopathy: immunoglobulin G3 and clinical correlates. Am Heart J. 2002;143:1076–84.
132. Latif N, et al. Frequency and specificity of antiheart antibodies in patients with dilated cardiomyopathy detected using SDS-PAGE and western blotting. J Am Coll Cardiol. 1993;22:1378–84.
133. Wolff PG, et al. Laminin distribution and autoantibodies to laminin in dilated cardiomyopathy and myocarditis. Am Heart J. 1989;117:1303–9.
134. Portig I, et al. Antibodies against stress proteins in sera of patients with dilated cardiomyopathy. J Mol Cell Cardiol. 1997;29:2245–51.
135. Schultheiss HP, et al. Immunological analysis of auto-antibodies against the adenine nucleotide translocator in dilated cardiomyopathy. J Mol Cell Cardiol. 1985;17:603–17.
136. Schulze K, et al. Antibodies to ADP-ATP carrier--an autoantigen in myocarditis and dilated cardiomyopathy-impair cardiac function. Circulation. 1990;81:959–69.
137. Caforio AL, et al. High frequency of circulating anti-heart and anti-intercalated disc autoantibodies: evidence for autoimmunity in idiopathic recurrent acute pericarditis. Heart. 2010;96:779–84.
138. Störk S, et al. Stimulating autoantibodies directed against the cardiac beta1-adrenergic receptor predict increased mortality in idiopathic cardiomyopathy. Am Heart J. 2006;152:697–704.
139. Staudt A, et al. Potential role of humoral immunity in cardiac dysfunction of patients suffering from dilated cardiomyopathy. J Am Coll Cardiol. 2004;44:829–36.
140. Staudt A, et al. Fc(gamma) receptors IIa on cardiomyocytes and their potential functional relevance in dilated cardiomyopathy. J Am Coll Cardiol. 2007;49:1684–92.
141. Caforio AL, et al. Passive transfer of affinity-purified anti-heart autoantibodies (AHA) from sera of patients with myocarditis induces experimental myocarditis in mice. Int J Cardiol. 2015;179:166–77.
142. Mahon NG, Murphy RT, Macrae C, Caforio A, Elliott PM, Mckenna WJ. Echocardiographic screening in asymptomatic relatives of dilated cardiomyopathy patients reveals preclinical disease. Ann Intern Med. 2005;143:108–15.
143. Bornholz B, et al. A standardised FACS assay based on native, receptor transfected cells for the clinical diagnosis and monitoring of β1-adrenergic receptor autoantibodies in human heart disease. Clin Chem Lab Med. 2015;54:683–91. https://doi.org/10.1515/cclm-2015-0603.
144. Jahns R. Autoantibodies directed against cardiac troponin I—friend or foe? (Editorial). Eur J Heart Fail. 2010;12:645–8.
145. Sekhri V, et al. Cardiac sarcoidosis: a comprehensive review. Arch Med Sci. 2011;7(4):546–54.

146. Caforio A, Adler Y, Agostini C, Allanore Y, Anastasakis A, Arad M, Böhm M, Charron P, Pm E, Eriksson U, Felix S, Garcia-Pavia P, Hachulla E, Heymans S, Imazio M, Klingel K, Marcolongo R, Matucci Cerinic M, Pantazis A, Plein S, Poli V, Rigopoulos A, Seferovic P, Shoenfeld Y, Zamorano J, Linhart A. Diagnosis and management of myocardial involvement in systemic immune-mediated diseases: a position statement of the ESC working group on myocardial and pericardial disease. Eur Heart J. 2017;38:2649–62.
147. Japanese Circulation Society (JCS) Joint Working Group. Guidelines for diagnosis and treatment of myocarditis. Circ J. 2011;75:734–43.
148. Warren KG, et al. Intravenous synthetic peptide MBP8298 delayed disease progression in an HLA class II-defined cohort of patients with progressive multiple sclerosis: results of a 24-month double-blind placebo-controlled clinical trial and 5 years of follow-up treatment. Eur J Neurol. 2006;13(8):887–95.
149. Tzartos SJ, et al. Antigen-specific apheresis of pathogenic autoantibodies from myasthenia gravis sera. Ann N Y Acad Sci. 2008;1132:291–9.
150. Bygren P, et al. Goodpasture's syndrome treated with staphylococcal protein A immunoadsorption. Lancet. 1985;2:1295–6.
151. Palmer A, et al. Treatment of systemic lupus erythematosus by extracorporeal immunoadsorption. Lancet. 1988;2:272.
152. Neubert K, et al. The proteasome inhibitor bortezomib depletes plasma cells and protects mice with lupus-like disease from nephritis. Nat Med. 2008;14:748–55.
153. Jahns R, et al. A new cyclic receptor-peptide prevents development of heart dilatation and failure induced by antibodies activating cardiac beta1-adrenergic receptors. Circulation. 2005;112(suppl II)
154. Ungerer M, et al. First administration of COR-1 in man—a cyclic peptide which neutralizes anti-beta1-receptor antibodies in heart failure. Circulation. 2010;122(21 Supplement):A 19730.
155. Felix SB, et al. Hemodynamic effects of immunoadsorption and subsequent immunoglobulin substitution in dilated cardiomyopathy: three-month results from a randomized study. J Am Coll Cardiol. 2000;35(6):1590–8.
156. Staudt A, et al. Immunohistological changes in dilated cardiomyopathy induced by immunoadsorption therapy and subsequent immunoglobulin substitution. Circulation. 2001;103:2681–6.
157. Felix SB, et al. Immunoadsorption therapy in dilated cardiomyopathy. Expert Rev Cardiovasc Ther. 2015;13:145–52.
158. Ameling S, et al. Myocardial gene expression profiles and cardiodepressant autoantibodies predict response of patients with dilated cardiomyopathy to immunoadsorption therapy. Eur Heart J. 2013;34:666–75.
159. Afanasyeva M, et al. Autoimmune myocarditis: cellular mediators of cardiac dysfunction. Autoimmun Rev. 2004;3(7–8):476–86.
160. Shi Y, et al. Regulatory T cells protect mice against coxsackievirus-induced myocarditis through the transforming growth factor beta-coxsackie-adenovirus receptor pathway. Circulation. 2010;121(24):2624–34.
161. Baldeviano GC, et al. Interleukin-17A is dispensable for myocarditis but essential for the progression to dilated cardiomyopathy. Circ Res. 2010;106(10):1646–55.
162. Kong YC, et al. Opportunistic autoimmune disorders potentiated by immune-checkpoint inhibitors anti-CTLA-4 and anti-PD-1. Front Immunol. 2014;5:206.
163. Läubli H, et al. Acute heart failure due to autoimmune myocarditis under pembrolizumab treatment for metastatic melanoma. J Immunother Cancer. 2015;21(3):11.
164. Sellier-Leclerc AL, et al. Fulminant viral myocarditis after rituximab therapy in pediatric nephrotic syndrome. Pediatr Nephrol. 2013;28(9):1875–9.
165. Toscano G, et al. Rituximab in recurrent idiopathic giant cell myocarditis after heart transplantation: a potential therapeutic approach. Transpl Int. 2014;27(5):e38–42. https://doi.org/10.1111/tri.12270.

166. Kulkarni HS, et al. Rituximab and cytokine release syndrome. Case Rep Oncol. 2012;5(1):134–41.
167. Zanotti-Cavazzoni SL, et al. Cardiac dysfunction in severe sepsis and septic shock. Curr Opin Crit Care. 2009;15(5):392–7.
168. Marchand L, et al. Dilated cardiomyopathy revealing cushing disease: a case report and literature review. Medicine (Baltimore). 2015;94(46):e2011.
169. Bybee KA, et al. Stress-related cardiomyopathy syndromes. Circulation. 2008;118(4): 397–409.
170. Caforio AL, et al. Acute biopsy-proven lymphocytic myocarditis mimicking Takotsubo cardiomyopathy. Eur J Heart Fail. 2009;11:428–31.

Myocarditis in Systemic Immune-Mediated Diseases

11

Alida L. P. Caforio, Renzo Marcolongo, Anna Baritussio, Loira Leoni, Chun-Yan Cheng, and Sabino Iliceto

11.1 Introduction

Systemic immune-mediated diseases (SIDs) are a miscellaneous group of clinical conditions that share an immunological pathogenesis and include autoimmune, granulomatous, vasculitic, and autoinflammatory diseases [1, 2]. Cardiac involvement in SIDs, though frequently underestimated or unrecognized, is rather common and can produce severe clinical pictures with adverse prognosis [3–5]. Myocarditis is a feature of SIDs, though also coronary vessels, cardiac valves, and pericardium can be involved [1].

Both systemic and organ-specific autoimmune diseases are characterized by aberrant cellular and/or humoral immune responses to self-antigens in genetically predisposed individuals. Autoantibodies (AAbs) can trigger systemic tissue inflammation and organ damage via immune complex formation, as in systemic lupus erythematosus (SLE), or may affect a target organ or tissue, resulting, in autoimmune myocarditis, in major arrhythmia and/or heart failure [6–15].

A. L. P. Caforio (✉) · A. Baritussio · C.-Y. Cheng
Cardiology, Department of Cardiological, Thoracic and Vascular Sciences and Public Health, University of Padova, Padova, Italy

Cardioimmunology Outpatient Clinic, University of Padova, Padova, Italy
e-mail: alida.caforio@unipd.it; anna.baritussio@gmail.com, anna.baritussio@aopd.veneto.it; 073047chengchunyan@163.com

R. Marcolongo
Cardioimmunology Outpatient Clinic, University of Padova, Padova, Italy

Haematology and Clinical Immunology Unit, Department of Medicine, University of Padova, Padova, Italy
e-mail: renzo.marcolongo@tiscali.it

L. Leoni · S. Iliceto
Cardiology, Department of Cardiological, Thoracic and Vascular Sciences and Public Health, University of Padova, Padova, Italy
e-mail: loira.leoni@gmail.com, loira.leoni@aopd.veneto.it; sabino.iliceto@unipd.it

A. L. P. Caforio (ed.), *Myocarditis*, https://doi.org/10.1007/978-3-030-35276-9_11

Besides antibody-mediated autoimmunity, an aberrant cellular immune response can also exert a determinant role in the pathogenesis of some SIDs, such as in sarcoidosis, where cardiac involvement, frequently silent or unrecognized for a long time, can suddenly manifest with a life-threatening arrhythmia [1–3]. In addition, the heart can be a target in some aggressive cell-mediated systemic vasculitis, such as eosinophilic granulomatosis with polyangiitis (EGPA) and other *A*nti-*N*eutrophilic *C*ytoplasmic *A*utoantibody (ANCA)-associated vasculitis (AAV) [1, 2].

Autoinflammatory syndromes (AS) are a mixed group of genetically determined inflammatory syndromes caused by aberrant activation of innate immunity, which does not involves AAbs nor autoreactive T cells. In AS, acute inflammatory response can be triggered by both pathogen (PAMP) or disease associated (DAMP) pattern of recognition receptors, which promote the release of interleukin-1 (IL-1) eventually leading to inflammasome formation [1, 2]. Mediterranean fever (MF) may seldom cause pericarditis; recently, also idiopathic recurrent pericarditis, a common complication of acute pericarditis, which responds to the IL1 inhibitor anakinra, has been interpreted as a possible AS [1, 2]. Conversely, myocardial involvement is uncommon in AS, though the possible role of IL1-induced inflammasome activation in fulminant myocarditis is debated [16]. Finally, a clear-cut distinction between AS and autoimmune diseases is not always possible since they are both part of a unique immunopathogenic spectrum [1, 2].

This chapter will focus on myocardial inflammation in SIDs that, if not promptly recognized and adequately treated, eventually evolves to dilated cardiomyopathy (DCM) or non-dilated hypokinetic cardiomyopathy [17–20]. Furthermore, since diagnosis and management of myocarditis in SIDs are still poorly debated in medical literature, leading to late diagnosis and/or under-treatment, proper multidisciplinary teamwork, and cardiological approach to these patients will be also briefly addressed [15, 21–25].

11.2 General Approach to Diagnosis

Clinical presentation and frequency of myocardial involvement may vary greatly among SIDs, requiring distinct considerations according to the specific disease. Consequently, cardiological work-up should be clinically oriented and individually tailored [1].

Myocarditis in SIDs, as in its isolated form, can have a variable clinical presentation, ranging from unexplained dyspnea, to palpitations, chest pain (with or without serum troponin elevation), syncope, arrhythmia, acute or chronic congestive heart failure, cardiogenic shock, and aborted sudden cardiac death [20]. Furthermore, SIDs, due to chronic inflammation and prolonged corticosteroid therapy, are usually characterized by accelerated coronary artery disease (CAD) as well as diffuse microvascular dysfunction [26]. Consequently, in SIDs an underlying coronary ischemic disorder should always be suspected and ruled out by appropriate non-invasive or invasive diagnostic procedures [20, 26, 27].

Regardless to its etiology, increased serum troponin may be indicative of myocardial involvement, though it is well known that myocarditis can occur also in the absence of troponin release [20]. Other serum biomarkers, such as natriuretic peptides (NT-pro BNP or BNP), should be assessed, in keeping with current international heart failure guidelines, when cardiac involvement is suspected [20, 28].

Myocarditis can be associated with new unexplained abnormal findings on standard 12-lead electrocardiogram (ECG) or 24 h-ECG Holter monitoring, thus they should always be part of the diagnostic work up in SIDs [1, 20] (Table 11.1).

Standard trans-thoracic echocardiography (TTE) with Doppler analysis is also essential in the detection of cardiac structure and function abnormalities, including pericardial and valve involvement; it should be readily performed in SIDs when cardiac involvement is suspected, though its findings may turn out to be non-specific [1, 20, 29–31]. Subclinical myocardial involvement can be detected by advanced ultrasound methods, such as deformation imaging, and valve involvement by trans-esophageal echocardiography (TEE) and 3D imaging [32–39]. Doppler assessment of tricuspid and pulmonary regurgitation gradients is key for non-invasive diagnosis of pulmonary hypertension (PH), a frequent and ominous complication of several SIDs [39, 40].

Cardiac magnetic resonance (CMR) should be carried out when myocarditis is suspected and to differentiate it from non-inflammatory myocardial infiltration [20]. In addition, CMR with tissue characterization sequences (T1 and T2 weighted imaging) and late gadolinium enhancement (LGE), together with multi-parametric mapping, may contribute to define non-ischemic inflammatory myocardial involvement and to monitor response to treatment. The typical subepicardial-mid-myocardial LGE pattern seen in some SIDs usually allows differential diagnosis from CAD. LGE and T1 mapping can also identify early changes in systemic sclerosis (SSc) [41–43] and rheumatoid arthritis (RA) [44–46], where LGE pattern has also been shown to correlate with disease activity.

Computed tomography (CT) can be particularly useful to show coronary and aortic calcification, as in severe RA [46], coronary CT may be used to screen patients with at low/intermediate risk of coronary artery disease, and can integrate TTE in PH work-up [40].

Table 11.1 Myocarditis in SIDs: cardiovascular "red flags" in the absence of known non-inflammatory causes

• Effort or rest dyspnea
• Bilateral ankle edema
• Palpitations
• Chest pain (with or without serum troponin elevation)
• Syncope and major arrhythmias
• Recent onset acute heart failure or unexpected appearance of chronic congestive heart failure
• Cardiogenic shock and aborted sudden cardiac death
• Elevation of serum troponin
• Elevation of natriuretic peptides (NT-pro BNP or BNP)
• New abnormal findings on standard 12-lead electrocardiogram (ECG), 24 h-ECG Holter monitoring, or standard echocardiography

Positron emission tomography with 2-deoxy-2-fluoro-D-glucose (FDG-PET) is particularly useful to detect inflammation in specific organs, such as in cardiac sarcoidosis [3, 47], and may offer non-invasive quantification of myocardial blood flow, revealing microvascular dysfunction and impaired coronary flow reserve, and predicting adverse outcome [48]. Whenever possible, sophisticated and expensive second-step cardiac tests, such as CMR and FDG-PET, should be performed in institutional centers experienced in rare cardiac disease assessment.

Endomyocardial biopsy (EMB) is the gold standard and the sine qua non for the diagnosis of myocarditis. Primarily, EMB provides differentiation between infectious and non-infectious myocarditis by means of histological, immunohistochemical, and molecular tools [20, 49–54]; secondly, besides identifying inflammation, EMB may reveal a non-inflammatory myocardial diseases such as cardiac amyloidosis [49–54]. In SIDs, EMB may be particularly useful when both invasive and non-invasive findings suggest non-ischemic myocardial involvement, or when there is an unexplained and/or sudden change in cardiac status and clinical decision-making requires histological confirmation. EMB may also foster critical treatment decisions based on histopathological results, particularly in eosinophilic myocarditis, sarcoidosis, and in giant cell myocarditis (GCM). In experienced hands, EMB has a low rate of complication (0–0.8% of serious events) and sampling errors [55–58]. Histological and immunohistochemical investigation requires at least three myocardial tissue samples from the right or left ventricle; they should be immediately fixed in 4% buffered formaldehyde for all histological and immunohistochemical staining and for special stains of storage diseases. Furthermore, at least two additional myocardial samples (fixed in RNA later or snap-frozen in liquid nitrogen and stored at −80 °C) should be obtained for molecular analyses, including cardiotropic viruses and bacteria, by reverse transcription (RT-) polymerase chain reaction (PCR) detection [20, 49]. Finally, EMB has a significant clinical value only if myocardial samples are taken, processed, and evaluated by specifically trained pathologists from certified institutional laboratories [1].

11.3 General Principles of Management

Due to heterogeneity in clinical presentations and variable frequency of cardiac and myocardial involvement in different SIDs it is impossible to outline a common management flow chart (Table 11.2). However, despite lack of robust evidence-base for management of affected patients, some general principles can be addressed.

Aggressive and prolonged immunosuppressive therapy (IT), frequently including corticosteroids, may be needed as background in SIDs, particularly at disease onset or in flares [15, 23]. IT has to be personalized, according to clinical presentation, disease activity, involvement of vital organs, and the presence of comorbidities, since clinical response is variable and disease evolution may be unpredictable. IT is finely tuned to achieve the lowest level of disease activity along with minimal drug toxicity, i.e., treat-to-target strategy [59]. Myocarditis in SIDs may lead to irreversible organ damage and is associated with poor survival, thus it is an indication to a more intensive IT [1, 3, 47, 60–71].

Table 11.2 Diversity of cardiac involvement in SIDs

Cardiac involvement	Presentation/clinical frequency
Systemic lupus erythematosus	Pericarditis 30%, myocarditis 1%, valvular involvement 10%, endocarditis <1%
Systemic sclerosis	Reduced left ventricular ejection fraction (LVEF) 5%, diastolic dysfunction 30%, reduced right ventricular ejection fraction (RVEF) 5–10%, pericarditis 10–20%, reports on myocarditis
Rheumatoid arthritis	Main complication: accelerated atherosclerosis; cardiomyopathy or myocarditis 3–30%, all cardiac structures may be affected
Sjögren syndrome	Reports on valvulopathies, pericardial effusion, arrhythmias
Inflammatory myopathies	Myocarditis in up to 30% of autopsies
Mixed connective tissue disease	Ischemic heart disease and myocarditis (case reports)
Sarcoidosis	Clinical (arrhythmias) 5–7%; granulomas in autopsy 20–30%
Eosinophilic granulomatosis with polyangiitis	Endomyocarditis, endomyocardial fibrosis up to 60%, cardiomyopathy 20%
Granulomatosis with polyangiitis	Pericarditis 35%, coronary arteritis 12%, cardiomyopathy 30%, arrhythmias 6%, valvular lesions 6%
Takayashu arteritis	Myocarditis is uncommon, can cause heart failure even in the absence of systemic hypertension or valvulopathy
Kawasaki disease	Ischemic heart disease; myocarditis is evident in 50–70% of patients during the acute phase of the disease
Spondyloarthritis	Cardiovascular disease as leading cause of death 36% in psoriatic arthritis, valvular disease 1–34%, anecdotally myocardits
Myasthenia gravis	Reports on cardiomyopathy, giant cell myocarditis
Autoinflammatory diseases	Pericarditis, fulminant myocarditis? (anecdotal, case reports)

Main IT complications include organ toxicity (e.g., liver, kidney, bone marrow, etc.) and a higher incidence of acquired infections and/or reactivation of latent or opportunistic infections. In addition, the prolonged use of corticosteroids is associated with adverse cardiovascular and metabolic side effects [72]. Therefore, steroid-sparing strategies are preferred, especially if prolonged IT is required. Finally, teratogenic and oncogenic effects of some immunosuppressants, e.g., methotrexate or mycophenolate mofetil, should be minimized and active screening programs are advisable in this high-risk population.

11.4 Myocarditis in Specific SIDs

11.4.1 Systemic Lupus Erythematosus (SLE)

SLE is a multisystemic autoimmune disease characterized by polymorphic clinical features and protean symptoms, which can be misleading and delay the diagnosis (Table 11.3) [73]. SLE pathogenesis is predominantly mediated by the deposition of immune complexes and complement proteins in virtually every organ and tissue producing inflammation. Joints, serous membranes, skin, and kidneys are more

Table 11.3 Updated American College of Rheumatology Classification diagnostic Criteria for SLE [77]

Criterion[a]	Definition
1. Malar rash	Fixed, flat, or raised erythema over the malar eminences, tending to spare the nasolabial folds
2. Discoid rash	Erythematous raised patches with adherent keratotic scaling and follicular plugging (older lesions may demonstrate atrophic scarring)
3. Photosensitivity	Skin rash as a result of unusual reaction to sunlight, by patient history or physician observation
4. Oral ulcers	Oral or nasopharyngeal ulceration, usually painless, observed by a physician
5. Arthritis	Nonerosive arthritis involving at least 2 peripheral joints, characterized by tenderness, swelling, or effusion
6. Serositis	(A) Pleuritis: Convincing history of pleuritic pain or rub heard by a physician or evidence of pleural effusion *or* (B) Pericarditis: Documented by ECG or rub or evidence of pericardial effusion
7. Renal disorder	(A) Persistent proteinuria >0.5 g/day or > 3+ if quantitation not performed *or* (B) Cellular casts: May be red blood cell, hemoglobin, granular, tubular, or mixed
8. Neurologic disorder	(A) Seizures: In the absence of offending drugs or known metabolic derangements (e.g., uremia, ketoacidosis, electrolyte imbalance) *or* (B) Psychosis: In the absence of offending drugs or known metabolic derangements (e.g., uremia, ketoacidosis, electrolyte imbalance)
9. Hematologic disorder	(A) Hemolytic anemia: With reticulocytosis *or* (B) Leukopenia: < 4000/mm^3 total on =2 occasions *or* (C) Lymphopenia: < 1500/mm^3 on =2 occasions *or* (D) Thrombocytopenia: < 100,000/mm^3 in the absence of offending drugs
10. Immunologic disorder	(A) Anti-DNA: Antibody to native DNA in abnormal titer *or* (B) Anti-Sm: Presence of antibody to Smith (Sm) nuclear antigen *or* (C) Positive finding of antiphospholipid antibodies based on (1) an abnormal serum level of IgG or IgM anticardiolipin antibodies, (2) a positive test result for lupus anticoagulant using a standard method, or (3) a false-positive serologic test for syphilis known to be positive for =6 months and confirmed by *Treponema pallidum* immobilization or fluorescent treponemal antibody absorption tests
11. Antinuclear antibody (ANA)	An abnormal titer of antinuclear antibody by immunofluorescence or an equivalent assay at any point in time and in the absence of drugs known to be associated with drug-induced lupus syndrome

ECG electrocardiogram, *Ig* immunoglobulin, *SLE* systemic lupus erythematosus
[a]SLE can be diagnosed if any 4 or more of the following 11 criteria are present, serially or simultaneously, during any interval of observation

frequently involved. Over 50% of SLE patients show some degree of heart involvement, ranging from pericarditis, which is the most common, even if frequently asymptomatic, cardiac complication in SLE, to the pathognomonic Libman–Sacks endocarditis, coronary artery involvement, and myocarditis [74, 75]. In SLE-related myocarditis, granular complement and immunoglobulin tissue deposits are evident at autopsy and EMB. Compared to postmortem studies of the sixties, reporting myocarditis in up to 57% of SLE patients, nowadays, SLE myocarditis appears to be far less frequent at autopsy (up to 8%) possibly in relation to better immunosuppressive regimens [15, 72]. Yet, myocarditis has been recently reported as the first clinical manifestation in 58.6% of a cohort of 29 SLE patients [76].

Clinical presentation of SLE myocarditis is non-specific and can be difficult to recognize, particularly when SLE diagnosis is not yet clearly established [77, 78]. It should be suspected when an unexplained increase in troponin I and/or NT-pro BNP [79], global or segmental hypo-kinesis on TTE are noticed in SLE patients. CMR imaging may detect abnormalities even at pre-clinical SLE stages, showing a non-ischemic pattern of myocardial LGE and/or edema [79]. Since accelerated atherosclerosis is well known to occur in SLE, CAD must be ruled out [26, 27].

EMB, applying PCR for the detection of infectious agents, may be useful for differential diagnosis of SLE myocarditis, since SLE patients are at high risk of infection due equally to a primary SLE-associated immunodeficiency [80] and/or to IT [20, 80]. Furthermore, EMB can differentiate SLE myocarditis from the rare chloroquine/hydroxychloroquine-induced cardiomyopathy [78, 81].

SLE myocarditis requires a prompt treatment with high-dose corticosteroids, usually in combination with a steroid-sparing immunosuppressive agent, such as azathioprine, mycophenolate mofetil, and/or high-dose intravenous immunoglobulin (HDIV-Ig) [60].

11.4.2 Systemic Sclerosis (SSc)

SSC is a rare immune-mediated disease with a progressive and irreversible chronic evolution, which is characterized by the generalized thickening of the skin and other soft tissues due to increased collagen deposition (Table 11.4) [82]. Microcirculatory vasculopathy is another typical histological feature. SSc is almost invariably a serious disease, which severely impairs patient quality of life and has a relentless progression with a fatal outcome [82]. SSc represents a major challenge for involved physicians. A definitive and comprehensive therapy for SSc is still lacking, although some clinical manifestations (i.e., digital ulceration, and gastro-esophageal reflux, pulmonary hypertension, renal crisis) are nowadays, at least in part, treatable [82].

In SSc, early myocardial involvement is frequent and often clinically occult/indolent, but when it becomes symptomatic, the prognosis is poor [1]. However, since cardiopulmonary symptoms can be also related to other, non-primary cardiac causes, such as lung interstitial fibrosis, concomitant pulmonary hypertension and/or coronary artery disease, and renal insufficiency, an early referral to a cardiologist for a complete diagnostic work-up should always be encouraged even in

Table 11.4 Systemic sclerosis (SSc) 2013 ACR/EULAR classification [83]

Item[a]	Sub-item(s)	Weight/ score
Skin thickening of the fingers of both hands extending proximal to the metacarpophalangeal joints *(sufficient criterion)*	–	9
Skin thickening of the fingers *(only count the higher score)*	Puffy fingers Sclerodactyly of the fingers (distal to the metacarpophalangeal joints but proximal to the proximal interphalangeal joints)	2 4
Fingertip lesions *(only count the higher score)*	Digital tip ulcers Fingertip pitting scars	2 3
Telangiectasia	–	2
Abnormal nailfold capillaries	–	2
Pulmonary arterial hypertension and/or interstitial lung disease *(maximum score is 2)*	Pulmonary arterial hypertension Interstitial lung disease	2 2
Raynaud's phenomenon	–	3
SSc-related autoantibodies (anticentromere, anti-topoisomerase I [anti-Scl-70], anti-RNA polymerase III) *(maximum score is 3)*	Anticentromere Anti-topoisomerase I Anti-RNA polymerase III	3

[a]These criteria are applicable to any patient to include in an SSc study. The criteria are not applicable to patients with skin thickening sparing the fingers or having a scleroderma-like disorder that better explains their manifestations (e.g., nephrogenic sclerosing fibrosis, generalized morphea, eosinophilic fasciitis, scleredema diabeticorum, scleromyxedema, erythromyalgia, porphyria, lichen sclerosis, graft-versus-host disease, diabetic cheiroarthropathy). The total score is determined by adding the maximum weight (score) in each category. Patients with a total score of ≥9 are classified as having definite SSc

asymptomatic and newly diagnosed patients [20, 61–64, 83–90, 91]. Actually, pulmonary hypertension (PH) should always be carefully searched in SSc [40].

Primary myocardial involvement in SSc is mainly linked to dysfunction and/or structural damage of the cardiac microvascular bed, leading to repeated focal ischemic injury and progressive myocardial fibrosis [84], but it can also be secondary to a SSc-related generalized myositis involving the myocardium [85].

Standard 12 lead ECG is abnormal in 50% of patients, the most common abnormality being left bundle branch block (16%), followed by first-degree (8%), or advanced atrioventricular (A-V) blocks (<2%) [89].

As for SLE, myocarditis should be suspected in SSc patients with unexplained increased (more than threefold) CPK or troponin [91], left ventricular systolic dysfunction (LSVD) and/or diastolic dysfunction (LVDD) [86–88], non-ischemic abnormal CMR tissue patterns [64]. In these patients EMB should be considered, to rule out myocardial infections possibly associated with IT [20, 61, 64, 85].

LSVD is the hallmark of primary SSc myocardial involvement [86], and can be easily detected by routine TTE, while advanced echocardiography techniques (i.e., tissue-Doppler and speckle-tracking strain analysis) can be useful in detection of heart failure with preserved ejection fraction (HFpEF) [87, 88] and LVDD [87, 88].

Twenty-four hour-ECG Holter monitoring may detect supraventricular and/or ventricular arrhythmias; QTc prolongation may be associated with life-threatening tachyarrhythmias [90]. SSc is perceived as having a high arrhythmic burden, with a 5% sudden death rate in patients with both skeletal and cardiac muscle disease [92].

SSc myocarditis usually requires prompt and aggressive IT [20, 60–63], while heart failure, arrhythmia, and conduction disturbances should be treated according to current international guidelines [28, 93].

11.4.3 Rheumatoid Arthritis (RA)

RA is a chronic autoimmune inflammatory disease with a worldwide diffusion, mainly affecting small joints, but frequently presenting also with extra-articular and systemic clinical manifestations.

RA is linked to a high risk of cardiovascular disease (CVD) and heart failure, resulting in premature morbidity and mortality, and reduced life expectancy compared to subjects without RA [94]. Positive AAbs status, joint pain severity, and conventional risk factors are strongly associated with increased CVD risk [94].

At present, accelerated atherosclerosis is considered a main complication, resulting from the cumulative effect of chronic systemic inflammation, oxidative stress, prolonged anti-inflammatory therapy, and classical CVD risk factors [95]. All cardiac structures can be affected in RA resulting in pericarditis (common, but symptomatic in less than 1%), myocarditis, myocardial fibrosis, arrhythmia, CAD including coronaritis, valvular disease (usually a single valve, resulting mainly in regurgitation and rarely in stenosis), PH, and cardiomyopathy [96–98]. A focal lymphocytic, diffuse necrotizing, or granulomatous myocarditis can be found in 3–30% of RA patients [96–98] with a predilection for the left ventricle. Myocardial granulomas are morphologically identical to subcutaneous RA nodules [96]. Recent CMR-based studies suggest that RA myocarditis may be more prevalent than previously suspected, even in asymptomatic patients, but more correlative data with EMB are needed [45]. Since RA patients have a high burden of CVD, mainly because of disease chronicity and accelerated atherosclerosis [94, 95], a multidisciplinary management including a cardiologist is always indicated.

11.4.4 Inflammatory Myopathies (IMs)

IMs are a heterogeneous group of diseases primarily affecting skeletal muscle, including dermatomyositis, polymyositis, necrotizing autoimmune myositis, inclusion-body myositis, and overlap myositis [98].

Besides "idiopathic" forms, IMs can be triggered by a viral infection or may be linked to a hidden malignancy. IMs are chronic diseases that can affect both adult and children, producing the progressive weakening of skeletal muscles, with a possible impairment of respiration and swallowing [99]. Diagnostic work-up of IMs includes skeletal muscle biopsy, to detect distinguishing histological features in every specific form, electromyography, muscle MR, determination of serum level of muscle enzymes (creatine kinase, aldolase, LDH), and specific AAbs (anti-tRNA-synthetase) [100].

Cardiac involvement in IMs is often clinically occult in most patients, but it may be suspected by non-invasive cardiovascular methods [63, 100, 101] and is usually related to bad outcome [101, 102]. Myocarditis occurs in up to 30% of autopsied patients, with or without concomitant coronary or vessel vasculitis [100].

Both biopsy-proven lymphocytic and GCM may be found in IM patients, with or without myositis-specific (anti- tRNA-synthetase) AAbs [67, 103–105], with negative prognostic implications [68, 104, 105]. Myocardial ischemia (due to coronary vasculitis), pericardial, or valve disease may also occur [101]. Cardiovascular mortality ranges from 5 to 17%, most frequently caused by myocardial infarction, heart failure, and myocarditis [101].

Cardiological diagnostic work-up is identical to that of clinically suspected myocarditis in other SIDs [67, 100, 101, 105]. Standard treatment of IMs includes corticosteroids in combination with methotrexate, azathioprine, mycophenolate mofetil, cyclosporine A, cyclophosphamide, and HDIV-Ig. The concomitant occurrence of myocarditis is an indication to the intensification of standard IT [68, 101, 103–105].

11.4.5 Primary Sjögren Syndrome (PSS)

PSS is a chronic autoimmune disease, most frequently affecting middle-aged women, which causes the development of a typical exocrinopathy, producing xerostomia and xerophthalmia, and dryness of mucous membranes [106]. In more than one-third of cases, PSS also involves extra glandular sites, such as lungs, kidneys, and joints, and fatigue is one of the most common symptoms [106].

The diagnosis of PSS requires either the histological evidence of focal lymphocytic infiltrates in minor salivary glands or the presence of serum anti-SSA/SSB AAbs (50 to 90% of patients), thought they are not specific for primary SS since they are found also in SLE and other connectivitis [106].

Only few isolated cases of clinically suspected myocarditis have been described in primary SS, one of which associated with a cryoglobulinemic vasculitis [107, 108]. An echocardiographic study in 107 consecutive primary SS patients without cardiac symptoms and 112 healthy controls, matched for age and gender, has shown a higher prevalence of valvulopathies, pericardial effusion, higher systolic pulmonary pressure, LVDD [109].

Congenital heart block (CHB) is seldom associated (2% of cases) with maternal AAbs against SSA (Ro) or SSB (La) proteins (neonatal lupus syndrome) [110]. Some infants with CHB, usually young (less than 2 year-old), or older (greater than 10 year-old), may develop endomyocardial fibroelastosis leading sometimes to heart failure despite early pacemaker implantation [111, 112]. This encourages a long follow-up of CHB children of mothers with anti-SSA/SSB AAbs. Long follow-up of CHB children of mothers with anti-SSA/SSB AAbs is recommended [111, 112].

11.4.6 Mixed Connective Tissue Disease (MCTD)

This uncommon SIDs are characterized by overlapping clinical features of SLE, SSc, and IMs. In the absence of pulmonary involvement, MCTD usually has a relatively benign evolution. However, as for other SIDs, recent evidence suggests that cardiac involvement in MCTD is associated with poor prognosis [113]. Besides ischemic heart disease, leading mortality causes in MCTD also include myocarditis, which is probably an expression of the myositis-like background frequently associated to MCTD [114]. As for SLE, MTCD related myocarditis requires IT with prednisone usually in combination with a steroid-sparing immunosuppressive agent [115].

11.4.7 Sarcoidosis

Sarcoidosis is a multiorgan immune-mediated granulomatous disease of unknown origin, frequently pauci/asymptomatic, which may affect both sexes and people of from different ethnic groups (with a more severe evolution in blacks), mainly in the first three decades of life, and which can mimic other diseases (i.e., tuberculosis, lymphoma, etc.) [3]. Multiple environmental and occupational factors may trigger the disease and host factors seem equally to play a crucial role [116]. The diagnosis of sarcoidosis is based upon the histological evidence of typical CD4 rich, non-caseating, or necrotizing granulomas in involved tissues, and is reinforced by other clinical and non-invasive diagnostic findings [3, 47].

It commonly presents with hilar lymphadenopathy, pulmonary infiltration, dry cough, fever, fatigue, and weight loss. Kidney (nephrolithiasis), arthritis, enlarged superficial lymph nodes, and skin (e.g., *erythema nodosum*, *lupus pernio*, Löfgren syndrome), salivary, meningeal, neurological, and ocular (Heerfordt syndrome) involvement can be also observed [117, 118]. In patients with active sarcoidosis, serum angiotensin converting enzyme can be increased, along with calcium and phosphate blood levels and urinary excretion.

Heart involvement can be found in up to 7% of patients [47], but it is often underestimated or unrecognized: autopsy studies reported myocardial granulomas in 20–30% of patients. Sarcoid granulomas may involve any site of the heart, although left ventricular free wall, posterior interventricular septum, papillary muscles, right ventricle, and the atria are most frequently affected (figure AM thinned IVS, PLAX). The extension of myocardial granulomatosis is directly related to bad prognosis [3]. In Japanese patients heart involvement accounts for 50–85% of the deaths compared to 13–20% in Caucasians, confirming that racial factors may play a role in disease expression [3].

Cardiac sarcoidosis may occur at any time and does not always correlate with other extra cardiac locations. It should be suspected when a patient with known sarcoidosis develops conduction blocks, tachyarrhythmia, congestive cardiac failure, pericarditis, or DCM. However, sudden death can be the starting and only clinical expression of cardiac sarcoidosis, particularly in patients aged over 40 years while "idiopathic" A-V block of various degrees and ventricular tachycardia in apparently healthy subjects are other possible starting manifestations of the disease [47, 117, 118].

Other possible clinical manifestations of cardiac sarcoidosis include unexplained brady-tachyarrhythmia, heart failure signs and symptoms, LVDD and/or LVSD on echocardiography or CMR, and/or abnormal tissue patterns on CMR or FDG-PET uptake [3, 47, 117, 118], and unexplained steroid-responsive cardiomyopathy [3, 47, 117, 118]. Arrhythmogenic right ventricular cardiomyopathy should be considered in differential diagnosis [47, 117, 118].

Non-invasive imaging is indicated in all patients with suspected cardiac sarcoidosis and the definitive diagnosis of cardiac involvement requires a combined approach, often including CMR and PET. EMB may be of clinical value, but, since in sarcoidosis the myocardium is involved in a patchy fashion, its sensitivity may be decreased by sampling error. Yet, when positive, EMB provides histological and etiological differential diagnosis from idiopathic GCM and other infectious granulomatous forms (e.g., mycobacteria, Bartonella henselae, Toxoplasma gondii, and Yersinia) [3].

Corticosteroids are the treatment gold standard also for cardiac sarcoidosis [3, 47], and they can be effectively combined with other immunosuppressive drugs (Table 11.5). However, response to medical therapy is variable and cardiac transplantation sometimes becomes the only option.

Even if corticosteroids may improve A-V node recovery or reverse it transiently, pacemaker therapy is often needed [3, 93, 119]. Internal cardioverter defibrillator (ICD) implantation may be considered earlier in patients with cardiac sarcoidosis who had hemodynamically compromising sustained ventricular arrhythmia or aborted cardiac arrest, if survival >1 year with good functional status can be expected. The most effective antiarrhythmic drugs are β-blockers and amiodarone. Catheter ablation of ventricular arrhythmia is usually considered after an ICD implantation or failure of antiarrhythmic drug therapy. Primary and secondary sudden cardiac death prevention should be in keeping with current international guidelines [93, 119].

Table 11.5 Pharmacological management of cardiac sarcoidosis [3, 47, 119]

	Drug schedules	Notes
Corticosteroids	• Pulse of iv methylprednisolone (500 mg daily) • Oral prednisone (initial dose ~ 1 mg/kg/day) • Prednisone is gradually tapered to a maintenance therapy (5–10 mg/die) for 6–9 months	• Gold standard therapy • Optimal dose and duration to be personalized
Disease-modifying-anti-rheumatic drugs (DMARDs) and standard IT	• Hydroxychloroquine (400 mg/daily) • Methotrexate (10–20 mg weekly) • Azathioprine (100–150 mg daily) • Mycophenolate mofetil (1.0–2.0 gr daily) • Pulse of iv cyclophosphamide (500–1000 mg every 3–4 weeks)	• IT alone or in combination with steroids indicated in aggressive cardiac sarcoidosis
Biological agents	• Infliximab • Adalimumab • Rituximab	• Off-label may be considered in refractory subjects

11.4.8 Eosinophilic Granulomatosis with Polyangiitis (EGPA, Formerly Churg–Strauss Syndrome)

EGPA is a rare eosinophilic-rich, necrotizing granulomatous vasculitis often involving the respiratory tract and predominantly affecting small to medium vessels (Table 11.6) [4, 120, 121]. The clinical presentation of the disease is characterized by a classical triad including asthma, allergic rhinitis, and marked peripheral blood eosinophilia [121, 122].

EGPA belongs to the spectrum of AAV, although ANCA positivity (30–40% of cases) is lower than in other AAV [5, 65, 122]. Indeed, two major clinical subsets have been identified, an ANCA-positive EGPA, with features of small-vessel vasculitis, and an ANCA-negative one, in which organ damage is mainly mediated by tissue eosinophilic infiltration [4, 122].

Multiple immunocompetent cells take part in the pathogenesis of EGPA, including Th1, Th2, Th17 cells, and activated B cells producing ANCA [4]. EGPA can be triggered by the exposure to allergens or drugs, but a genetic background has been also recognized [4, 122].

Table 11.6 Eosinophilic granulomatosis with polyangiits (EGPA): classification criteria by the 2012 Chapel Hill Consensus conference and the 1990 American College of Rheumatology (ACR) [120, 121]

1990 ACR classification criteria [120]	EGPA (Churg–Strauss syndrome): at least four of these six criteria are positive[a]
	Asthma
	Eosinophilia >10%
	Neuropathy (mono or poly)
	Pulmonary infiltrates, non-fixed
	Paranasal sinus abnormality
	Extravascular eosinophils
2012 CHCC statements for the definition of EGPA [121]	Eosinophil-rich and necrotizing granulomatous inflammation often involving the respiratory tract and necrotizing vasculitis predominantly affecting small to medium vessels and associated with asthma and eosinophilia
	Nasal polyps are common
	ANCA is more frequent when glomerulonephritis is present. 100% with documented necrotizing glomerulonephritis have ANCA
	Limited expressions of EGPA confined to the upper or lower respiratory tract may occur
	Granulomatous and nongranulomatous extravascular inflammation, such as nongranulomatous eosinophil-rich inflammation of lungs, myocardium, and gastrointestinal tract, is common

[a]Three overlapping EGPA phases of EGPA:

- Phase 1, nonallergic eosinophilic asthma and other allergy symptoms, such as rhinosinusitis and/or nasal polyposis, are the defining feature
- Phase 2, tissue and blood eosinophilia
- Phase 3, eosinophilic tissue infiltration, small-vessel eosinophilic vasculitis, eosinophilic granulomas

Myocardial involvement in EGPA can take the features of either endomyocarditis/endomyocardial fibrosis (up to 60% of cases, with endocavitary thrombosis in about 10%), and inflammatory cardiomyopathy (up to 20%), which is typically associated with high eosinophilic cell count and the absence of ANCA [5, 66].

In EGPA associated myocarditis long-term prognosis is poor [4], leading to a restrictive cardiomyopathy or DCM [4, 66], which is an independent risk factor for death [5].

Cardiac screening should include laboratory assessment (CK-MB and troponin) and ECG, echocardiography, and CMR. Echocardiography and/or CMR can detect regional wall-motion abnormalities, pericardial effusion (20% of cases), and intracavitary thrombi [5, 66]. Tissue characterization by CMR may show features suggestive for myocarditis and myocardial fibrosis. Coronary abnormalities should be ruled out by coronary angiography. EMB may provide diagnosis of EGPA myocarditis, particularly in ANCA-negative patients with early and/or predominant cardiac involvement [66]. Diagnostic work-up should be aimed to the identification of other causes of hypereosinophilic syndromes with possible heart involvement (toxic, infectious/parasitic, clonal, hypersensitivity) [123, 124].

The standard therapeutic approach to EGPA is based on high-dose corticosteroids plus immunosuppressive agents, including cyclophosphamide [65, 66]. Recent studies seem to suggest also the efficacy of rituximab, an anti CD20 monoclonal antibody, and of mepolizumab, an anti-IL-5 monoclonal antibody.

11.4.9 Granulomatosis with Polyangiitis (GPA, Formerly Wegener's Granulomatosis)

GPA is a rare necrotizing granulomatous AAV, predominantly affecting small to medium vessels, which usually involves the upper and lower respiratory tract, but any other organ, including kidneys and central nervous system (CNS), can be affected (Table 11.7) [120, 121].

Cardiac manifestations, such as pericarditis (35% of cases), coronary arteritis (12%), cardiomyopathy (30%), arrhythmias (6%), and valvular lesions (6%), have been reported [125]. However, the extent and type of cardiac involvement are still poorly defined. Between 1957 and 2005, the French Vasculitis Study Group included 1108 patients with systemic necrotizing vasculitides, among them 311 patients with GPA [126]. Cardiac involvement was diagnosed in 13% of GPA subjects; a multivariate analysis identified age, renal, and cardiac failure as independent negative prognostic factors [126]. Conversely, in the Vasculitis Clinical Research Consortium longitudinal multicenter cohort study including 517 GPA patients, cardiac involvement was found in only 3.3% of GPA subjects and was not associated with a higher rate of relapse or premature death [125]. In a meta-analysis of long-term follow-up data from 4 European clinical trials including 535 newly diagnosed AAV patients, of whom 53% GPA cases, cardiovascular involvement, found in a minority (5.7%) of patients, was independently associated with a higher risk of relapse [127].

Table 11.7 Granulomatosis with polyangiitis (GPA): classification criteria by the 2012 Chapel Hill Consensus conference and the 1990 American College of Rheumatology (ACR) [120, 121]

1990 ACR criteria for GPA (Wegener's granulomatosis) classification [120]	GPA is defined by the presence of at least two of the following four criteria
	Abnormal urinary sediment (red cell casts or greater than five red blood cells per high power field)
	Abnormal chest-X ray (nodules, cavities, or fixed infiltrates)
	Oral ulcers or nasal discharge
	Granulomas at tissue biopsy
2012 CHCC statements for GPA definition [121]	Necrotizing granulomatous inflammation and necrotizing vasculitis associated with antineutrophil cytoplasmic antibody (ANCA)
	Predominantly small to medium vessels (e.g., capillaries, venules, arterioles, arteries, and veins) are affected
	The upper and lower respiratory tract is usually involved
	Necrotizing glomerulonephritis is common
	Ocular vasculitis and pulmonary capillaritis with hemorrhage are frequent

In the absence of immunosuppressive treatment, the outcome of GPA is nearly always fatal [127]. In recent years, the combination of classical immunosuppressive drugs, such as cyclophosphamide, with biologic agents such as rituximab, has remarkably improved GPA prognosis [128]. Since cardiovascular GPA involvement may predict poor prognosis and/or higher risk of relapse [126, 127], an upgraded immunosuppressive regimen may be considered [128].

11.4.10 Other Primary Vasculitides

Myocarditis can occur also in patients with Takayasu arteritis (TA), an uncommon vasculitis of great/medium size arteries, usually affecting young women [129]. In TA patients, the occurrence of myocarditis can cause heart failure even in the absence of systemic hypertension or valvulopathy. Myocarditis in TA arteritis seems to respond to IT [130].

Finally, in Kawasaki disease or mucocutaneous lymph-node syndrome, a vasculitis of medium size arteries affecting children in the first 2 years of life, myocarditis is evident in 50–70% of patients during the acute phase of the disease [131].

11.4.11 Myasthenia Gravis (MG)

MG is both an AAbs and a helper T-cell mediated autoimmune disease, often associated with thymic hyperplasia or thymoma and, less frequently (up to 8%), with autoimmune thyroid diseases, RA and SLE. MG affects patients of either sex, at any age [69]. Diagnosis is established by patient history, characterized by fluctuating muscular weakness involving ocular and bulbar muscles, producing seeing, speech, chewing, deglutition, and breathing impairment, respectively. Less frequently, also nuchal or limb muscles are involved, with difficulty in maintaining head posture and increasing arm and leg weakness.

Electromyography and detection of AAbs interfering with the acetylcholine receptor (AChR) are key elements for diagnosis [69]. Patients without anti-AChR AAbs often have AAbs against the muscle-specific receptor tyrosine kinase and other postsynaptic neuromuscular junction components. In addition, AAbs against striated muscular antigens, such as anti-titin, anti-ryanodine, and anti-Kv 1.4 AAbs, can be detected almost exclusively in thymoma patients [132]. In Japanese patients, anti-Kv 1.4 AAbs specifically correlate with severe MG, myasthenia crisis, myocarditis, and ECG abnormalities [133].

Cardiac involvement in MG may include Takotsubo or stress induced cardiomyopathy, myocarditis, abnormal ECG findings, such as QT-prolongation, anticholinesterase induced A-V block, and sudden cardiac death [133]. Heart rate variability is disturbed, due to autonomic dysfunction [134]. Since coronary arteries dilate in response to acetylcholine, cases of diffuse coronary spasm associated with anticholinesterase therapy have been reported [135]. Nevertheless, there is no association between MG and CAD. Takotsubo is typically observed during myasthenia crisis episodes, older patients being at a higher risk [136]. Myocarditis typically affects thymoma-related elderly MG patients and is associated with skeletal muscle cross-reactive striational anti-heart AAbs [133]; diagnosis is often delayed because heart failure symptoms may be misinterpreted. Biopsy-proven GCM may be associated with MG and carries a worse prognosis, compared to other forms of myocarditis [70, 71]. The threshold for suspecting GCM should be low in MG, particularly in elderly patients and in those with skeletal muscle cross-reactive striational anti-heart AAbs. When GCM is suspected, particularly if life-threatening heart failure and/or arrhythmias are present, EMB should be promptly carried out [20, 50, 119] in order to start as soon as possible an adequate IT, according to the patient's age and the clinical condition [20, 70, 71].

11.4.12 Spondyloarthritis (SA)

SA is a heterogeneous family of rheumatic, chronic inflammatory conditions primarily affecting joints, ligaments, tendon insertions (enthesitis), and axial skeleton causing functional impairment and deformities.

SA is associated with increased cardiovascular morbidity and mortality, though the contributory role of CVD risk factors and of anti-inflammatory treatment needs to be further defined [137]. In psoriatic arthritis, CVD is the leading cause of death (36.2%) and the death risk is 1.3 times greater than in the general population.

Cardiovascular symptoms are present in 10% of SA patients and clinical presentations may include CAD, valvular disease, mainly aortitis and aortic insufficiency (1–34%), conduction defects and, anecdotally, myocarditis [137–139]. An association between disease activity and CVD risk has been suggested in SA, but statin therapy is still under scrutiny [140].

11.4.13 Autoinflammatory Syndromes (AS)

This is still an incompletely outlined group of systemic inflammatory diseases, characterized by recurrent fever, elevation of acute phase reactants such as CRP, but usually lacking high AAbs titer or antigen-specific T cells (Table 11.8) [141]. Monogenic AS, including MF, tumor necrosis factor receptor-associated periodic fever syndrome (TRAPS) and other less frequent syndromes (e.g., cryopyrin-associated periodic syndrome—CAPS-, and Hyper-IgD syndrome—HIDS -), have a typical genetic hereditary profile and usually start early in life. They commonly involve the skin, serous membranes, joints, gastrointestinal tract, eyes and, less frequently, the nervous system; complications include severe inflammatory anemia and AA amyloidosis, which usually does not affect the heart [141]. Occasionally, MF and TRAPS may cause recurrent pericarditis, while clinically suspected myocarditis has been only anecdotally reported in TRAPS [142].

Multifactorial AS, including adult-onset Still's disease (AOSD) or systemic-onset juvenile idiopathic arthritis (sJIA), apparently lack a typical genetic profile and usually start later in life. Macrophage activation syndrome can occur in patients with AOSD/sJIA. Other well-known immune-mediated disorders, such as Bechet's disease and inflammatory bowel disease, are nowadays interpreted as overlapping conditions between AS and autoimmune diseases [141, 143]. A neutrophilic myocarditis can be an uncommon complication of AOSD, Behçet and Crohn's disease, while GCM has been reported in association with both Crohn and Bechet's diseases [142, 144–146].

Table 11.8 Autoinflammatory syndromes (AS)

Monogenic syndromes
• Familial Mediterranean fever (FMF)
• Tumor necrosis factor receptor-associated periodic syndrome (TRAPS)
• Hyper-IgD syndrome (HIDS)
• Cryopyrin-associated periodic syndromes (CAPS): Familial cold autoinflammatory syndrome, Muckle–Wells syndrome, Neonatal onset multisystem inflammatory disease/chronic infantile neurologic cutaneous arthropathy syndrome (NOMID/CINCA)
• Juvenile systemic granulomatosis (Blau syndrome, early onset sarcoidosis)
• Syndrome of pyogenic arthritis, pyoderma gangrenosum, and acne (PAPA syndrome, PAPAS, PAPGA syndrome)
• Majeed syndrome
• Deficiency of interleukin-1 receptor antagonist (DIRA)
• Mevalonic aciduria
Nonhereditary or polygenic disorders
• Adult-onset Still's disease (AOSD) and systemic-onset juvenile idiopathic arthritis (sJIA)
• Syndrome of periodic fever, aphthous stomatitis, pharyngitis, and adenitis (PAPAS, PFAPA syndrome)
• Schnitzler syndrome
• Other proposed autoinflammatory diseases: Behçet's disease, psoriatic arthritis, Crohn's disease, Sweet's syndrome, relapsing polychondritis, urticarial vasculitis, etc.

Due to positive response to anakinra, an anti-IL1 receptor antagonist, recurrent idiopathic pericarditis has been recently interpreted as a disease belonging to the spectrum of AS. Similarly, the encouraging clinical response to anakinra, reported in a case of fulminant myocarditis seems to suggest a putative role of inflammasome in the pathogenesis at least in these cases [16].

11.5 Conclusions

Myocardial tissue is frequently involved in clinical and pathological evolution of SIDs, adding a significant negative burden to their prognosis. Actually, in SIDs, myocarditis can either be an early clinical manifestation or have a silent and long-time unrecognized evolution. For these reasons, standard clinical management of SIDs patients should always include an initial cardiological screening at diagnosis and a regular follow-up once cardiac involvement is recognized.

References

1. Caforio A, Adler Y, Agostini C, Allanore Y, Anastasakis A, Arad M, Böhm M, Charron P, Elliott PM, Eriksson U, Felix SB, Garcia-Pavia P, Hachulla E, Heymans S, Imazio M, Klingel K, Marcolongo R, Matucci Cerinic M, Pantazis A, Plein S, Poli V, Rigopoulos A, Seferovic P, Shoenfeld Y, Zamorano JL, Linhart A. Diagnosis and management of myocardial involvement in systemic immune-mediated diseases: A position statement of the ESC Working Group on Myocardial and Pericardial Disease. Eur Heart J. 2017;38:2649–62.
2. McGonagle D, McDermott MF. A proposed classification of the immunological diseases. PLoS Med. 2006;3:1242–7.
3. Kusano KF, Satomi K. Diagnosis and treatment of cardiac sarcoidosis. Heart. 2016;102:184–90.
4. Mahr A, Moosig F, Neumann T, Szczeklik W, Taillé C, Vaglio A, Zwerina J. Eosinophilic granulomatosis with polyangiitis (Churg-Strauss): evolutions in classification, etiopathogenesis, assessment and management. Curr Opin Rheumatol. 2014;26:16–23.
5. Comarmond C, Pagnoux C, Khellaf M, Cordier JF, Hamidou M, Viallard JF, Maurier F, Jouneau S, Bienvenu B, Puéchal X, Aumaître O, Le Guenno G, Le Quellec A, Cevallos R, Fain O, Godeau B, Seror R, Dunogué B, Mahr A, Guilpain P, Cohen P, Aouba A, Mouthon L, Guillevin L, French Vasculitis Study Group. Clinical characteristics and long-term followup of the 383 patients enrolled in the French vasculitis study group cohort. Arthritis Rheum. 2013;65:270–81.
6. Mann DL. The emerging role of innate immunity in the heart and vascular system: for whom the cell tolls. Circ Res. 2011;108:1133–45.
7. Eriksson U, Ricci R, Hunziker L, Kurrer MO, Oudit GY, Watts TH, Sonderegger I, Bachmaier K, Kopf M, Penninger JM. Dendritic cell-induced heart failure requires essential cooperation between adaptive and innate immunity. Nat Med. 2003;9:1484–9.
8. Mills KH. TLR-dependent T cell activation in autoimmunity. Nat Rev Immunol. 2011;11:807–22.
9. Ciccacci C, Perricone C, Ceccarelli F, Rufini S, Di Fusco D, Alessandri C, Spinelli FR, Cipriano E, Novelli G, Valesini G, Borgiani P, Conti F. A multilocus genetic study in a cohort of Italian SLE patients confirms the association with STAT4 gene and describes a new association with HCP5 gene. PLoS One. 2014;9:e111991.
10. Meder B, Rühle F, Weis T, Homuth G, Keller A, Franke J, Peil B, Lorenzo Bermejo J, Frese K, Huge A, Witten A, Vogel B, Haas J, Völker U, Ernst F, Teumer A, Ehlermann P, Zugck C,

Friedrichs F, Kroemer H, Dörr M, Hoffmann W, Maisch B, Pankuweit S, Ruppert V, Scheffold T, Kühl U, Schultheiss HP, Kreutz R, Ertl G, Angermann C, Charron P, Villard E, Gary F, Isnard R, Komajda M, Lutz M, Meitinger T, Sinner MF, Wichmann HE, Krawczak M, Ivandic B, Weichenhan D, Gelbrich G, El-Mokhtari NE, Schreiber S, Felix SB, Hasenfuß G, Pfeufer A, Hübner N, Kääb S, Arbustini E, Rottbauer W, Frey N, Stoll M, Katus HA. A genome-wide association study identifies 6p21 as novel risk locus for dilated cardiomyopathy. Eur Heart J. 2014;35:1069–77.

11. Camporeale A, Poli V. IL-6, IL-17 and STAT3: a holy trinity in auto-immunity? Front Biosci (Landmark Ed). 2012;17:2306–26.
12. Wahren-Herlenius M, Dörner T. Immunopathogenic mechanisms of systemic autoimmune disease. Lancet. 2013;382:819–31.
13. Mackern-Oberti JP, Llanos C, Vega F, Salazar-Onfray F, Riedel CA, Bueno SM, Kalergis AM. Role of dendritic cells in the initiation, progress and modulation of systemic autoimmune diseases. Autoimmun Rev. 2015;14:127–39.
14. Suurmond J, Diamond B. Autoantibodies in systemic autoimmune diseases: specificity and pathogenicity. J Clin Invest. 2015;125:2194–202.
15. Cho JH, Feldman M. Heterogeneity of autoimmune diseases: pathophysiologic insights from genetics and implications for new therapies. Nat Med. 2015;21:730–8.
16. Cavalli G, Dinarello CA. Anakinra therapy for non-cancer inflammatory diseases. Front Pharmacol. 2018;9:1157.
17. Richardson P, McKenna W, Bristow M, Maisch B, Mautner B, O'Connell J, Olsen E, Thiene G, Goodwin J, Gyarfas I, Martin I, Nordet P. Report of the 1995 World Health Organization/International Society and Federation of Cardiology Task Force on the definition and classification of cardiomyopathies. Circulation. 1996;93:841–2.
18. Pinto YM, Elliott PM, Arbustini E, Adler Y, Anastasakis A, Böhm M, Duboc D, Gimeno J, de Groote P, Imazio M, Heymans S, Klingel K, Komajda M, Limongelli G, Linhart A, Mogensen J, Moon J, Pieper PG, Seferovic PM, Schueler S, Zamorano JL, Caforio AL, Charron P. Proposal for a revised definition of dilated cardiomyopathy, hypokinetic non-dilated cardiomyopathy, and its implications for clinical practice: a position statement of the ESC working group on myocardial and pericardial diseases. Eur Heart J. 2016;37:1850–8.
19. Elliott P, Andersson B, Arbustini E, Bilinska Z, Cecchi F, Charron P, Dubourg O, Kuhl U, Maisch B, McKenna WJ, Monserrat L, Pankuweit S, Rapezzi C, Seferovic P, Tavazzi L, Keren A. Classification of the cardiomyopathies: a position statement from the European Society of Cardiology Working Group on Myocardial and Pericardial Diseases. Eur Heart J. 2008;29:270–6.
20. Caforio AL, Pankuweit S, Arbustini E, Basso C, Gimeno-Blanes J, Felix SB, Fu M, Heliö T, Heymans S, Jahns R, Klingel K, Linhart A, Maisch B, McKenna W, Mogensen J, Pinto YM, Ristic A, Schultheiss HP, Seggewiss H, Tavazzi L, Thiene G, Yilmaz A, Charron P, Elliott PM, European Society of Cardiology Working Group on Myocardial and Pericardial Diseases. Current state of knowledge on aetiology, diagnosis, management, and therapy of myocarditis: a position statement of the European Society of Cardiology Working Group on Myocardial and Pericardial Diseases. Eur Heart J. 2013;34:2636–48.
21. Kania G, Blyszczuk P, Stein MS, Valaperti A, Germano D, Dirnhofer S, Hunziker L, Matter CM, Eriksson U. Heart-infiltrating prominin 1+/CD133+ progenitor cells represent the cellular source of TGF-β-mediated cardiac fibrosis in experimental autoimmune myocarditis. Circ Res. 2009;105:462–70.
22. Miao CG, Xiong YY, Yu H, Zhang XL, Qin MS, Song TW, Du CL. Critical roles of microRNAs in the pathogenesis of systemic sclerosis: new advances, challenges and potential directions. Int Immunopharmacol. 2015;28:626–33.
23. Dinarello CA, Simon A, van der Meer JW. Treating inflammation by blocking interleukin-1 in a broad spectrum of diseases. Nat Rev Drug Discov. 2012;11:633–52.
24. Heymans S, Corsten MF, Verhesen W, Carai P, van Leeuwen RE, Custers K, Peters T, Hazebroek M, Stöger L, Wijnands E, Janssen BJ, Creemers EE, Pinto YM, Grimm D, Schürmann N, Vigorito E, Thum T, Stassen F, Yin X, Mayr M, de Windt LJ, Lutgens E, Wouters K, de

Winther MP, Zacchigna S, Giacca M, van Bilsen M, Papageorgiou AP, Schroen B. Macrophage microRNA-155 promotes cardiac hypertrophy and failure. Circulation. 2013;128:1420–32.
25. Valaperti A, Nishii M, Germano D, Liu PP, Eriksson U. Vaccination with Flt3L-induced CD8α+ dendritic cells prevents CD4+ T helper cell-mediated experimental autoimmune myocarditis. Vaccine. 2013;31:4802–11.
26. Faccini A, Kaski JC, Camici PG. Coronary microvascular dysfunction in chronic inflammatory rheumatoid diseases. Eur Heart J. 2016;37:1799–806.
27. Agewall S, Beltrame JF, Reynolds HR, Niessner A, Rosano G, Caforio AL, De Caterina R, Zimarino M, Roffi M, Kjeldsen K, Atar D, Kaski JC, Sechtem U, Tornvall P, WG on Cardiovascular Pharmacotherapy. ESC working group position paper on myocardial infarction with non-obstructive coronary arteries. Eur Heart J. 2016;38(3):143–53. pii: ehw149.
28. Ponikowski P, Voors AA, Anker SD, Bueno H, Cleland JG, Coats AJ, Falk V, González-Juanatey JR, Harjola VP, Jankowska EA, Jessup M, Linde C, Nihoyannopoulos P, Parissis JT, Pieske B, Riley JP, Rosano GM, Ruilope LM, Ruschitzka F, Rutten FH, van der Meer P, McMurray JJ, Aboyans V, Achenbach S, Agewall S, Al-Attar N, Atherton JJ, Bauersachs J, Camm JA, Carerj S, Ceconi C, Coca A, Elliott P, Erol Ç, Ezekowitz J, Fernández-Golfín C, Fitzsimons D, Guazzi M, Guenoun M, Hasenfuss G, Hindricks G, Hoes AW, Iung B, Jaarsma T, Kirchhof P, Knuuti J, Kolh P, Konstantinides S, Lainscak M, Lancellotti P, Lip GY, Maisano F, Mueller C, Petrie MC, Piepoli MF, Priori SG, Torbicki A, Tsutsui H, van Veldhuisen DJ, Windecker S, Yancy C, Zamorano JL, Authors/Task Force Members; Document Reviewers Filippatos G. 2016 ESC Guidelines for the diagnosis and treatment of acute and chronic heart failure: the Task Force for the diagnosis and treatment of acute and chronic heart failure of the European Society of Cardiology (ESC). Developed with the special contribution of the Heart Failure Association (HFA) of the ESC. Eur Heart J. 2016;37(27):2129–200. pii: ehw128.
29. Chow PC, Ho MH, Lee TL, Lau YL, Cheung YF. Relation of arterial stiffness to left ventricular structure and function in adolescents and young adults with pediatric-onset systemic lupus erythematosus. J Rheumatol. 2007;34:1345–52.
30. Corrao S, Argano C, Pistone G, Messina S, Calvo L, Perticone F. Rheumatoid arthritis affects left ventricular mass: systematic review and meta-analysis. Eur J Intern Med. 2015;26:259–67.
31. Sasson Z, Rasooly Y, Chow CW, Marshall S, Urowitz MB. Impairment of left ventricular diastolic function in systemic lupus erythematosus. Am J Cardiol. 1992;69:1629–34.
32. Chung HT, Huang YL, Yeh KW, Huang JL. Subclinical deterioration of left ventricular function in patients with juvenile-onset systemic lupus erythematosus. Lupus. 2015;24:263–72.
33. Leal GN, Silva KF, França CM, Lianza AC, Andrade JL, Campos LM, Bonfá E, Silva CA. Subclinical right ventricle systolic dysfunction in childhood-onset systemic lupus erythematosus: insights from two-dimensional speckle-tracking echocardiography. Lupus. 2015;24:613–20.
34. Rosenbaum E, Krebs E, Cohen M, Tiliakos A, Derk CT. The spectrum of clinical manifestations, outcome and treatment of pericardial tamponade in patients with systemic lupus erythematosus: a retrospective study and literature review. Lupus. 2009;18:608–12.
35. Adler Y, Charron P, Imazio M, Badano L, Barón-Esquivias G, Bogaert J, Brucato A, Gueret P, Klingel K, Lionis C, Maisch B, Mayosi B, Pavie A, Ristić AD, Sabaté Tenas M, Seferovic P, Swedberg K, Tomkowski W, Achenbach S, Agewall S, Al-Attar N, Angel Ferrer J, Arad M, Asteggiano R, Bueno H, Caforio AL, Carerj S, Ceconi C, Evangelista A, Flachskampf F, Giannakoulas G, Gielen S, Habib G, Kolh P, Lambrinou E, Lancellotti P, Lazaros G, Linhart A, Meurin P, Nieman K, Piepoli MF, Price S, Roos-Hesselink J, Roubille F, Ruschitzka F, Sagristŕ Sauleda J, Sousa-Uva M, Uwe Voigt J, Luis Zamorano J, European Society of Cardiology (ESC). 2015 ESC Guidelines for the diagnosis and management of pericardial diseases: The Task Force for the Diagnosis and Management of Pericardial Diseases of the European Society of Cardiology (ESC)Endorsed by: The European Association for Cardio-Thoracic Surgery (EACTS). Eur Heart J. 2015;36:2921–64.
36. Yiu KH, Wang S, Mok MY, Ooi GC, Khong PL, Lau CS, Tse HF. Relationship between cardiac valvular and arterial calcification in patients with rheumatoid arthritis and systemic lupus erythematosus. J Rheumatol. 2011;38:621–7.

37. Zuily S, Regnault V, Selton-Suty C, Eschwège V, Bruntz JF, Bode-Dotto E, De Maistre E, Dotto P, Perret-Guillaume C, Lecompte T, Wahl D. Increased risk for heart valve disease associated with antiphospholipid antibodies in patients with systemic lupus erythematosus: meta-analysis of echocardiographic studies. Circulation. 2011;124:215–24.
38. Roldan CA, Tolstrup K, Macias L, Qualls CR, Maynard D, Charlton G, Sibbitt WL Jr. Libman-sacks endocarditis: detection, characterization, and clinical correlates by three-dimensional transesophageal echocardiography. J Am Soc Echocardiogr. 2015;28:770–9.
39. Rudski LG, Lai WW, Afilalo J, Hua L, Handschumacher MD, Chandrasekaran K, Solomon SD, Louie EK, Schiller NB. Guidelines for the echocardiographic assessment of the right heart in adults: a report from the American Society of Echocardiography endorsed by the European Association of Echocardiography, a registered branch of the European Society of Cardiology, and the Canadian Society of Echocardiography. J Am Soc Echocardiogr. 2010;23: 685–713.
40. Galiè N, Humbert M, Vachiery JL, Gibbs S, Lang I, Torbicki A, Simonneau G, Peacock A, Vonk Noordegraaf A, Beghetti M, Ghofrani A, Gomez Sanchez MA, Hansmann G, Klepetko W, Lancellotti P, Matucci M, McDonagh T, Pierard LA, Trindade PT, Zompatori M, Hoeper M, Aboyans V, Vaz Carneiro A, Achenbach S, Agewall S, Allanore Y, Asteggiano R, Paolo Badano L, Albert Barberà J, Bouvaist H, Bueno H, Byrne RA, Carerj S, Castro G, Erol Ç, Falk V, Funck-Brentano C, Gorenflo M, Granton J, Iung B, Kiely DG, Kirchhof P, Kjellstrom B, Landmesser U, Lekakis J, Lionis C, Lip GY, Orfanos SE, Park MH, Piepoli MF, Ponikowski P, Revel MP, Rigau D, Rosenkranz S, Völler H, Luis ZJ. 2015 ESC/ERS Guidelines for the diagnosis and treatment of pulmonary hypertension: the Joint Task Force for the Diagnosis and Treatment of Pulmonary Hypertension of the European Society of Cardiology (ESC) and the European Respiratory Society (ERS): Endorsed by: Association for European Paediatric and Congenital Cardiology (AEPC), International Society for Heart and Lung Transplantation (ISHLT). Eur Heart J. 2016;37:67–119.
41. Hachulla AL, Launay D, Gaxotte V, de Groote P, Lamblin N, Devos P, Hatron PY, Beregi JP, Hachulla E. Cardiac magnetic resonance imaging in systemic sclerosis: a cross-sectional observational study of 52 patients. Ann Rheum Dis. 2009;68:1878–84.
42. Allanore Y, Meune C. Primary myocardial involvement in systemic sclerosis: evidence for a microvascular origin. Clin Exp Rheum. 2010;28:S48–53.
43. Barison A, Gargani L, De Marchi D, Aquaro GD, Guiducci S, Picano E, Cerinic MM, Pingitore A. Early myocardial and skeletal muscle interstitial remodelling in systemic sclerosis: insights from extracellular volume quantification using cardiovascular magnetic resonance. Eur Heart J Cardiovasc Imaging. 2015;16:74–80.
44. Mavrogeni S, Karabela G, Stavropoulos E, Gialafos E, Sfendouraki E, Kyrou L, Kolovou G. Imaging patterns of heart failure in rheumatoid arthritis evaluated by cardiovascular magnetic resonance. Int J Cardiol. 2013;168:4333–5.
45. Ntusi NA, Piechnik SK, Francis JM, Ferreira VM, Matthews PM, Robson MD, Wordsworth PB, Neubauer S, Karamitsos TD. Diffuse myocardial fibrosis and inflammation in rheumatoid arthritis: insights from CMR T1 mapping. JACC Cardiovasc Imaging. 2015;8:526–36.
46. Paccou J, Renard C, Liabeuf S, Kamel S, Fardellone P, Massy ZA, Brazier M, Mentaverri R. Coronary and abdominal aorta calcification in rheumatoid arthritis: relationships with traditional cardiovascular risk factors, disease characteristics, and concomitant treatments. J Rheumatol. 2014;41:2137–44.
47. Hamzeh N, Steckman DA, Sauer WH, Judson MA. Pathophysiology and clinical management of cardiac sarcoidosis. Nat Rev Cardiol. 2015;12:278–88.
48. Herzog BA, Husmann L, Valenta I, Gaemperli O, Siegrist PT, Tay FM, Burkhard N, Wyss CA, Kaufmann PA. Long-term prognostic value of 13N ammonia myocardial perfusion positron emission tomography added value of coronary flow reserve. J Am Coll Cardiol. 2009;54:150–6.
49. Leone O, Veinot JP, Angelini A, Baandrup UT, Basso C, Berry G, Bruneval P, Burke M, Butany J, Calabrese F, d'Amati G, Edwards WD, Fallon JT, Fishbein MC, Gallagher PJ, Halushka MK, McManus B, Pucci A, Rodriguez ER, Saffitz JE, Sheppard MN, Steenbergen C, Stone JR, Tan C, Thiene G, van der Wal AC, Winters GL. 2011 consensus statement on

endomyocardial biopsy from the Association for European Cardiovascular Pathology and the Society for Cardiovascular Pathology. Cardiovasc Pathol. 2012;21:245–74.
50. Cooper LT, Baughman KL, Feldman AM, Frustaci A, Jessup M, Kuhl U, Levine GN, Narula J, Starling RC, Towbin J, Virmani R. The role of endomyocardial biopsy in the management of cardiovascular disease: a scientific statement from the American Heart Association, the American College of Cardiology, and the European Society of Cardiology Endorsed by the Heart Failure Society of America and the heart failure Association of the European Society of cardiology. Eur Heart J. 2007;28:3076–93.
51. Ardehali H, Howard DL, Hariri A, Qasim A, Hare JM, Baughman KL, Kasper EK. A positive endomyocardial biopsy result for sarcoid is associated with poor prognosis in patients with initially unexplained cardiomyopathy. Am Heart J. 2005;150:459–63.
52. Austin BA, Duffy B, Tan C, Rodriguez ER, Starling RC, Desai MY. Comparison of functional status, electrocardiographic, and echocardiographic parameters to mortality in endomyocardial-biopsy proven cardiac amyloidosis. Am J Cardiol. 2009;103:1429–33.
53. Baccouche H, Mahrholdt H, Meinhardt G, Merher R, Voehringer M, Hill S, Klingel K, Kandolf R, Sechtem U, Yilmaz A. Diagnostic synergy of non-invasive cardiovascular magnetic resonance and invasive endomyocardial biopsy in troponin-positive patients without coronary artery disease. Eur Heart J. 2009;30:2869–79.
54. Thurberg BL, Fallon JT, Mitchell R, Aretz T, Gordon RE, O'Callaghan MW. Cardiac microvascular pathology in Fabry disease: evaluation of endomyocardial biopsies before and after enzyme replacement therapy. Circulation. 2009;119:2561–7.
55. Yilmaz A, Kindermann I, Kindermann M, Mahfoud F, Ukena C, Athanasiadis A, Hill S, Mahrholdt H, Voehringer M, Schieber M, Klingel K, Kandolf R, Böhm M, Sechtem U. Comparative evaluation of left and right ventricular endomyocardial biopsy: differences in complication rate and diagnostic performance. Circulation. 2010;122:900–9.
56. Kindermann I, Kindermann M, Kandolf R, Klingel K, Bültmann B, Müller T, Lindinger A, Böhm M. Predictors of outcome in patients with suspected myocarditis. Circulation. 2008;118:639–48.
57. Caforio AL, Calabrese F, Angelini A, Tona F, Vinci A, Bottaro S, Ramondo A, Carturan E, Iliceto S, Thiene G, Daliento L. A prospective study of biopsy-proven myocarditis: prognostic relevance of clinical and aetiopathogenetic features at diagnosis. Eur Heart J. 2007;28:1326–33.
58. Holzmann M, Nicko A, Kühl U, Noutsias M, Poller W, Hoffmann W, Morguet A, Witzenbichler B, Tschöpe C, Schultheiss HP, Pauschinger M. Complication rate of right ventricular endomyocardial biopsy via the femoral approach: a retrospective and prospective study analyzing 3048 diagnostic procedures over an 11-year period. Circulation. 2008;118:1722–8.
59. Smolen JS. Treat-to-target: rationale and strategies. Clin Exp Rheumatol. 2012;30:S2–6.
60. Tincani A, Rebaioli CB, Taglietti M, Shoenfeld Y. Heart involvement in systemic lupus erythematosus, anti-phospholipid syndrome and neonatal lupus. Rheumatology. 2006;45:iv8–13.
61. Pieroni M, De Santis M, Zizzo G, Bosello S, Smaldone C, Campioni M, De Luca G, Laria A, Meduri A, Bellocci F, Bonomo L, Crea F, Ferraccioli G. Recognizing and treating myocarditis in recent-onset systemic sclerosis heart disease: potential utility of immunosuppressive therapy in cardiac damage progression. Semin Arthritis Rheum. 2014;43:526–33.
62. Liangos O, Neure L, Kühl U, Pauschinger M, Sieper J, Distler A, Schwimmbeck PL, Braun J. The possible role of myocardial biopsy in systemic sclerosis. Rheumatology. 2000;39:674–9.
63. Mueller KA, Mueller II, Eppler D, Zuern CS, Seizer P, Kramer U, Koetter I, Roecken M, Kandolf R, Gawaz M, Geisler T, Henes JC, Klingel K. Clinical and histopathological features of patients with systemic sclerosis undergoing endomyocardial biopsy. PLoS One. 2015;10:e0126707.
64. Pingitore A, Guiducci S, Conforti ML, De Marchi D, Gargani L, Moggi-Pignone A, Randone SB, Lombardi M, Picano E, Matucci-Cerinic M. Early detection of myocardial and pulmonary oedema with MRI in an asymptomatic systemic sclerosis patient: successful recovery with pulse steroid. Rheumatology. 2013;52:1920–1.
65. Moosig F, Bremer JP, Hellmich B, Holle JU, Holl-Ulrich K, Laudien M, Matthis C, Metzler C, Nölle B, Richardt G, Gross WL. A vasculitis centre based management strategy leads to

improved outcome in eosinophilic granulomatosis and polyangiitis (Churg–Strauss, EGPA): monocentric experiences in 150 patients. Ann Rheum Dis. 2013;72:1011–117.
66. Brucato A, Maestroni S, Masciocco G, Ammirati E, Bonacina E, Pedrotti P. Cardiac involvement in Churg-Strauss syndrome. G Ital Cardiol. 2015;16:493–500.
67. Allanore Y, Vignaux O, Arnaud L, Puéchal X, Pavy S, Duboc D, Legmann P, Kahan A. Effects of corticosteroids and immunosuppressors on idiopathic inflammatory myopathy related myocarditis evaluated by magnetic resonance imaging. Ann Rheum Dis. 2006;65:249–52.
68. Ali MS, Mba BI, Husain AN, Ciftci FD. Giant cell myocarditis: a life-threatening disorder heralded by orbital myositis. BMJ Case Rep. 2016;23:2016.
69. Berrih-Aknin S, Le Panse R. Myasthenia gravis: a comprehensive review of immune dysregulation and etiological mechanisms. J Autoimmun. 2014;52:90–100.
70. Kon T, Mori F, Tanji K, Miki Y, Kimura T, Wakabayashi K. Giant cell polymyositis and myocarditis associated with myasthenia gravis and thymoma. Neuropathology. 2013;33: 281–7.
71. Joudinaud TM, Fadel E, Thomas-de-Montpreville V, Mussot S, Flecher EM, Dartevelle PG. Fatal giant cell myocarditis after thymoma resection in myasthenia gravis. J Thorac Cardiovasc Surg. 2006;131:494–5.
72. Bulkley BH, Roberts WC. The heart in systemic lupus erythematosus and the changes induced in it by corticosteroid therapy. A study of 36 necropsy patients. Am J Med. 1975;58:243–64.
73. D'Cruz D, Khamashta M, Hughes GRV. Cardiovascular manifestations of systemic lupus erythematosus. In: Wallace DJ, Hahn BH, editors. Dubois' lupus erythematosus. Philadelphia: Lippincott William and Wilkins; 2002. p. 645.
74. Lee-Kirsch MA, Gong M, Chowdhury D, Senenko L, Engel K, Lee YA, de Silva U, Bailey SL, Witte T, Vyse TJ, Kere J, Pfeiffer C, Harvey S, Wong A, Koskenmies S, Hummel O, Rohde K, Schmidt RE, Dominiczak AF, Gahr M, Hollis T, Perrino FW, Lieberman J, Hübner N. Mutations in the gene encoding the 3′-5′ DNA exonuclease TREX1 are associated with systemic lupus erythematosus. Nat Genet. 2007;39:1065–7.
75. Morita M, Stamp G, Robins P, Dulic A, Rosewell I, Hrivnak G, Daly G, Lindahl T, Barnes DE. Gene-targeted mice lacking the Trex1 (DNase III) 30/50 DNA exonuclease develop inflammatory myocarditis. Mol Cell Biol. 2004;24:6719–27.
76. Thomas G, Cohen Aubart F, Chiche L, Haroche J, Hié M, Hervier B, et al. Lupus myocarditis: initial presentation and Longterm outcomes in a multicentric series of 29 patients. J Rheumatol. 2017;44:24–32.
77. Hochberg MC. Updating the American College of Rheumatology revised criteria for the classification of systemic lupus erythematosus. Arthritis Rheum. 1997;40:1725.
78. Jain D, Halushka MK. Cardiac pathology of systemic lupus erythematosus. J Clin Pathol. 2009;62:584–92.
79. Mavrogeni S, Bratis K, Markussis V, Spargias C, Papadopoulou E, Papamentzelopoulos S, Constadoulakis P, Matsoukas E, Kyrou L, Kolovou G. The diagnostic role of cardiac magnetic resonance imaging in detecting myocardial inflammation in systemic lupus erythematosus. Differentiation from viral myocarditis. Lupus. 2013;22:34–43.
80. Perazzio SF, Granados Á, Salomão R, Silva NP, Carneiro-Sampaio M, Andrade LE. High frequency of immunodeficiency-like states in systemic lupus erythematosus: a cross-sectional study in 300 consecutive patients. Rheumatology. 2016;55(9):1647–55. pii: kew227.
81. Yogasundaram H, Putko BN, Tien J, Paterson DI, Cujec B, Ringrose J, Oudit GY. Hydroxychloroquine-induced cardiomyopathy: case report, pathophysiology, diagnosis, and treatment. Can J Cardiol. 2014;30:1706–15.
82. Denton CP, Khanna D. Systemic sclerosis. Lancet. 2017;390:1685–99.
83. van den Hoogen F, Khanna D, Fransen J, Johnson SR, Baron M, Tyndall A, Matucci-Cerinic M, Naden RP, Medsger TA Jr, Carreira PE, Riemekasten G, Clements PJ, Denton CP, Distler O, Allanore Y, Furst DE, Gabrielli A, Mayes MD, van Laar JM, Seibold JR, Czirjak L, Steen VD, Inanc M, Kowal-Bielecka O, Müller-Ladner U, Valentini G, Veale DJ, Vonk MC, Walker UA, Chung L, Collier DH, Csuka ME, Fessler BJ, Guiducci S, Herrick A, Hsu VM, Jimenez S, Kahaleh B, Merkel PA, Sierakowski S, Silver RM, Simms RW, Varga J, Pope JE. 2013

classification criteria for systemic sclerosis: an American College of Rheumatology/European League against Rheumatism collaborative initiative. Arthritis Rheum. 2013;65:2737–47.
84. Venalis P, Kumánovics G, Schulze-Koops H, Distler A, Dees C, Zerr P, Palumbo-Zerr K, Czirják L, Mackevic Z, Lundberg IE, Distler O, Schett G, Distler JH. Cardiomyopathy in murine models of systemic sclerosis. Arthritis Rheumatol. 2015;67:508–16.
85. Carette S, Turcotte J, Mathon G. Severe myositis and myocarditis in progressive systemic sclerosis. J Rheumatol. 1985;12:997–9.
86. Allanore Y, Meune C, Vonk MC, Airo P, Hachulla E, Caramaschi P, Riemekasten G, Cozzi F, Beretta L, Derk CT, Komócsi A, Farge D, Balbir A, Riccieri V, Distler O, Chialà A, Del Papa N, Simic KP, Ghio M, Stamenkovic B, Rednic S, Host N, Pellerito R, Zegers E, Kahan A, Walker UA, Matucci-Cerinic M, EUSTAR co-authors. Prevalence and factors associated with left ventricular dysfunction in the EULAR scleroderma trial and research group (EUSTAR) database of patients with systemic sclerosis. Ann Rheum Dis. 2010;69:218–21.
87. Meune C, Avouac J, Wahbi K, Cabanes L, Wipff J, Mouthon L, Guillevin L, Kahan A, Allanore Y. Cardiac involvement in systemic sclerosis assessed by tissue-Doppler echocardiography during routine care: A controlled study of 100 consecutive patients. Arthritis Rheum. 2008;58:1803–9.
88. Yiu KH, Schouffoer AA, Marsan NA, Ninaber MK, Stolk J, Vlieland TV, Scherptong RW, Delgado V, Holman ER, Tse HF, Huizinga TW, Bax JJ, Schuerwegh AJ. Left ventricular dysfunction assessed by speckle-tracking strain analysis in patients with systemic sclerosis: relationship to functional capacity and ventricular arrhythmias. Arthritis Rheum. 2011;63:3969–78.
89. Morelli S, Sgreccia A, Ferrante L, Barbieri C, Bernardo ML, Perrone C, De Marzio P. Relationship between electrocardiographic and echocardiographic findings in systemic sclerosis (scleroderma). Int J Cardiol. 1996;57:151–60.
90. Kostis JB, Seibold JR, Turkevich D, Masi AT, Grau RG, Mesdger TA Jr, Steen VD, Clements PJ, Szydlo L, D'Angelo WA. Prognostic importance of cardiac arrhythmias in systemic sclerosis. Am J Med. 1988;84:1007–15.
91. Avouac J, Meune C, Chenevier-Gobeaux C, Borderie D, Lefevre G, Kahan A, Allanore Y. Cardiac biomarkers in systemic sclerosis: contribution of high-sensitivity cardiac troponin in addition to N-terminal pro-brain natriuretic peptide. Arthritis Care Res. 2015;67:1022–30.
92. Follansbee WP, Zerbe TR, Medsger TA. Cardiac and skeletal muscle disease in systemic sclerosis (scleroderma): a high risk association. Am Heart J. 1993;125:194–203.
93. Priori SG, Blomström-Lundqvist C, Mazzanti A, Blom N, Borggrefe M, Camm J, Elliott PM, Fitzsimons D, Hatala R, Hindricks G, Kirchhof P, Kjeldsen K, Kuck KH, Hernandez-Madrid A, Nikolaou N, Norekvål TM, Spaulding C, Van Veldhuisen DJ, Authors/Task Force Members; Document Reviewers. 2015 ESC Guidelines for the management of patients with ventricular arrhythmias and the prevention of sudden cardiac death: the Task Force for the Management of Patients with Ventricular Arrhythmias and the Prevention of Sudden Cardiac Death of the European Society of Cardiology (ESC). Endorsed by: Association for European Paediatric and Congenital Cardiology (AEPC). Eur Heart J. 2015;36:2793–867.
94. Wright K, Crowson CS, Gabriel SE. Cardiovascular comorbidity in rheumatic diseases: a focus on heart failure. Heart Fail Clin. 2014;10:339–52.
95. Avouac J, Meune C, Chenevier-Gobeaux C, Dieudé P, Borderie D, Lefevre G, Kahan A, Allanore Y. Inflammation and disease activity are associated with high circulating cardiac markers in rheumatoid arthritis independently of traditional cardiovascular risk factors. J Rheumatol. 2014;41:248–55.
96. Lebowitz WB. The heart in rheumatoid arthritis (rheumatoid disease):a clinical and pathological study of sixty-two cases. Ann Intern Med. 1963;58:102–23.
97. Roldan CA, DeLong C, Qualls CR, Crawford MH. Characterization of valvular heart disease in rheumatoid arthritis by transesophageal echocardiography and clinical correlates. Am J Cardiol. 2007;100:496–502.
98. Pappas DA, Taube JM, Bathon JM, Giles JT. A 73-year-old woman with rheumatoid arthritis and shortness of breath. Arthritis Rheum. 2008;59:892–9.
99. Atluri RB. Inflammatory myopathies. Mo Med. 2016;113(2):127–30.

100. Dalakas MC. Inflammatory muscle diseases. N Engl J Med. 2015;372:1734–47.
101. Zhang L, Wang GC, Ma L, Zu N. Cardiac involvement in adult polymyositis or dermatomyositis: a systematic review. Clin Cardiol. 2012;35:686–91.
102. Danko K, Ponyi A, Constantin T, Borgulya G, Szegedi G. Long-term survival of patients with idiopathic inflammatory myopathies according to clinical features: a longitudinal study of 162 cases. Medicine. 2004;83:35–42.
103. Sharma K, Orbai AM, Desai D, Cingolani OH, Halushka MK, Christopher-Stine L, Mammen AL, Wu KC, Zakaria S. Brief report: antisynthetase syndrome-associated myocarditis. J Card Fail. 2014;20:939–45.
104. Kwon OH, Kim MN, Kim SA, Seok HY, Park SM, Kim BJ, Kim CH, Shim WJ, Shim JS, Lee MG. Fulminant lymphocytic myocarditis associated with orbital myositis and diaphragmatic paralysis. Cardiovasc Pathol. 2016;25:55–8.
105. Dieval C, Deligny C, Meyer A, Cluzel P, Champtiaux N, Lefevre G, Saadoun D, Sibilia J, Pellegrin JL, Hachulla E, Benveniste O, Hervier B. Myocarditis in patients with Antisynthetase syndrome: prevalence, presentation, and outcomes. Medicine. 2015;94:e798.
106. Luciano N, Valentini V, Calabrò A, Elefante E, Vitale A, Baldini C, Bartoloni E. One year in review 2015: Sjögren's syndrome. Clin Exp Rheumatol. 2015;33:259–71.
107. Yoshioka K, Tegoshi H, Yoshida T, Uoshima N, Kasamatsu Y. Myocarditis and primary Sjögren's syndrome. Lancet. 1999;354:128–9.
108. Kau CK, Hu JC, Lu LY, Tseng JC, Wang JS, Cheng HH. Primary Sjögren's syndrome complicated with cryoglobulinemic glomerulonephritis, myocarditis, and multi-organ involvement. J Formos Med Assoc. 2004;103:707–10.
109. Vassiliou VA, Moyssakis I, Boki KA, Moutsopoulos HM. Is the heart affected in primary Sjögren's syndrome? An echocardiographic study. Clin Exp Rheumatol. 2008;26:109–12.
110. Llanos C, Izmirly PM, Katholi M, Clancy RM, Friedman DM, Kim MY, Buyon JP. Recurrence rates of cardiac manifestations associated with neonatal lupus and maternal/fetal risk factors. Arthritis Rheum. 2009;60:3091–7.
111. Moak JP, Barron KS, Hougen TJ, Wiles HB, Balaji S, Sreeram N, Cohen MH, Nordenberg A, Van Hare GF, Friedman RA, Perez M, Cecchin F, Schneider DS, Nehgme RA, Buyon JP. Congenital heart block: development of late-onset cardiomyopathy, a previously underappreciated sequela. J Am Coll Cardiol. 2001;37:238–42.
112. Villain E, Coastedoat-Chalumeau N, Marijon E, Boudjemline Y, Piette JC, Bonnet D. Presentation and prognosis of complete atrioventricular block in childhood, according to maternal antibody status. J Am Coll Cardiol. 2006;48:1682–7.
113. Aringer M, Steiner G, Smolen JS. Does mixed connective tissue disease exist? Yes. Rheum Dis Clin North Am. 2005;31:411–20.
114. Ungprasert P, Wannarong T, Panichsillapakit T, Cheungpasitporn W, Thongprayoon C, Ahmed S, Raddatz DA. Cardiac involvement in mixed connective tissue disease: a systematic review. Int J Cardiol. 2014;171:326–30.
115. Figliozzi S, Rizzo S, Cheng C, Iliceto S, Basso C, ALP C, Marcolongo R. Biopsy proven lymphocytic myocarditis with heart failure and troponin release in a middle-aged female with mixed connective tissue disease. JACC Case Rep. 2019;1(2):171–4.
116. Lazarus A. Sarcoidosis: epidemiology, etiology, pathogenesis, and genetics. Dis Mon. 2009 Nov;55(11):649–60.
117. Baughman RP, Grutters JC. New treatment strategies for pulmonary sarcoidosis: antimetabolites, biological drugs, and other treatment approaches. Lancet Respir Med. 2015;2015(3):813–22.
118. Facco M, Cabrelle A, Teramo A, Olivieri V, Gnoato M, Teolato S, Ave E, Gattazzo C, Fadini GP, Calabrese F, Semenzato G, Agostini C. Sarcoidosis is a Th1/Th17 multisystem disorder. Thorax. 2011;66:144–50.
119. Birnie DH, Sauer WH, Bogun F, Cooper JM, Culver DA, Duvernoy CS, Judson MA, Kron J, Mehta D, Cosedis Nielsen J, Patel AR, Ohe T, Raatikainen P, Soejima K. HRS expert consensus statement on the diagnosis and management of arrhythmias associated with cardiac sarcoidosis. Heart Rhythm. 2014;11:1305–23.

120. Leavitt RY, Fauci AS, Bloch DA, Michel BA, Hunder GG, Arend WP, Calabrese LH, Lie FJF, Lightfoot RW Jr, Masi AT, McShane DJ, Mills JA, Stevens MB, Wallace SL, Zvaifler NJ. The American College of Rheumatology 1990 criteria for the classification of Wegener's granulomatosis. Arthritis Rheum. 1990;33:1101–7.
121. Jennette JC, Falk RJ, Bacon PA, Basu N, Cid MC, Ferrario F, Flores-Suarez LF, Gross WL, Guillevin L, Hagen EC, Hoffman GS, Jayne DR, Kallenberg CG, Lamprecht P, Langford CA, Luqmani RA, Mahr AD, Matteson EL, Merkel PA, Ozen S, Pusey CD, Rasmussen N, Rees AJ, Scott DG, Specks U, Stone JH, Takahashi K, Watts RA. 2012 revised International Chapel Hill Consensus Conference nomenclature of vasculitides. Arthritis Rheum. 2013;65:1–11.
122. Vaglio A, Buzio C, Zwerina J. Eosinophilic granulomatosis with polyangiitis (Churg–Strauss): state of the art. Allergy. 2013;68:261–73.
123. Bleeker JS, Syed FF, Cooper LT, Weiler CR, Tefferi A, Pardanani A. Treatment-refractory idiopathic hypereosinophilic syndrome: pitfalls and progress with use of novel drugs. Am J Hematol. 2012;87:703–6.
124. Nutman TB. Evaluation and differential diagnosis of marked, persistent eosinophilia. Immunol Allergy Clin North Am. 2007;27:529–49.
125. McGeoch L, Carette S, Cuthbertson D, Hoffman GS, Khalidi N, Koening CL, Langford CA, McAlear CA, Moreland L, Monach PA, Seo P, Specks U, Ytterberg SR, Merkel PA, Pagnoux C, Vasculitis Clinical Research Consortium. Cardiac involvement in granulomatosis with polyangiitis. J Rheumatol. 2015;42:1209–12.
126. Guillevin L, Pagnoux C, Seror R, Mahr A, Mouthon L, Le Toumelin P, French Vasculitis Study Group (FVSG). The five-factor score revisited: assessment of prognoses of systemic necrotizing vasculitides based on the French Vasculitis Study Group (FVSG) cohort. Medicine. 2011;90:19–27.
127. Walsh M, Flossmann O, Berden A, Westman K, Höglund P, Stegeman C, Jayne D, European Vasculitis Study Group. Risk factors for relapse of antineutrophil cytoplasmic antibody-associated vasculitis. Arthritis Rheum. 2012;64:542–8.
128. Guillevin L, Pagnoux C, Karras A, Khouatra C, Aumaître O, Cohen P, Maurier F, Decaux O, Ninet J, Gobert P, Quémeneur T, Blanchard-Delaunay C, Godmer P, Puéchal X, Carron PL, Hatron PY, Limal N, Hamidou M, Ducret M, Daugas E, Papo T, Bonnotte B, Mahr A, Ravaud P, Mouthon L, French Vasculitis Study Group. Rituximab versus azathioprine for maintenance in ANCA-associated vasculitis. N Engl J Med. 2014;371:1771–80.
129. Mavrogeni S, Manoussakis MN. Myocarditis and subclavian stenosis in Takayasu arteritis. Int J Cardiol. 2011;148:223–4.
130. Talwar KK, Chopra P, Narula J, Shrivastava S, Singh SK, Sharma S, et al. Myocardial involvement and its response to immunosuppressive therapy in nonspecific aortoarteritis. Int J Cardiol. 1988;21(3):323–34.
131. Newburger JW, et al. Diagnosis, treatment, and long-term management of Kawasaki disease: a statement for health professionals from the committee on rheumatic fever, endocarditis and Kawasaki disease, council on cardiovascular disease in the young, American Heart Association. Circulation. 2004;110:2747–71.
132. Suzuki S, Utsugisawa K, Yoshikawa H, Motomura M, Matsubara S, Yokoyama K, Nagane Y, Maruta T, Satoh T, Sato H, Kuwana M, Suzuki N. Autoimmune targets of heart and skeletal muscles in myasthenia gravis. Arch Neurol. 2009;66:1334–8.
133. Suzuki S, Baba A, Kaida K, Utsugisawa K, Kita Y, Tsugawa J, Ogawa G, Nagane Y, Kuwana M, Suzuki N. Cardiac involvements in myasthenia gravis associated with anti-Kv1.4 antibodies. Eur J Neurol. 2014;21:223–30.
134. Peric S, Rakocevic-Stojanovic V, Nisic T, Pavlovic S, Basta I, Popovic S, Damjanovic S, Lavrnic D. Cardiac autonomic control in patients with myasthenia gravis and thymoma. J Neurol Sci. 2011;307:30–3.
135. Comerci G, Buffon A, Biondi-Zoccai GG, Ramazzotti V, Romagnoli E, Savino M, Rebuzzi AG, Biasucci LM, Loperfido F, Crea F. Coronary vasospasm secondary to hypercholinergic crisis: an iatrogenic cause of acute myocardial infarction in myasthenia gravis. Int J Cardiol. 2005;103:335–7.

136. Bansal V, Kansal MM, Rowin J. Broken heart syndrome in myasthenia gravis. Muscle Nerve. 2011;44:990–3.
137. Gensler LS. Axial spondyloarthritis: the heart of the matter. Clin Rheumatol. 2015;34:995–8.
138. Przepiera-Bedzak H, Brzosko I, Peregud-Pogorzelska M, Wódecki M. Brzosko MCardiovascular manifestations of seronegative inflammatory spondyloarthropathies. Ann Acad Med Stetin. 2010;56:62–5.
139. Klingberg E, Sveälv BG, Täng MS, Bech-Hanssen O, Forsblad-d'Elia H, Bergfeldt L. Aortic regurgitation is common in ankylosing spondylitis - time for routine echocardiography evaluation? Am J Med. 2015;128:1244–50.
140. van der Valk FM, Bernelot Moens SJ, Verweij SL, Strang AC, Nederveen AJ, Verberne HJ, Nurmohamed MT, Baeten DL, Stroes ES. Increased arterial wall inflammation in patients with ankylosing spondylitis is reduced by statin therapy. Ann Rheum Dis. 2016;75(10):1848–51. https://doi.org/10.1136/annrheumdis-2016-209176.
141. Kastner DL, Aksentijevich I, Goldbach-Mansky R. Autoinflammatory disease reloaded: a clinical perspective. Cell. 2010;140:784–90.
142. Trost S, Rosé CD. Myocarditis and sacroiliitis: 2 previously unrecognized manifestations of tumor necrosis factor receptor associated periodic syndrome. J Rheumatol. 2005;32:175–7.
143. Hedayatfar A. Behçet's disease: autoimmune or autoinflammatory? J Ophthalmic Vis Res. 2013;8:291–3.
144. Higashihara M, Mori M, Takeuchi A, Ogita T, Miyamoto T, Okimoto T. Myocarditis in Behcet's disease--a case report and review of the literature. J Rheumatol. 1982;9:630–3.
145. Maeda S, Tamur A, Zaizen H, Takahashi N. Behçet's disease complicated by giant-cell myocarditis. Intern Med. 2014;53:1721.
146. Savage E, Wazir T, Drake M, Cuthbert R, Wright G. Fulminant myocarditis and macrophage activation syndrome secondary to adult-onset Still's disease successfully treated with Tocilizumab. Rheumatology. 2014;53:1352–3.

Giant Cell and Hypersensitivity Myocarditis

12

Yahaira Ortiz Gonzalez and Leslie T. Cooper

12.1 Historical Background

Giant cell myocarditis (GCM) is an uncommon inflammatory disease of the myocardium that is usually rapidly progressive and carries a high mortality [1]. Hypersensitivity myocarditis (HSM) shares some histological features and a generally poor prognosis with GCM. Because of their rarity and rapidly progressive clinical course, both disorders are frequently undiagnosed until autopsy or heart transplantation. This chapter will first review our current understanding of the typical and rare clinical and histological features of these disorders. The second part of this chapter will link pathogenesis and the gaps in the knowledge of HSM and GCM mechanisms with proposals for translational studies to pioneer better management strategies.

GCM was first described by Sergius Saltykow, a pathologist in Basel, Switzerland, in a fatal case of myocarditis in a man with abdominal infection [2]. The first case demonstrated representative features of the disorder including rapid clinical deterioration and typical histology of diffuse myocardial inflammation with multinucleated giant cells and myocyte necrosis [2]. Until the 1970s, GCM and idiopathic granulomatous myocarditis (or cardiac sarcoidosis, CS) were terms used interchangeably to describe a group of myocarditis with giant cells [3]. In 1975 a landmark paper argued that the histology of GCM was histologically distinct from CS (idiopathic granulomatous myocarditis) and should be distinguished by the greater number of eosinophils, prominent necrosis, and the absence of granuloma [4]. The terms GCM and CS attempt to define uniform histological categories, but the diseases actually overlap in a minority of cases. Recently a multicenter team characterized this intermediate form of myocarditis with histological features of both CS and GCM and an intermediate risk of death or heart transplantation [5]. The prevalence of GCM

Y. O. Gonzalez · L. T. Cooper (✉)
Department of Cardiovascular Medicine, Mayo Clinic in Florida, Jacksonville, FL, USA
e-mail: Gonzalez.Yahaira@mayo.edu; cooper.leslie@mayo.edu

A. L. P. Caforio (ed.), *Myocarditis*, https://doi.org/10.1007/978-3-030-35276-9_12

is known from referral center autopsy and heart biopsy registries and has been estimated to be around 0.007% of deaths [6–8] or 0.4% of native heart biopsies [9, 10].

HSM was classically described in the context of an adverse drug reaction to sulfonamides. French and Weller reported autopsy findings from 126 cases of fatal interstitial myocarditis in patients exposed to sulfonamides. Histologic evaluation showed a distinct pattern of mononuclear cell, especially eosinophils, infiltration predominantly located in the perivascular region, and lack of significant myocardial necrosis (Fig. 12.1) [11, 12]. Eosinophilic infiltration was also observed in other organs such as lungs, liver, and kidneys [12]. They developed an experimental model to recapitulate the disease by intraperitoneal delivery of sulfa-containing medications and could cause similar interstitial myocarditis. Other medications and the smallpox vaccine have been linked to hypersensitivity myocarditis including those listed on Table 12.1 [11, 13–15].

Despite a lack of necrosis, HSM has a poor prognosis with a 46.3% rate of death, ventricular assist device use, or transplantation at 120 days compared to other forms of eosinophilic myocarditis (Fig. 12.2) [16]. The distinction between GCM and HSM is challenging because occasionally some of the same

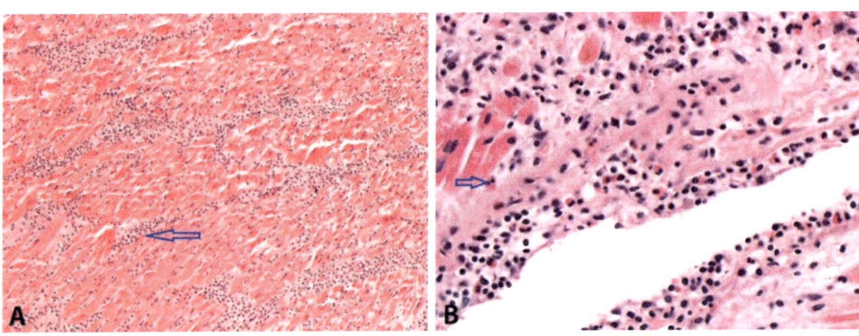

Fig. 12.1 Photomicrography of the myocardium. (**a**) A "roadmap" pattern of perivascular mixed inflammation with eosinophils (arrow) (H&E, 100×); (**b**) Higher power view of perivascular inflammation showing small round lymphocytes, histiocytes, and eosinophils with bilobed nuclei (arrow) (H&E, 400×). Courtesy of Dr. Natraj Katta. Katta et al. [11]

Table 12.1 List of some of the medications that can cause hypersensitivity myocarditis

Medications associated with hypersensitivity myocarditis	
Sulfonamides	Phenytoin
Clozapine	Carbamazepine
Dobutamine	Cephalosporin
Methyldopa	Digoxin
Penicillin	Isoniazid
Spironolactone	Hydrochlorothiazide
Chlorthalidone	Sulfadiazine

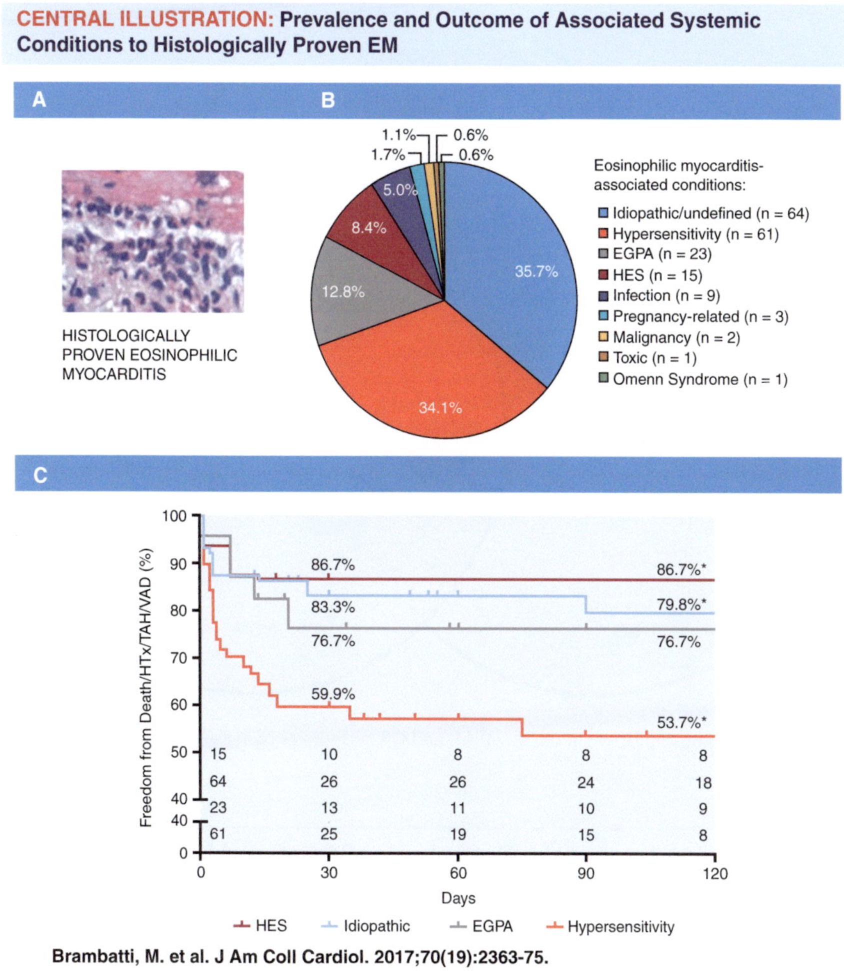

Fig. 12.2 Kaplan-Meier survival free from death, heart transplantation, total artificial heart, and long-term left ventricular assist device of different forms of eosinophilic myocarditis. *HES* Hypereosinophilic syndrome, *EGPA* Eosinophilic granulomatous polyangiitis

medications that cause HSM can cause GCM with features of systemic hypersensitivity [17]. This observation has led to the hypothesis that some cases of HSM might be an early form of GCM before giant cells have time to form in the lesions. In experimental GCM, giant cells appear after about 2 weeks. Both disorders are characterized by high rates of heart failure, ventricular arrhythmias, and hemodynamic instability [17, 18]. Based on these observations, we propose a paradigm to describe the current relationships between GCM, HSM, and CS (Fig. 12.3).

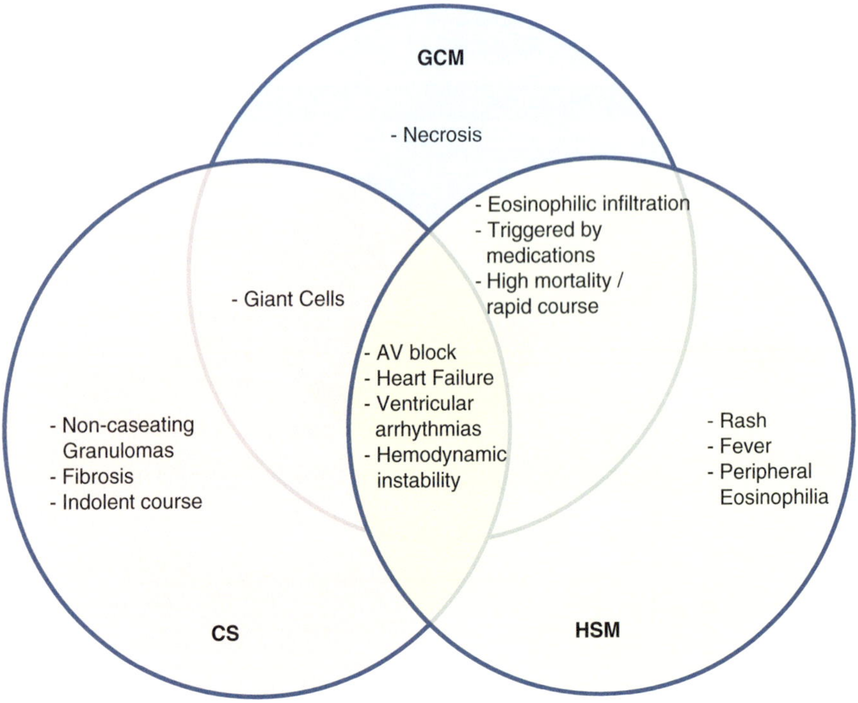

Fig. 12.3 Relationship between GCM, HSM, and CS

12.2 Comparison of the Pathology of GCM and HSM

The gross cardiac pathology of GCM often reveals increased heart weight associated with biventricular dilatation; however, recent onset and clinically fulminant cases may have left ventricular wall thickening and normal sized chambers due to extensive inflammation and edema [6]. Small pericardial effusions are common, but rarely associated with tamponade physiology. Rare findings include epicardial inflammatory polyps filled with giant cells, shown in Fig. 12.4, and occasionally cardiac free wall rupture [6]. Recently a more benign form of GCM was described in an isolated atrial form. The atria can be severely dilated and thickened with preserved ventricular function as shown in the cardiac MRI in Fig. 12.5 [19, 20]. The gross pathology of HSM also features a dilated heart, but accompanied by eosinophil rich infiltrates in other organs such as the liver. Intracavitary thrombi are relatively common in HSM due to the pro-thrombotic major basic protein that is released from degranulated eosinophils [13, 21].

Histologically, idiopathic GCM is characterized by the presence of multinucleated giant cells, diffuse infiltration of lymphocytic inflammatory cells, and myocardial necrosis. Fibrosis is usually absent or mild and granulomas are absent. The

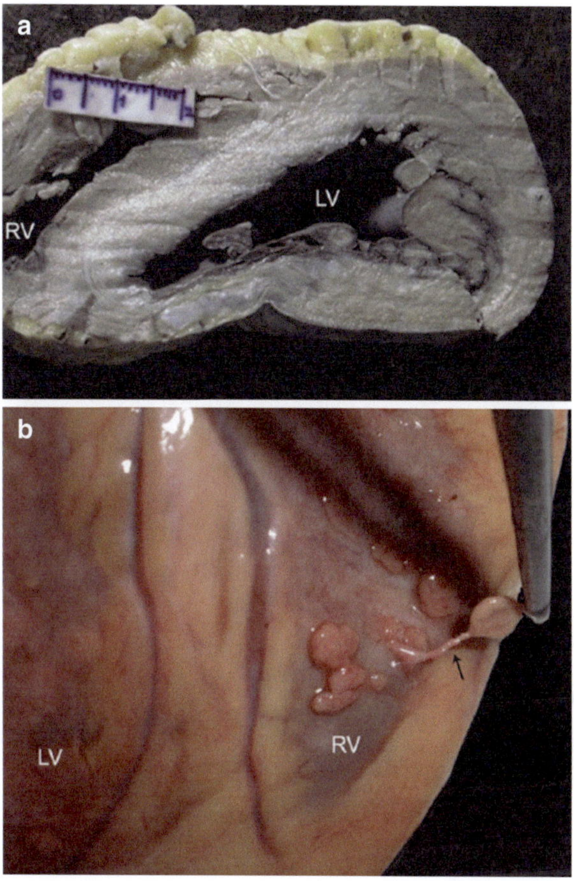

Fig. 12.4 Gross anatomy of giant cell myocarditis. (**a**) Biventricular dilatation with multifocal nontransmural glistening gray-white foci of fibrosis in the posterior wall. (**b**) The arrow shows exudates on the posterior surface of the right ventricle. Obtained from Vaideeswar and Cooper [6]

giant cells are frequently found near the edges of active inflammatory lesions [22]. Autopsies of cases with idiopathic GCM have shown areas of necrosis with giant cells at the margins that seem to be contiguous with myocardial cell fibers, suggesting the possibility of the giant cells being derived from myocytes [4]. When giant cells are present in the center of noncaseating granulomas, granulomatous diseases such as sarcoidosis, tuberculosis, and fungal myocarditis should be considered. Aschoff bodies in rheumatic carditis, granulomatosis with polyangiitis, Whipple's disease, and foreign body reactions around ventricular assist devices or pacemaker leads may have giant cells embedded in interstitial granulomas [23–25]. In CS there is more fibrosis, while in GCM there is a greater number of eosinophils and diffuse pattern of inflammatory cells as shown in Fig. 12.6 [3]. After immunosuppression, histological improvement occurs gradually first with disappearance of eosinophils, giant cells, and lastly the lymphocytic infiltration [26]. In contrast, the classic histology of HSM is a perivascular, eosinophil rich, lesions with little necrosis. Other eosinophil rich lesions such as the endocardial process typical of idiopathic hypereosinophilic syndrome should be considered [22].

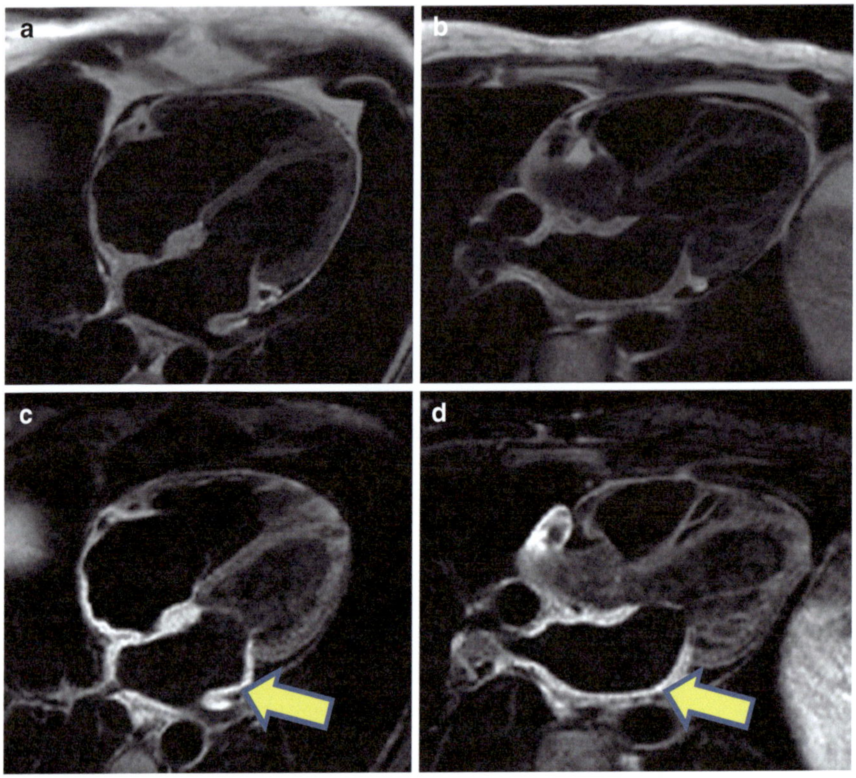

Fig. 12.5 Cardiac MRI findings in atrial giant cell myocarditis. T2 weighted imaging with end diastolic four-chamber view (**a**) and 3-chamber (**b**) with marked bi-atrial thickening and enlargement. T2 weighted spectral adiabatic inversion recovery sequence imaging with end diastolic four-chamber (**c**) and 3-chamber (**d**) showing marked edema of atria (tissue enhancement labeled by yellow arrow) without ventricular involvement. (Obtained from Larsen et al. [19])

12.3 Clinical Presentation

HSM and GCM are both associated with heart failure and ventricular arrhythmias. Most patients with GCM present with progressive heart failure symptoms over several weeks. GCM usually affects younger individuals with a mean age of about 42 years old without gender difference [10]. The older age of subjects in one report, the GCM Treatment Trial, was due to a more fulminant course in younger screened subjects who either received a VAD/transplant or died before enrollment [27]. These data suggest that the clinical course can be slightly less aggressive in older patients. The time from symptom onset to diagnosis was 1.2 ± 4.4 months for GCM [3]. The most common presenting symptoms observed in the Multicenter GCM study group were heart failure symptoms with shortness of breath, decrease in exercise tolerance, and peripheral edema in 75% of the patients; syncope, palpitations, and

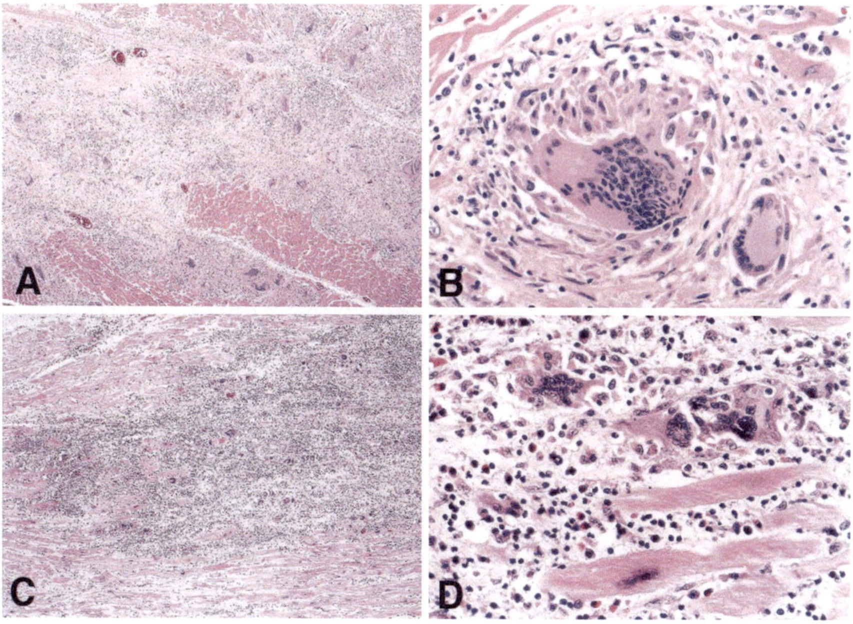

Fig. 12.6 (**a**) Cardiac sarcoidosis characterized by granulomas (H&E ×60). (**b**) High-power magnification showing well-formed non-necrotizing granulomas composed of epithelioid histiocytes and giant cells embedded in the collagenous stroma. Mononuclear cells and fibroblast surround the granulomas (H&E ×400). (**c**) Idiopathic GCM showing widespread necrosis of myocytes by a dense cellular infiltrate (H&E ×100) (**d**) High-power magnification of idiopathic GCM displaying giant cells, lymphocytes, histiocytes, eosinophils, and damaged myocytes (H&E ×400). Obtained from Okura et al. [3]

sudden cardiac death in 14% of the patients; chest pain or electrocardiographic changes suggestive of acute coronary syndrome in 6% of the patients; and complete heart block in 5% [1]. A common cause of death in patients with GCM and HSM is refractory ventricular tachycardia [21, 28]. Extracorporeal membrane oxygenation (ECMO) with LV venting has been used as a short-term support strategy for patients who develop a non-perfusing rhythm [29].

Several extracardiac features and exceptions to the typical cardiac presentation of GCM are worth noting. Twenty percent of cases are associated with features of autoimmunity in other organs, most commonly inflammatory bowel disease. At the time of diagnosis, inflammation can be found in other organs including skeletal muscles and liver in about 10% of cases in our experience. In children with GCM (younger than 19 years) only females had extracardiac inflammation [30]. Myasthenia gravis may be present sometimes associated with thymoma, the one tumor associated with GCM. There have been no families described with multiple affected family members and no genes associated with disease risk. There are no clusters of cases to suggest a particular pathogen or toxic exposure. In the cases of isolated atrial GCM, findings include mitral and tricuspid regurgitation, atrial mural thrombus, and atrial fibrillation [19].

Similar to GCM, patients with HSM present with shortness of breath (47.5%), chest pain (35.5%), and fever (54.2%) [16]. In contrast to GCM, HSM seems to affect a slightly younger population with median age of 35 years. There is usually a history of recent new drug exposure or a vaccine, particularly smallpox vaccines. Peripheral eosinophilia is common, present in 63.5% of cases, whereas it is rare in GCM [21]. Sometimes a skin rash or elevated transaminases from hepatitis will suggest hypersensitivity and a target for biopsy to confirm the diagnosis [13, 21]. Thus the classic HSM presentation would be dyspnea or chest pain with tachycardia and nonspecific electrocardiogram changes [11, 13, 28]. The history of recent new drug or vaccine, presence of a rash, eosinophilia, and other features of hypersensitivity would lead towards advanced imaging and biopsy. A careful investigation for intracardiac thrombus is indicated as venous and arterial thrombi appear to be more common in the presence of degranulating eosinophils.

12.4 Diagnosis

EMB for diagnosis of suspected GCM and HSM should be considered in patients with rapidly progressive heart failure despite guideline directed medical therapy [31, 32]. Endomyocardial biopsy (EMB) for GCM has over 80% sensitivity compared to CS or routine lymphocytic myocarditis that is only 20–30%, due to the diffuse inflammation of the myocardium compared to heterogeneous distribution in the latter disease [33]. In the case of GCM, repeated endomyocardial biopsies and left ventricular tissues biopsies increase the sensitivity from 68% to 93% [34, 35]. There are no studies to date reporting the sensitivity of EMB for HSM. Thus the recommendation for biopsy for suspected HSM is based on expert opinion (Level C) [36].

Biopsy technique is important to get an acceptable sensitivity. In 2007 the American Heart Association, American College of Cardiology, and European Society of Cardiology (AHA/ACCF/ESC) published a scientific statement recommending to obtain 5–10 samples from more than one region of the right ventricular septum and to place the samples in 10% neutral formalin solution [36, 37]. With special stains and gene chip analysis, infiltrative diseases, viral genomes, and inflammatory diseases can be quantitated. EMB is indicated as a class I recommendation (level of evidence B) for the unexplained new onset heart failure of less than 2 weeks duration associated with hemodynamic compromise or in the setting of ventricular arrhythmias or AV block that does not respond to medical therapy [36]. In the setting of unexplained heart failure symptoms associated with dilated cardiomyopathy and a suspected allergic reaction with eosinophilia, EMB is a class IIa indication [36].

EMB risk varies with user experience and technique. In an analysis of the United States Nationwide Inpatient Sample database the rate of cardiac tamponade requiring pericardiocentesis was higher in patients without heart transplant at a rate of

0.7% versus 0.19% in post-heart transplant patients [38]. In addition, the rate of perforation seemed to be higher in females (0.94%) compared to males (0.53%) [38]. In experienced centers using flexible, softer bioptomes, the risks are lower. Single center studies have reported risk of tamponade requiring surgical intervention in about 0.58–0.64% of cases and no reported deaths [39, 40]. Large series from Germany and Italy reported a 0.01% risk of death and 0.04–0.4% risk of perforation when performed by an experienced operator [41].

When biopsy is non-diagnostic or infeasible, cardiac magnetic resonance (CMR) can be used as a noninvasive diagnostic tool to suggest the diagnosis of myocarditis [42]. CMR may aid in the identification of myocarditis but tissue is needed to confirm diagnosis especially in the case of GCM. Although CMR seems like a practical first approach studies are often limited by the hemodynamic instability of the patients.

In 2018, the Consensus Criteria for CMR in myocardial inflammation, known as the Lake Louise Criteria, was updated to reflect the use of novel mapping modalities that allows for higher sensitivity and diagnostic accuracy compared to the original criteria (proposed in 2009). The updated Lake Louise Criteria provides strong evidence for acute myocarditis when there is presence of at least of one criterion of each of the following two categories:

- myocardial edema demonstrated by either T2 mapping or T2 weighted images with increased signal intensity;
- or non-ischemic myocardial injury by abnormal T1, extracellular volume fraction (ECV), or late gadolinium enhancement.

Other supportive criteria for the diagnosis of acute myocarditis include presence of effusion in cine images or abnormal LGE, or regional or global systolic left ventricular dysfunction [42].

In the recent years, studies have demonstrated greater diagnostic accuracy for acute myocarditis (<14 days of symptoms) with the use of newer CMR modalities such as native T1 mapping, T2 mapping, and ECV [42, 43]. In the MyoRacer trial, in which CMR techniques were compared to EMB as the diagnostic standard, T1 mapping had the highest diagnostic accuracy (81%) as shown in Fig. 12.7 [43]. Similar results have been observed across different studies as shown in a meta-analysis of 22 CMR studies [44]. The hierarchical receiver-operator curves and areas under the curve (AUC) comparing their diagnostic performance are as follows: T1 mapping (AUC: 0.95; 95% CI: 0.93–0.97), T2 mapping (AUC: 0.88; 95% CI: 0.85–0.91), ECV (AUC: 0.81; 95% CI: 0.78–0.85), T2 weighted imaging (AUC: 0.80; 95% CI: 0.76–0.83), early gadolinium enhancement (AUC: 0.78; 95% CI: 0.74–0.81), late gadolinium enhancement (AUC: 0.89; 95% CI: 0.86–0.92), and the Lake Louise Criteria 2009 (AUC: 0.81; 95% CI: 0.77–0.84) [44].

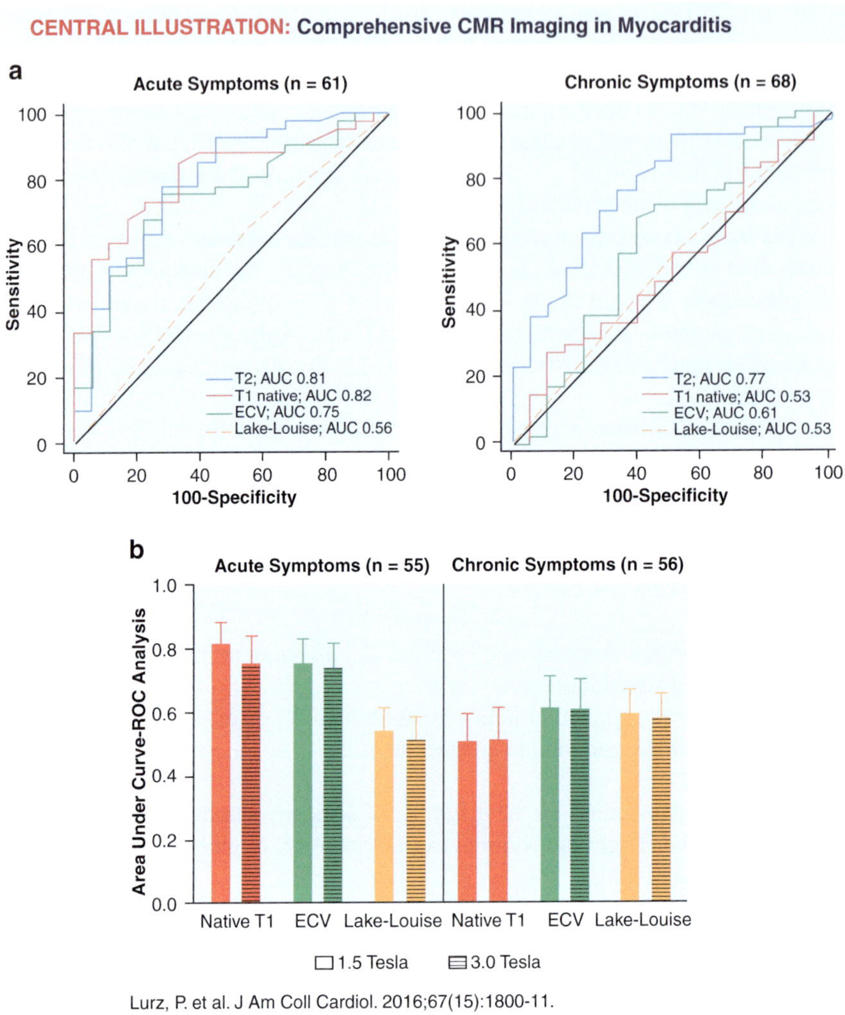

Fig. 12.7 (**a**) Per the receiver-operator curves (ROCs) on 1.5-T imaging, in patients with acute symptoms (left), the AUCs were significantly higher for native T_1 ($p = 0.002$), ECV ($p = 0.04$), and T_2 ($p = 0.001$) as compared with LLC, with no significant differences between mapping techniques. In patients with chronic symptoms (right), the AUC for T_2 mapping was superior to LLC ($p = 0.002$) and native T_1 ($p = 0.04$). (**b**) The comparison of receiver-operator analyses on 1.5- versus 3-T imaging showed no significant differences between field strength. *AUC* area under the curve, *CMR* cardiac magnetic resonance, *ECV* extracellular volume fraction, *LLC* Lake Louise criteria. (Obtained from Lurz et al. [43])

12.5 Therapies

The survival of patients with GCM is about 3 months from symptom onset to death or transplant without immunosuppression. The median time from admission to death, long-term mechanical circulatory support, or total artificial heart was about

3 days (IQR: 1–9 days) for HSM [21]. Survival for GCM and HSM likely increases with early use of immunosuppressive therapy. In a study by Kandolin et al., in the era of immunosuppression, among 32 patients with GCM, five patients died and ten underwent transplantation for a median survival of 11 months from symptom onset (1–66 months) [34]. GCM patients who undergo heart transplantation have a similar survival as those who have transplant for dilated cardiomyopathy [45].

12.6 Immunosuppressive Treatment

Randomized treatment trials for GCM and HSM are infeasible due to the rarity of the disease and rapid clinical course. However, case series and one prospective trial for GCM suggest that combination immunosuppressive therapy that includes cyclosporine may improve transplant-free survival in GCM. The prospective GCM treatment trial attempted to randomize patients with GCM and less than 3 months from symptom onset to either an active treatment arm (muromonab-CD3, cyclosporine, and steroids) or a usual care arm (prednisone, azathioprine, or no immunosuppression at investigator's discretion). Although 60 patients with suspected and proven GCM were referred to the investigators during the 5 year enrollment window, 36 received VAD, transplant or died (with histologic confirmation of GCM) before they could be enrolled. Of the remaining 24 diagnosed by biopsy and eligible, 12 signed consent and 11 completed the trial or a prospective registry for the subjects who refused randomization. After 2 years of enrollment only eight patients were registered and all subjects chose the registry with defined treatment, muromonab-CD3 5 mg/day for 10 days and cyclosporine titrated to target levels of 150–300 ng/ml for 1 year. For the first 3 days of treatment muromonab-CD3 was preceded by IV solumedrol 10 mg/kg followed by a prednisone taper for 1 year [27]. The average trough CSA level was 169 ng/ml at 1 month and 126 ng/ml at 6 months. One patient died within the year from respiratory complications (autopsy demonstrated no inflammation in the heart) and two underwent heart transplantation. Compared to matched historical controls diagnosed by biopsy and treated with prednisone or no immunosuppression, survival free of transplantation was improved at 1 year with immunosuppressive therapy. One subject died of biopsy-proven recurrent GCM after stopping all immunosuppressive after 1 year. On follow-up biopsy after 4 weeks of treatment there was marked reduction in inflammatory cells and an increase in fibrosis. The serious adverse effects reported from therapy included transient renal insufficiency due to treatment with cyclosporine that improved with substitution to sirolimus [26, 27]. Sirolimus has also been shown to be beneficial as an adjunctive therapy in post-heart transplant recurrence of GCM [46]. Figure 12.8 shows the histologic improvement in GCM after 30 days of immunosuppression therapy [47].

Kandolin et al. reported a retrospective study of GCM patients treated with combination immunosuppressive therapy that included corticosteroids, azathioprine, and cyclosporine or mycophenolate mofetil ± gamma globulin and muromonab. Survival was 85% at 14 months of follow up. The most common adverse therapeutic effects reported in this study included renal insufficiency, lymphocytopenia, pancreatitis, muscular weakness, weight gain, and insomnia [34].

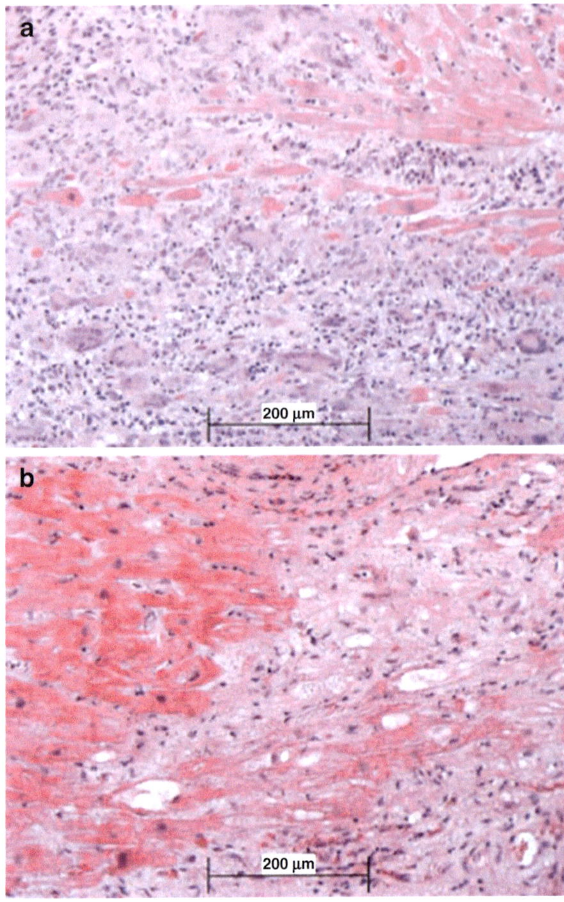

Fig. 12.8 Histological findings of giant cell myocarditis (**a**) with diffuse myocardial inflammation and presence of giant cells that (**b**) improve after 30 days of immunosuppressive therapy with some replacement fibrosis. Obtained from Cooper et al. [27]

A retrospective study of 46 patients with GCM treated with triple immunosuppressive therapy (most patients treated with prednisone, azathioprine, and cyclosporine) showed an improved 1 year transplant-free survival of 80% and 5 year transplant-free survival of 58% which is slightly higher than that reported by the multicenter GCM study group [8]. The excellent transplant-free survival in this population may in part be related to the relatively preserved left ventricular ejection fraction of 41% and low New York Heart Association (NYHA) classification, primarily I and II.

In contrast to GCM, treatment of hypersensitivity myocarditis consists of withdrawing the offending agent if known and support with guideline directed therapies. Immunosuppressive therapy with corticosteroids, sometimes with cyclosporine, alemtuzumab, mepolizumab, and interferon gamma has been used with anecdotal success [14, 48]. In some instances when eosinophilia is due to dobutamine, myocarditis may improve with substation of milrinone or mechanical circulatory support (MCS) [49].

12.7 Mechanical Circulatory Support

All patients with recent onset cardiomyopathy should receive treatment according to current heart failure guidelines [50–52]. Unfortunately due to the acute onset of disease and common deterioration to hemodynamic instability, GCM and HSM patients may not tolerate optimization of medical treatment and instead may require single or multiple inotropes or MCS. In this clinical scenario, we advocate for early EMB and referral to a medical center with expertise at transplantation. Case series and case reports of patients with GCM support surgical MCS with either left ventricular assist device (LVAD), biventricular support, or percutaneous temporary MCS (Impella, ECMO) as a bridge to transplantation or recovery [29, 53–58]. In an older series, patients who had LVAD for GCM prior to transplantation had a lower survival 57% at 30 days and 29% at 1 year compared to the 93% survival in patients who underwent transplantation without LVAD support [53]. The poor prognosis of the GCM treated mostly without immunosuppression is also demonstrated in a French registry study of 13 patients with GCM, 11 received ECMO, one received biventricular support, and one received LVAD. All of the patients either died (4) or received transplantation (9) [59]. Few of these patients had EMB diagnosis or immunosuppression prior to transplant.

Mechanical unloading of the left ventricle in the setting of GCM or HSM may decrease inflammation and increase the chance of successful bridge to transplantation or recovery [60]. This effect could be less with peripheral VA ECMO since the increased afterload from retrograde perfusion without venting can cause LV dilatation from increased wall stress [57, 61]. Strategies to lessen this impact include use of an Impella or an intra-aortic balloon pump for offloading of the ventricle. One case report of a patient with GCM with a left ventricular Impella 5.0 was placed for 39 days along with standard heart failure therapy and immunosuppression with steroids and azathioprine. Decreased inflammation was noted on biopsies at 2 weeks and 4 weeks. The offloading effects were eradicated after explantation of Impella despite continuation of immunosuppression therapy [57]. The balance of risks and benefits from immunosuppressive therapy for GCM or HSM after MCS needs to be individualized [29].

12.8 Transplantation

Transplantation should be considered for GCM patients who fail to respond to guideline directed care and immunosuppression. The estimated survival of GCM patients in the early 1990s–2000s before transplantation was 69% at 1 year, 58% at 2 years, and 52% at 5 years [34]. The cumulative survival post-heart transplant for GCM patients was 94%, 82%, and 68%, at 1, 5, and 10 years, respectively [45]. An analysis performed on the United Network for Organ Sharing Registry (UNOS) demonstrated no difference in death or allograft loss among GCM patients who had undergone heart transplantation compared to other forms of cardiomyopathy or dilated cardiomyopathy, but these patients did have a higher risk of acute rejection [45]. Recurrence of GCM in the allograft has been reported in up to 25% of patients' post-heart transplant [34]. The range of time to recurrence of GCM following transplant is from 3 weeks to 9 years. Anecdotally, the earlier and more aggressive recurrences occurred in patients under age 20 [62]. Most recurrences are detected on routine surveillance biopsy and respond to a bolus and taper of corticosteroids. Recurrence associated with allograft dysfunction is more serious and rarely can lead to loss of the allograft. Management is not certain, but case reports and our experience in native heart GCM suggest that one dose of Campath can be highly effective at improving LV function. Utilization of individual institution's protocol may be used as a guide for the frequency of EMB along with echocardiography, electrocardiogram, and history and physical. In the case of HSM and eosinophilic myocarditis there may be an increased risk of acute cellular rejection in patients with HSM prior to transplantation compared to those patients without HSM, but no difference in survival [63, 64].

12.9 Pathogenesis and Proposal for Future Investigations

The discussion of pathogenesis usually precedes the clinical aspects of disease in this type of review. We chose to move this section to the end because so little is known and the gaps in our mechanistic knowledge are what can best direct translational studies to impact the burden of these clinically important and immune-mediated diseases.

GCM is usually an autoimmune disorder [1, 23, 24]. In the Multicenter Giant Cell Myocarditis Study Group the autoimmune disorder mostly associated with GCM was ulcerative colitis in 8% of the patients. Other autoimmune disorders associated with GCM in less than 2% of the cases included optic neuritis, fibromyalgia, hyperthyroidism, hypothyroidism, and cryofibrinogenemia [1]. Single case reports have shown an association of GCM with coxsackie B2 [65], parvovirus B19 [66], and human herpesvirus [67].

The experimental model of GCM in Lewis rats develops after immunization with human cardiac myosin in complete Freud's adjuvant. The experimental disease is mediated by T lymphocytes and improves with calcineurin inhibitors or anti-T cell monoclonal antibodies. Corticosteroids alone do not improve outcome in this model. The histology is identical to human disease [68]. In one clinical study, GCM was associated with autoantibodies against cardiac myosin that bind to the beta-adrenergic receptors and induce cAMP protein kinase activity [69, 70].

The mechanism of ventricular tachycardia in GCM is associated with altered trafficking of desmosomal proteins, similar to the changes observed in arrhythmogenic right ventricular cardiomyopathy (ARVC). Plakophillin and plakoglobin can translocate to the cytosol as shown in Fig. 12.9 [71]. The loss of desmosomal proteins at the cell junctions may provide a substrate for ventricular arrhythmias.

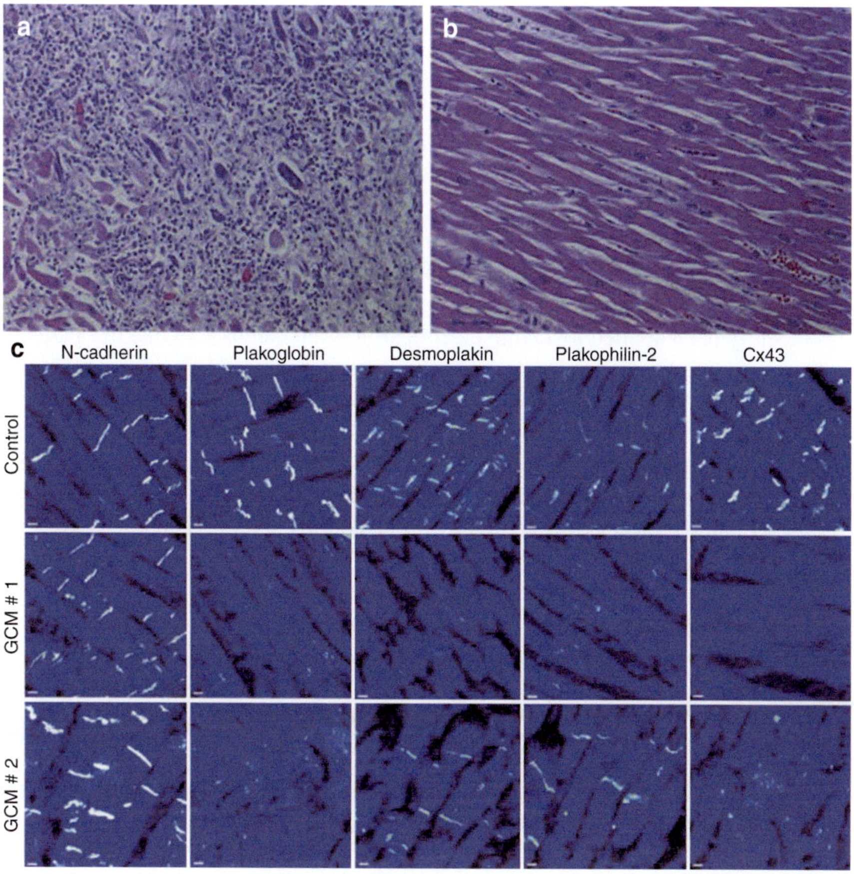

Fig. 12.9 (**a**) Microscopic appearance of the myocardium from a patient with GCM, showing severe destruction of cardiac myocytes (hematoxylin–eosin, magnification ×20). (**b**) Normal-appearing myocardium from the same patient, showing no apparent inflammatory or degenerative changes (hematoxylin–eosin, magnification ×20). (**c**) Representative confocal immunofluorescence images of control myocardium and myocardium from two patients with GCM. Specific immunoreactive signal for plakoglobin was significantly depressed in both cases compared with controls, as was signal for the major gap junction protein Cx43. Expression of other desmosomal proteins, including desmoplakin and plakophilin-2, varied, but signal for the nondesmosomal adhesion protein N-cadherin was present in all GCM cases analyzed and indistinguishable from controls. GCM indicates giant cell myocarditis; Cx43, connexin43 [71]

Eosinophilic myocarditis begins with infiltration of eosinophils into the myocardium and the release of myotoxic proteins including major basic protein from the eosinophilic granules. The eosinophilic infiltration occurs mainly in the perivascular areas. The major basic proteins and eosinophilic cationic proteins activate mast cells and subsequently cause myocyte necrosis and late fibrosis [14, 72]. Activated mast cells release histamine, cytokines, leukotrienes, and prostaglandins resulting in increased vascular permeability and vasodilation [73]. Tissue factor is also released from eosinophilic granules and can promote thrombosis and systemic embolization. Risk factors for HSM have not been identified.

The substantial gaps in our mechanistic knowledge suggest several prime areas for near-term translational research. The first for both GCM and HSM is to define factors associated with disease susceptibility. There is not one unique trigger or environmental exposure that links the known clinical cases. However, the development of relatively large and diverse cardiomyopathy databases allows for newer artificial intelligence algorithms to be applied to define subtle factors and collections of factors that could yield at novel risk profiles. A similar kind of technique has recently been applied to a large electrocardiogram database to identify patients with undiagnosed cardiomyopathy [74].

The genetic contributions to GCM and HSM disease risk are also ripe for investigation with newer whole genome sequencing linked to transcriptomic profiles. Such multi-platform integrated data has been used to define risk of dementia [75]. Finally, more pathway specific treatments based on immunophenotype may lower the rates of side effects associated with corticosteroids and lower long-term risk of cardiomyopathy [76].

References

1. Cooper LT Jr, Berry GJ, Shabetai R. Idiopathic giant-cell myocarditis--natural history and treatment. Multicenter Giant Cell Myocarditis Study Group Investigators. N Engl J Med. 1997;336(26):1860–6.
2. Saltykow S. Uber diffuse myokarditis. Virchows Archiv fur Pathologische Anatomie. 1905;182:1–39.
3. Okura Y, et al. A clinical and histopathologic comparison of cardiac sarcoidosis and idiopathic giant cell myocarditis. J Am Coll Cardiol. 2003;41(2):322–9.
4. Davies M, Pomerance A, Teare R. Idiopathic giant cell myocarditis—a distinctive clinico-pathological entity. Br Heart J. 1975;37:192–5.
5. Maleszewski JJ, Larsen BT, Castonguay MC, Youg RK, Cooper LT, Halushka MK. Is there an intermediate diagnostic category between sarcoidosis and idiopathic giant cell myocarditis? Lab Investig. 2014;94:90A–5A.
6. Vaideeswar P, Cooper LT. Giant cell myocarditis: clinical and pathological features in an Indian population. Cardiovasc Pathol. 2013;22(1):70–4.
7. Okada R, Wakafuji S. Myocarditis in autopsy. Heart Vessels Suppl. 1985;1:23–9.
8. Ekstrom K, et al. Long-term outcome and its predictors in giant cell myocarditis. Eur J Heart Fail. 2016;18(12):1452–8.
9. Winters GL, Costanzo-Nordin MR. Pathological findings in 2300 consecutive endomyocardial biopsies. Mod Pathol. 1991;4(4):441–8.
10. Cooper LT Jr, ElAmm C. Giant cell myocarditis. Diagnosis and treatment. Herz. 2012;37(6):632–6.
11. Katta N, Balla S, Aggarwal K. Clozapine-induced hypersensitivity myocarditis presenting as sudden cardiac death. Autops Case Rep. 2016;6(4):9–13.
12. Fench A, Weller C. Interstitial myocarditis following the clinical and experimental use of sulfonamide drugs. Am J Pathol. 1942;18:122.
13. Fenoglio JJ Jr, McAllister HA Jr, Mullick FG. Drug related myocarditis. I. Hypersensitivity myocarditis. Hum Pathol. 1981;12(10):900–7.

14. Cheung CC, et al. Eosinophilic myocarditis. Am J Med Sci. 2017;354(5):486–92.
15. Engler RJ, et al. A prospective study of the incidence of myocarditis/pericarditis and new onset cardiac symptoms following smallpox and influenza vaccination. PLoS One. 2015;10(3):e0118283.
16. Brambatti M, et al. Eosinophilic myocarditis: characteristics, treatment, and outcomes. J Am Coll Cardiol. 2017;70(19):2363–75.
17. Daniels PR, et al. Giant cell myocarditis as a manifestation of drug hypersensitivity. Cardiovasc Pathol. 2000;9(5):287–91.
18. Burke AP, et al. Hypersensitivity myocarditis. Arch Pathol Lab Med. 1991;115(8):764–9.
19. Larsen BT, et al. Atrial giant cell myocarditis: a distinctive clinicopathologic entity. Circulation. 2013;127(1):39–47.
20. Law KK, et al. Echocardiographic features of atrial myocarditis with giant cells: a case report. J Am Soc Echocardiogr. 2004;17(10):1073–6.
21. Brambatti M, et al. Eosinophilic myocarditis characteristics, treatment, and outcomes. J Am Coll Cardiol. 2017;70(19):2363–75.
22. Cooper LT Jr. Acute heart failure due to fulminant and giant cell myocarditis. Herz. 2006;31(8):767–70.
23. Blauwet LA, Cooper LT. Idiopathic giant cell myocarditis and cardiac sarcoidosis. Heart Fail Rev. 2013;18(6):733–46.
24. Mitoff PR, et al. Giant cell myocarditis in a patient with a spondyloarthropathy after a drug hypersensitivity reaction. Can J Cardiol. 2013;29(9):1138 e7–8.
25. Cooper LT Jr. Giant cell and granulomatous myocarditis. Heart Fail Clin. 2005;1(3):431–7.
26. Maleszewski JJ, et al. Long-term risk of recurrence, morbidity and mortality in giant cell myocarditis. Am J Cardiol. 2015;115(12):1733–8.
27. Cooper LT, et al. Usefulness of immunosuppression for Giant cell myocarditis. Am J Cardiol. 2008;102(11):1535–9.
28. Taliercio CP, Olney BA, Lie JT. Myocarditis related to drug hypersensitivity. Mayo Clin Proc. 1985;60(7):463–8.
29. Ammirati E, et al. Giant cell myocarditis successfully treated with antithymocyte globuline and extracorporeal membrane oxygenation for 21 days. J Cardiovasc Med (Hagerstown). 2016;17(Suppl 2):e151–3.
30. Cooper LT. Giant cell myocarditis in children. Prog Pediatr Cardiol. 2007;24(1):47–9.
31. Bozkurt B, et al. Current diagnostic and treatment strategies for specific dilated cardiomyopathies: a scientific statement from the American Heart Association. Circulation. 2016;134(23):e579–646.
32. Caforio AL, et al. Current state of knowledge on aetiology, diagnosis, management, and therapy of myocarditis: a position statement of the European Society of Cardiology Working Group on Myocardial and Pericardial Diseases. Eur Heart J. 2013;34(33):2636–48. 2648a-2648d.
33. Shields RC, et al. The role of right ventricular endomyocardial biopsy for idiopathic giant cell myocarditis. J Card Fail. 2002;8(2):74–8.
34. Kandolin R, et al. Diagnosis, treatment, and outcome of giant-cell myocarditis in the era of combined immunosuppression. Circ Heart Fail. 2013;6(1):15–22.
35. Stiermaier T, et al. Biventricular endomyocardial biopsy in patients with suspected myocarditis: feasibility, complication rate and additional diagnostic value. Int J Cardiol. 2017;230:364–70.
36. Cooper LT, et al. The role of endomyocardial biopsy in the management of cardiovascular disease. Eur Heart J. 2007;28(24):3076–93.
37. Stone JR, et al. Recommendations for processing cardiovascular surgical pathology specimens: a consensus statement from the Standards and Definitions Committee of the Society for Cardiovascular Pathology and the Association for European Cardiovascular Pathology. Cardiovasc Pathol. 2012;21(1):2–16.
38. Shah Z, et al. National trends and procedural complications from endomyocardial biopsy: results from the National inpatient sample, 2007-2014. Cardiology. 2018;141(3):125–31.
39. Bennett MK, et al. Evaluation of the role of endomyocardial biopsy in 851 patients with unexplained heart failure from 2000-2009. Circ Heart Fail. 2013;6(4):676–84.

40. Slawek S, et al. Endomyocardial biopsy via the femoral access - still safe and valuable diagnostic tool. BMC Cardiovasc Disord. 2016;16(1):222.
41. Chimenti C, Frustaci A. Contribution and risks of left ventricular endomyocardial biopsy in patients with cardiomyopathies: a retrospective study over a 28-year period. Circulation. 2013;128(14):1531–41.
42. Ferreira VM, et al. Cardiovascular magnetic resonance in nonischemic myocardial inflammation: expert recommendations. J Am Coll Cardiol. 2018;72(24):3158–76.
43. Lurz P, et al. Comprehensive cardiac magnetic resonance imaging in patients with suspected myocarditis: the MyoRacer-trial. J Am Coll Cardiol. 2016;67(15):1800–11.
44. Kotanidis CP, et al. Diagnostic accuracy of cardiovascular magnetic resonance in acute myocarditis: a systematic review and meta-analysis. JACC Cardiovasc Imaging. 2018;11(11):1583–90.
45. Elamm CA, et al. Heart transplantation in giant cell myocarditis: analysis of the united network for organ sharing registry. J Card Fail. 2017;23(7):566–9.
46. Patel AD, et al. Sirolimus for recurrent giant cell myocarditis after heart transplantation: a unique therapeutic strategy. Am J Ther. 2018;26(5):600–3.
47. Cooper LT Jr, et al. Usefulness of immunosuppression for giant cell myocarditis. Am J Cardiol. 2008;102(11):1535–9.
48. Bleeker JS, et al. Treatment-refractory idiopathic hypereosinophilic syndrome: pitfalls and progress with use of novel drugs. Am J Hematol. 2012;87(7):703–6.
49. Grabellus F, et al. Resolved hypersensitivity myocarditis after ventricular circulatory assist. Ann Thorac Surg. 2003;76(6):2102–4.
50. Yancy CW, et al. 2017 ACC/AHA/HFSA focused update of the 2013 ACCF/AHA guideline for the management of heart failure: a report of the American College of Cardiology/American Heart Association task force on clinical practice guidelines and the Heart Failure Society of America. J Am Coll Cardiol. 2017;70(6):776–803.
51. Yancy CW, et al. 2016 ACC/AHA/HFSA focused update on new pharmacological therapy for heart failure: an update of the 2013 ACCF/AHA guideline for the management of heart failure: a report of the American College of Cardiology/American Heart Association task force on clinical practice guidelines and the Heart Failure Society of America. J Am Coll Cardiol. 2016;68(13):1476–88.
52. Ponikowski P, et al. 2016 ESC guidelines for the diagnosis and treatment of acute and chronic heart failure. Rev Esp Cardiol (Engl Ed). 2016;69(12):1167.
53. Brilakis ES, et al. Survival outcomes of patients with giant cell myocarditis bridged by ventricular assist devices. ASAIO J. 2000;46(5):569–72.
54. Eid SM, et al. Resolution of giant cell myocarditis after extended ventricular assistance. Arch Pathol Lab Med. 2009;133(1):138–41.
55. Marelli D, et al. Support with the BVS 5000 assist device during treatment of acute giant-cell myocarditis. Tex Heart Inst J. 2003;30(1):50–6.
56. Stoica SC, et al. Ventricular assist surprise: giant cell myocarditis or sarcoidosis? J Thorac Cardiovasc Surg. 2003;126(6):2072–4.
57. Tschope C, et al. Mechanical unloading by fulminant myocarditis: LV-IMPELLA, ECMELLA, BI-PELLA, and PROPELLA concepts. J Cardiovasc Transl Res. 2018;12(2):116–23.
58. Annamalai SK, et al. The Impella microaxial flow catheter is safe and effective for treatment of myocarditis complicated by cardiogenic shock: an analysis from the global cVAD registry. J Card Fail. 2018;24(10):706–10.
59. Montero S, et al. Fulminant giant-cell myocarditis on mechanical circulatory support: management and outcomes of a French multicentre cohort. Int J Cardiol. 2018;253:105–12.
60. Cooper LT, Zehr KJ. Biventricular assist device placement and immunosuppression as therapy for necrotizing eosinophilic myocarditis. Nat Clin Pract Cardiovasc Med. 2005;2(10):544–8.
61. Schrage B, et al. Unloading of the left ventricle during venoarterial extracorporeal membrane oxygenation therapy in cardiogenic shock. JACC Heart Fail. 2018;6(12):1035–43.
62. Singh TP, et al. Total lymphoid irradiation: new therapeutic option for refractory giant cell myocarditis. J Heart Lung Transplant. 2004;23(4):492–5.

63. Takkenberg JJ, et al. Eosinophilic myocarditis in patients awaiting heart transplantation. Crit Care Med. 2004;32(3):714–21.
64. Kanai-Yoshizawa S, et al. Hypersensitivity myocarditis and outcome after heart transplantation. J Heart Lung Transplant. 2013;32(5):553–9.
65. Meyer T, et al. Giant cell myocarditis due to Coxsackie B2 virus infection. Cardiology. 1997;88(3):296–9.
66. Dennert R, et al. Giant cell myocarditis triggered by a parvovirus B19 infection. Int J Cardiol. 2009;134(1):115–6.
67. Drut RM, Drut R. Giant-cell myocarditis in a newborn with congenital herpes simplex virus (HSV) infection: an immunohistochemical study on the origin of the giant cells. Pediatr Pathol. 1986;6(4):431–7.
68. Kodama M, et al. A novel experimental model of giant cell myocarditis induced in rats by immunization with cardiac myosin fraction. Clin Immunol Immunopathol. 1990;57(2):250–62.
69. Li Y, et al. Mimicry and antibody-mediated cell signaling in autoimmune myocarditis. J Immunol. 2006;177(11):8234–40.
70. Mascaro-Blanco A, et al. Consequences of unlocking the cardiac myosin molecule in human myocarditis and cardiomyopathies. Autoimmunity. 2008;41(6):442–53.
71. Asimaki A, et al. Altered desmosomal proteins in granulomatous myocarditis and potential pathogenic links to arrhythmogenic right ventricular cardiomyopathy. Circ Arrhythm Electrophysiol. 2011;4(5):743–U240.
72. Ogbogu PU, Rosing DR, Horne MK 3rd. Cardiovascular manifestations of hypereosinophilic syndromes. Immunol Allergy Clin N Am. 2007;27(3):457–75.
73. Schnyder B, Brockow K. Pathogenesis of drug allergy--current concepts and recent insights. Clin Exp Allergy. 2015;45(9):1376–83.
74. Attia ZI, et al. Screening for cardiac contractile dysfunction using an artificial intelligence-enabled electrocardiogram. Nat Med. 2019;25(1):70–4.
75. Ebbert MTW, et al. Conserved DNA methylation combined with differential frontal cortex and cerebellar expression distinguishes C9orf72-associated and sporadic ALS, and implicates SERPINA1 in disease. Acta Neuropathol. 2017;134(5):715–28.
76. Myers JM, et al. Cardiac myosin-Th17 responses promote heart failure in human myocarditis. JCI Insight. 2016;1(9):e85851.

13 Myocarditis in Children

Giuseppe Limongelli, Daniele Masarone, Emanuele Monda, Augusto Esposito, Marta Rubino, and Giuseppe Pacileo

13.1 Definition

According to WHO/ISFC criteria [1], myocarditis is "An inflammatory disease of the myocardium diagnosed by established histological, immunological and immunohistochemical criteria".

Established histological Dallas [2] criteria define myocarditis as follows: "Histological evidence of inflammatory infiltrates within the myocardium associated with myocyte degeneration and necrosis of non-ischaemic origin". The histological diagnosis of myocarditis includes different forms, classified according to the type of inflammatory cell infiltrate: lymphocytic, eosinophilic, giant cell myocarditis, and cardiac sarcoidosis.

Although most cases are asymptomatic or pauci-symptomatic, myocarditis remains a challenging and potentially life-threatening disease. It represents an important cause of morbidity and mortality in children, due to disease complications (i.e., life-threatening arrhythmias and cardiogenic shock in the acute phase; cardiac dysfunction and dilated cardiomyopathy, chronic evolution of the disease).

G. Limongelli (✉)
Paediatric Cardiology, Department of Translational Medical Sciences, Vanvitelli University, Naples, Italy

Heart Failure Unit, AORN Colli, Naples, Italy

Institute of Cardiovascular Sciences, University College of London, London, UK
e-mail: limongelligiuseppe@libero.it

D. Masarone · E. Monda · A. Esposito · M. Rubino · G. Pacileo
Paediatric Cardiology, Department of Translational Medical Sciences, Vanvitelli University, Naples, Italy

Heart Failure Unit, AORN Colli, Naples, Italy
e-mail: danielemasarone@libero.it; emanuelemonda@me.com; augustoesposito1990@gmail.com; rubinomarta@libero.it; gpacileo58@gmail.com

A. L. P. Caforio (ed.), *Myocarditis*, https://doi.org/10.1007/978-3-030-35276-9_13

13.2 Epidemiology

The incidence of paediatric myocarditis is estimated to be 1.95 of 100,000 patients/year. Nevertheless, the true incidence is difficult to determine. Indeed, on the one hand, disease presentation is often with no symptoms (subclinical myocarditis). On the other hand, imaging and laboratory tests are not so specific, and endomyocardial biopsy (EMB) is not performed in most cases. Moreover, symptoms are frequently not specific, sometimes masquerading as respiratory and gastrointestinal infections [3–6].

In children, all ages can be affected by the disease, but two incidence peaks have been shown to occur: in infants aged <1 year and in teenagers [7]. No particular race predilection has been reported. Boys aged 6–15 years seem to have a higher risk than girls, and the risk difference increases with age [8].

Myocarditis is a frequent cause of sudden death, dilated cardiomyopathy and heart failure in children. Sudden death in the paediatric population is commonly associated with myocarditis; in an autopsy study performed at a single paediatric centre, sudden death occurred in 57% of autopsied patients with a diagnosis of myocarditis [9]. Similarly, myocarditis accounts for 30–35% of children with dilated cardiomyopathy phenotypes in the Australian [10] and North American [11] Paediatric Cardiomyopathy Registries.

13.3 Aetiology

Myocarditis may result from infectious or non-infectious causes. From an etiologic perspective, myocarditis cases usually fall into 1 of the following 3 main categories (Table 13.1):

- Infectious myocarditis;
- Immune-mediated myocarditis;
- Toxic myocarditis.

13.3.1 Infectious Myocarditis

Infectious myocarditis presumably accounts for most myocarditis cases and can be caused by viruses, bacteria, fungi, protozoa and helminths, with some differences based on geographic location. In the western world the main causes of paediatric myocarditis are viral, while, in developing nations, infectious myocarditis is most often associated with rheumatic fever, Chagas' disease or AIDS.

13.3.1.1 Virus

More than 50% of paediatric acute myocarditis in North America and Europe are caused by cardiotropic viruses and the main agents identified are enterovirus, adenovirus, influenza viruses, human herpesvirus-6 (HHV-6), Epstein–Barr virus, cytomegalovirus, hepatitis C virus, and parvovirus B19.

Table 13.1 Aetiology of myocarditis in children

Infectious myocarditis
Virus
RNA viruses: Coxsackieviruses A and B, echoviruses, polioviruses, influenza A and B viruses, respiratory syncytial virus, mumps virus, measles virus, rubella virus, hepatitis C virus, dengue virus, yellow fever virus, Chikungunya virus, Junin virus, Lassa fever virus, rabies virus, human immunodeficiency virus-1; DNA viruses: Adenoviruses, parvovirus B19, cytomegalovirus, human herpesvirus-6, Epstein–Barr virus, varicella-zoster virus, herpes simplex virus, variola virus, vaccinia virus
Bacteria
Staphylococcus, Streptococcus, Pneumococcus, Meningococcus, Gonococcus, Salmonella, Corynebacterium diphtheriae, Haemophilus influenzae, Mycobacterium (tuberculosis), Mycoplasma pneumoniae, Brucella
Spirochateal
Borrelia (Lyme disease), Leptospira (Weil disease)
Protozoal
Trypanosoma cruzi, Toxoplasma gondii, Entamoeba, Leishmania
Parasitic
Trichinella spiralis, Echinococcus granulosus, Taenia solium
Rickettsial
Coxiella burnetii (Q fever), R. rickettsii (Rocky Mountain spotted fever), R. tsutsugamuschi
Fungal
Aspergillus, Actinomyces, Blastomyces, Candida, Coccidioides, Cryptococcus, Histoplasma, Mucormycoses, Nocardia, Sporothrix
Immune-mediated myocarditis
Allergens
Drugs: Penicillin, cefaclor, colchicine, furosemide, isoniazid, lidocaine, tetracycline, sulfonamides, phenytoin, phenylbutazone, methyldopa, thiazide diuretics, amitriptyline. Tetanus toxoid, vaccines, serum sickness
Alloantigens
Heart transplant rejection
Autoantigens
Infection-negative lymphocytic, infection-negative giant cell associated with autoimmune or immune-oriented disorders: Systemic lupus erythematosus, rheumatoid arthritis, Churg-Strauss syndrome, Kawasaki's disease, inflammatory bowel disease, scleroderma, polymyositis, myasthenia gravis, insulin-dependent diabetes mellitus, thyrotoxicosis, sarcoidosis, Wegener's granulomatosis, rheumatic heart disease (rheumatic fever)
Toxic myocarditis
Drugs
Amphetamines, anthracyclines, cocaine, cyclophosphamide, ethanol, fluorouracil, lithium, catecholamines, hemetine, interleukin-2, trastuzumab, clozapine
Heavy metals
Copper, iron, lead
Miscellaneous
Scorpion sting, snake, and spider bites, bee and wasp stings, carbon monoxide, inhalants, phosphorus, arsenic, sodium azide
Hormones
Phaeochromocytoma, vitamins: Beriberi
Physical agents
Radiation, electric shock

Enteroviruses (most commonly coxsackie B viruses) are responsible for up to 25% of viral myocarditis [12]. Enteroviruses gain access to human hosts via the gastrointestinal or respiratory tracts; the heart is a secondary target. Coxsackie B viruses and some adenoviruses exhibit tropism for cardiomyocytes via a common transmembrane receptor, the coxsackievirus and adenovirus receptor (CAR) [13–15].

Human immunodeficiency virus (HIV) is also associated with myocarditis, in particular in developing nations. The infection is often asymptomatic, but HIV myocarditis may cause systolic and diastolic dysfunction in paediatric patients. Moreover, some drugs used in active antiretroviral therapy (HAART) regimens, like Zidovudine, are cardiotoxic themselves [16].

13.3.1.2 Bacteria

Bacterial myocarditis can be caused by many kinds of bacteria such as Staphylococcus aureus, streptococcus, pneumococcus, and Neisseria meningitidis. Even Borrelia burgdorferi, the spirochete responsible of Lyme disease, can result in both acute and chronic myocarditis and it is an important cause in childhood. A recent study of 207 children with early disseminated Lyme disease found that 16% had mild to fulminant myocarditis, 42% had advanced atrioventricular block [17].

Although full recovery is the norm, Lyme carditis sometimes persists and may lead to chronic heart failure.

13.3.1.3 Acute Rheumatic Fever

Acute rheumatic fever results from an autoimmune response to infection with the group A streptococcus. The illness is characterized by varying degrees of inflammation of the joints and the heart, typically manifesting as polyarthritis and valvular regurgitation. Cardiac involvement during acute rheumatic fever can result in rheumatic heart disease, which can cause heart failure and premature mortality. The highest incidence is observed in children aged 5–15 years. It is a rare cause of heart disease in the USA and in Europe, but it is still a frequent cause of heart disease in developing countries, since antibiotics are not routinely administered for pharyngitis and compliance is low.

13.3.1.4 Protozoa

Chagas' disease is the most important cause of acquired cardiomyopathy in Latin America and is caused by Trypanosoma cruzi [18].

The clinical course of Chagas' disease is usually divided into an acute and a chronic phase. Symptoms during the acute phase include fever, inflammation at the inoculation site, unilateral palpebral oedema, enlarged lymph nodes and splenomegaly. Severe acute disease occurs in less than 1% of patients and includes manifestations such as acute myocarditis, pericardial effusion and meningoencephalitis. This phase usually resolves spontaneously in 2–4 months, after which the patients remain chronically infected if untreated. Up to 70% of patients will never have symptoms, the remainder develop chronic cardiac disease with progressive cardiomegaly, arrhythmia, thromboembolic events and heart failure [19, 20]. This chronic phase is thought to be associated with persistent inflammation [21], and development of cardiac fibrosis [22, 23].

13.3.2 Immune-Mediated Myocarditis

The main subtypes of immune-mediated myocarditis are autoimmune myocarditis and myocarditis related to drug hypersensitivity.

Autoimmune myocarditis may occur as an isolated entity, in which the primary, and usually only, target organ is the heart. Also, several systemic autoimmune diseases may affect heart tissues, generating myocarditis in the context of a broader autoimmune phenomenon. Myocarditis is most frequently associated with systemic lupus erythematosus, but it may also occur in association with Sjögren's syndrome, vasculitides and polymyositis [24–26].

Drugs hypersensitivity reactions can affect the heart and cause myocarditis. They usually occur within 8 weeks from the introduction of the drug, but may develop at any time. The most commonly responsible agents are antiepileptics, antimicrobials, allopurinol and sulfonamides. This syndrome usually resolves with administration of corticosteroids and the interruption of the drug; however, some patients may have a prolonged course.

13.3.3 Toxic Myocarditis

In addition to infectious agents and immune-mediate causes, a wide variety of substances can cause myocardial injury. In some cases, the tissue damage is acute, transient and associated with the presence of an inflammatory infiltrate with myocyte necrosis. In other cases, the damaging agents can cause chronic changes with histological evidence of fibrosis and the development of dilated or restrictive cardiomyopathy [27]. Many chemical and pharmacological substances can cause myocardial damage and cardiac dysfunction, such as amphetamines, anthracyclines, cocaine and clozapine. Moreover, different physical agents (e.g., radiation) can cause direct myocardial damage.

13.4 Pathogenesis

13.4.1 Viral Myocarditis

Our understanding of the pathophysiology of viral myocarditis mostly stems from studies of rodent models in which susceptible strains of mice are infected with a cardiotropic virus such as coxsackievirus B. The virus is resumed in the cell by endothelial receptors, in particular the coxsackie-adenovirus receptor (CAR) [28, 29].

In addition to CAR, coxsackievirus serotypes B1, B3 and B5 use the decay acceleration factor, while adenoviruses use αv integrins109 [30, 31] as coreceptors for viral entry. This knowledge makes us able to define a first difference, since the binding to the decay acceleration factor increases viral virulence in coxsackievirus B infections.

Coxsackie-adenovirus receptor is highly expressed in the brain and heart, with a peak in the perinatal period with a subsequent and gradual decrease in relation to age [32]. In fact, in the prenatal heart, CAR is detected on the whole surface of cardiac myocytes, while in the adult heart CAR is predominantly at the intercalated disks [33]. The expression level and CAR position in infants and children may help to explain the high susceptibility of this population to coxsackievirus B3-mediated myocarditis (CVB3). Understanding these mechanisms completely subverted the idea of a myocarditis as a typically autoimmune pathology in which the presence of autoantibodies directed against the heart proteins of myocytes was the correct pathogenetic mechanism [34]. However, the lack of myocardial damage observed in CAR knockout mice has suggested a primary mechanism in viral myocarditis in the course of the studies and at least in the acute phase of a strictly inflammatory and not autoimmune type [35].

Therefore, the duration and degree of the innate immune response to viral infection play a crucial role in the development of myocarditis. A variety of inflammation mediators, including cytokines such as tumour necrosis factor (TNF), nitric oxide, toll-like receptors and complement are increased. These mediators do not seem to play a unique role. In fact, a mouse model has shown an increase in TNF levels, not only with a decrease in viral load but also with an exaggerated immune response and a late mortality. Nitric oxide not only inhibits viral replication but also contributes to the development of cardiomyopathy by worsening myocardial injury [36, 37]. Toll-like receptors and myeloid-88 differentiation factor (MyD88), an adaptive molecule for toll-like receptors, minimize viral replication in the heart [38], but MyD88 appears to significantly influence the severity of myocardial inflammation [39, 40]. The complement cascade amplifies both the innate and the adaptive immune response, increasing the susceptibility to autoimmune myocarditis and the progression to chronic DCM. In other words, the massive activation of the immune system appears as a negative predictive factor in long-term prognosis.

However, the innate immune system cannot always build up an effective immune response by itself. Viruses that escape the innate immune system replicate, producing viral proteins that cause direct damage to the myocardium [41]. Coxsackievirus B3 infection in mice with severe combined immunodeficiency induces myocardial damage [42]. The picornavirus 2A protease has been shown to inhibit protein synthesis of host cells, and the 2A protease CVB3 cleaves host protein dystrophin, which may induce cardiomyopathy.

In addition to their proteolytic activity in the myocytes, the CVB3 2A and 3C proteases may induce apoptosis, resulting in further cardiomyocytic injury [43, 44].

Inhibition of these viral proteases could be a new target in the treatment of viral-induced myocarditis. We can therefore conclude that a pathogenetic mechanism of direct damage is added, or substituted, to the acute activation damage of the immune system (Fig. 13.1).

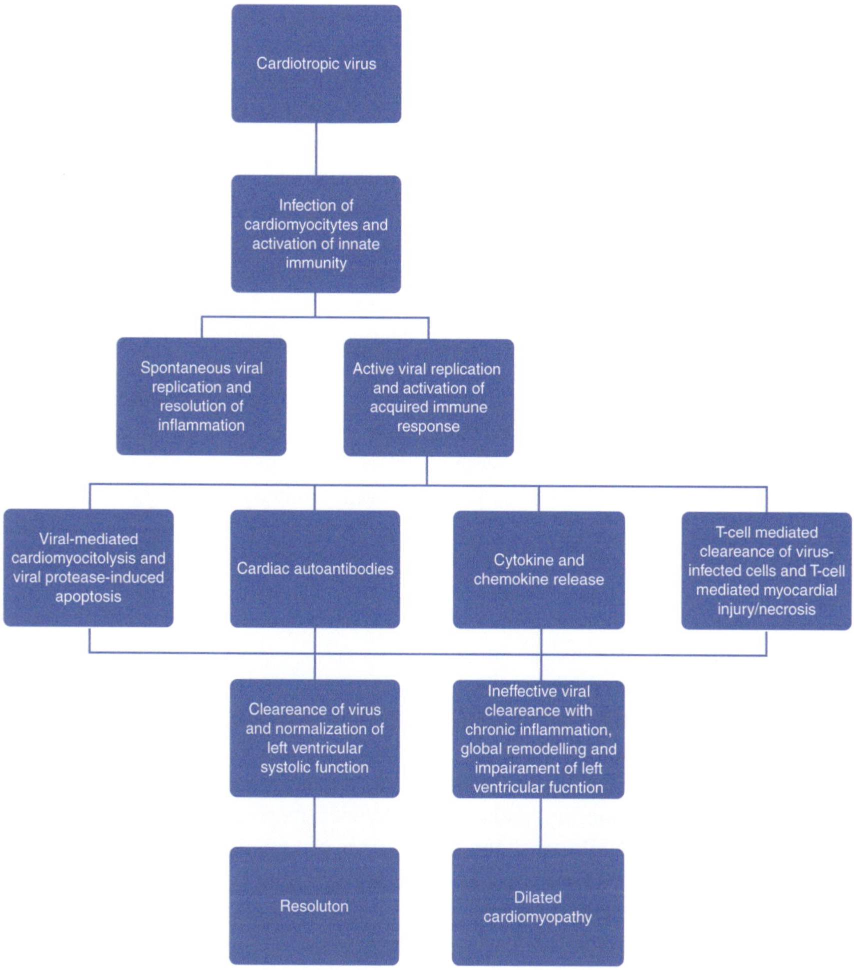

Fig. 13.1 Pathogenesis of viral myocarditis

13.4.2 Autoimmune Myocarditis

Autoimmune myocarditis, exemplified by giant cell myocarditis, usually occurs without an identified trigger such as a viral infection, although viral infection can amplify naturally occurring autoantibodies and autoreactive T cells [45].

In the pathogenesis of this form of myocarditis a central role is played by mononuclear cells, in particular monocytes, macrophages and T lymphocytes that represent more than 60% of the inflammatory infiltrate observed in the myocardium.

In keeping with this, the inhibition of the monocyte chemoattractant 1 protein and of inflammatory protein of 1α macrophages reduces the severity and prevalence of myocarditis [46, 47]. The types of T helper cells 1 and 2 (Th1 and Th2) secrete cytokines such as TNF and interleukins, which are associated with the development of autoimmune myocarditis within 6–12 h of viral infection in sensitive mice. The T helper cell of type 17 (TH17) produces interleukin-17, which drives the development of severe autoimmune myocarditis in mice with γ-interferon deficiency [48]. Inhibition of T-cell proliferation and activation in mice attenuate the immune response and decrease the severity of myocarditis. In addition, CD4 + T lymphocytes play a critical role in the induction of autoimmune myocarditis, not only for the production of key cytokines but also for the production of antibodies and autoantibodies. In autoimmune myocarditis after CVB3 infection, they develop antibodies against multiple cardiac antigens, including epitopes of cardiac myosin. Autoantibodies can actually precede the development of the disease. In particular, antibodies to β-1 cardiac adrenergic receptors [49, 50] were found in the serum of patients with myocarditis and DCM, and the removal of β-1 circulating antibody adrenergic antibody in patients with DCM by immunoadsorption improved cardiac function [51]. The possibility of exploiting the serum autoantibody demonstration to identify therapeutic targets before the occurrence of irreversible cardiac lesions remains open.

13.5 Clinical Presentation

The clinical presentation of acute myocarditis in children varies according to age [52]. Typically, infants have non-specific symptoms (malaise, fever, poor appetite, poor weight gain or irritability) and signs (tachypnea, respiratory distress and tachycardia). Symptoms in children older than 2 years of age, in whom "ischemic-like presentation" is common, include chest and/or abdominal pain; dyspnoea, fatigue, cough and oedema are also common [3].

Children, particularly infants, often have a more fulminant presentation than adults and may require advanced circulatory and respiratory support in early stages of their disease [53].

Despite the "critical" presentation, many patients with fulminant myocarditis, when promptly treated, will recover entirely with a good prognosis.

13.6 Diagnostic Approach

Because of the highly variable clinical presentation, ranging from mild and non-specific symptoms to cardiogenic shock, and the limited availability of diagnostic tools, the evaluation of children with suspected myocarditis represents a difficult challenge in clinical cardiology.

According to the recent ESC position statement diagnosis of definite myocarditis is obtained only with endomyocardial biopsy (Table 13.2). However, a diagnosis of clinically suspected myocarditis may be obtained with the first line and second line tests.

Table 13.2 Diagnostic criteria of clinically suspected myocarditis

Clinical presentation
Acute chest pain, pericarditic, or pseudo-ischaemic
New-onset (days up to 3 months) or worsening of dyspnoea at rest or exercise, and/or fatigue, with or without left and/or right heart failure signs
Subacute/chronic (>3 months) or worsening of dyspnoea at rest or exercise, and/or fatigue, with or without left and/or right heart failure signs
Palpitation, and/or unexplained arrhythmia symptoms and/or syncope, and/or aborted sudden cardiac death
Unexplained cardiogenic shock
Laboratory
Elevated TnT/TnI
Rest or dynamic electrocardiogram
Newly abnormal 12 lead ECG and/or Holter and/or stress testing, any of the following: I to III-degree atrioventricular block, or bundle branch block, ST/T wave change (ST elevation or non-ST elevation, T wave inversion), sinus arrest, ventricular tachycardia or fibrillation and asystole, atrial fibrillation, reduced R wave height, intraventricular conduction delay (widened QRS complex), abnormal Q waves, low voltage, frequent premature beats, supraventricular tachycardia
Functional and structural abnormalities on cardiac imaging
New, otherwise unexplained left ventricular function abnormality (including incidental finding in apparently asymptomatic subjects): Regional, wall motion or global systolic or diastolic function abnormality, with or without ventricular dilatation, with or without increased wall thickness, with or without pericardial effusion, with or without endocavitary thrombi
Tissue characterization by cardiac magnetic resonance
Oedema and/or LGE of classical myocarditic pattern

Modified from [54]. Clinically suspected myocarditis if ≥1 clinical presentation and ≥1 diagnostic criteria from different categories, in the absence of: (1) angiographically detectable coronary artery disease (coronary stenosis ≥ 50%); (2) known pre-existing cardiovascular disease or extra-cardiac causes that could explain the syndrome (e.g. valve disease, congenital heart disease, hyperthyroidism, etc.). Suspicion is higher with higher number of fulfilled criteria. If the patient is asymptomatic ≥2 diagnostic criteria should be met.

13.7 First Line Test

13.7.1 Laboratory

Laboratory findings of myocarditis can include leucocytosis, elevated erythrocyte sedimentation rate and C reactive protein [55]. Cardiac biomarkers, such as creatine kinase, troponin T and troponin I, may be elevated (indicating myocardial damage), with reported sensitivity and specificity of troponin I, respectively, of 34% and 89% [56].

In fulminant myocarditis laboratory features of multi-organ failure (elevated serum urea nitrogen, creatinine, and liver enzymes) may be present [57].

Viral serology is of limited utility in the diagnosis of viral myocarditis because the prevalence of circulatory IgG antibodies for cardiotropic viruses in the general population is high in the absence of viral heart disease [58, 59].

On the other hand, serum cardiac autoantibodies (i.e., antibodies of IgG class, which are shown to be cardiac and disease-specific for myocarditis) can be used as biomarkers for identifying patients in whom (in the absence of active infection of the myocardium) immunosuppression and immunomodulation may be useful [60, 61].

13.7.2 Electrocardiogram

Electrocardiogram (ECG) is usually abnormal in myocarditis though ECG signs are neither specific or sensitive. ECG can vary from non-specific T wave and ST-segment changes to ST-segment elevation like in acute myocardial infarction [62].

Atrioventricular block may be present due to mild left dilatation or more frequently related to Lyme disease, cardiac sarcoidosis or giant cell myocarditis [63]. QRS duration higher than 120 msec was found to be an independent predictor of death and cardiac transplantation, while Q waves and repolarization abnormalities were unrelated to the outcome or immunohistological features of inflammation on EMB [64].

13.7.3 Echocardiography

The echocardiogram is the most useful, widely available and low-cost test for patients with acute myocarditis. Echocardiography provides immediate data on cardiac morphology and structure, chamber volumes/diameters, wall thickness, ventricular systolic/diastolic function and pulmonary pressure.

Typically, patients with acute myocarditis often show poorly functioning left ventricle with minimal dilation, with or without regional wall motion abnormalities [65]. There may be ventricular thickening secondary to myocardial oedema (particularly in giant cell myocarditis), and left atrial enlargement may not be prominent, even when mitral regurgitation is present.

Newer imaging techniques such as tissue Doppler imaging or speckle tracking echocardiography may detect "pre-clinical" left ventricular dysfunction [66] (Fig. 13.2); however, their routine use in clinical practice remains to be determined.

13.8 Second Level Investigations

13.8.1 Cardiovascular Magnetic Resonance

Cardiac magnetic resonance (CMR) represents an essential tool for the investigation of myocarditis in children.

CMR represents the gold standard for evaluation of left ventricular diameters/volumes, systolic function and wall motion abnormalities. In addition, CMR has the unique potential to characterize cardiac tissue and therefore detect the intracellular and interstitial oedema, hyperemia and, in more severe cases, cellular necrosis and fibrosis [67].

CMR findings in myocarditis may vary depending on the time elapsed from onset of symptoms to CMR assessment.

In the acute phase, the T2-weighted sequences can detect the extent and severity of cardiac inflammation and can distinguish acute or chronic myocarditis [68].

In the subacute/chronic phase, late gadolinium enhancement (LGE) can detect myocardial fibrosis, and in children two common patterns of myocardial damage

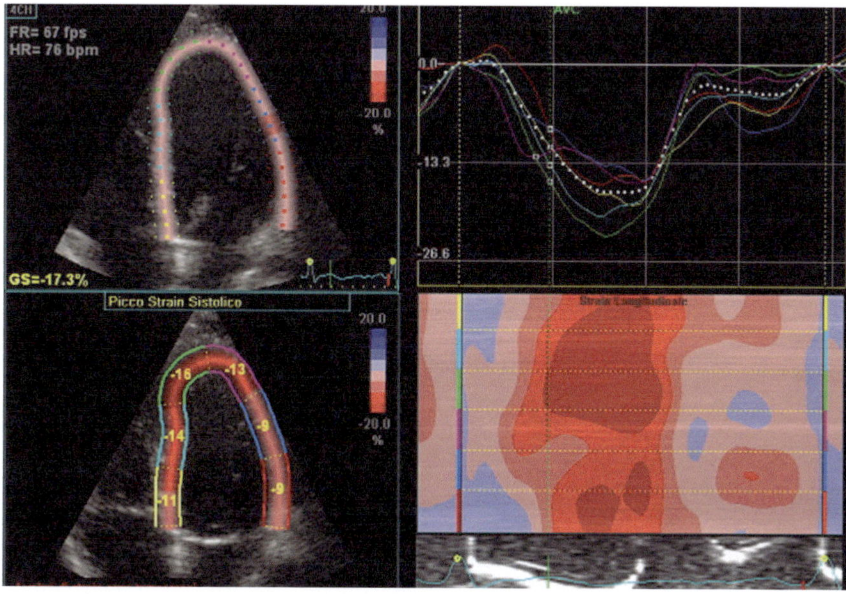

Fig. 13.2 2D STE measurement of longitudinal strain in apical 4-chamber view in a patient with myocarditis

have been described: an intramural, rim-like pattern in the septal wall and a subepicardial (patchy) distribution in the left ventricle lateral wall [69].

13.8.2 Endomyocardial Biopsy

Endomyocardial biopsy (EMB) represents the gold standard for the diagnosis of definite myocarditis according to Dallas criteria [70] and for differential diagnosis between myocarditis and dilated cardiomyopathies.

According to Dallas criteria myocarditis is defined as the presence of a cellular inflammatory infiltration in direct association with myocyte necrosis without typical features of ischemic necrosis while inflammation is defined by immunohistochemical detection of focal or diffuse mononuclear infiltrates (T lymphocytes and macrophages) with 14 cells/mm^2, in addition to enhanced expression of human leucocyte antigen class II molecules.

Despite more evidence indicates that clinical utility of Dallas criteria is limited by many factors (i.e., sampling error, variation in expert interpretation, variance with other markers of viral infection and immune activation in the heart and variance with treatment outcomes) they are still useful for detecting a subset of patients with cellular myocarditis [71].

However, it is necessary to underscore that biopsy samples of the right ventricle must be analysed not only by routine haematoxylin-eosin staining (to detect cellular infiltration and myocyte necrosis) but a fresh frozen sample should also be obtained for PCR analysis (for detecting common viral causes of myocarditis). According to the scientific statement of American Heart Association/American College of Cardiology/European Society of Cardiology accepted indication to EBM are clinical scenarios according to fulminant myocarditis, and in acute heart failure unresponsive to usual care within 1–2 weeks [72].

13.9 Therapeutic Approach

13.9.1 Conventional Therapy

13.9.1.1 Haemodynamically Unstable Patients

Patient in shock requires aggressive therapy to increase oxygen delivery while minimizing consumption. Intubation with mechanical ventilation is necessary to reduce the oxygen consumption of the respiratory muscles, also favouring alveolar recruitment as a result of positive pressure ventilation [73].

In patients with systemic congestion, diuretic therapy should be initiated preferring continuous infusions when intermittent administration has not led to adequate diuresis [74]. Inotropes (Table 13.3) are used to increase stroke volume and cardiac output [75]. Although increased inotropism results in improved cardiac output and blood pressure, the final result is increased myocardial oxygen consumption and demand [76]. The failing myocardium has a limited contractile reserve, and haemodynamic collapse can occur with high-dose inotropic support in this setting. When acute heart failure does not respond to aggressive medical management, mechanical circulatory support must be considered.

In general, ventricular assist devices are used as a bridge to transplantation, since prolonged support periods may be needed. However, recovery from acute, including fulminant, myocarditis is often rapid, then ECMO or short-term use of ventricular assist device is more appropriate [77]. Arrhythmia prevention is a crucial component in the management of all patients with acute heart failure. For this purpose, first-line measures are the maintenance of normal serum electrolyte concentration of and use of the lowest effective doses of inotropes.

For treatment of ventricular tachycardia, as well as refractory atrial tachycardias amiodarone is commonly used [78].

Table 13.3 Common inotropes used in acute heart failure in children

Inotropes	Type of administration	Dose
Dobutamine	Continuous infusion	2.5–10 μg/kg/min
Epinephrine	Continuous infusion	0.01–0.1 μg/kg/min
Epinephrine	Intermittent bolus	0.01 μg/kg
Milrinone	Continuous infusion	0.5–1 μg/kg/min
Levosimendan	Continuous infusion	0.05–0.2 μg/kg/min

The gradual weaning of intravenous therapies is indicated following the improvement of end-organ perfusion. In this phase, inotropes are stopped, and intravenous diuretics are changed into oral forms. Finally, therapy with "disease-modifying drugs" (i.e., beta blockers and ACE inhibitors) is started with a gradual dose up-titration during follow-up.

13.9.1.2 Haemodynamically Stable Patients

Asymptomatic patients without left ventricular systolic dysfunction do not require pharmacologic therapy but only a careful follow-up.

Asymptomatic patients with left ventricular dysfunction may require disease-modifying drugs until complete recovery of systolic function is achieved.

13.9.2 Specific Therapy

Besides the conventional heart failure regimen, specific treatment strategies have been proposed targeting the presence of viral infection or inflammation.

13.9.2.1 Antiviral Therapy

Interferon-beta treatment has been proposed as a potential therapy to eliminate enteroviral and adenoviral genomes in patients with left ventricular systolic dysfunction.

In an open-label pilot study including 22 adult patients with chronic heart failure and enterovirus or adenovirus persistence, treatment with interferon-beta has been shown to eliminate viral genome and to improve left ventricular systolic function [79]. More recently a prospective, placebo-controlled randomized multicentre study has demonstrated that interferon-beta treatment is associated with viral elimination or substantial decrease of viral load, resulting in improved functional performance (i.e., NYHA class, quality of life) of the patients [80]. Despite these encouraging results, more data in support of a specific risk/benefit ratio are needed for routinely use of interferon-beta particularly in children with viral myocarditis.

13.9.2.2 Immunomodulation/Immunosuppression

Myocardial inflammatory processes due to autoimmunity may persist even after complete elimination of the virus from the myocardium and require immunosuppressive treatment to prevent the onset of inflammatory cardiomyopathy (ICM). High dose intravenous immunoglobulins (IVIG) have been proposed as a complementary therapy to improve left ventricular systolic function in patients with virus-negative myocarditis/ICM [81]; however, more recent trials have revealed that treatment with intravenous immunoglobulin in children was not effective [82]. A recent Cochrane systematic review concludes that IVIG therapy may be beneficial in a select group of children beyond the neonatal period who have viral encephalitis with myocarditis [83].

Immunoadsorption is a therapeutic concept currently under discussion; the rationale is to lower cardiotoxic antibodies in the patient's plasma, and extract antibodies and immune complexes from the heart as well [84]. Despite some positive results, the clinical utility of immunoadsorption is still under debate [85].

Immunosuppressive therapy has been proposed as valuable resource in the management of chronic virus-negative myocarditis/inflammatory cardiomyopathy [86].

However, its role in children with myocarditis remains controversial [87]. While some recent studies have shown improvement in left ventricular systolic function and NYHA class symptoms among children treated with corticosteroids and other immunosuppressive agents, like cyclosporine, others found no differences in outcome [88, 89]. However, it is commonly accepted that immunosuppression with corticosteroids, cyclosporine or muromonab-CD3 is useful in giant cell and active virus-negative lymphocytic myocarditis [90].

13.9.2.3 Physical Activity Limitation

Due to arrhythmic risk, physical activity is contraindicated for at least 6 months in all patients with myocarditis. In patients with reduced systolic function, physical activity may be resumed after complete left ventricular recovery and the demonstration of no arrhythmias at 24-h ECG Holter monitoring and stress testing.

References

1. Richardson P, McKenna W, Bristow M, Maisch B, Mautner B, O'Connell J, Olsen E, Thiene G, Goodwin J, Gyarfas I, Martin I, Nordet P. Report of the 1995 World Health Organization/International Society and Federation of Cardiology Task Force on the definition and classification of cardiomyopathies. Circulation. 1996;93:841–2.
2. Aretz HT, Billingham ME, Edwards WD, Factor SM, Fallon JT, Fenoglio JJ Jr, Olsen EG, Schoen FJ. Myocarditis: a histopathologic definition and classification. Am J Cardiovasc Pathol. 1985;1:1–10.
3. Canter CE, Simpson KE. Diagnosis and treatment of myocarditis in children in the current era. Circulation. 2014;129:115–28.
4. Freedman SB, Haladyn JK, Floh A, Kirsch JA, Taylor G, Thull-Freedman J. Pediatric myocarditis. Emergency department clinical findings and diagnostic evaluation. Pediatrics. 2007;120:1278–85.
5. Durani Y, Egan M, Baffa J, Selbst SM, Nagar AL. Pediatric myocarditis: presenting clinical characteristics. Am J Emerg Med. 2009;27:942–7.
6. Verma NA, Zheng XT, Harris MU, Cadichon SB, Melin-Aldana H, Khetsuriani N, Oberste MS, Shulman ST. Outbreak of coxsackievirus B1 myocarditis in neonates. Clin Infect Dis. 2009;49:759–63.
7. Ghelani SJ, Spaeder MC, Pastor W, Spurney CF, Klugman D. Demographics, trends, and outcomes in pediatric acute myocarditis in the United States, 2006 to 2011. Circ Cardiovasc Qual Outcomes. 2012;5:622–7.
8. Anita A, Essi P, Sipilä JOT, Jouni P, Paivi R, Ville K. Occurrence and features of childhood myocarditis: a nationwide study in Finland. J Am Heart Assoc. 2017;6(11):e005306.
9. Webber SA, Boyle GJ, Jaffe R, Pickering RM, Beerman LB, Fricker FJ. Role of right ventricular endomyocardial biopsy in infants and children with suspected or possible myocarditis. Br Heart J. 1994;72:360–3.
10. Daubeney PE, Nugent AW, Chondros P, Carlin JB, Colan SD, Cheung M, Davis AM, Chow CW, Weintraub RG, National Australian Childhood Cardiomyopathy Study. Clinical features and outcomes of childhood dilated cardiomyopathy: results from a national population-based study. Circulation. 2006;114:2671–8.

11. Towbin JA, Lowe AM, Colan SD, Sleeper LA, Orav EJ, Clunie S, Messere J, Cox GF, Lurie PR, Hsu D, Canter C, Wilkinson JD, Lipshultz SE. Incidence, causes, and outcomes of dilated cardiomyopathy in children. JAMA. 2006;296:1867–76.
12. Fairley CK, Ryan M, Wall PG, Weinberg J. The organisms reported to cause infective myocarditis and pericarditis in England and Wales. J Infect. 1996;32:223–5.
13. Freimuth P, Philipson L, Carson SD. The coxsackievirus and adenovirus receptor. Curr Top Microbiol Immunol. 2008;323:67–87.
14. Pinkert S, et al. Prevention of cardiac dysfunction in acute coxsackievirus B3 cardiomyopathy by inducible expression of a soluble coxsackievirus-adenovirus receptor. Circulation. 2009;120:2358–66.
15. Blailock ZR, Rabin ER, Melnick JL. Adenovirus myocarditis in mice. An electron microscopic study. Exp Mol Pathol. 1968;9:84–96.
16. Pollack A, Kontorovich AR, Fuster V, Dec GW. Viral myocarditis—diagnosis, treatment options, and current controversies. Nat Rev Cardiol. 2015;12:670–80.
17. Singh P, Hemal A, Agarwal S, Kumar D. Cardiac manifestations in HIV infected children. Indian J Pediatr. 2015;82:230–4. https://doi.org/10.1007/s12098-014-1481-9.
18. Costello JM, Alexander ME, Greco KM, Perez-Atayde AR, Laussen PC. Lyme carditis in children: presentation, predictive factors, and clinical course. Pediatrics. 2009;123(5):e835–41.
19. Higuchi Mde L, Benvenuti LA, Martins Reis M, et al. Pathophysiology of the heart in Chagas' disease: current status and new developments. Cardiovasc Res. 2003;60:96–107.
20. Tostes S Jr, Bertulucci Rocha-Rodrigues D, de Araujo Pereira G, et al. Myocardiocyte apoptosis in heart failure in chronic Chagas' disease. Int J Cardiol. 2005;99:233–7.
21. Zacks MA, Wen J-J, Vyatkina G, et al. An overview of chagasic cardiomyopathy: pathogenic importance of oxidative stress. An Acad Bras Cienc. 2005;77:695–715.
22. Cardoni RL, Antunez MI, Morales C, et al. Release of reactive oxygen species by phagocytic cells in response to live parasites in mice infected with Trypanosoma cruzi. Am J Trop Med Hyg. 1997;56:329–34.
23. Leon JS, Wang K, Engman DM. Captopril ameliorates myocarditis in acute experimental Chagas disease. Circulation. 2003;107:2264–9.
24. Cihakova D, Rose NR. Pathogenesis of myocarditis and dilated cardiomyopathy. Adv Immunol. 2008;99:95–114.
25. Busteed S, et al. Myocarditis as a prognostic indicator in systemic lupus erythematosus. Postgrad Med J. 2004;80(944):366–7.
26. Levin MD, Zoet-Nugteren SK, Markusse HM. Myocarditis and primary Sjogren's syndrome. Lancet. 1999;354(9173):128–9.
27. Ansari A, Maron BJ, Berntson DG. Drug-induced toxic myocarditis. Tex Heart Inst J. 2003;30(1):76–9.
28. Kaur T, Mishra B, Saikia UN, Sharma M, Bahl A, Ratho RK. Expression of coxsackievirus and adenovirus receptor and its cellular localization in myocardial tissues of dilated cardiomyopathy. Exp Clin Cardiol. 2012;17(4):183–6.
29. Tracy S, Hofling K, Pirruccello S, et al. Group B coxsackievirus myocarditis and pancreatitis: connection between viral virulence phenotypes in mice. J Med Virol. 2000;62:70–81.
30. Bergelson JM, Cunningham JA, Droguett G, et al. Isolation of a common receptor for Coxsackie B viruses and adenoviruses 2 and 5. Science (New York, NY). 1997;275:1320–3.
31. Wickham TJ, Filardo EJ, Cheresh DA, et al. Integrin alpha v beta 5 selectively promotes adenovirus mediated cell membrane permeabilization. J Cell Biol. 1994;127:257–64.
32. Kashimura T, Kodama M, Hotta Y, et al. Spatiotemporal changes of coxsackievirus and adenovirus receptor in rat hearts during postnatal development and in cultured cardiomyocytes of neonatal rat. Virchows Arch. 2004;444:283–92.
33. Martino TA, Petric M, Brown M, et al. Cardiovirulent coxsackieviruses and the decay-accelerating factor (CD55) receptor. Virology. 1998;244:302–14.
34. Fechner H, Noutsias M, Tschoepe C, et al. Induction of coxsackievirus-adenovirus-receptor expression during myocardial tissue formation and remodeling: identification of a cell-to-cell contact-dependent regulatory mechanism. Circulation. 2003;107:876–82.

35. Shi Y, Chen C, Lisewski U, et al. Cardiac deletion of the Coxsackievirus-adenovirus receptor abolishes Coxsackievirus B3 infection and prevents myocarditis in vivo. J Am Coll Cardiol. 2009;53:1219–26.
36. Huber SA. Autoimmunity in coxsackievirus B3 induced myocarditis. Autoimmunity. 2006;39:55–61.
37. Huang CH, Vallejo JG, Kollias G, et al. Role of the innate immune system in acute viral myocarditis. Basic Res Cardiol. 2009;104:228–37.
38. Szalay G, Sauter M, Hald J, et al. Sustained nitric oxide synthesis contributes to immunopathology in ongoing myocarditis attributable to interleukin-10 disorders. Am J Pathol. 2006;169:2085–93.
39. Hardarson HS, Baker JS, Yang Z, et al. Toll-like receptor 3 is an essential component of the innate stress response in virus-induced cardiac injury. Am J Phys. 2007;292:H251–8.
40. Fuse K, Chan G, Liu Y, et al. Myeloid differentiation factor-88 plays a crucial role in the pathogenesis of Coxsackievirus B3-induced myocarditis and influences type I interferon production. Circulation. 2005;112:2276–85.
41. Fairweather D, Frisancho-Kiss S, Njoku DB, et al. Complement receptor 1 and 2 deficiency increases coxsackievirus B3-induced myocarditis, dilated cardiomyopathy, and heart failure by increasing macrophages, IL-1beta, and immune complex deposition in the heart. J Immunol. 2006;176:3516–24.
42. Lamphear BJ, Yan R, Yang F, et al. Mapping the cleavage site in protein synthesis initiation factor eIF-4 gamma of the 2A proteases from human Coxsackievirus and rhinovirus. J Biol Chem. 1993;268:19200–3.
43. Xiong D, Yajima T, Lim BK, et al. Inducible cardiac-restricted expression of enteroviral protease 2A is sufficient to induce dilated cardiomyopathy. Circulation. 2007;115:94–102.
44. Chau DH, Yuan J, Zhang H, et al. Coxsackievirus B3 proteases 2A and 3C induce apoptotic cell death through mitochondrial injury and cleavage of eIF4GI but not DAP5/p97/NAT1. Apoptosis. 2007;12:513–24.
45. Goser S, Ottl R, Brodner A, et al. Critical role for monocyte chemoattractant protein-1 and macrophage inflammatory protein-1alpha in induction of experimental autoimmune myocarditis and effective anti-monocyte chemoattractant protein-1 gene therapy. Circulation. 2005;112:3400–7.
46. Rangachari M, Mauermann N, Marty RR, et al. T-bet negatively regulates autoimmune myocarditis by suppressing local production of interleukin 17. J Exp Med. 2006;203:2009–19.
47. Haga T, Suzuki J, Kosuge H, et al. Attenuation of experimental autoimmune myocarditis by blocking T cell activation through 4-1BB pathway. J Mol Cell Cardiol. 2009;46:719–27.
48. Hayward SL, Bautista-Lopez N, Suzuki K, et al. CD4 T cells play major effector role and CD8 T cells initiating role in spontaneous autoimmune myocarditis of HLA-DQ8 transgenic IAb knockout nonobese diabetic mice. J Immunol. 2006;176:7715–25.
49. Caforio AL, Mahon NJ, Tona F, et al. Circulating cardiac autoantibodies in dilated cardiomyopathy and myocarditis: pathogenetic and clinical significance. Eur J Heart Fail. 2002;4:411–7.
50. Caforio AL, Mahon NJ, McKenna WJ. Cardiac autoantibodies to myosin and other heart-specific autoantigens in myocarditis and dilated cardiomyopathy. Autoimmunity. 2001;34:199–204.
51. Wallukat G, Morwinski M, Kowal K, et al. Autoantibodies against the beta-adrenergic receptor in human myocarditis and dilated cardiomyopathy: beta-adrenergic agonism without desensitization. Eur Heart J. 1991;12(Suppl D):178–81.
52. Blauwet LA. Myocarditis. Prog Cardiovasc Dis. 2010;52:274–88.
53. Kyto V, Saukko P, Lignitz E, et al. Diagnosis and presentation of fatal myocarditis. Hum Pathol. 2005;36:1003–7.
54. Caforio AL, Pankuweit S, Arbustini E, European Society of Cardiology Working Group on Myocardial and Pericardial Diseases, et al. Current state of knowledge on aetiology, diagnosis, management, and therapy of myocarditis: a position statement of the European Society of Cardiology Working Group on Myocardial and Pericardial Diseases. Eur Heart J. 2013;34:2636–48. https://doi.org/10.1093/eurheartj/eht210.

55. Bioesborek PS, Beek AM, Germans T, Niesen HW, van Rossum AC. Diagnosis of myocarditis: current state and future perspectives. Int J Cardiol. 2015;191:211–9.
56. Smith SC, Ladenson JH, Mason JW, Jaffe AS. Elevations of cardiac troponin I associated with myocarditis. Experimental and clinical correlates. Circulation. 1997;95(1):163–8.
57. Ginsberg F. Fulminant myocarditis. Crit Care Clin. 2013;29(3):465–83.
58. Liu P, Martino T, Opavsky MA, Penninger J. Viral myocarditis: balance between viral infection and immune response. Can J Cardiol. 1996;12:935–43.
59. Baboonian C, Treasure T. Meta-analysis of the association of enteroviruses with human heart disease. Heart. 1997;78:539–43.
60. Caforio AL, Calabrese F, Angelini A, Tona F, Vinci A, Bottaro S, Ramondo A, Carturan E, Iliceto S, Thiene G, Daliento L. A prospective study of biopsy-proven myocarditis: prognostic relevance of clinical and aetiopathogenetic features at diagnosis. Eur Heart J. 2007;28:1326–33.
61. Maisch B, Bültmann B, Factor S, Gröne H-J, Hufnagel G, Kawamura K, Kühl U, Olsen EJ, Pankuweit S, Virmani R, McKenna W, Richardson PJ, Thiene G, Schultheiss HP, Sekiguchi M. World Heart Federation consensus conferences's definition of inflammatory cardiomyopathy (myocarditis): report from two expert committees on histology and viral cardiomyopathy. Heartbeat. 1999;4:3–4.
62. Cooper LT Jr. Myocarditis. N Engl J Med. 2009;360:1526–38.
63. Chien SJ, Liang CD, Lin IC, Lin YJ, Huang CF. Myocarditis complicated by complete atrioventricular block: nine years' experience in a medical center. Pediatr Neonatol. 2008;49(6):218–22.
64. Ukena C, Mahfoud F, Kindermann I, Kandolf R, Kindermann M, Bohm M. Prognostic electrocardiographic parameters in patients with suspected myocarditis. Eur J Heart Fail. 2011;13:398–405.
65. Pinamonti B, Alberti E, Cigalotto A, et al. Echocardiographic findings in myocarditis. Am J Cardiol. 1988;62:285–91.
66. Leitman M, Vered Z, Tyomkin V, Macogon B, Moravsky G, Peleg E, Copel L. Speckle tracking imaging in inflammatory heart diseases. Int J Cardiovasc Imaging. 2018;34(5):787–79.
67. Abdel-Aty H, Boye P, Zagrosek A, et al. Diagnostic performance of cardiovascular magnetic resonance in patients with suspected acute myocarditis: comparison of different approaches. J Am Coll Cardiol. 2005;45:1815–22.
68. Aletras AH, Kellman P, Derbyshire JA, Arai AE. ACUT2E TSE SSFP: a hybrid method for T2-weighted imaging of edema in the heart. Magn Reson Med. 2008;59:229–35.
69. Friedrich MG, Sechtem U, Schulz-Menger J, Holmvang G, Alakija P, Cooper LT, White JA, Abdel-Aty H, Gutberlet M, Prasad S, Aletras A, Laissy JP, Paterson I, Filipchuk NG, Kumar A, Pauschinger M, Liu P, International Consensus Group on Cardiovascular Magnetic Resonance in Myocarditis. Cardiovascular magnetic resonance in myocarditis: A JACC White Paper. J Am Coll Cardiol. 2009;53(17):1475–87.
70. Leone O, Veinot JP, Angelini A, Baandrup UT, Basso C, Berry G, Bruneval P, Burke M, Butany J, Calabrese F, d'Amati G, Edwards WD, Fallon JT, Fishbein MC, Gallagher PJ, Halushka MK, McManus B, Pucci A, Rodriguez ER, Saffitz JE, Sheppard MN, Steenbergen C, Stone JR, Tan C, Thiene G, van der Wal AC, Winters GL. 2011 consensus statement on endomyocardial biopsy from the Association for European Cardiovascular Pathology and the Society for Cardiovascular Pathology. Cardiovasc Pathol. 2012;21:245–74.
71. Baughman KL. Diagnosis of myocarditis: death of Dallas criteria. Circulation. 2006;113(4):593–5.
72. Cooper LT, Baughman KL, Feldman AM, et al. The role of endomyocardial biopsy in the management of cardiovascular disease: a scientific statement from the American Heart Association, the American College of Cardiology, and the European Society of Cardiology endorsed by the Heart Failure Society of America and the Heart Failure Association of the European Society of Cardiology. Eur Heart J. 2007;28:3076–93.
73. Duncan BW, Bohn DJ, Atz AM, French JW, Laussen PC, Wessel DL. Mechanical circulatory support for the treatment of children with acute fulminant myocarditis. J Thorac Cardiovasc Surg. 2001;122:440.

74. Lowrie L. Diuretic therapy of heart failure in infants and children. Prog Pediatr Cardiol. 2000;12(1):45–55.
75. Maack C, Eschenhagen T, Hamdani N, Heinzel FR, Lyon AR, Manstein DJ, Metzger J, Papp Z, Tocchetti CG, Yilmaz MB, Anker SD, Balligand JL, Bauersachs J, Brutsaert D, Carrier L, Chlopicki S, Cleland JG, de Boer RA, Dietl A, Fischmeister R, Harjola VP, Heymans S, Hilfiker-Kleiner D, Holzmeister J, de Keulenaer G, Limongelli G, Linke WA, Lund LH, Masip J, Metra M, Mueller C, Pieske B, Ponikowski P, Ristic A, Ruschitzka F, Seferovic PM, Skouri H, Zimmermann WH, Mebazaa A. Treatments targeting inotropy. Eur Heart J. 2018;40:3626. https://doi.org/10.1093/eurheartj/ehy600.
76. Masarone D, Valente F, Rubino M, Vastarella R, Gravino R, Rea A, Russo MG, Pacileo G, Limongelli G. Pediatric heart failure: a practical guide to diagnosis and management. Pediatr Neonatol. 2017;58(4):303–12.
77. Rajagolpal SK, Almond CS, Laussen PC, Rycus PT, Wypij D, Thiagarajan RR. Extracorporeal membrane oxygenation for the support of infants, children, and young adults with acute myocarditis: a review of the Extracorporeal Life Support Organization registry. Crit Care Med. 2010;38:382.
78. Bink-Boelkens MT. Pharmacologic management of arrhythmias. Pediatr Cardiol. 2000;21:508.
79. Kühl U, Pauschinger M, Schwimmbeck PL, Seeberg B, Lober C, Noutsias M, Poller W, Schultheiss HP. Interferon-beta treatment eliminates cardiotropic viruses and improves left ventricular function in patients with myocardial persistence of viral genomes and left ventricular dysfunction. Circulation. 2003;107(22):2793–8.
80. Schultheiss HP, Piper C, Sowade O, Waagstein F, Kapp JF, Wegscheider K, Groetzbach G, Pauschinger M, Escher F, Arbustini E, Siedentop H, Kuehl U. Betaferon in chronic viral cardiomyopathy (BICC) trial: Effects of interferon-β treatment in patients with chronic viral cardiomyopathy. Clin Res Cardiol. 2016;105(9):763–73.
81. Druncker NA, Colan SD, Lewis AB, Beiser AS, Wessel DL, Takahashi M, Baker AL, Perez-Atayde AR, Newbunger JW. Gamma-globulin treatment of acute myocarditis in the pediatric population. Circulation. 1994;89(1):252–7.
82. English RF, Janosky JE, Ettedgui JA, Webber SA. Outcomes for children with acute myocarditis. Cardiol Young. 2004;14(5):488–93.
83. Robinson J, Hartling L, Vandermeer B, Klassen TP. Intravenous immunoglobulin for presumed viral myocarditis in children and adults. Cochrane Database Syst Rev. 2015;(5):CD004370. https://doi.org/10.1002/14651858.CD004370.pub3.
84. Schultheiss HP, Kühl U, Cooper LT. The management of myocarditis. Eur Heart J. 2011;32(21):2616–25.
85. Müller J, Wallukat G, Dandel M, Bieda H, Brandes K, Spiegelsberger S, Nissen E, Kunze R, Hetzer R, Muller J. Immunoglobulin adsorption in patients with idiopathic dilated cardiomyopathy. Circulation. 2000;101(4):385–91.
86. Frustaci A. Immunosuppressive therapy in myocarditis. Circ J. 2015;79(1):4–7. https://doi.org/10.1253/circj.CJ-14-1192. Epub 2014 Dec 2.
87. Maisch B, Pankuweit S. Current treatment options in (peri)myocarditis and inflammatory cardiomyopathy. Herz. 2012;37(6):644–56. Review.
88. Bergmann KRP. Myocarditis and pericarditis in the pediatric patient: validated management strategies. Emerg Med Pract. 2015;12(7):1–22.
89. Aziz KU, Patel N, Sadullah T, Tasneem H, Thawerani H, Talpur S. Acute viral myocarditis: role of immunosuppression: a prospective randomised study. Cardiol Young. 2010;20(5):509–15.
90. Cooper LT Jr, Hare JM, Tazelaar HD, Edwards WD, Starling RC, Deng MC, et al. Usefulness of immunosuppression for giant cell myocarditis. Am J Cardiol. 2008;102:1535–9.

Immunosuppressive Therapy in Myocarditis: Lessons from Clinical Trials and Future Perspectives

14

Andrea Frustaci and Cristina Chimenti

14.1 Introduction

Myocarditis is an inflammatory disease of the heart caused by viral, bacterial and fungal infection, systemic diseases, autoimmune dysregulation, drugs, and toxins. From the clinical point of view it ranges from subclinical poorly symptomatic forms to life threatening arrhythmias, cardiogenic shock, and sudden death.

Although in about 40% of cases acute myocarditis may resolve spontaneously [1], in the remaining patients it evolves to a chronic phase as a consequence of an abnormal immune response, with ventricular dilation, reduced contractility, and clinical progression to heart failure [2].

Despite the advancement of diagnostic techniques in defining the etiology of myocarditis a specific standardized treatment is not yet available. This is mainly related to the still unknown mechanisms regulating the normal or abnormal host immune response, leading either to virus elimination and spontaneous resolution of the inflammatory process or to an immune mediated damage persisting with or without viral clearance. In addition, the type of infectious agent and its prevalent mechanism of cell damage (i.e., directly cytopathic or immune-mediated) may also affect the evolution of myocardial inflammation.

In particular, the use of immunosuppressive treatment for lymphocytic myocarditis is still controversial, both in children [3, 4] and in adults [5, 6] presenting with either cardiac arrhythmias [7] or heart failure [8]. Indeed, in the absence of specific markers of eligibility for this treatment, a large trial by Mason et al. [6] in the past produced misleading results, showing no survival improvement in

A. Frustaci (✉) · C. Chimenti
Department of Cardiovascular, Respiratory, Nephrologic,
Geriatric and Anaesthesiologic Sciences, La Sapienza University, Rome, Italy

IRCCS L. Spallanzani, Rome, Italy
e-mail: biocard@inmi.it; cristinachimenti@libero.it

A. L. P. Caforio (ed.), *Myocarditis*, https://doi.org/10.1007/978-3-030-35276-9_14

myocarditis patients treated with immunosuppressive drugs versus placebo. For this reason the use of immunosuppressive therapy is still confined to the treatment of eosinophilic [9], granulomatous [10], giant-cell [11], and drug hypersensitivity myocarditis, i.e., due to clozapine [12], beta-blockers [13], clomipramine [14], as well as lymphocytic myocarditis associated with connective tissue diseases [15] or with the rejection of a transplanted heart. Wojnicz et al. [16] in a randomized placebo-controlled study suggested that an up-regulation of HLA antigens in the myocardial tissue of patients with lymphocytic myocarditis may identify a homogeneous subgroup of inflammatory dilated cardiomyopathy sustained by autoimmune mechanisms of damage, and may represent a marker of susceptibility to the treatment. However, in this study, the presence of viral genome in the myocardium was not investigated.

Our group in retrospective and prospective studies identified the characteristics of patients who are responders to immunosuppressive therapy and the cellular and molecular mechanisms of cardiac recovery after immunosuppression.

14.2 Retrospective Study

In a retrospective study, the virologic and immunologic profiles of patients with active lymphocytic myocarditis and chronic heart failure, responders and non-responders to immunosuppressive therapy, were analyzed [17]. Forty-one patients with a histological diagnosis of active myocarditis and characterized by a progressive heart failure with an ejection fraction (EF) of less than 40%, lasting over 6 months in spite of conventional supportive therapy were studied. All patients were similar in terms of duration and severity of cardiac disease, histological findings, and poor responsiveness to full supportive therapy. They received immunosuppressive therapy including 1 mg/kg/day prednisone for 4 weeks followed by 0.33 mg/kg/day for 5 months and 2 mg/kg/day azathioprine for 6 months. Patients were classified as responders if they had a decrease of at least one NYHA class and an improvement in EF $\geq$10% compared to baseline measures and as non-responders if NYHA class and EF failed to improve or deteriorated or in the presence of major events, including cardiogenic shock, heart transplantation, or cardiac death. Among the 41 patients, 21 responded with a prompt improvement of EF and showed evidence of healed myocarditis at control biopsy. Conversely, 20 patients failed to respond, and 12 of them remained stable, 3 underwent a cardiac transplantation, and 5 died, showing an histologic evolution toward a dilated cardiomyopathy. Retrospective PCR on frozen endomyocardial samples and evaluation of circulating cardiac autoantibodies on patients sera showed that non-responders had a high prevalence of viral genomes in the myocardium (85%) and no detectable autoantibodies in the serum, whereas 90% of responders were positive for autoantibodies, with only 3 (15%) presenting viral genomes on PCR analysis. Among the non-responders the myocardial persistence of enterovirus and adenovirus or their combination was associated with the worst clinical outcome. These data indicate that the absence of cardiac viral genomes is a prerequisite for the clinical use of immunosuppression, and suggest a potential impact of antiviral agents for patients with virus-positive inflammatory cardiomyopathy. Interestingly, serology for cardiotropic viruses failed to predict the presence of viral genome in the myocardium. This result, also confirmed in a recent study [18], suggests that this tool cannot be used as an alternative to endomyocardial tissue PCR to diagnose viral myocarditis.

14.3 Prospective Study

To confirm the retrospective results in a prospective manner, we performed a randomized, double-blind, placebo-controlled single center trial enrolling patients with myocarditis and chronic heart failure and submitting all patients with no evidence at PCR of a myocardial viral infection to immunosuppressive treatment [19]. Eighty-five patients were treated with prednisone 1 mg/kg/day for 4 weeks followed by 0.33 mg/kg/day for 5 months and azathioprine 2 mg/kg/day for 6 months (43 patients, Group 1) or placebo (42 patients, Group 2) in addition to conventional therapy for heart failure. Primary outcome was 6-month improvement in left ventricular function. Group 1 showed a significant improvement of left ventricular ejection fraction (LVEF) and a significant decrease in left ventricular dimensions and volumes compared to baseline. Specifically, 38 out of 43 patients on immunosuppressive therapy (88%) showed an improvement of cardiac function and dimensions. The remaining five patients maintained a stable clinical picture and cardiac function parameters. Remarkably, even patients with severe advanced disease (LVEDD up to 90 mm and LVEF up to 20%) significantly improved, being able to resume their previous work. The duration of heart failure did not correlate with the extent of recovery. At 6 month follow-up none of Group 2 patients showed improvement of LVEF, that, conversely, significantly worsened compared with baseline. In particular, 35/42 Group 2 patient (83%) showed further impairment of cardiac function while the remaining 7 patients remained stable. No major adverse reaction was seen as a result of immunosuppression. Histological analysis showed an active myocarditis with diffuse inflammatory infiltrates associated with focal necrosis of the adjacent myocytes (meeting the Dallas criteria) with interstitial and focal replacement fibrosis in most of left and right ventricular specimens from all patients. The infiltrates included mainly activated T cells (CD45ROpositive, CD3positive) with moderate amount of cytotoxic lymphocytes (CD8positive) and macrophages (CD68positive).

Morphometric analysis showed no differences in terms of extent of fibrosis and amount of inflammatory cells between Group 1 and Group 2 patients. Control histology at 1 and 6 month showed, in the 38 Group 1 patients who improved with immunosuppression, a healed myocarditis with disappearance of inflammatory infiltrates associated with interstitial and focal replacement fibrosis. In the five Group 1 patients who did not improve, myocardial inflammation reduced or disappeared in the control biopsies but some degenerative changes of cardiomyocytes were observed. In Group 2 patients, control biopsies were not dissimilar from baseline, showing persistence of myocarditis as well as expansion of interstitial and replacement fibrosis.

The results of this trial confirmed the positive impact of immunosuppression on recovery of LV function in a high rate (88%) of patients with virus-negative inflammatory cardiomyopathy. Remarkably a striking improvement occurred even in patients with extreme LV dilatation and dysfunction. In this group of patients myocardial inflammation was most likely the result of an immune-mediated injury towards segregated (i.e., myosin) or new antigens shared with viral components (i.e., antigenic mimicry). In this regard responders to immunosuppressive therapy showed an upregulation of human histocompatibility complex (HLA) expression on myocardial tissue, presumably related to autoantigen presentation in cardiomyocytes. Specifically, overexpression of toll-like receptor 4 in cardiomyocytes of patients with inflammatory cardiomyopathy predicts response to immunosuppressive therapy [20].

Efficacy of immunosuppressive therapy in virus-negative inflammatory cardiomyopathy has been confirmed by further and larger studies [21] showing long-term control of myocardial inflammation as well as persistently improved cardiac contractility over time.

Lack of response in 12% of cases suggests the presence of not screened viruses or mechanisms of damage and inflammation not susceptible to immunosuppression. With regard to undetected viral genomes, metagenomic assessment of the myocardial virome, including DNA and RNA extraction from PCR-negative endomyocardial biopsies and use of GS-FLX platform, may identify new infectious agents and provide indications for a more selective administration of immunosuppressive therapy.

Definition of gene expression profiles in endomyocardial tissue and peripheral lymphocytes of patients with various types of myocarditis/inflammatory cardiomyopathy may allow in the next future a precise characterization and a specific treatment of the disease through a careful molecular analysis of peripheral blood samples.

14.4 Cellular Mechanisms of Cardiac Recovery

Cell mechanisms of cardiac recovery in patients with inflammatory cardiomyopathy treated with immunosuppression were analyzed, including cell death, activation of cell proliferation, and reconstitution of myofibrillar cell content [22] to clarify the impact of cell repair vs cell proliferation or the possible contribute of cell death inhibition. The responders, all showing the presence of circulating cardiac autoantibodies and absence of viral genomes in the myocardium at PCR analysis, and 10 non-responders, characterized by worsening of left ventricular dysfunction, absence of circulating cardiac autoantibodies, and presence of myocardial viral genomes [17] were retrospectively studied in order to analyze the cellular events associated with the opposite clinical outcome. Transmission electron microscopy studies showed in all patients, before treatment, large cytoplasmic areas that were apparently empty or filled with fine granular material, as a result of the reduced myofibrillar content (myofibrillolysis). After 6 month immunosuppressive treatment, in responders, myofibrillar mass and architecture recovered, while in myocytes of non-responders there was a further reduction in myofibrillar content. Further evidence of a strong activation of contractile protein synthesis comes, in responding patients, from molecular biology studies of alpha and beta isoforms of myosin heavy chain (MHC). The increased expression of α-MHC and inhibition of β-MHC synthesis with an enhanced α/β MHC ratio after effective treatment strongly suggest gene activation of fetal protein isoforms that typically become operative in the process of cell repair. Apoptotic and necrotic cell death in cardiomyocytes were greater in baseline biopsies of responders and non-responders than in controls, showing that myocyte loss is an important mechanism of myocardial damage in myocarditis with cardiac dysfunction. Importantly, after 6 months of effective immunosuppressive therapy, apoptosis and necrosis decreased by 85% and 62%, respectively, while they further increased by 42% and 46%, respectively, in follow-up biopsies of non-responders. The number of cycling myocytes in baseline myocardial tissue of both responders and non-responders was greater than in controls and significantly increased after immunosuppression in both groups suggesting that in chronic myocarditis, as in other forms of heart failure, there is an activation of myocyte regeneration in the attempt to compensate cell loss. Thus, our study suggests that recovery of cardiac function in patients with myocarditis responding to immunosuppression is associated with remarkable cellular events, including strong inhibition of cell degeneration and death, activation of cell proliferation, and mostly newly synthesized contractile elements.

14.5 Conclusion

Immunosuppressive therapy is an important resource in the management of chronic virus-negative inflammatory cardiomyopathy. Lack of identification of new or unconventional viral agents remains a major limit of this therapeutic approach explaining the minor cohort of non-responders. Future objective will be the development of molecular programs (i.e., metagenomic assessment of myocardial virome) able to assess elusive genome sequences.

Source of Funding The study has been supported by AIFA grant "Multicenter randomized study on the efficacy of immunosuppression in patients with virus-negative inflammatory cardiomyopathy" (FARM12JCXN) and by European Project ERA-CVD "Transnational Research Projects on Cardiovascular Diseases"(JTC 2016 IKDT-IGCM).

References

1. Dec GW Jr, Palacios IF, Fallon JT, Aretz HT, Mills J, Lee DC, Johnson RA. Active myocarditis in the spectrum of acute dilated cardiomyopathies: clinical features, histologic correlates, and clinical outcome. N Engl J Med. 1985;312:885–90.
2. Caforio AL, Pankuweit S, Arbustini E, Basso C, Gimeno-Blanes J, Felix SB, Fu M, Heliö T, Heymans S, Jahns R, Klingel K, Linhart A, Maisch B, McKenna W, Mogensen J, Pinto YM, Ristic A, Schultheiss HP, Seggewiss H, Tavazzi L, Thiene G, Yilmaz A, Charron P, Elliott PM, European Society of Cardiology Working Group on Myocardial and Pericardial Diseases. Current state of knowledge on aetiology, diagnosis, management, and therapy of myocarditis: a position statement of the European Society of Cardiology Working Group on Myocardial and Pericardial Diseases. Eur Heart J. 2013;34(33):2636–48, 2648a-2648d.
3. Matitiau A, Perez-Atayde A, Sanders SP, Sluysmans T, Parness IA, Spevak PJ, Colan SD. Infantile dilated cardiomyopathy. Relation of outcome to left ventricular mechanics, hemodynamics, and histology at the time of presentation. Circulation. 1994;90:1310–8.
4. Lee KJ, McCrindle BW, Bohn DJ, Wilson GJ, Taylor GP, Freedom RM, Smallhorn JF, Benson LN. Clinical outcomes of acute myocarditis in childhood. Heart. 1999;82:226–33.
5. Parrillo JE, Cunnion RE, Epstein SE, Parker MM, Suffredini AF, Brenner M, Schaer GL, Palmeri ST, Cannon RO III, Alling D. A prospective, randomized, controlled trial of prednisone for dilated cardiomyopathy. N Engl J Med. 1989;321:1061–8.
6. Mason JW, O'Connell JB, Herskowitz A, Rose NR, McManus BM, Billingham ME, Moon TE. A clinical trial of immunosuppressive therapy for myocarditis: the Myocarditis Treatment Trial Investigators. N Engl J Med. 1995;333:269–75.
7. Chimenti C, Calabrese F, Thiene G, Pieroni M, Maseri A, Frustaci A. Inflammatory left ventricular microaneurysms as a cause of apparently idiopathic ventricular tachyarrhythmias. Circulation. 2001;104:168–73.
8. Feldman AM, McNamara D. Myocarditis. N Engl J Med. 2000;343:1388–98.
9. Frustaci A, Gentiloni N, Chimenti C, Natale L, Gasbarrini G, Maseri A. Necrotizing myocardial vasculitis in Churg-Strauss syndrome: clinicohistologic evaluation of steroids and immunosuppressive therapy. Chest. 1998;114:1484–9.
10. Badorff C, Schwimmbeck PL, Kühl U, Gerhold M, Stein H, Schultheiss HP. [Cardiac sarcoidosis: diagnostic validation by endomyocardial biopsy and therapy with corticosteroids]. Z Kardiol. 1997;86:9–14.
11. Cooper LT Jr, Berry GJ, Shabetai R. Idiopathic giant-cell myocarditis—natural history and treatment. Multicenter Giant Cell Myocarditis Study Group Investigators. N Engl J Med. 1997;336:1860–6.
12. Pieroni M, Cavallaro R, Chimenti C, Smeraldi E, Frustaci A. Clozapine-induced hypersensitivity myocarditis. Chest. 2004;126(5):1703–5.
13. Frustaci A, Verardo R, Sale P, Toscano F, Critelli G, Russo MA, Chimenti C. Hypersensitivity myocarditis induced by beta-blockers: an unexpected cause of abrupt deterioration in hypertrophic cardiomyopathy. Intensive Care Med. 2007;33(10):1848–9. Epub 2007 Jun 26. No abstract available.
14. Frustaci A, Ferilli FA, Chimenti C. Hypersensitivity myocarditis and necrotizing coronary vasculitis by clomipramine causing steroid-sensitive cardiogenic shock. Circ Cardiovasc Imaging. 2019;12:e008736.
15. Frustaci A, Gentiloni N, Caldarulo M. Acute myocarditis and left ventricular aneurysm as presentations of systemic lupus erythematosus. Chest. 1996;109:282–4.
16. Wojnicz R, Nowalany-Kozielska E, Wojciechowska C, Glanowska G, Wilczewski P, Niklewski T, Zembala M, Polonski L, Rozek MM, Wodniecki J. Randomized, placebo-controlled study for immunosuppressive treatment of inflammatory dilated cardiomyopathy: two-year follow-up results. Circulation. 2001;104:39–45.
17. Frustaci A, Chimenti C, Calabrese F, Pieroni M, Thiene G, Maseri A. Immunosuppressive therapy for active lymphocytic myocarditis: virological and immunologic profile of responders versus nonresponders. Circulation. 2003;107:857–63.

18. Mahfoud F, Gartner B, Kindermann M, Ukena C, Gadomski K, Klinkel K. Virus serology in patients with suspected myocarditis: utility or futility? Eur Heart J. 2011;32:897–903.
19. Frustaci A, Russo MA, Chimenti C. Randomized study on the efficacy of immunosuppressive therapy in patients with virus-negative inflammatory cardiomyopathy: the TIMIC study. Eur Heart J. 2009;30:1995–2002.
20. Chimenti C, Verardo R, Scopelliti F, Grande C, Petrosillo N, De Paulis R, Frustaci A. Myocardial expression of Toll-like receptor 4 predicts the response to immunosuppressive therapy in patients with virus-negative cardiomyopathy. Eur J Heart Fail. 2017;19:915–25.
21. Escher F, Kuhl U, Lassner D, Poller W, Pieske B, Tschope C, Schultheiss HP. Long-term outcome of patients with virus-negative chronic myocarditis or inflammatory cardiomyopathy after immunosuppressive therapy. Clin Res Cardiol. 2016;105(12):1011–20.
22. Frustaci A, Chimenti C, Pieroni M, Salvatori L, Morgante E, Sale P, Ferretti E, Petrangeli E, Gulino A, Russo MA. Cell death, proliferation and repair in human myocarditis responding to immunosuppressive therapy. Mod Pathol. 2006;19:755–65.

Immunomodulation and Immunoadsorption in Inflammatory Dilated Cardiomyopathy

15

Bishwas Chamling, Stephanie Könemann, Marcus Dörr, and Stephan B. Felix

15.1 Introduction

Dilated cardiomyopathy (DCM) is characterized by dilatation and impaired contractility of the left ventricle or both ventricles which result in progressive heart failure [1, 2] that cannot be explained by abnormal loading conditions or the extent of ischaemic injury [3]. Heart failure is not only one of the most common causes for high morbidity and mortality worldwide but also represents a substantial economic burden for patients as well as the health care system. Despite recent improvements in therapy, large clinical trials have shown that DCM still accounts for 30–40% of all heart failure cases requiring heart transplantation [4].

DCM is a heterogeneous disease with a multifactorial aetiology [3, 5] which may include idiopathic, familial, genetic, autoimmune, viral or toxic genesis. Moreover, various gene mutations have been reported to be associated with DCM ranging from genes that are related to cytoskeletal/sarcolemmal proteins, nuclear envelope, sarcomere and transcriptional coactivator proteins to genes related to encoding contractile sarcomeric proteins [2]. Altogether about 20–35% of DCM cases are considered to be familial [2]. Myocarditis is another common cause of DCM. In addition to systemic inflammatory diseases, in particular, viral infections may induce myocardial inflammation. Myocardial cell infiltrates of $CD4^+$, $CD8^+$ T- lymphocytes and monocytes/macrophages are frequently detected in endomyocardial biopsies (EMBs) of patients with myocarditis due to viral infections [6]. Myocardial inflammation may become chronic and cause myocardial dysfunction which resembles the

B. Chamling · S. Könemann · M. Dörr · S. B. Felix (✉)
Department of Internal Medicine B, Cardiology, University Medicine Greifswald, Greifswald, Germany

DZHK (German Centre for Cardiovascular Research), Partner Site Greifswald, Greifswald, Germany
e-mail: Bishwas.Chamling@med.uni-greifswald.de; Stephanie.Koenemann@med.uni-greifswald.de; Marcus.Doerr@med.uni-greifswald.de; Stephan.Felix@med.uni-greifswald.de

A. L. P. Caforio (ed.), *Myocarditis*, https://doi.org/10.1007/978-3-030-35276-9_15

clinical phenotype of DCM and is called inflammatory dilated cardiomyopathy (DCM) [6]. While almost every form of myocardial injury involves inflammatory activation, the term 'inflammatory cardiomyopathies' refers to a diverse group of disorders leading to myocardial dysfunction. Their manifestation ranges from reversible forms to those involving chronic remodelling and eventually resulting in DCM. Hence, inflammatory DCM is defined by the presence of inflammatory cells in association with left ventricular (LV) dilatation and reduced ejection fraction [6, 7]. For a subset of affected patients, there seems to be an association between myocarditis, inflammatory DCM and DCM [6, 8–10]. Immunohistochemistry of EMBs is particularly meaningful since evidence of myocardial inflammation is associated with poor outcome in patients with suspected myocarditis [11].

Lymphocytic myocarditis is the most common cause of inflammatory DCMs in developed countries [12]. While parvovirus B19 (PVB19) can be detected in >50% of the German patients these viruses are rare in the USA [13], where adenoviruses and enteroviruses are the most commonly found pathogens irrespective of the patient's age [14]. Nevertheless, it should also be mentioned that a broad array of other infectious pathogens including bacteria and parasites as well as autoimmune disorders, toxins and hypersensitivity can lead to inflammatory DCMs [6].

In addition to disturbances of the cellular immune system, abnormalities of the humoral immunity represent another important factor in the development of myocarditis and DCM. Antibodies against various epitopes have been identified in patients with myocarditis and DCM [15]. For instance, anti β-1 adrenergic receptor autoantibodies are found in up to 60% of patients with DCM, but only in 10–13% of all cases of ischaemic cardiomyopathy [16]. In DCM patients with end-stage-heart failure, these autoantibodies can be found in more than 80% of cases suggesting their involvement in disease progression [16].

15.2 Clinical Manifestations and Diagnosis

The clinical presentation of myocarditis is described in detail in Chap. 2. Patients with inflammatory cardiomyopathy have symptoms that are similar to other types of cardiomyopathies or heart failure. Inflammatory DCM, which is frequently first diagnosed as the result of chronic myocarditis, however, can manifest very differently in each individual. These manifestations can range from typical heart failure symptoms like fatigue, peripheral oedema, precordial chest pain, syncope, palpitations and decreased exercise tolerance to ventricular arrhythmias or a complete heart block. Routine clinical diagnostics include case history, electrocardiogram (ECG), chest X-ray, clinical laboratory testing, echocardiography, cardiac MRI, cardiopulmonary exercise tests, cardiac catheterization including coronary angiography, laevocardiography and EMB which represents the gold standard for diagnosis of myocardial inflammation [6]. According to the position paper of the European Society of Cardiology (ESC) myocardial inflammation is characterized by ≥14 leucocytes/mm^2 including up to 4 monocytes/mm^2 in the presence of $CD3^+$ T-lymphocytes ≥7 cells/mm^2 whereby inflammatory DCM is defined as myocarditis in association with cardiac dysfunction [6]. Other clinical diagnostics like CT scan and genetic testing/screening can be applied if indicated.

15.3 Pathogenesis of Inflammatory Dilated Cardiomyopathy

As stated above, both experimental and clinical data indicate that both viral infection and inflammatory processes may be involved in the pathogenesis of myocarditis and DCM [6, 8–10, 17–23]. Viral persistence or chronic myocarditis is associated with progression of ventricular cardiac dysfunction [24] known as inflammatory DCM which is a frequent non-genetic cause of DCM [4, 6, 25]. Virus-induced myocardial damage and host immune responses aiming to resist and fight against the virus explain the pathology of inflammatory DCM [26]. Depending on genetic susceptibility of the patient, microbial agents can trigger autoimmunity [6, 27] leading to chronic autoantigen-driven myocardial inflammation and eventually end-stage heart failure [22]. In other words, progression from myocarditis to inflammatory DCM and DCM may occur in patients with immunohistologically confirmed persistence of myocardial inflammation where the infective microbial agents could not be eliminated successfully or in patients with persisting myocardial inflammation despite successful elimination of the microbial agents presenting as autoreactive myocarditis as shown in Fig. 15.1 [6].

Several mechanisms that are involved in the autoimmune response and in myocardial injury are being discussed as causal factors for myocardial inflammation.

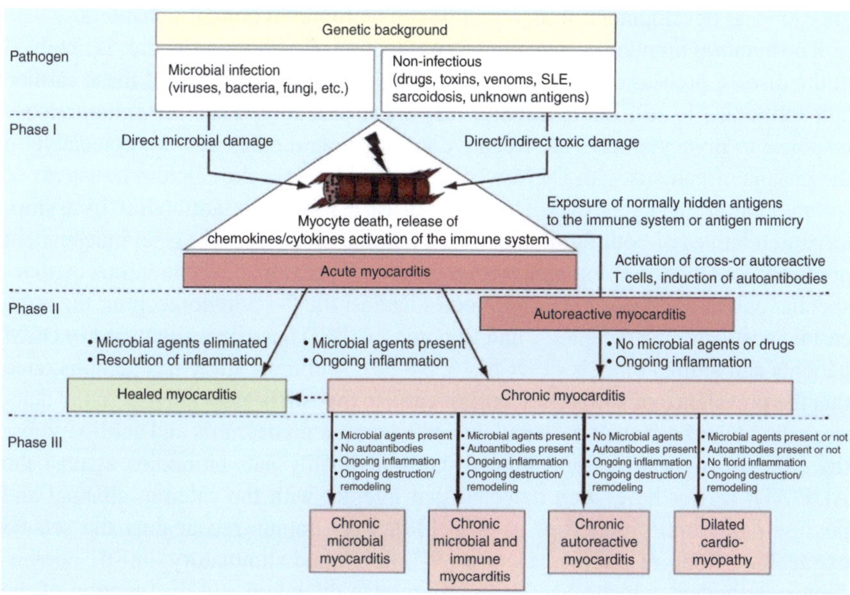

Fig. 15.1 Pathogenetic mechanisms involved in myocarditis and progression to dilated cardiomyopathy (reproduced from Oxford University Press) [6]

Both exogenous as well as endogenous factors including viral infection and damage associated molecular patterns (DAMPs) cause primary myocardial injury with exposure of cardiac autoantigens and consecutive autoimmune response. This induction of cardiac autoimmunity leads to secondary myocardial damage causing severe deterioration of cardiac function [15].

Direct virus-induced myocardial injury and the following pathological inflammatory response are mainly documented by animal experiments. In such experimental models it has been shown that the virus enters the myocardium using receptor complexes, such as the common receptor for coxsackie and adenoviruses [28]. The fact that activated autoreactive T-lymphocytes may mediate myocardial damage has already been disclosed in an experimental model of autoimmune myocarditis induced by myosin [29] through TLRs [30]. The innate immune system gets activated via toll-like receptors (TLRs), especially TLR-3 and TLR-4. Type-1 interferon is then released as an attempt to clear the virus after an activation of natural killer cells and macrophages [30]. Such activation of the innate immune system subsequently leads to proliferation of B- and T-cells of the cellular and humoral immune system thus attacking viral as well as myocardial proteins such as myosin in an autoimmune fashion [30]. Likewise, dendritic cells, loaded with a heart-specific self-peptide, induce $CD4^+$ T-cell-mediated myocarditis in mice; this finding demonstrates that exposure of cardiac proteins as antigens to the immune system induces cardiac injury mediated by autoimmune mechanisms [27]. In summary, inflammatory cells activated by intracellular cardiac proteins which are released during virus-induced injury may lead to autoimmune myocarditis [31]. Details regarding the involvement of the cellular and humoral immune system in the progression and development of myocarditis can be found in previous chapters.

The humoral immune system with its production of cardiac antibodies is involved in the disease process as well [6, 15]. Although the functional role of these cardiac autoantibodies is still under debate, they most probably reflect an inflammatory response to myocyte necrosis. Negative inotropic antibodies that are detectable in the plasma of patients with DCM were shown to decrease the calcium transients of isolated cardiomyocytes [32]. Detection of cardiac-specific antibodies in asymptomatic relatives of both familial and non-familial DCM patients is an independent predictor for DCM development within the next 5 years [6, 33]. Numerous cardiac-specific autoantibodies such as antibodies against the β-1 adrenoreceptor, the muscarinic acetylcholine receptor-2 and troponin I (cTNI) have been identified in DCM patients and animal models of DCM [6, 34–36]. A clinical study has demonstrated that the prevalence of antibodies against cardiac myosin is associated with the deterioration of cardiac function in patients with chronic myocarditis and cardiomyopathy [37]. In myocarditis and dilated cardiomyopathy autoantibodies against the ADP/ATP carrier have been detected that interact with the calcium channel and possess cardiotoxic properties as well [38]. Rats immunized against the second extracellular loop of the β-1 receptor [34], developed stimulatory anti-β1 adrenoceptor antibodies, which resulted in progressive dilatation and dysfunction of the LV resembling the clinical phenotype of DCM. Importantly, isogenic transfer of stimulatory anti-β1 adrenoceptor antibodies from cardiomyopathic into healthy rats reproduced the DCM phenotype. These data provide evidence that anti-β1 adrenoceptor antibodies might be causative for DCM. In addition, antibodies against cTNI were shown to be responsible for the development of DCM in programmed cell death-1 (PD-1) immunoinhibitory co-receptor deficient mice [35]. Furthermore, immunization of mice against cTNI causes a severe autoimmune myocarditis eventually leading to cardiac fibrosis and heart failure [36]. The pathophysiological role of cardiac autoantibodies in the development of cardiac dysfunction of DCM patients has been investigated by clinical intervention studies [32, 39].

15.4 Immunomodulation and Immunoadsorption as Treatment Options

Until now, there is no specific evidence-based therapy available for the treatment of DCM. According to the guidelines, drug treatment of DCM is identical to that of other causes of heart failure. Angiotensin converting enzyme (ACE) blockers or angiotensin-receptor-neprilysin inhibitors (ARNI), beta blockers, mineralocorticoid receptor antagonists and diuretics are still the standard drugs that are used in DCM. If pharmacotherapy or interventions like resynchronisation devices remain ineffective, left ventricular assist device (LAVD) [40] or heart transplantation currently remains the only therapeutic option [41]. There are, however, a few novel treatment options which may be a promising therapeutic alternative or supportive measure for patients with DCM. Depending on the aetiology of inflammation and cardiac dysfunction, different specific therapeutic procedures may be applicable. Apart from cases with fulminant myocarditis, abrupt onset and profound hemodynamic instability where intensive care treatment with intravenous inotropes, vasopressors and even mechanical circulatory support is required [42], the therapy of inflammatory DCM may be generally divided into immunomodulating and immunoadsorption (IA) therapy regardless of their specific inflammatory aetiology based on the current state of knowledge.

15.4.1 Immunomodulation

Immunomodulation refers to the alteration of an immune response caused by various agents of the cellular or the humoral immune systems to a desired level. This may include antiviral therapy, immunosuppression or the application of intravenous immunoglobulins. The aetiology of myocarditis and its respective treatment with antiviral and immunosuppressive therapy are the focus of other chapters and are therefore not being discussed here in detail. In this chapter we focus on the potential role of immunomodulation for the treatment of inflammatory DCM.

Since the production of innate interferons was shown to be associated with clinical recovery it seems possible that exogenous interferons may be protective in chronic viral diseases [43, 44]. Clearance of cardiotropic viruses as well as improvement of left ventricular ejection fraction (LVEF) could be achieved by IFN-β1a treatment in patients with persistence of viral genome and LV dysfunction, in an uncontrolled, open-label phase II study [44]. Later the same group demonstrated that both spontaneous IFN-β production in response to infection and IFN-β administration over 6 months were associated with effective enterovirus clearance and improved outcome [43]. In another clinical phase II trial, Betaferon in chronic viral cardiomyopathy (BICC) patients with enterovirus-, adenovirus- and parvovirus B19-positive genomes were treated with either IFNβ-1b or placebo. This trial confirmed that the immunomodulatory IFNβ-1b treatment is safe and well-tolerated [45] and improves effective virus clearance or reduction of virus load in patients with chronic viral cardiomyopathy. Furthermore, IFNβ-1b treatment leads to an improvement of quality-of-life, New York Heart Association class (NYHA) functional class as well as patient global assessment [45]. These results have to be confirmed by a large randomized phase III study. A randomized study should also investigate the effects of IFNβ-1b on LV function.

Immunosuppressive therapy for inflammatory DCM is another therapeutic option. The first prospective, randomized, controlled trial investigating prednisone for the treatment of 60 DCM patients with myocardial inflammation and 62 without inflammation showed that this treatment option had only marginal clinical benefits [46]. Likewise, the myocarditis treatment trial (MTT), in which the Dallas criteria [47] and LVEF (<45%) were used as inclusion criteria showed no benefit of immunosuppression (cyclosporine/prednisolone) versus placebo [48]. The primary endpoint, a change in LVEF at week 28 after immunosuppressive treatment (prednisone and either cyclosporine or azathioprine) in addition to conventional therapy was not reached in this trial [48]. While the use of immunosuppression as a general strategy does not seem to be effective per se [48], there may be a subset of patients with inflammatory DCM and immunohistologically proven myocarditis that show a long-term benefit with improvement of LV systolic function under immunosuppressive therapy [49]. The monocentric tailored immunosuppression in inflammatory DCM (TIMIC) placebo-controlled study aimed to analyse the efficacy of immunosuppressive therapy with prednisone and azathioprine in 85 patients with heart failure for more than 6 months and immunohistochemical evidence of active lymphocytic but virus-negative myocarditis [50]. Whereas the control group showed no improvement of LV function, the intervention group exhibited not only a significant increase of the LVEF from 27% at baseline to 46% after 6 months but also a significant decrease of the LV end-diastolic volume. In addition, the NYHA functional class improved significantly [50]. These findings should, however, be confirmed by a multicentre trial.

Both clinically as well as experimentally, the application of intravenous immunoglobulin (IVIG) has been proven to be beneficial in various inflammatory settings [51, 52]. Treatment with IVIG relies on a broad therapeutic approach and influences the immune system through various mechanisms. The beneficial effects of IVIG in autoantibody-mediated diseases can be explained by neutralization, accelerated clearance, prevention of Fcγ receptor binding [51] and reduction in autoantibody production [53]. Application of IVIG exerts both proinflammatory as well as anti-inflammatory effects, as shown in sepsis and in viral myocardial inflammation [54,

55]. Proinflammatory effects comprise the activation of both immune cells and the complement system leading to opsonisation of the infective agents, i.e. one of the most important first line events of defence [54]. Similarly, anti-inflammatory effects of IVIG comprise release of anti-inflammatory cytokines like the interleukin receptor antagonist (IL-1RA) and interleukin (IL)-8 and inhibition of the production of proinflammatory cytokines like IL-1 and IL-6 during the process of neutralization of bacterial and other toxins [55]. Interestingly, positive effects of high-dose IVIG are achieved by modulation of regulatory T-cells, macrophages and myeloid dendritic cells in those diseases which are caused by hyperactivity of cellular immunity [52]. In patients with congestive heart failure, IVIG induced an anti-inflammatory net effect resulting from a change in the balance between inflammatory and anti-inflammatory cytokines, which correlated with improvement of LVEF [56]. In contrast, a prospective placebo-controlled clinical trial using IVIG in recent-onset DCM or myocarditis with a LVEF <40% and a disease history of less than 6 months showed no additional beneficial effects on LV function and functional capacity. Moreover, the event free survival rate was not significantly improved either [57].

Currently, any treatment beyond standard heart failure therapy should be driven by aetiology and based on results of randomized studies. Considering all published data, more randomized, controlled, multicentre trials are required to evaluate immunosuppressive, immune-modulating or antiviral therapies for treatment of DCM and inflammatory DCM.

15.4.2 Immunoadsorption Therapy

Effective removal of pathogenic substances, especially specific antibodies and circulating immune complexes from plasma of patients can be achieved by IA therapy which substantially differs from pharmacotherapy where pharmacologically active substances are added to the system. IA as a distinct form of therapeutic apheresis has been proven to be an effective method of treating autoantibody induced diseases. In autoimmune diseases such as Goodpasture syndrome and lupus erythematosus removal of circulating antibodies by unspecific IA has been successfully applied [58, 59].

Several systems have been designed to selectively and efficiently remove pathogenic substances. In previous studies different IA systems using specific anti-β1-AR antibody binding peptide columns (Coraffin®, Affina Immuntechnik) [60], non-specific sheep antihuman immunoglobulin G (IgG) columns (Ig-Thersaorb®, PlasmaSelect) [61] or staphylococcal protein A-agarose columns (Immunosorba®, Fresenius HemoCare) were applied. For IA, the anticoagulated patient's blood is separated into plasma and blood cells by a plasma separation device (Fig. 15.2). The plasma continuously gained in this manner is transferred to the adsorbers that bind antibodies and immune complexes. Two adsorbers are used in order to increase adsorption capacity and thereby the effectiveness and time efficiency of the method. During the treatment, the two adsorbers work alternately. While one is adsorbing, the other one is being desorbed, and vice versa. Plasma freed from antibodies is

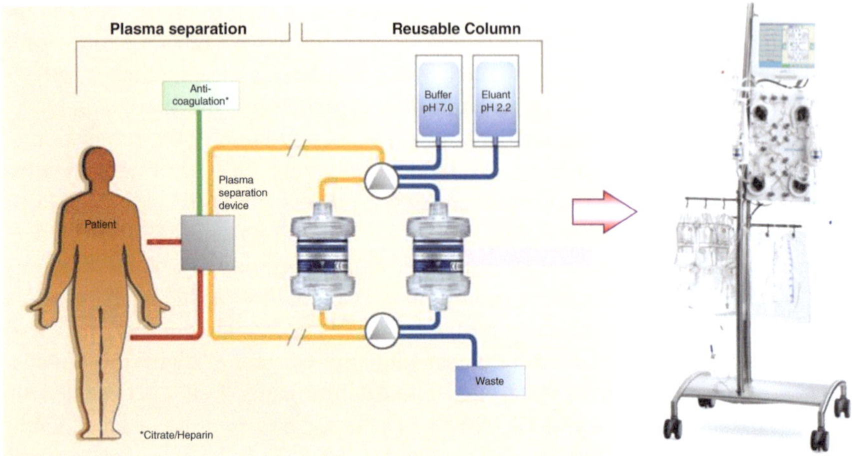

Fig. 15.2 Principle of IA with double adsorber (modified with permission from Fresenius Medical Care)

re-transfused to the patient and the adsorber is washed out with eluates and buffer. Thereafter, antibodies can be adsorbed again in the next cycle.

The potential role of cardiac autoantibodies in the development and progression of cardiac dysfunction in DCM led to the hypothesis that their removal might result in an improvement of haemodynamics and a reduction in myocardial inflammation of affected patients. Although an initial uncontrolled pilot study included only nine patients with DCM and severe heart failure (Cardiac index [CI] < 2.5 L/min/m^2, LVEF <25%; NYHA class III-IV) who received IA on 5 consecutive days, it could be demonstrated that the removal of circulating antibodies from the plasma of these patients by anti-IgG columns resulted in a significant improvement of functional cardiac parameters like cardiac output and systemic vascular resistance [62]. Another open-controlled pilot study included 18 patients with DCM and severe LV systolic dysfunction (LVEF <30%, CI < 2.5 L/min/m^2) as well as severe symptoms of heart failure (NYHA class III–IV). All patients were on stable oral medication. In this study, IA was followed by subsequent intravenous substitution of IgG (IA/IgG) to reduce infection risk following IgG depletion. This intervention was performed in 4 courses at monthly intervals and induced an haemodynamic improvement which persisted after 3 months with a significant increase in stroke volume by 30% and a concomitant increase in LVEF as well as symptom relief in the treatment group, whereas LV function and symptoms did not change in the control group [63]. A proof-of-principle-study showed for the first time that cardiodepressant antibodies can be removed from the plasma of DCM patients by IA and that an early haemodynamic improvement among these patients, as shown by an increase in cardiac index, correlated with the cardiodepressant effect of the antibodies on isolated rat cardiomyocytes [32]. Moreover, detection of such negative inotropic antibodies in patients' plasma before IA was shown to be of predictive value for short- as well as for long-term positive outcome [64]. Another study investigated the effect of IA/IgG on plasma nt-BNP and nt-ANP levels in 15 DCM patients with severe heart failure (LVEF <35%). Four courses of IA/IgG therapy were performed at monthly intervals for 3 months and the results showed not only a significant improvement of LVEF, but also a reduction of LV dimension and of plasma nt-BNP level [65]. A novel potential mechanism hinting towards an interaction of immunoglobulins obtained from DCM patients with cardiomyocytes was proposed in an experimental study, using isolated rat cardiomyocytes. This study indicated that the interaction of immunoglobulins obtained from DCM patients with cardiomyocytes implements the binding of DCM–IgG–F(ab′)$_2$ to their cardiac antigens—but that the Fc part may trigger the negative inotropic effects via a newly detected Fcγ receptor on cardiomyocytes [66]. This cross-linking between the F(ab′)$_2$ of DCM-IgG directed against various cardiac antigens and the simultaneous binding of the Fc part of DCM-IgG might explain why autoantibodies directed against various cardiac antigens are able to induce the same functional effects [66].

Finally, the question arises whether IA/IgG also has an impact on myocardial inflammation. This was determined in another randomized controlled study that included 25 patients exhibiting signs of myocardial inflammation (lymphocytes >2.4 cells/mm^2) in EMBs and severe LV dysfunction (LVEF <30%). Immunohistochemistry was obtained from EMBs at baseline and after 3 months. In comparison to controls, four courses of IA/IgG at monthly intervals not only improved LVEF but also significantly mitigated myocardial inflammation within 3 months as shown by a significant reduction of CD3$^+$, CD4$^+$ and CD8$^+$ cells and a concomitant decrease of HLA class II expression, another maker for myocardial inflammation [61]. In addition, a link between cellular and humoral immunity has been demonstrated since IA/IgG therapy was associated with a decrease of activated T-cells and an increase of regulatory T-cells [67, 68].

Whereas initial studies performed IA/IgG in four courses at monthly intervals, a subsequent study showed that one course of IA treatment with protein A, using an improved treatment protocol for IgG3 reduction, induces an improvement of LV function over a period of 6 months, comparable to that achieved with the initial protocol [69]. Usually, IA is followed by intravenous immunoglobulin (IVIG) substitution to prevent infectious complications that might arise after the depletion of circulating IgG [63]. However, high doses of IVIG may be associated with adverse events in subjects with autoimmune diseases [70]. Therefore it is of interest whether IA without IgG substitution might be safe and effective as well. A prospective case-control study that included 34 patients with DCM and NYHA class II–IV, LVEF <29% and an evidence of elevated levels of β1-adrenerge receptor autoantibodies was able to show that one course of IA without substitution of IgG was safe and significantly improved LVEF and NYHA class after 1 year [71].

In the majority of heart failure patients, regardless of the underlying aetiology, cardiac antibodies can be detected in the myocardium which might contribute to disease progression [72]. In 71% of all patients with end-stage heart failure, immunoglobulin G out of which 48% belonged to subtype IgG3 was localized in the sarcolemma of cardiomyocytes [72]. Interestingly, the beneficial haemodynamic effects of IA/IgG therapy in DCM patients may depend on the efficacy of the removal of IgG-3 subclass antibodies [69, 73].

Taken together, the functional role of cardiac autoantibodies in patients with symptomatic heart failure due to DCM has already been investigated by several uncontrolled and open-controlled, randomized studies where the removal of serum IgG from the plasma of DCM patients by IA/IgG resulted in an increase of LVEF [74], cardiac index [32] and exercise capacity [74]. Besides an improvement in cardiac functional and morphological parameters or symptoms relief several other uncontrolled pilot and open-controlled studies confirmed the positive effects of IA therapy including a decrease in clinical biomarkers related to heart failure [32, 62, 63, 69, 71, 73, 75–78] and an improvement in endothelial function [79]. Two clinical studies were able to show a long-term effect of IA regarding improvement of cardiac function and symptoms [71, 80], out of which one study could even show a reduced rate of heart transplantations and requirement of ventricular assist devices during a follow-up of up to 14.7 years [80].

Although IA represents an innovative therapeutic option for patients with DCM as well as inflammatory cardiomyopathy, a solid mechanism for the improvement of LV function was not discovered yet. It should also be noted that the response of DCM patients to IA treatment shows a wide inter-individual variability regarding changes in cardiac function after intervention. Thus, about 60% of all DCM patients treated with IA are considered as responders (improvement of LVEF ≥20 relative and ≥5% absolute 6 months after IA/IgG) [39]. Genetic factors such as Fcγ-receptors polymorphism might partly explain this variability. In addition, it was shown that shorter disease duration and severe impairment of LV function were associated with better results after IA treatment including a greater increase in LVEF [76]. While anti-β1-AR-autoantibodies have been associated with the development and progression of DCM it has been reported that haemodynamic improvement is independent of the presence of anti-β1-AR-autoantibodies in DCM patients. Thus, both patients with and without the proof of anti-β1-AR-autoantibodies showed similar results which might suggest that the beneficial effects of IA are at least not solely associated with the elimination of anti-β1-AR-autoantibodies [32, 81]. There are, however, also reports indicating indirect effects of the selective elimination of anti-β1-AR-autoantibodies leading to an improvement of cardiac performance by decreasing oxidative stress which may be functionally relevant [82].

In search of a predictive marker to distinguish between responders and non-responders it was found that the negative inotropic activity of patient's antibodies in combination with the gene expression patterns of their endomyocardial biopsies at baseline predicted their response to IA therapy [83]. Nevertheless, a marker that may be used in the daily routine to reliably identify patients who may profit from this expensive and invasive treatment procedure is still not in sight. Moreover, while the current data indicate that IA is a promising new therapeutic approach for the removal of cardiotropic antibodies of patients with DCM as well as inflammatory DCM, this novel therapeutic intervention needs to be verified in a large randomized placebo controlled, and prospective multicentre clinical trial. A corresponding study is currently underway and soon to be completed (http://clinicaltrials.gov/show/NCT00558584).

15.5 Summary

DCM is a very heterogeneous disease with various aetiologies. Several mechanisms known to be involved in the autoimmune response and in myocardial injury are being discussed as causal factors. Considering all the sparse data, in addition to standard heart failure therapy individualized and aetiology driven therapy seems to be the best option. More randomized, controlled, multicentre trials are required to evaluate all novel therapeutic options for treatment of DCM and inflammatory cardiomyopathy such as immunomodulation or IA. At present, IA is still at an experimental stage and its application in the clinical routine may be recommended after the evaluation of the ongoing double-blind, placebo-controlled large multicentre trial investigating the effects of IA/IgG therapy.

References

1. Pinto YM, Elliott PM, Arbustini E, Adler Y, Anastasakis A, Bohm M, et al. Proposal for a revised definition of dilated cardiomyopathy, hypokinetic non-dilated cardiomyopathy, and its implications for clinical practice: a position statement of the ESC working group on myocardial and pericardial diseases. Eur Heart J. 2016;37(23):1850–8.
2. Maron BJ, Towbin JA, Thiene G, Antzelevitch C, Corrado D, Arnett D, et al. Contemporary definitions and classification of the cardiomyopathies: an American Heart Association scientific statement from the council on clinical cardiology, heart failure and transplantation committee; quality of care and outcomes research and functional genomics and translational biology interdisciplinary working groups; and council on epidemiology and prevention. Circulation. 2006;113(14):1807–16.
3. Richardson P, McKenna W, Bristow M, Maisch B, Mautner B, O'Connell J, et al. Report of the 1995 World Health Organization/International Society and Federation of Cardiology Task Force on the definition and classification of cardiomyopathies. Circulation. 1996;93(5):841–2.
4. Haas J, Frese KS, Peil B, Kloos W, Keller A, Nietsch R, et al. Atlas of the clinical genetics of human dilated cardiomyopathy. Eur Heart J. 2015;36(18):1123–35a.
5. Mestroni L, Rocco C, Gregori D, Sinagra G, Di Lenarda A, Miocic S, et al. Familial dilated cardiomyopathy: evidence for genetic and phenotypic heterogeneity. Heart Muscle Disease Study Group. J Am Coll Cardiol. 1999;34(1):181–90.
6. Caforio AL, Pankuweit S, Arbustini E, Basso C, Gimeno-Blanes J, Felix SB, et al. Current state of knowledge on aetiology, diagnosis, management, and therapy of myocarditis: a position statement of the European Society of Cardiology Working Group on Myocardial and Pericardial Diseases. Eur Heart J. 2013;34(33):2636–48, 48a-48d.
7. Elliott P, Andersson B, Arbustini E, Bilinska Z, Cecchi F, Charron P, et al. Classification of the cardiomyopathies: a position statement from the European Society of Cardiology Working Group on Myocardial and Pericardial Diseases. Eur Heart J. 2008;29(2):270–6.
8. Dec GW Jr, Palacios IF, Fallon JT, Aretz HT, Mills J, Lee DC, et al. Active myocarditis in the spectrum of acute dilated cardiomyopathies. Clinical features, histologic correlates, and clinical outcome. N Engl J Med. 1985;312(14):885–90.

9. Feldman AM, McNamara D. Myocarditis. N Engl J Med. 2000;343(19):1388–98.
10. Cooper LT Jr. Myocarditis. N Engl J Med. 2009;360(15):1526–38.
11. Kindermann I, Kindermann M, Kandolf R, Klingel K, Bultmann B, Muller T, et al. Predictors of outcome in patients with suspected myocarditis. Circulation. 2008;118(6):639–48.
12. Sagar S, Liu PP, Cooper LT Jr. Myocarditis. Lancet. 2012;379(9817):738–47.
13. Kuhl U, Pauschinger M, Noutsias M, Seeberg B, Bock T, Lassner D, et al. High prevalence of viral genomes and multiple viral infections in the myocardium of adults with "idiopathic" left ventricular dysfunction. Circulation. 2005;111(7):887–93.
14. Bowles NE, Ni J, Kearney DL, Pauschinger M, Schultheiss HP, McCarthy R, et al. Detection of viruses in myocardial tissues by polymerase chain reaction. Evidence of adenovirus as a common cause of myocarditis in children and adults. J Am Coll Cardiol. 2003;42(3):466–72.
15. Kaya Z, Leib C, Katus HA. Autoantibodies in heart failure and cardiac dysfunction. Circ Res. 2012;110(1):145–58.
16. Dandel M, Wallukat G, Potapov E, Hetzer R. Role of beta(1)-adrenoceptor autoantibodies in the pathogenesis of dilated cardiomyopathy. Immunobiology. 2012;217(5):511–20.
17. Bowles NE, Richardson PJ, Olsen EG, Archard LC. Detection of Coxsackie-B-virus-specific RNA sequences in myocardial biopsy samples from patients with myocarditis and dilated cardiomyopathy. Lancet. 1986;1(8490):1120–3.
18. Kandolf R. Virus etiology of inflammatory cardiomyopathy. Dtsch Med Wochenschr. 2004;129:2187–92.
19. Liu PP, Mason JW. Advances in the understanding of myocarditis. Circulation. 2001;104(9):1076–82.
20. Magnani JW, Dec GW. Myocarditis: current trends in diagnosis and treatment. Circulation. 2006;113(6):876–90.
21. Pauschinger M, Bowles NE, Fuentes-Garcia FJ, Pham V, Kuhl U, Schwimmbeck PL, et al. Detection of adenoviral genome in the myocardium of adult patients with idiopathic left ventricular dysfunction. Circulation. 1999;99(10):1348–54.
22. Heymans S, Eriksson U, Lehtonen J, Cooper LT Jr. The quest for new approaches in myocarditis and inflammatory cardiomyopathy. J Am Coll Cardiol. 2016;68(21):2348–64.
23. Rose NR. Viral myocarditis. Curr Opin Rheumatol. 2016;28(4):383–9.
24. Kuhl U, Pauschinger M, Seeberg B, Lassner D, Noutsias M, Poller W, et al. Viral persistence in the myocardium is associated with progressive cardiac dysfunction. Circulation. 2005;112(13):1965–70.
25. Bozkurt B, Colvin M, Cook J, Cooper LT, Deswal A, Fonarow GC, et al. Current diagnostic and treatment strategies for specific dilated cardiomyopathies: a scientific statement from the American Heart Association. Circulation. 2016;134(23):e579–646.
26. Miteva K, Van Linthout S, Volk HD, Tschope C. Immunomodulatory effects of mesenchymal stromal cells revisited in the context of inflammatory cardiomyopathy. Stem Cells Int. 2013;2013:353097.
27. Eriksson U, Ricci R, Hunziker L, Kurrer MO, Oudit GY, Watts TH, et al. Dendritic cell-induced autoimmune heart failure requires cooperation between adaptive and innate immunity. Nat Med. 2003;9(12):1484–90.
28. Bergelson JM, Cunningham JA, Droguett G, Kurt-Jones EA, Krithivas A, Hong JS, et al. Isolation of a common receptor for Coxsackie B viruses and adenoviruses 2 and 5. Science. 1997;275(5304):1320–3.
29. Smith SC, Allen PM. Myosin-induced acute myocarditis is a T cell-mediated disease. J Immunol. 1991;147(7):2141–7.
30. Zhang P, Cox CJ, Alvarez KM, Cunningham MW. Cutting edge: cardiac myosin activates innate immune responses through TLRs. J Immunol. 2009;183(1):27–31.
31. Rose NR. Viral damage or 'molecular mimicry'-placing the blame in myocarditis. Nat Med. 2000;6(6):631–2.
32. Felix SB, Staudt A, Landsberger M, Grosse Y, Stangl V, Spielhagen T, et al. Removal of cardiodepressant antibodies in dilated cardiomyopathy by immunoadsorption. J Am Coll Cardiol. 2002;39(4):646–52.

33. Caforio AL, Mahon NG, Baig MK, Tona F, Murphy RT, Elliott PM, et al. Prospective familial assessment in dilated cardiomyopathy: cardiac autoantibodies predict disease development in asymptomatic relatives. Circulation. 2007;115(1):76–83.
34. Jahns R, Boivin V, Hein L, Triebel S, Angermann CE, Ertl G, et al. Direct evidence for a beta 1-adrenergic receptor-directed autoimmune attack as a cause of idiopathic dilated cardiomyopathy. J Clin Invest. 2004;113(10):1419–29.
35. Okazaki T, Tanaka Y, Nishio R, Mitsuiye T, Mizoguchi A, Wang J, et al. Autoantibodies against cardiac troponin I are responsible for dilated cardiomyopathy in PD-1-deficient mice. Nat Med. 2003;9(12):1477–83.
36. Goser S, Andrassy M, Buss SJ, Leuschner F, Volz CH, Ottl R, et al. Cardiac troponin I but not cardiac troponin T induces severe autoimmune inflammation in the myocardium. Circulation. 2006;114(16):1693–702.
37. Lauer B, Schannwell M, Kuhl U, Strauer BE, Schultheiss HP. Antimyosin autoantibodies are associated with deterioration of systolic and diastolic left ventricular function in patients with chronic myocarditis. J Am Coll Cardiol. 2000;35(1):11–8.
38. Schultheiss HP, Kuhl U, Janda I, Melzner B, Ulrich G, Morad M. Antibody-mediated enhancement of calcium permeability in cardiac myocytes. J Exp Med. 1988;168(6):2105–19.
39. Felix SB, Beug D, Dorr M. Immunoadsorption therapy in dilated cardiomyopathy. Expert Rev Cardiovasc Ther. 2015;13(2):145–52.
40. Fukunaga N, Rao V. Left ventricular assist device as destination therapy for end stage heart failure: the right time for the right patients. Curr Opin Cardiol. 2018;33(2):196–201.
41. Ponikowski P, Voors AA, Anker SD, Bueno H, Cleland JGF, Coats AJS, et al. 2016 ESC guidelines for the diagnosis and treatment of acute and chronic heart failure. Rev Esp Cardiol (Engl Ed). 2016;69(12):1167.
42. McCarthy RE 3rd, Boehmer JP, Hruban RH, Hutchins GM, Kasper EK, Hare JM, et al. Long-term outcome of fulminant myocarditis as compared with acute (nonfulminant) myocarditis. N Engl J Med. 2000;342(10):690–5.
43. Kuhl U, Lassner D, von Schlippenbach J, Poller W, Schultheiss HP. Interferon-beta improves survival in enterovirus-associated cardiomyopathy. J Am Coll Cardiol. 2012;60(14):1295–6.
44. Kuhl U, Pauschinger M, Schwimmbeck PL, Seeberg B, Lober C, Noutsias M, et al. Interferon-beta treatment eliminates cardiotropic viruses and improves left ventricular function in patients with myocardial persistence of viral genomes and left ventricular dysfunction. Circulation. 2003;107(22):2793–8.
45. Schultheiss HP, Piper C, Sowade O, Waagstein F, Kapp JF, Wegscheider K, et al. Betaferon in chronic viral cardiomyopathy (BICC) trial: effects of interferon-beta treatment in patients with chronic viral cardiomyopathy. Clin Res Cardiol. 2016;105(9):763–73.
46. Parrillo JE, Cunnion RE, Epstein SE, Parker MM, Suffredini AF, Brenner M, et al. A prospective, randomized, controlled trial of prednisone for dilated cardiomyopathy. N Engl J Med. 1989;321(16):1061–8.
47. Aretz HT. Myocarditis: the Dallas criteria. Hum Pathol. 1987;18(6):619–24.
48. Mason JW, O'Connell JB, Herskowitz A, Rose NR, McManus BM, Billingham ME, et al. A clinical trial of immunosuppressive therapy for myocarditis. The Myocarditis Treatment Trial Investigators. N Engl J Med. 1995;333(5):269–75.
49. Wojnicz R, Nowalany-Kozielska E, Wojciechowska C, Glanowska G, Wilczewski P, Niklewski T, et al. Randomized, placebo-controlled study for immunosuppressive treatment of inflammatory dilated cardiomyopathy: two-year follow-up results. Circulation. 2001;104(1):39–45.
50. Frustaci A, Russo MA, Chimenti C. Randomized study on the efficacy of immunosuppressive therapy in patients with virus-negative inflammatory cardiomyopathy: the TIMIC study. Eur Heart J. 2009;30(16):1995–2002.
51. Tha-In T, Bayry J, Metselaar HJ, Kaveri SV, Kwekkeboom J. Modulation of the cellular immune system by intravenous immunoglobulin. Trends Immunol. 2008;29(12):608–15.
52. Tjon AS, van Gent R, Jaadar H, Martin van Hagen P, Mancham S, van der Laan LJ, et al. Intravenous immunoglobulin treatment in humans suppresses dendritic cell function via stimulation of IL-4 and IL-13 production. J Immunol. 2014;192(12):5625–34.

53. Aukrust P, Yndestad A, Ueland T, Damas JK, Froland SS, Gullestad L. The role of intravenous immunoglobulin in the treatment of chronic heart failure. Int J Cardiol. 2006;112(1):40–5.
54. Nimmerjahn F, Ravetch JV. Anti-inflammatory actions of intravenous immunoglobulin. Annu Rev Immunol. 2008;26:513–33.
55. Maisch B, Pankuweit S. Current treatment options in (peri)myocarditis and inflammatory cardiomyopathy. Herz. 2012;37(6):644–56.
56. Gullestad L, Aass H, Fjeld JG, Wikeby L, Andreassen AK, Ihlen H, et al. Immunomodulating therapy with intravenous immunoglobulin in patients with chronic heart failure. Circulation. 2001;103(2):220–5.
57. McNamara DM, Holubkov R, Starling RC, Dec GW, Loh E, Torre-Amione G, et al. Controlled trial of intravenous immune globulin in recent-onset dilated cardiomyopathy. Circulation. 2001;103(18):2254–9.
58. Bygren P, Freiburghaus C, Lindholm T, Simonsen O, Thysell H, Wieslander J. Goodpasture's syndrome treated with staphylococcal protein A immunoadsorption. Lancet. 1985;2(8467):1295–6.
59. Palmer A, Gjorstrup P, Severn A, Welsh K, Taube D. Treatment of systemic lupus erythematosus by extracorporeal immunoadsorption. Lancet. 1988;2(8605):272.
60. Wallukat G, Muller J, Hetzer R. Specific removal of beta1-adrenergic autoantibodies from patients with idiopathic dilated cardiomyopathy. N Engl J Med. 2002;347(22):1806.
61. Staudt A, Schaper F, Stangl V, Plagemann A, Bohm M, Merkel K, et al. Immunohistological changes in dilated cardiomyopathy induced by immunoadsorption therapy and subsequent immunoglobulin substitution. Circulation. 2001;103(22):2681–6.
62. Dorffel WV, Felix SB, Wallukat G, Brehme S, Bestvater K, Hofmann T, et al. Short-term hemodynamic effects of immunoadsorption in dilated cardiomyopathy. Circulation. 1997;95(8):1994–7.
63. Felix SB, Staudt A, Dorffel WV, Stangl V, Merkel K, Pohl M, et al. Hemodynamic effects of immunoadsorption and subsequent immunoglobulin substitution in dilated cardiomyopathy: three-month results from a randomized study. J Am Coll Cardiol. 2000;35(6):1590–8.
64. Staudt A, Staudt Y, Dorr M, Bohm M, Knebel F, Hummel A, et al. Potential role of humoral immunity in cardiac dysfunction of patients suffering from dilated cardiomyopathy. J Am Coll Cardiol. 2004;44(4):829–36.
65. Staudt A, Staudt Y, Hummel A, Empen K, Dorr M, Trimpert C, et al. Effects of immunoadsorption on the nt-BNP and nt-ANP plasma levels of patients suffering from dilated cardiomyopathy. Ther Apher Dial. 2006;10(1):42–8.
66. Staudt A, Eichler P, Trimpert C, Felix SB, Greinacher A. Fc(gamma) receptors IIa on cardiomyocytes and their potential functional relevance in dilated cardiomyopathy. J Am Coll Cardiol. 2007;49(16):1684–92.
67. Bulut D, Scheeler M, Wichmann T, Borgel J, Miebach T, Mugge A. Effect of protein A immunoadsorption on T cell activation in patients with inflammatory dilated cardiomyopathy. Clin Res Cardiol. 2010;99(10):633–8.
68. Bulut D, Creutzenberg G, Mugge A. The number of regulatory T cells correlates with hemodynamic improvement in patients with inflammatory dilated cardiomyopathy after immunoadsorption therapy. Scand J Immunol. 2013;77(1):54–61.
69. Staudt A, Dorr M, Staudt Y, Bohm M, Probst M, Empen K, et al. Role of immunoglobulin G3 subclass in dilated cardiomyopathy: results from protein A immunoadsorption. Am Heart J. 2005;150(4):729–36.
70. Schmaldienst S, Mullner M, Goldammer A, Spitzauer S, Banyai S, Horl WH, et al. Intravenous immunoglobulin application following immunoadsorption: benefit or risk in patients with autoimmune diseases? Rheumatology (Oxford). 2001;40(5):513–21.
71. Muller J, Wallukat G, Dandel M, Bieda H, Brandes K, Spiegelsberger S, et al. Immunoglobulin adsorption in patients with idiopathic dilated cardiomyopathy. Circulation. 2000;101(4):385–91.

72. Youker KA, Assad-Kottner C, Cordero-Reyes AM, Trevino AR, Flores-Arredondo JH, Barrios R, et al. High proportion of patients with end-stage heart failure regardless of aetiology demonstrates anti-cardiac antibody deposition in failing myocardium: humoral activation, a potential contributor of disease progression. Eur Heart J. 2014;35(16):1061–8.
73. Staudt A, Bohm M, Knebel F, Grosse Y, Bischoff C, Hummel A, et al. Potential role of autoantibodies belonging to the immunoglobulin G-3 subclass in cardiac dysfunction among patients with dilated cardiomyopathy. Circulation. 2002;106(19):2448–53.
74. Herda LR, Trimpert C, Nauke U, Landsberger M, Hummel A, Beug D, et al. Effects of immunoadsorption and subsequent immunoglobulin G substitution on cardiopulmonary exercise capacity in patients with dilated cardiomyopathy. Am Heart J. 2010;159(5):809–16.
75. Staudt A, Hummel A, Ruppert J, Dorr M, Trimpert C, Birkenmeier K, et al. Immunoadsorption in dilated cardiomyopathy: 6-month results from a randomized study. Am Heart J. 2006;152(4):712.e1–6.
76. Staudt A, Herda LR, Trimpert C, Lubenow L, Landsberger M, Dorr M, et al. Fcgamma-receptor IIa polymorphism and the role of immunoadsorption in cardiac dysfunction in patients with dilated cardiomyopathy. Clin Pharmacol Ther. 2010;87(4):452–8.
77. Doesch AO, Mueller S, Konstandin M, Celik S, Kristen A, Frankenstein L, et al. Effects of protein A immunoadsorption in patients with chronic dilated cardiomyopathy. J Clin Apher. 2010;25(6):315–22.
78. Pokrovsky SN, Ezhov MV, Safarova MS, Saidova MA, Shitov VN, Afanasieva MI, et al. Ig apheresis for the treatment of severe DCM patients. Atheroscler Suppl. 2013;14(1):213–8.
79. Bulut D, Scheeler M, Niedballa LM, Miebach T, Mugge A. Effects of immunoadsorption on endothelial function, circulating endothelial progenitor cells and circulating microparticles in patients with inflammatory dilated cardiomyopathy. Clin Res Cardiol. 2011;100(7):603–10.
80. Dandel M, Wallukat G, Englert A, Lehmkuhl HB, Knosalla C, Hetzer R. Long-term benefits of immunoadsorption in beta(1)-adrenoceptor autoantibody-positive transplant candidates with dilated cardiomyopathy. Eur J Heart Fail. 2012;14(12):1374–88.
81. Mobini R, Staudt A, Felix SB, Baumann G, Wallukat G, Deinum J, et al. Hemodynamic improvement and removal of autoantibodies against beta1-adrenergic receptor by immunoadsorption therapy in dilated cardiomyopathy. J Autoimmun. 2003;20(4):345–50.
82. Schimke I, Muller J, Priem F, Kruse I, Schon B, Stein J, et al. Decreased oxidative stress in patients with idiopathic dilated cardiomyopathy one year after immunoglobulin adsorption. J Am Coll Cardiol. 2001;38(1):178–83.
83. Ameling S, Herda LR, Hammer E, Steil L, Teumer A, Trimpert C, et al. Myocardial gene expression profiles and cardiodepressant autoantibodies predict response of patients with dilated cardiomyopathy to immunoadsorption therapy. Eur Heart J. 2013;34(9):666–75.

Clinical Management and Follow-Up of Myocarditis Patients on Immunosuppressive Therapy

16

Renzo Marcolongo, Anna Baritussio, Silvia Gianstefani, Chun-Yan Cheng, Sabino Iliceto, and Alida L. P. Caforio

16.1 Cardioimmunology: A New Perspective in Cardiology

The immune response (IR) results from a complex sequence of cellular and molecular interactions taking place in virtually every organ and body tissue, thus preserving host integrity via internal environment regulation and counteraction to external threats. Therefore, it is not surprising that, when constitutionally imbalanced or deranged by external triggers, both the innate and adaptive arms of the IR may contribute to the onset of systemic immune-mediated diseases (SIDs), namely autoimmune/autoinflammatory and other general immune-mediated disorders, and organ-specific autoimmune diseases (OSAD).

The heart interlaces with the immune system close connections and the presence of resident immune cells in the human cardiovascular system is now generally acknowledged [1]. In myocardial tissue, functional role of the immune cells falls well beyond simple protective purposes, contributing to homeostatic regulation. Notably, among resident cardiac immune cells, macrophages exert their influence

R. Marcolongo (✉)
Haematology and Clinical Immunology Unit, Department of Medicine, University of Padua, Padua, Italy

Cardioimmunology Outpatient Clinic, University of Padua, Padua, Italy
e-mail: renzo.marcolongo@tiscali.it

A. Baritussio · S. Gianstefani · C.-Y. Cheng · A. L. P. Caforio
Cardioimmunology Outpatient Clinic, University of Padua, Padua, Italy

Department of Cardiological, Thoracic and Vascular Sciences and Public Health, University of Padua, Padua, Italy
e-mail: anna.baritussio@gmail.com; silviagians@yahoo.it; 073047chengchunyan@163.com; alida.caforio@unipd.it

S. Iliceto
Department of Cardiological, Thoracic and Vascular Sciences and Public Health, University of Padua, Padua, Italy
e-mail: sabino.iliceto@unipd.it

A. L. P. Caforio (ed.), *Myocarditis*, https://doi.org/10.1007/978-3-030-35276-9_16

on physiological development and remodelling of myocardial tissue. They also establish tight connections with conduction fibres, endocardial and pericardial membranes, endothelial cells and coronary vessels. Thus, in normal conditions, local immunity contributes to the regulation of physiological turnover of cardiac cells and the interstitial matrix. However, cardiac immune cells become even more important in the cardiac injury-repair phenomenon after myocardial infarction (e.g., cardiac fibrosis and ventricular dilatation) and following cardiac inflammatory, infective, metabolic and/or toxic injuries.

In the circulatory system, besides vascular inflammation underlying atherogenesis or leading to the onset of vasculitis syndromes, altered IR plays a key role in both initiation and progression of autoimmune myocarditis (AM) and inflammatory dilated cardiomyopathy (DCM) [2, 3]. Similarly, other well-known cardiac inflammatory conditions such as rheumatic fever, which still accounts for a high heart disease burden in underdeveloped countries, or idiopathic recurrent pericarditis, a common clinical problem, result from altered IR in either its autoimmune or autoinflammatory features [4, 5]. Actually, in addition to adaptive immunity, immunopathogenic reactions taking place in cardiac and pericardial tissues may involve innate immunity and activation of pathogen associated (PAMP) or disease associated (DAMP) molecular pattern of recognition receptors, eventually leading to interleukin-1 (IL-1) driven inflammasome formation [6, 7].

Genetic and environmental factors can equally influence expression of the host IR. For example, infection can damage myocardial tissue producing inflammation, which, in genetically susceptible individuals, becomes persistent and shifts to chronic AM/DCM [3]. In particular, following aggression by specific infectious agents, such as coxsackie B3 virus and adenovirus, myocardial myosin and other cardiac antigenic proteins (e.g., β1-adrenergic receptors, adenine nucleotide translocator, sarcoplasmic reticulum ATPase, etc.) may become targets of autoimmune aggression eventually leading to AM/DCM [8]. Therefore, a complete diagnostic workup of AM/DCM should always include endomyocardial biopsy (EMB) in order to provide histological and immunohistological evidence of myocardial inflammation/necrosis and, at the same time, to assess the presence of viral genomes in myocytes by molecular techniques, mainly polymerase chain reaction (PCR) [9, 10]. In experimental models, both cell and antibody-mediated IR arms may contribute to myocardial autoimmunity development. Actually, organ-specific anti-heart autoantibodies (AHA) can be detected in peripheral blood of AM/DCM patients and their symptom-free family members by indirect immunofluorescence (IIFL) technique, thus providing indirect evidence of its immunological and genetic background [11–13]. It has also been suggested that, in a subset of patients with AM/DCM, AHA may play a direct pathogenic role [14, 15].

Even though AM/DCM is frequently observed as isolated cardiac disease, it may also belong to the clinical picture of some SIDs, often with bad prognostic implications. In particular, the appearance of myocarditis may unexpectedly complicate clinical evolution of anti-neutrophilic antibodies-related vasculitides (i.e., eosinophilic granulomatosis with polyangiitis and granulomatosis with polyangiitis), sarcoidosis and connective tissue diseases (i.e., systemic lupus erythematosus, systemic sclerosis, Sjögren disease, rheumatoid arthritis and autoimmune inflammatory myopathies) [16]. Furthermore, lymphocytic AM can also accompany common OSAD, like type 1 diabetes, while giant cell myocarditis (GCM) can be associated with myasthenia gravis secondary to thymic hypertrophy/thymoma [17, 18]. Recently, aggressive inflammatory myocarditis has been reported following selective blockade of cytotoxic T lymphocyte antigen (CTLA4) and programmed cell death protein-1 (PD-1) or its ligand (PD-1 L) that are part of some anticancer treatments (i.e., immune checkpoint inhibition). Although precise mechanisms remain uncertain, immune checkpoint inhibition-associated myocarditis seems linked to uncontrolled elicitation of autoreactive cardiac T cells in patients with subclinical autoimmunity [19, 20].

The ever-growing knowledge that is rapidly gathering around cardiac immunity clearly contributes to outline a new field of research and clinical investigation in cardiology, namely *cardioimmunology*, which opens new perspectives and possibility in diagnosis and treatment of cardiovascular diseases.

16.2 Immunosuppressive Therapy: Definition and Clinical Purposes

The immune system consists of a capillary network of lymphatic tissues, organs and vessels, equally distributed in every body district, which are made of specialized cell clusters with different and well-defined functions. In response to specific stimulation and signals, immune cells and their mediators can also easily migrate from a body district to another by both lymphatic and blood circulation. Consequently, host IR flexibly adapts itself to ever-changing interactions with the external environment that, in turn, exerts its epigenetic influence on the immune system. Structural complexity of IR per se along with host genetic predisposition and environmental triggers may occasionally give origin to dysfunctional responses that produce immune-mediated diseases [21].

In the last decades, immunological research and transplantation medicine provided deeper insight into human IR physiology and pathology, enabling development of innovative therapeutic approaches to transplant rejection, SIDs and OSAD [22]. Nevertheless, classical immunosuppressive drugs, such as corticosteroids, antimetabolites, calcineurin or mTor inhibitors, and some biological agents, such as high-dosage i.v. immunoglobulins (HDIVIG), still represent an effective initial therapeutic approach to SIDs and OSAD.

Immunosuppressive therapy (IT) can be defined as a balanced inhibition of the host IR, intentionally induced by means of drugs, biological agents (e.g., HDIVIG, polyclonal antithymocyte globulins, monoclonal antibodies) and/or physical procedures (e.g., plasma exchange, photopheresis, immunoadsorption, etc.), with the purpose to prevent or control harmful/undesired reactions.

Common clinical indications to IT, besides SIDs, OSAD and graft rejection, also include graft vs host disease and generalized allergic/hypersensitivity disorders. IT can be addressed to different biological and functional targets, such as immune cell reproduction, recruitment, trafficking, interaction and mediator release, as well as cytokines, their receptors and complement proteins. In addition to inactivation of the pathogenic cell framework underlying abnormal immune reactivity, IT is also intended to provide an anti-inflammatory action. According to circumstances and severity of the clinical picture, IT can be more or less aggressive or specific. IT needs to be constantly adapted and monitored in every patient with the purpose of preserving an acceptable level of immunocompetency and minimizing drug toxicity and/or adverse effects. Thus, IT schedules may vary considerably from patient to patient, ranging from intensive, multiple/sequential drug administration in critical situations, to long-term monotherapy to maintain disease remission, i.e., personalized treat-to-target approach [23].

16.3 Immunosuppressive Therapy: Preparatory Patient Workup (Safety Checklist)

IT should be started only following histological confirmation of AM/DCM diagnosis and after accurate exclusion of other known causes of inflammatory cardiomyopathy, particularly viral infection. If available, detection of serum AHA by IIFL is recommended to provide further evidence of autoimmune involvement [11].

In our experience, a preparatory diagnostic workup, namely the *Safety Checklist*, in biopsy-proven AM/DCM patients eligible to IT should include blood and instrumental tests that are summarized in Table 16.1. The *Safety Checklist* is intended to rule out potential general and individual risks related to IT; some tests should also be part of a regular follow-up in these patients. Patients who are candidates to IT should be screened for common latent infections (e.g., viral hepatitis B and C, human papilloma virus, HIV, EBV, CMV active infection, borreliosis, toxoplasmosis, trypanosomiasis cruzi, typical and atypical mycobacterial infections, toxocara canis in eosinophilic myocarditis, Campylobacter jejuni, etc.) or hidden malignancy (e.g., in situ prostatic or cervical malignancy, etc.).Thus, the *Safety Checklist* in female patients should include gynaecological inspection along with cervical smear to rule out in situ malignancy or Human Papilloma Virus (HPV) infection; screening mammography and pregnancy test should be carried out if appropriate. Male patients should be checked for serum prostatic specific antigen (PSA) levels. Patients presenting serum paraprotein should undergo haematological evaluation before starting IT. Additional clinical tests can be planned according to specific patients' needs. As a rule, before starting IT with potentially cytotoxic drugs, patients in reproductive age should be offered the possibility of semen/oocyte preservation.

Finally, immunosuppressive drugs should always be prescribed with caution in patients with impaired liver and/or kidney function, specific drug allergy/intolerance, concomitant primary immunodeficiency, major psychiatric disorders and history of alcohol or drug abuse.

Table 16.1 Preparatory clinical workup before starting immunosuppressive therapy (*Safety Checklist*)

Clinical and instrumental procedures
• Echocardiography
• Standard ECG
• 24 h Holter ECG
• Chest X-ray
• Complete abdominal ultrasound scan (selected patients, depending on patient's history)
• Dental inspection
• Gynaecological inspection/cervical smear examination
• Screening mammography when indicated
Laboratory tests
• Complete cell blood count
• ESR/CRP
• Renal and liver function
• Fasting glycaemia
• Complete urinalysis
• Serum immunoglobulin level
• Serological scrutiny for latent infections (see above), including tests for HBV, HCV, HIV, CMV, EBV, tuberculosis (Quantiferon), Borreliosis, toxoplasmosis, etc.
• NT-ProBNP/BNP
• Troponin
• Basic serum amylase and mutations of TMPT (if azathioprine is planned)
• Pregnancy test when indicated
• Serum PSA (male patients)

16.4 Immunosuppressive Therapy in Autoimmune Myocarditis

Current clinical studies support the efficacy of IT in disassembling the immunological framework that fuels cardiac inflammation and myocardial damage in AM/DCM, enabling stable cardiac function recovery [24–26]. Furthermore, IT reduces life-threatening arrhythmias and prevents chronic progression to DCM. Thus, in AM/DCM patients presenting with early severe/worsening myocardial dysfunction and/or life-threatening arrhythmia, or in those who do not respond readily to conventional cardiovascular therapy, IT should not be delayed. Nevertheless, fulminant myocarditis, besides aggressive cardiovascular therapy and mechanical circulatory support, deserves attentive discrimination before starting IT since its evolution may vary considerably from patient to patient and spontaneous recovery can be observed more frequently than in chronic/subacute cases [27].

Most published clinical trials and retrospective studies on IT in AM/DCM are based on the administration of a gradually decreasing dose of prednisone in combination with either azathioprine or cyclosporine over 6 months on average [24–26]. Overall, they suggest that in patients with biopsy-proven, non-infectious AM/DCM without specific contraindications, IT is an effective and safe option to control myocardial inflammation, leading to lasting recovery of cardiac function, and reduction of concurrent arrhythmia.

Corticosteroids, and in particular prednisone and methylprednisolone, are still mainstay of IT. They affect function and trafficking of immune cells by both inhibiting their migration to inflammation sites and reducing capillary permeability to proinflammatory mediators [28]. Prednisone and methylprednisolone, at a dose >1 mg/kg/day, seem particularly effective to induce a deep immunosuppressive effect and a rapid regression of myocardial inflammation. Pulse i.v. methylprednisolone, at a daily dose of 1 g can be administered in life-threatening AM as attack therapy [29]. Corticosteroids are equally efficient in controlling acute myocardial necrosis caused by eosinophilic cell infiltration in both isolated and SIDs associated primary eosinophilic myocarditis [30].

In patients who are non-responsive or intolerant to azathioprine or cyclosporine, and in specific myocarditis forms (e.g., primary eosinophilic myocarditis), alternative immunosuppressive agents, such as mycophenolate mofetil and methotrexate, can be equally employed [31, 32].

In both isolated AM/DCM and SIDs associated myocarditis, monoclonal antibodies (MoAbs) targeting specific cells (i.e., rituximab—anti-CD20 MoAb—for B lymphocytes, muromonab—anti-OKT3 MoAb—for T lymphocytes) and cytokines or their receptors (i.e., mepolizumab for IL-5 and anakinra for IL-1 receptor) have been added to standard IT with promising results. In particular, efficacy of anakinra has been occasionally reported in fulminant myocarditis, while rituximab has been successfully administered to a patient with recurrent GCM after heart transplantation [33–37].

In uncontrolled studies, infusion of HDIVIG was able to improve both myocardial function and survival in AM/DCM patients where standard IT was contraindicated [38]. T cell depletion by the infusion of rabbit derived antithymoglobulin, though effective, should be considered with caution in patients with aggressive, steroid-resistant GCM, due to the risk of systemic adverse reactions and appearance of severe leukopenia or thrombocytopenia [39, 40]. Selective removal of plasma immunoglobulins in patients with AM/DCM by immunoadsorption, an extracorporeal blood purification technique, followed by replacement with pool-derived immunoglobulins, showed promising results. In particular, removal of IgG3 directed against anti-β1-adrenergic receptors produced long-lasting hemodynamic improvement in patients with DCM. However, though relatively rapid and safe, immunoadsorption in AM/DCM is still under investigation [41].

Current clinical data do not provide conclusive indication about the optimal duration of IT in AM/DCM. According to expert consensus, whereas immunosuppression should be life-long in GCM, optimal IT length is yet undefined in chronic lymphocytic AM with stable recovery of cardiac function. Actually, in lymphocytic AM, azathioprine, an antimetabolite interfering with purine synthesis with good steroid sparing action, is usually started at the dose of 2 mg/kg/day p.o. in combination with oral prednisone at about 1 mg/kg/day and then continued for 6 months [24–26]. Yet, it is worth emphasizing that azathioprine takes several weeks before reaching its full therapeutic activity. In addition, since general experience acquired in SIDs and other conditions suggests that long-term treatment (i.e., >6 months) with azathioprine is particularly useful in maintaining stable remission, this can also be hypothesized for AM/DCM [42]. Azathioprine is considered to be safe even in pregnant women and in paediatric patients; anyway, before starting treatment, it is advisable to test patient peripheral blood for thiopurine methyltransferase (TPMT) mutation to prevent the appearance of secondary leukopenia/agranulocytosis [43]. Severe myelosuppression can be also observed following concomitant administration of azathioprine and allopurinol [44].

Cyclosporine A, a calcineurin inhibitor, represents a possible alternative in patients who are intolerant to azathioprine. It is usually given as oral therapy, at a dose ranging from 2 to 4 mg/kg/day, in combination with prednisone at about 1 mg/kg/day; in selected clinical situations, such as GCM, cyclosporine can also be effectively associated with azathioprine [45, 46]. Yet, despite its proven efficacy in lymphocytic AM, cyclosporine is not as easy to handle as azathioprine due to its numerous drug interactions and adverse effects. Finally, at least at the beginning, patients on cyclosporine require regular monitoring of its blood concentration to adjust therapeutic dose.

Although not yet standardized in primary AM/DCM treatment, mycophenolate mofetil, a selective and reversible inhibitor of inosine monophosphate dehydrogenase, seems to be promising in patients who show poor response to first line treatment or who are intolerant to azathioprine [31].

Methotrexate, a folic acid analogue interfering with nucleic acid synthesis acting as disease-modifying anti-rheumatic agent, can be administered at low dose (7.5–20 mg per week) either p.o. or by subcutaneous injection. Methotrexate alters mononuclear cell function and mediator release, particularly pro-inflammatory/pro-atherosclerotic cytokines such as IL-1, IL-6 and tumour necrosis factor-α (TNF-α). Methotrexate is generally well tolerated and its adverse effects are usually mild and dose-dependent; they include leukopenia, hepatic toxicity, mucosal toxicity (stomatitis), secondary infections and, very uncommonly, allergic reactions (skin rash, pneumonitis). Concomitant weekly administration of folic acid partially prevents methotrexate adverse effects. Methotrexate is frequently part of therapeutic schedules in SIDs, such as systemic lupus erythematosus, rheumatoid arthritis, sarcoidosis, eosinophilic granulomatosis with polyangiitis, systemic hyper-eosinophilic syndromes, etc., where myocarditis can be part of the clinical picture [47].

16.5 The Cardioimmunology Outpatient Clinic: Myocarditis Patient Follow-Up and Coaching

Diagnosis and treatment of AM/DCM require close inter-professional partnership involving cardiologists, pathologists, radiologists, immunologists, rheumatologists and other experienced healthcare personnel [48]. However, a truly effective teamwork should also include the patient and his/her caregivers.

Following histological diagnosis and after completing the *Safety Checklist*, similarly to transplanted patients, AM/DCM patients who start IT should enter a long-term follow-up in a dedicated *cardioimmunology outpatient clinic/day-service*. Given the peculiarity of AM/DCM and its treatment, cardiologists and physicians involved in AM/DCM patient follow-up should receive specific training, with particular attention to IT and patient education. Actually, if not appropriately and efficiently managed in collaboration with patients and/or their caregivers, both disease itself and IT can cause serious and disabling complications or potentially lethal harms. For patients with AM/DCM, everyday life means to cope with new limitations (involving family relationships, sexual life, work, school, physical activity, etc.), along with disease-related risks and the complexity of a self-managed multidrug treatment. Thus, physicians and professionals who treat AM/DCM patients require good relational attitude in order to establish a solid and empathic therapeutic relationship. Actually, patients and their carers can be proficiently helped to cope with their condition by providing them with the basic knowledge and skills related to self-management of disease and treatment.

Therapeutic Patient Education (TPE) is a specific educational technique aimed at patient's empowerment [49, 50]. According to a systematic health education model, TPE starts with the correct identification of patient's perspective, including his/her knowledge and concerns about disease and treatment, and needs (*educational diagnosis*). This entails that healthcare professionals who take care of AM/DCM patients have to learn how to listen and interpret correctly both verbal and non-verbal messages of their patients. This also applies to caregivers and, in particular, to parents of paediatric patients; adolescent patients can deserve even more attention and dedication. When necessary, psychological consultation and emotional support should be assured to the patient. Then, when indicated and after having acquired patient's consent, it will be possible to define a shared personalized therapeutic-educational plan (*educational/therapeutic objective agreement*), addressing specific points and indications related to the patient's participation. In practice, the *educational/therapeutical objective agreement* should clearly specify therapeutic tasks assigned to the patient, with particular regard to the accomplishment of safety issues (*safety agreement*) and treatment goals. TPE learning contents, including drug safety, hygienic rules, prevention of infectious complications, level and type of physical activity, nutrition, contraception and general lifestyle, should be taught in plain non-technical language (*patient/caregiver's teaching*) by physicians and nurses with specific expertise. Subsequently, patient's understanding, knowledge and home practice should be carefully checked, and his/her questions, problems or concerns should be readily addressed to find out and amend possible misunderstandings/mistakes (*patient's knowledge and skill assessment*). This is particularly important immediately after hospital discharge when patients start to self-manage a multidrug treatment schedule including a number of potentially dangerous medications, such as immunosuppressive drugs, antiarrythmics, diuretics and anticoagulants.

In conclusion, doctors should learn to work *with* rather than *for* their patients. Indeed, successful implementation of *Clinical Risk Management* in AM/DCM

Table 16.2 Key points for immunosuppressive therapy (IT) in AM/DCM

1. Biopsy-proven diagnosis of infection-negative AM/DCM
2. Careful selection of IT candidates (safety check list)
3. Personalized IT regimen
4. Therapeutic patients' education (TPE) to IT safety and disease self-management in everyday life
5. Close/ceaseless interdisciplinary teamwork

requires both fully aware consent and efficient participation of patients and/or their caregivers [51]. In this perspective, skilful professional expertise in both cardioimmunology and patients' coaching are equally essential, non-negotiable conditions to cope with and treat AM/DCM (Table 16.2).

References

1. Swirski K, Nahrendor M. Cardioimmunology: the immune system in cardiac homeostasis and disease. Nat Rev Immunol. 2018;18:733–44.
2. Libby P. Inflammation in atherosclerosis. Nature. 2002;420(6917):868–74.
3. Caforio A, Pankuweit S, Charron P, Cooper L, Basso C, Felix S, Fu M, Gimeno R, Helio T, Heymans S, Jahns R, McKenna WJ, Klingel K, Linhart A, Maisch B, Mogensen J, Monserrat L, Pinto Y, Ristic A, Schultheiss HP, Seggewiss H, Tavazzi L, Yilmaz A, Elliott P. Current state of knowledge on aetiology, diagnosis, management and therapy of myocarditis: a position statement of the European Society of Cardiology Working Group on myocardial and pericardial diseases. Eur Heart J. 2013;34(33):2636–48.
4. Cunningham MW. Rheumatic fever, autoimmunity, and molecular mimicry: the streptococcal connection. Int Rev Immunol. 2014;33:314–29.
5. Imazio M, Gaita F. Acute and recurrent pericarditis. Cardiol Clin. 2017;35(4):505–13.
6. Toldo S, Kannan H, Bussani R, Anzini M, Sonnino C, Sinagra G, Merlo M, Mezzaroma E, De-Giorgio F, Silvestri F, Van Tassell BW, Baldi A, Abbate A. Formation of the inflammasome in acute myocarditis. Int J Cardiol. 2014;171(3):e119–21.
7. Cantarini L, Lopalco G, Selmi C, Napodano S, De Rosa G, Caso F, Costa L, Iannone F, Rigante D. Autoimmunity and autoinflammation as the yin and yang of idiopathic recurrent acute pericarditis. Autoimmun Rev. 2015;14(2):90–7.
8. Caforio ALP, Grazzini M, Mann JM, Keeling PJ, Bottazzo GF, McKenna WJ, Schiaffino S. Identification of the alpha and beta myosin heavy chain isoforms as major autoantigens in dilated cardiomyopathy. Circulation. 1992;85:1734–42.
9. Leone O, Veinot JP, Angelini A, Baandrup UT, Basso C, Berry G, Bruneval P, Burke M, Butany J, Calabrese F, d'Amati G, Edwards WD, Fallon JT, Fishbein MC, Gallagher PJ, Halushka MK, McManus B, Pucci A, Rodriguez ER, Saffitz JE, Sheppard MN, Steenbergen C, Stone JR, Tan C, Thiene G, van der Wal AC, Winters GL. 2011 consensus statement on endomyocardial biopsy from the Association for European Cardiovascular Pathology and the Society for Cardiovascular Pathology. Cardiovasc Pathol. 2012;21:245–74.
10. Caforio ALP, Calabrese F, Angelini A, Tona F, Vinci A, Bottaro S, Ramondo A, Carturan E, Iliceto S, Thiene G, Daliento L. A prospective study of biopsy-proven myocarditis: prognostic relevance of clinical and etiopathogenetic features at diagnosis. Eur Heart J. 2007;28(11):1326–33.
11. Caforio ALP, Bonifacio E, Stewart JT, Neglia D, Parodi O, Bottazzo GF, McKenna WJ. Novel organ-specific circulating cardiac autoantibodies in dilated cardiomyopathy. J Am Coll Cardiol. 1990;15:1527–34.

12. Caforio ALP, Keeling PJ, Zachara E, Mestroni L, Camerini F, Mann JM, Bottazzo GF, McKenna WJ. Evidence from family studies for autoimmunity in dilated cardiomyopathy. Lancet. 1994;344:773–7.
13. Caforio ALP, Mahon NG, Baig KM, Tona F, Murphy RT, Elliott PM, McKenna WJ. Prospective familial assessment in dilated cardiomyopathy: cardiac autoantibodies predict disease development in asymptomatic relatives. Circulation. 2007;115:76–83.
14. Caforio ALP, Angelini A, Blank M, Shani A, Kivity S, Goddard G, Doria A, Bottaro S, Marcolongo R, Thiene G, Iliceto S, Shoenfeld Y. Passive transfer of affinity-purified anti-heart autoantibodies (AHA) from sera of patients with myocarditis induces experimental myocarditis in mice. Int J Cardiol. 2015;179:166–77.
15. Caforio ALP, Tona F, Bottaro S, Vinci A, Daliento L, Thiene G, Iliceto S. Clinical implications of anti-heart autoantibodies in myocarditis and dilated cardiomyopathy. Autoimmunity. 2008;41(1):35–45.
16. Caforio A, Adler Y, Agostini C, Allanore Y, Anastasakis A, Arad M, Böhm M, Charron P, Elliott PM, Eriksson U, Sb F, Garcia-Pavia P, Hachulla E, Heymans S, Imazio M, Klingel K, Marcolongo R, Matucci Cerinic M, Pantazis A, Plein S, Poli V, Rigopoulos A, Seferovic P, Shoenfeld Y, Jl Z, Linhart A. Diagnosis and management of myocardial involvement in systemic immune-mediated diseases: a position statement of the European Society of Cardiology Working Group on myocardial and pericardial disease. Eur Heart J. 2017;38:2649–62.
17. Eckel RH, Eisenbarth GS. Autoimmune diabetes inflames the heart. Sci Transl Med. 2012;4(138):138fs18.
18. Kandolin R, Lehtonen J, Salmenkivi K, Räisänen-Sokolowski A, Lommi J, Kupari M. Diagnosis, treatment, and outcome of giant-cell myocarditis in the era of combined immunosuppression. Circ Heart Fail. 2012;6:15–22.
19. Salem J-E, Manouchehri A, Moey M, Lebrun-Vignes B, Bastarache L, Pariente A, et al. Cardiovascular toxicities associated with immune checkpoint inhibitors: an observational, retrospective, pharmacovigilance study. Lancet Oncol. 2018;12:1579–89.
20. Müller OJ, Spehlmann ME, Frey N. Cardio-toxicity of checkpoint inhibitors. J Thorac Dis. 2018;10(Suppl 35):S4400–4.
21. Anaya JM, Ramirez-Santana C, Alzate MA, Molano-Gonzalez N, Rojas-Villarraga A. The autoimmune ecology. Front Immunol. 2016;7:139.
22. Floreth T, Bhorade SM, Ahya VN. Conventional and novel approaches to immunosuppression. Clin Chest Med. 2011;32(2):265–77.
23. Ford JA, Solomon DH. Challenges in implementing treat-to-target strategies in rheumatology. Rheum Dis Clin N Am. 2019;45(1):101–12.
24. Frustaci A, Russo MA, Chimenti C. Randomized study on the efficacy of immunosuppressive therapy in patients with virus-negative inflammatory cardiomyopathy: the {TIMIC} study. Eur Heart J. 2009;30:1995–2002.
25. Escher F, Kühl U, Lassner D, Poller W, Westermann D, Pieske B, Tschöpe C, Schultheiss HP. Long-term outcome of patients with virus-negative chronic myocarditis or inflammatory cardiomyopathy after immunosuppressive therapy. Clin Res Cardiol. 2016;105:1011–20.
26. Merken J, Hazebroek M, Van Paassen P, Verdonschot J, Van Empel V, Knackstedt C, Abdul Hamid M, Seiler M, Kolb J, Hoermann P, Ensinger C, Brunner-La Rocca HP, Poelzl G, Heymans S. Immunosuppressive therapy improves both short- and long-term prognosis in patients with virus-negative non-fulminant inflammatory cardiomyopathy. Circ Heart Fail. 2018;11(2):e004228.
27. Ginsberg F, Parrillo JE. Fulminant myocarditis. Crit Care Clin. 2013;29(3):465–83.
28. Fauci AS, Dale DC, Je B. Glucocorticoid therapy: mechanisms of action and clinical considerations. Ann Intern Med. 1976;84:304–15.
29. Ozawa H, Taoda A, Shinoda T, Yanagi H, Oki M, Takagi A. A case of Eosinophilic myocarditis associated with cardiogenic shock. Tokai J Exp Clin Med. 2017;42(4):156–9.
30. Kuchynka P, Palecek T, Masek M, Cerny V, Lambert L, Vitkova I, Linhart A. Current diagnostic and therapeutic aspects of eosinophilic myocarditis. Biomed Res. 2016;2016:2829583.

31. Thomas G, Cohen Aubart F, Chiche L, Haroche J, Hié M, Hervier B, Costedoat-Chalumeau N, Mazodier K, Ebbo M, Cluzel P, Cordel N, Ribes D, Chastre J, Schleinitz N, Veit V, Piette JC, Harlé JR, Combes A, Amoura Z. Lupus myocarditis: initial presentation and longterm outcomes in a multicentric series of 29 patients. J Rheumatol. 2017;44(1):24–32.
32. Campochiaro C, De Luca G, Sartorelli S, Tomelleri A, Esposito A, Candela C, Cavalli G, Dagna L. Efficacy and safety of methotrexate for the treatment of autoimmune virus-negative myocarditis: a case series. J Clin Rheumatol. 2018. https://doi.org/10.1097/RHU.0000000000000897.
33. Toscano G, Tartaro P, Fedrigo M, Angelini A, Marcolongo R. Rituximab in recurrent idiopathic giant cell myocarditis after heart transplantation: a potential therapeutic approach. Transpl Int. 2014;27(5):e38–42.
34. Perens G, Levi DS, Alejos JC, Wetzel GT. Muronomab-CD3 for pediatric acute myocarditis. Pediatr Cardiol. 2007;28(1):21–6.
35. Song T, Jones DM, Homsi Y. Therapeutic effect of anti-IL-5 on eosinophilic myocarditis with large pericardial effusion. BMJ Case Rep. 2017;24:2017.
36. Cheung CC, Constantine M, Ahmadi A, Shiau C, Chen LYC. Eosinophilic myocarditis. Am J Med Sci. 2017;354(5):486–92.
37. Cavalli G, Pappalardo F, Mangieri A, Dinarello CA, Dagna L, Tresoldi M. Treating life-threatening myocarditis by blocking Interleukin-1. Crit Care Med. 2016;44(8):e751–4.
38. Maisch B, Alter P. Treatment options in myocarditis and inflammatory cardiomyopathy: focus on i.v. immunoglobulins. Herz. 2018;43(5):423–30.
39. Suarez-Barrientos A, Wong J, Bell A, Lyster H, Karagiannis G, Banner NR. Usefulness of rabbit anti-thymocyte globulin in patients with Giant cell myocarditis. Am J Cardiol. 2015;116(3):447–51.
40. Deeks ED, Keating GM. Rabbit antithymocyte globulin (thymoglobulin): a review of its use in the prevention and treatment of acute renal allograft rejection. Drugs. 2009;69(11):1483–512.
41. Felix SB, Beug D, Dörr M. Immunoadsorption therapy in dilated cardiomyopathy. Expert Rev Cardiovasc Ther. 2015;13(2):145–52.
42. Sood R, Ansari S, Clark T, Hamlin PJ, Ford AC. Long-term efficacy and safety of azathioprine in ulcerative colitis. J Crohns Colitis. 2015;9(2):191–7.
43. Relling MV, Gardner EE, Sandborn WJ, Schmiegelow K, Pui C-H, Yee SW, Stein CM, Carrillo M, Evans WE, Klein TE. Clinical pharmacogenetics implementation consortium guidelines for thiopurine methyltransferase genotype and thiopurine dosing. Clin Pharmacol Ther. 2011;89(3):387–91.
44. Blaker PA, Arenas-Hernandez M, Smith MA, Shobowale-Bakre EA, Fairbanks L, Irving PM, Sanderson JD, Marinaki AM. Mechanism of allopurinol induced TPMT inhibition. Biochem Pharmacol. 2013;86(4):539–47.
45. Fahr A. Cyclosporin clinical pharmacokinetics. Clin Pharmacokinet. 1993;24(6):472–95.
46. Cooper LT Jr. Giant cell myocarditis: diagnosis and treatment. Herz. 2000;25(3):291–8.
47. Braun J, Rau R. An update on methotrexate. Curr Opin Rheumatol. 2009;21(3):216–23.
48. Caforio ALP, Marcolongo R, Jahns R, Fu M, Felix SB, Iliceto S. Immune-mediated and autoimmune myocarditis: clinical presentation, diagnosis and management. Heart Fail Rev. 2013;18(6):715–32.
49. W.H.O. Working Group, World Health Organization, Regional Office for Europe. Therapeutic Patient Education. Continuing education programs for healthcare providers in the field of prevention of chronic diseases. Geneva: WHO; 1998.
50. Aujoulat I, Marcolongo R, Bonadiman L, Deccache A. Reconsidering patient empowerment in chronic illness: a critique of models of self-efficacy and bodily control. Soc Sci Med. 2008;66(5):1228–39.
51. Marcolongo R, Bonadiman L, Gagnayre R. Gérer le risque clinique avec le patient: une contribution possible de l'éducation thérapeutique du patient. Gestion Hospitalière. 2008;477:417–22.

Antiviral Therapies: A Critical Reappraisal

17

Ahmed Elsanhoury, Sophie Van Linthout, and Carsten Tschöpe

17.1 Case Study

A 56-year-old female patient is recently diagnosed with heart failure (NYHA III). Coronary heart disease had been excluded by coronary angiography. Echocardiography and angiography showed a mildly dilated left ventricle (left ventricular end-diastolic diameter = 57 mm) with a significantly reduced systolic function (ejection fraction (EF): 29%) and absence of any valve disease. Cardiac function slightly improved after initiation of optimal medical symptomatic standard heart failure therapy. Cardiac MRI (cMRI) showed an acute myocarditis. Three months later, echocardiography showed no further improvement in EF but cMRI showed the development of cardiac fibrosis.

17.2 Introduction

Myocarditis is an inflammatory disorder of the myocardium induced by a wide variety of toxins and drugs (e.g., cocaine, check point inhibitors), and particularly by infectious agents, including bacteria, fungi, parasites, and most common cardiotropic viruses, as well as autoimmunity. Although most patients with acute myocarditis have a good prognosis when complete healing occurs, ongoing cardiac inflammation, e.g., due to cardiac viral persistence can cause severe heart failure with an impaired

A. Elsanhoury · S. Van Linthout · C. Tschöpe (✉)
BIH Center for Regenerative Therapies (BIHCRT)/Berlin-Brandenburg Center for Regenerative Therapies (BCRT), Charité University Medicine Berlin, Berlin, Germany

Department of Cardiology, Charité University Medicine Berlin, Humboldt-Universität zu Berlin, Berlin, Germany

DZHK (German Center for Cardiovascular Research), Partner Site Berlin, Berlin, Germany
e-mail: ahmed.elsanhoury@charite.de; sophie.van-linthout@charite.de; carsten.tschoepe@charite.de

A. L. P. Caforio (ed.), *Myocarditis*, https://doi.org/10.1007/978-3-030-35276-9_17

prognosis [1–3]. The pathogenesis of viral myocarditis is described to be associated, among others, with coxsackievirus B3 (CVB3), adenovirus (AV), human herpesvirus 6 (HHV-6), hepatitis C virus (HCV), human immunodeficiency virus (HIV), and influenza virus [3, 4]. Cardiotropic viruses typically spread from the lymphoid organs, which act as viral reservoirs, to the cardiomyocytes, a process, which is best understood for coxsackievirus-induced infection [5]. Persistent enterovirus (EV; most prominently CVB3) detection in the myocardium was found to be associated with worse clinical outcome in contrast to the patients who experience spontaneous clearance [6, 7]. Herpes viruses are lifelong persistent viruses that might get reactivated several years after childhood infection. The appearance of HHV-6 in the myocardial tissue may be due to reactivation [8, 9]. Although HHV-6 is a lymphotropic virus, it was shown to infect endothelial cells and cardiomyocytes and the chromosomally integrated form can be inherited through germline [10, 11]. Reactivation of chromosomally integrated HHV-6 (ciHHV-6) is frequently associated with myocarditis symptoms in addition to non-cardiac disorders [12]. The role of the vasculotropic virus parvovirus B19 (B19V) under these circumstances is still under discussion [13]. B19V commonly infects children ("Fifth disease") and is usually asymptomatic. Lethal outcomes of B19V infection are unusual. Nevertheless, rare examples of B19V induced hemophagocytic syndrome and myocarditis in infants and children are described [14–16]. So B19V infection is usually acquired in childhood, and persists lifelong in approximately 70% of adults and may belong to a cardiac bioportfolio. B19V DNA is found in the majority of chronic myocarditis in the absence of systemic infection, questioning whether this finding represents the cause of the disease. In the attempt to be able to differentiate between B19V persistence and acute infection or reactivation, some laboratories differentiate between B19V DNA and mRNA replicates. Whether the latter has a clinical significance is still under investigation [17]. However, in contrast to AV and CVB3 persistence, the finding of B19V DNA can be associated with endothelial dysfunction and impairment of endothelial repair [14, 15, 18, 19], but it was not associated with impaired prognosis [20, 21]. Therefore, B19V DNA persistence in the absence of systemic infection might be a bystander finding, without causing dilated inflammatory cardiomyopathy (DCMi).

17.3 Diagnosis

In general, either viral replication or viral protein expression from cardiotropic viruses can induce direct cellular dysfunction and trigger immune reactions within the cardiac tissue that usually involve cardiomyocytes, cardiac fibroblasts, and cardiac endothelial cells. The acute inflammatory reaction resolves spontaneously in 50–60% of patients [22, 23]. In the remainder, it results in various degrees of cardiac tissue destruction up to DCMi [2, 24] and subsequent dilated cardiomyopathy (DCM). The clinical presentation of viral-induced myocarditis/DCMi combines unspecific manifestations, e.g., dyspnea, fatigue, and peripheral oedema [2]. A differential diagnosis is unfeasible via noninvasive techniques: echocardiography and cardiac magnetic resonance imaging (cMRI) may detect acute inflammation, not

Table 17.1 Frequency distribution of cardiotropic viruses in the EMB specimens of suspected myocarditis patients in the European population [1]

B19V	CVB3	AV	HHV-6	EBV	HCV	B19V + HHV6	CVB3 + B19V
51.4%	9.4%	1.6%	21.6%	2%	0.8%	16.4%	5.5%

B19V parvovirus B19, *CVB3* coxsackievirus B3, *AV* adenovirus, *HHV-6* human herpesvirus 6, *EBV* Epstein–Barr virus, *HCV* hepatitis C virus

viral persistence [25]. Blood tests or the detection of antiviral antibodies are also insufficient [26]. In the chronic phase of the disease, cMRI is even not sensitive enough to exclude a still significant but low amount of cardiac inflammation, which can be associated with chronic cardiac viral persistence [27]. A clear-cut diagnosis of DCMi refractory to conservative treatments can only be achieved via endomyocardial biopsy (EMB; class IIa/C recommendation) [28]. Typically, > five specimens should be obtained and stored for histological, immunohistochemical, virological, and microbiological analysis. A study from Kühl et al. [1] described in 2005 the frequencies of cardiotropic viruses that might be associated with DCMi in the European population. Cardiotropic viral genomes were found in about 70% [29] of EMBs of patients with clinically suspected myocarditis. The rates of the individual viruses are shown in Table 17.1. However, it is important to mention that these frequencies are time- and geography-dependent.

17.4 Management of Inflammatory Cardiomyopathy

Currently, there is no specific treatment for myocarditis with viral persistence [22]. DCMi patients, typically presenting with heart failure symptoms, are treated with supportive heart failure therapies, including ß-adrenergic blockers, inhibitors of the renin–angiotensin–aldosterone system, and diuretics [30]. However, the aforementioned treatments do not interfere with the underlying virus-induced pathologic mechanisms. The specific treatment of DCMi is ought to be personalized, depending on the EMB analysis results. Patients, in whom EMB shows persistent cardiac inflammation with no evidence for viral genomes are expert-based recommended for weight-based immunosuppressive regimens, i.e., prednisone/azathioprine (Table 17.2) [26, 31, 38, 39]. Frustaci et al. [40] showed that chronic myocarditis patients with EMB-proven viral persistence are unlikely to respond to immune suppression treatment, in contrast to virus-negative patients, although multicenter data are still needed to corroborate this finding. This large group of patients needs to receive viral-specific therapies to prevent further deterioration of cardiac function. So far, no single antiviral agent is explicitly indicated for viral myocarditis. The off-label use of some medications established for other indications defines the current armamentarium against viral myocarditis. Data from clinical studies with some antivirals—described in the next sections—suggest that antiviral treatment should be started early enough before irreversible myocardial damage advances. However, the decision to use some of these drugs depends on the clinical scenario and the expertise of the clinician. They are not approved.

Table 17.2 Summary of endomyocardial biopsy-guided therapies[a]

EMB result	Treatment	Treatment regimen	Special considerations
Inflammation– virus–	Conventional treatment with symptomatic heart failure therapies including ARNI, ACE-I, ARBs, loop diuretics, and aldosterone antagonists	Lifelong treatment with the maximum tolerated doses	Genetic evaluation is recommended in case of cardiomyopathies and the therapy has to be adjusted accordingly
Inflammation+ virus–	Combined immunosuppressive therapy	Prednisone: 1 mg/kg/day for 1 month, tapered down to 0.33 mg/kg/day for 5 months Azathioprine: 2 mg/kg/day for 6 months [31]	Immunosuppression is contraindicated in case of EMB-evident CVB3 or adenovirus infection or RNA+ B19V
CVB3+ or adenovirus+	IFN-β-1b	4 MIU q.o.d for 6 months, via SC route	Dose titration using 2 MIU q.o.d for the first week is recommended [32]
mRNA+ B19V	Telbivudine	600 mg q.d for 6 months	DNA+/mRNA–B19V patients might benefit from immunosuppressive therapy [33–37]
mRNA+ ciHHV-6	Ganciclovir and valganciclovir	10-day course with 5 mg of IV ganciclovir q12h followed by 900 mg daily of valganciclovir p.o. for 6 months	To be proven in large-scale studies
HCV+	A combination therapy consisting of ombitasvir, paritaprevir, ritonavir, and dasabuvir	Two combination tablets (each containing 12.5 mg ombitasvir, 75 mg paritaprevir, and 50 mg ritonavir) q.d plus a single 250 mg dasabuvir tablet b.i.d	The regimen contains a CYP3A inhibitor; dose adjustment of some concomitant medications may be required
HIV+	A combination of 3 ARTs of different classes	As indicated in the products SmPC	Drug–drug interactions should be considered
Influenza A+ or influenza B+	Peramivir Oseltamivir	One time 300 mg IV dose 75 mg p.o. twice daily for 5 days	Immunosuppressive therapy is contraindicated

EMB endomyocardial biopsy, *ARNI* angiotensin receptor-neprilysin inhibitor, *ACE-I* angiotensin converting enzyme inhibitor, *ARBs* angiotensin receptor blockers, *IV* intravenous, *CVB3* coxsackievirus B3, *B19V* parvovirus B19, *IFN-β-1b* interferon beta-1b, *MIU* million international unit, *q.od* every other day, *SC* subcutaneous, *q.d* everyday, *ciHHV6* chromosomally integrated human herpes virus type 6, *q12h* every 12 h, *p.o.* oral, *HCV* human hepatitis C virus, *b.i.d.* twice daily, *HIV* human immunodeficiency virus, *SmPC* summary of product characteristics

[a]The treatment strategies presented are all experimental and should be employed only at highly specialized cardiomyopathy centers

17.5 Therapeutic Options for Virus-Associated Myocarditis/ Inflammatory Cardiomyopathy

Owing to the high rate of spontaneous remission and the experimental nature of the proposed treatments, the following interventions are suggested only in severe acute/ cardiogenic shock-like cases (e.g., influenza-associated myocarditis) or in DCM patients with symptoms persisting for 3 months or more.

17.5.1 Virus-Specific Therapies

17.5.1.1 Telbivudine

Basic Pharmacology

Telbivudine is an orally bioavailable thymidine nucleoside analogue that acts as hepatitis B virus (HBV) reverse transcriptase inhibitor via preferential inhibition of HBV second strand (DNA-dependent) compared with first strand (RNA-dependent) DNA synthesis [41], a mechanism that theoretically might interfere with the replication of the single stranded DNA genome of B19V. It can also exert anti-inflammatory properties. Telbivudine is marketed for the treatment of adults with chronic hepatitis B infection.

Therapeutic Rational

In cell culture, telbivudine was reported to exhibit endothelial- and cardio-protective pleiotropic effects [33]. Clinically, an off-label single-patient use approach in transcriptionally active B19V-associated myocarditis/DCMi leads to improvement of symptoms, cardiac function, and myocardial inflammation following a 6-month regimen with daily dose of 600 mg telbivudine on top of symptomatic heart failure treatments [33]. The clinical efficacy and safety of telbivudine as a treatment for transcriptionally active B19V-associated DCMi are currently under investigation in a randomized controlled study (PreTOPIC; EudraCT-Number: 2016–004825-17) [33]. In 2018, a study [34] that was conducted in the south-west of Germany on the EMBs of patients with unexplained cardiomyopathy described the association of transcriptionally active B19V with 21% of the cases and indicated telbivudine to a subset of patients who did not benefit from standard heart failure therapies. Despite the fact that telbivudine is prescribed off-label by various cardiology clinics to accelerate the recovery of some DCMi patients with high EMB B19V mRNA copy number, the role of both B19V and telbivudine in the aforementioned pathology is still uncertain and today represents an experimental approach.

Safety Considerations

The use of telbivudine in B19V DCMi patients follows the recommended dose for chronic hepatitis B treatment (600 mg/day). Severe adverse reactions to telbivudine are uncommon/rare at the 600 mg daily dose. Clinical and post-marketing studies showed that telbivudine is well tolerated, but myopathies and neuropathies may occur in a very small subset of patients; thus, monthly monitoring of the serum creatine kinase and creatinine levels is required [35, 36]. The single-patient use study did not result in any drug-related safety concerns or unexpected cardiac adverse events [33, 34]. Nevertheless, telbivudine should only be used under close monitoring at specialized myocarditis centers.

17.5.1.2 Viral DNA Polymerase Inhibitors: Ganciclovir and Valganciclovir

Basic Pharmacology

Ganciclovir is an acyclic guanosine nucleotide analogue that specifically inhibits viral DNA polymerase after intracellular conversion to a triphosphate form, a process that requires both viral and cellular kinases [42, 43]. Valganciclovir is an orally active valine ester prodrug of ganciclovir [42]. Both medications are indicated for cytomegalovirus (CMV) infections, but shown to be effective against HHV-6 [42, 44]. Moreover, ganciclovir and valganciclovir are also effective to prevent CMV, HHV-6, and Epstein Barr virus (EBV) infections in solid-organ transplant and immunocompromised patients [45, 46]. The clinical efficacy and the safety of both agents were established several years ago.

Therapeutic Rational

Conventional treatment of symptomatic HHV-6 infection consists of the antivirals ganciclovir, cidofovir, and foscarnet [47, 48]. Theoretically, the three can be used also against reactivated ciHHV-6 associated myocarditis. Valganciclovir is frequently used in HHV-6-associated conditions like limbic encephalitis and transplant complications. Several case reports have demonstrated that ciHHV-6 patients with encephalitis and chronic fatigue syndrome respond to ganciclovir and valganciclovir [49, 50]. Kühl et al. [12] treated six highly symptomatic heart failure patients with transcriptionally active HHV-6 using 5 mg ganciclovir every 12 h for 10 days, followed by a daily dose of 900 mg valganciclovir for 6 months. The antiviral therapy was reported to improve symptoms and cardiac function of all the patients, together with suppression of HHV-6 mRNA transcription. Three patients required prolonged therapy to maintain viral suppression. However, such therapy failed to clear HHV-6 from the myocardium.

Safety Considerations

The safety profiles of both ganciclovir and valganciclovir are similar. The most frequent adverse drug reactions following val–/ganciclovir are neutropenia, anemia, and diarrhea. Both medications were reported as safe and well tolerated in solid organ transplant patients [51]. There is limited information about the safety of val–/ganciclovir in HHV-6 associated myocarditis patients. The study from Kühl et al. [12] did not report any cardiologic or non-cardiologic adverse events. It is worth saying that the use of viral DNA polymerase inhibitors in HHV-6 associated myocarditis is yet to be proven in large-scale studies and should only be employed at highly specialized myocarditis centers.

17.5.1.3 Direct-Acting Antivirals

Basic Pharmacology

Direct-acting antivirals (DAAs) are molecules that target specific nonstructural proteins of HCV and result in the disruption of viral replication. DAAs include nonstructural proteins 3/4A (NS3/4A), protease inhibitors (PIs), NS5B nucleoside polymerase inhibitors (NPIs), NS5B non-nucleoside polymerase inhibitors (NNPIs), and NS5A inhibitors. DAAs are relatively new agents, representing a major advance in HCV treatment, with boceprevir and telaprivir being the first FDA approved DAAs on the market (May 2011) [52]. DAAs are far more efficient and well tolerated than interferon alpha (IFN-α) regarding HCV elimination. In combination, these DAA agents enabled IFN-free therapy with sustained virologic response (SVR) above 90% among patients with chronic HCV infection [53]. A treatment protocol that includes an oral combination of ombitasvir (NS5A inhibitor)/paritaprevir (NS3/4A inhibitor)/ritonavir (CYP3A inhibitor) together with an additional tablet of the NS5B NNPI dasabuvir achieved a SVR of 100% in HCV genotype-1 patients [54], which is the most prevalent HCV genotype in Europe [55]. Ritonavir boosts the plasma concentration of paritaprevir via the inhibition of CYP3A, a hepatic enzyme responsible for the oxidative metabolism of various molecules [56].

Therapeutic Rational

HCV infection has been reported in the EMBs of myocarditis and cardiomyopathy patients, where antiviral HCV therapies may have potential benefit, especially the new DAAs [57–59]. However, clinical information about the efficacy of DAAs in such patients is limited. Poller et al. [60] recently reported the outcomes of DAAs treatment in one critically ill HCV-positive patient who was listed for heart transplantation and did not tolerate IFN-α therapy. The patient received the ombitasvir, paritaprevir, ritonavir, and dasabuvir combination protocol for 12 weeks under close monitoring for possible adverse events. The treatment resulted in viral clearance, associated with significant improvement of NYHA functional class from III–IV before treatment to class II after viral clearance; heart transplantation became no longer necessary, suggesting a possible causal association of HCV with heart dysfunction.

Safety Consideration

Generally, DAAs are well tolerated by non-HF patients [61–64]. The new DAAs agents are highly virus-specific without cardiac side effects [65], in contrast to the classic anti-HCV IFN-α -based protocols that were not well tolerated in cardiomyopathy patients and had low SVR rates [60]. The ombitasvir/paritaprevir/ritonavir/dasabuvir combination is commonly associated with insomnia, anemia, pruritus, nausea, and vomiting. Moreover, ritonavir interferes with the metabolism of a wide range of medicinal products, being a CYP3A inhibitor. The study by Poller et al. [60] which employed the aforementioned combination in a critically ill HCV-associated heart failure patient reported that the treatment was well tolerated, except for severe hyponatremia and progressive weakness which required massive sodium substitution. The exact pharmacologic mechanism of this side effect is unknown but can be attributed to the interference of any of the drugs with the renal transporters. So far, the use of DAAs as specific treatments for HCV-associated cardiomyopathy is not proven yet and the data provided from a single study cannot conclude the safety and efficacy of those therapies in HCV-associated cardiomyopathy/myocarditis patients.

17.5.1.4 Antiretroviral Therapies

Basic Pharmacology

Antiretroviral therapies (ARTs) are composed of six classes that block HIV replication at different parts of the life cycle: (1) nucleoside reverse transcriptase inhibitors (NRTIs), which inhibit viral replication by competitive binding to reverse transcriptase, (2) nonnucleoside reverse transcriptase inhibitors (NNRTIs) that prevent viral replication by preventing addition of new nucleotides to the growing DNA chain, (3) integrase strand transfer inhibitors (INSTIs), which inhibit HIV replication by preventing integration of the viral genome into the host genome, (4) protease inhibitors that work by inhibiting viral maturation through inhibition of cleavage of polyproteins, (5) fusion inhibitors that inhibit the fusion of the viral envelope with the host cell membrane, and (6) CCR5 co-receptor antagonists which inhibits the process of HIV entry into CD4+ cells. Clinically, a combination of at least three ARTs from different classes is used in a personalized manner to control HIV infection, as the viral suitability to individual ARTs varies [66–68].

Therapeutic Rational

Heart diseases are frequently reported as causes of death in HIV patients [69, 70]. The heart failure hospitalization rate in HIV patients is double as high than in non-HIV patients [71]. Coronary heart disease, pericarditis, vascular diseases, and cardiomyopathies are frequently diagnosed in HIV patients [72–74]. HIV has been unambiguously linked to myocarditis and acquired cardiomyopathies [75, 76]. The exact mechanism that links HIV to cardiomyopathy is yet unknown. However, multiple pathologic mechanisms including direct viral infection of the myocardium and indirect cytokine, immune, ischemic and pharmacotoxic mechanisms have been described [73, 75, 77]. ARTs being potent agents to control HIV-infection have been shown to reduce the HIV-related events including cardiovascular diseases, especially when early initiated [78]. The use of ARTs correlated with reduced risk of cardiovascular damage, specifically systolic dysfunction [79] and has even been reported to improve left ventricular systolic function in pediatrics [80, 81]. A scientific statement from the American heart association stated that all HIV-associated cardiomyopathy patients with reduced EF are recommended to start or continue on ARTs therapy beside guideline directed heart failure therapies [82]. Aside from ARTs, patients with HIV were reported to have higher levels of cardiac autoantibodies, known markers of autoimmune myocarditis [83].

Safety Considerations

The increased access to ARTs is mirrored with a reduction in HIV-associated myocarditis and systolic dysfunction but it has also been described to shift HIV-associated cardiomyopathy towards diastolic dysfunction [79, 84]. Epidemiological studies advocate that diastolic dysfunction is the principal HIV-associated heart failure phenotype in the era of ARTs [85–87]. A pharmacotoxic mechanism may be involved. However, there are not enough data to draw a causal association between the use of ARTs and diastolic dysfunction. Zidovudine, a NRTI, is known to cause cardiomyopathy as a side effect via myocytes' mitochondrial damage and the disruption of the myocardial endothelial cell junctions [88, 89]. Clinicians should be aware of the interactions between individual ART agents and the concomitant medications, as ARTs exhibit a wide range of pharmacodynamic/−kinetic interactions with heart failure, anti-infective, and immune suppressant medications [90–92]. Heart transplantation HIV-patients are mostly affected from those interactions, which mandate careful drug use [93].

17.5.1.5 Neuraminidase Inhibitors

Basic Pharmacology

The neuraminidase inhibitors oseltamivir, zanamivir, and peramivir inhibit the release of influenza virions from the infected host cells, limiting the cycles of viral replication. These agents have activity against both influenza A and influenza B viruses [94]. Oseltamivir and zanamivir are administered during a 5- and 10-days course, via oral and inhalation route, respectively. Peramvivir is an intravenous single dose agent for emergency use [95].

Therapeutic Rational

Influenza-associated myocarditis is rarely reported. The frequency of such cases is controversial but appears to be generally low, and varies with season, place, and diagnostic criteria [96–102]. Influenza A and less commonly influenza B are associated with myocarditis [103–107]. Influenza A viral antigens and genetic material were detected in EMBs and autopsy samples from patients with myocarditis [99–101, 108]. The use of antivirals, especially neuraminidase inhibitors played a crucial role in halting the H1N1 influenza epidemic in 2009, and were found effective in reducing the influenza-associated complications including myocarditis. Morioka et al. [109] reported that oseltamivir treatment of 44 influenza infected infants aged <3 months in Japan prevented influenza-associated myocarditis. Interestingly, the H1N1 fatality rate in Japan was relatively low during the 2009 epidemic, owing to aggressive early therapy with neuraminidase inhibitors [109]. A case report by Geladari et al. described that early therapy with oseltamivir resulted in complete and full recovery of influenza B associated myocarditis [110]. Another case report described the successful treatment of influenza A associated fulminant myocarditis via single intravenous dose of peramivir [111]. Guillaume et al. discussed a series of four influenza B fulminant myocarditis cases and concluded that early antiviral therapy should be considered [112]. As a general observation, most of the reported cases received circulatory support therapy and extracorporeal membrane oxygenation (ECMO) support concomitantly to the antiviral therapy.

Safety Considerations

General side effects of neuraminidase inhibitors include nausea, vomiting, and bronchospasm in case of inhalation route [113]. The safety of these agents in myocarditis patients is not well established. The use of immune suppression therapy in influenza patients is controversial, and the data available about the use of neuraminidase inhibitors in influenza-associated myocarditis are very limited [114]. Further studies are necessary to warrant the use of antivirals in myocarditis-complicated influenza, to be equipped for any future influenza epidemic.

17.5.2 Immunomodulatory/Unspecific Antiviral Therapies

17.5.2.1 Interferons

Basic Pharmacology

Type I interferons (IFNs α, β, ω, and κ) are naturally occurring protein cytokines that signal through a common receptor complex composed of two transmembrane chains: IFN α/ß receptor 1 and 2 [115]. Activation of IFN receptors triggers a phosphorylation cascade, concluding in the transcription of a group of genes collectively known as IFN-stimulated genes [116]. IFN-α is secreted by human leukocytes while IFN-β is mainly secreted by fibroblasts. IFN-β1 is a human restricted subtype of the IFN-β, and is known to exert antiviral and immunoregulatory activities [117, 118]. The antiviral activities of IFNs include inhibition of viral replication and augmentation of MHC-I and -II antigen expression, facilitating viral antigen presentation and cellular immunity [115]. IFN-α has been shown to activate natural killer cells and cytotoxic T-cells [119–121]. It is important to highlight that IFNs are host targeting immune response modulators rather than direct antiviral agents. The unglycosylated recombinant form of IFN-β-1b [117] is used for the management of multiple sclerosis.

Therapeutic Rational

IFN-α was used for decades to counteract HCV infection up until the newly introduced directly acting antiviral agents (DAAs) took the lead in HCV treatment [53]. Moreover, the use of INF-α in HCV-associated myocarditis patients is limited by its side effects [65]. Accordingly, IFN-α will not be further discussed in this writing. IFN-β has been described to exhibit antiviral activity against CVB3 in vitro [122], and has been shown to be protective against murine CVB3-associated myocarditis [123]. Clinically, IFN-β serum levels are low in patients with persistent viral myocarditis, but significantly elevated in the serum of patients who spontaneously clear CVB3 infection [124]. In a pilot trial, Kühl et al. [125] followed the treatment of CVB3- and AV-associated DCMi patients with IFN-β-1b for 6 months and reported that the genomes of both viruses were totally cleared from the hearts of all treated patients, an outcome that was associated with significant clinical improvement [125, 126]. Later, the Betaferon® in chronic viral cardiomyopathy (BICC) placebo-controlled phase-II trial [32] concluded that 6 months treatment regimen with IFN-β-1b is of therapeutic value in EV and AV associated DCMi. The study described that the IFN-β-1b regimen induced viral clearance, symptomatic and cardiac function improvement. Symptomatic improvement was also reported in B19V-positive patients; however, viral clearance was not achieved [32]. It is worth mentioning that immunosuppression is contraindicated in EV and AV positive patients [28]. Those specific patients can be treated with IFN-β-1b. However, further trials are needed to support these first findings.

Safety Considerations

IFN-β-1b is primarily indicated for the management of multiple sclerosis employing a dose of 8 million international units (MIU) every other day via subcutaneous injection. The safety of IFN-β-1b has been demonstrated over the years, whereby the European Medicine Agency (EMA) safety assessment reports indorsed the use of IFN-β-1b in adults, with the exception of pregnant women and patients with known allergy to the recombinant protein.

The BICC trial demonstrated the safety of 6 months IFN-β-1b treatment in DCMi patients presenting with symptoms of heart failure and diastolic or systolic myocardial dysfunction. A significant overall clinical benefit was achieved and outweighed the potential risks [32]. The adverse events occurred at similar frequencies in both the active and the control groups [32, 127]. IFN-β-1b was well tolerated even by patients with severe systolic dysfunction (left ventricular ejection fraction below 35%). The study indicated that the treatment regimen did not result in any drug-related safety concerns or unexpected severe cardiac or non-cardiac adverse events [32]. Generally, the safety profile of IFN-β-1b in CVB3/AV associated DCMi patients is comparable to that known for multiple sclerosis indication. Drug-related adverse events include flu-like side effects, fatigue, and injection site reactions, usually occurring at the initial phase of the therapy. Reversible increase in transaminase levels (maximum AST/ALT values of 500/150 UI/L) is noticeable in patients receiving IFN-β-1b, which normalize after treatment cessation [127].

17.5.2.2 Immunoglobulins

Basic Pharmacology

Immunomodulatory treatment with intravenous immunoglobulins (IVIG): IgM, IgG, and IgA (IgGAM) interact with the immune system, regulate antiviral processes including complement system activation, pathogens' opsonization, and immune cell activation [128]. On the other side of the coin, IVIG exert anti-inflammatory effects via mediating anti-inflammatory cytokines production, e.g., IL8, inhibiting pro-inflammatory cytokines, e.g., IL-1 and IL-6, and reducing oxidative stress in addition to direct neutralization of viral proteins [129, 130].

Therapeutic Rationale

Immune-mediated mechanisms play a pivotal role in the pathogenesis of myocarditis/DCMi and are likely targets for IVIG therapy owing to its antiviral and immunomodulatory functions. A randomized controlled study (the IMAC study) on acute myocarditis patients without the knowledge of viral persistence showed no benefit from IVIG treatment [131]. However, in patients with viral persistence, the use of IVIG could be meaningful. Limited clinical studies and data from patient registries suggest IVIG for the treatment of AV-, B19V-, and CMV-associated DCMi. IVIG therapy was reported to clear AV and the associated myocardial inflammation at intermediate dose [132]. Complete elimination of B19V could not be achieved via IVIG but the associated inflammation was cleared. Pankuweit et al. [133] described that intravenous treatment with $\geq 2 \times 20$ g immunoglobulin reliably eliminated inflammation, and eradicated or only reduced the B19V load in about 50% of cases of B19V-associated myocarditis. In the event of severe B19V systemic infection, IVIG have been shown to reduce viral load and improve cardiac functions [134–136]. CMV was shown to be completely eradicated via high dose IVIG bolus [132, 135]. To this end, IVIG therapy can offer treatment option for persistent viral myocarditis, yet to be proven in large-scale clinical studies. Newly, a clinical trial (NTC00892112) investigating the efficacy of intravenous IgG to reduce B19V viral load in chronic B19V-positive cardiomyopathy patients with a B19V viral load above 200 copies/μg DNA has been completed. However, the results are not yet available.

Safety Considerations

Generally, the safety profile of IVIG is favorable. IVIG therapy is sometimes associated with mild side effects including flushing, headache, malaise, fever, chills, fatigue, and lethargy. Slow infusion rate and premedication with corticosteroids/antihistamines limit the side effects [137]. In line, the IMAC study reported only minor side effects, predominantly transient flulike symptoms or headache, which can be attributed to the immune system activation [131]. Severe side effects, e.g., renal failure and blood disorders were rarely reported [137, 138].

17.6 Conclusion

Viral infections are frequently associated with myocarditis and worse heart failure prognosis. Patients not responding to conventional heart failure therapies need to be biopsied for diagnostic analysis. The off-label use of several antivirals represents the current armamentarium against viral myocarditis. However, none of the proposed therapies is sufficiently studied to be declared as safe and effective in myocarditis patients. For that reason, all the aforementioned therapies should only be offered by experienced centers or on the basis of controlled studies. Recent single center experience suggests that selected patients with inflammatory cardiomyopathy and B19V persistence without signs of systemic active infection may gain a similar long lasting and safe benefit from immunosuppressive treatment, as do virus-negative individuals [37]. These results need further verification in a randomized controlled trial.

17.7 Case Study Answer

The case study described represents a typical indication for EMB for the diagnosis of suggested viral myocarditis, since the patient did not recover over time despite symptomatic heart failure therapy. Depending on the EMB-based diagnosis, different (anti-viral) therapies are suggested based on expert-based recommendations.

- After exclusion of viral persistence and if lymphocytic myocarditis is present, the use of immunosuppressive therapy in case of active inflammation ($\geq$14 leucocytes/mm^2 including up to 4 monocytes/mm^2 with the presence of CD3-positive T-lymphocytes $\geq$7 cells/mm^2) is permitted.
- CVB3/AV persistence suggests IFN-β treatment and prohibits the use of immunosuppressive agents.
- B19V transcriptional activity suggests experimental treatment with telbivudine or IV immune globulins.
- Active ciHHV-6 suggests ganciclovir and valganciclovir treatment.
- Defined HCV association suggests treatment with DAAs.
- HIV mandates anti-retroviral combination therapy without immune suppression.
- Influenza type A or B detection suggests the use of neuraminidase inhibitors.

References

1. Kuhl U, Pauschinger M, Noutsias M, Seeberg B, Bock T, Lassner D, et al. High prevalence of viral genomes and multiple viral infections in the myocardium of adults with "idiopathic" left ventricular dysfunction. Circulation. 2005;111(7):887–93.
2. Kuhl U, Schultheiss HP. Viral myocarditis. Swiss Med Wkly. 2014;144:w14010.
3. Trachtenberg BH, Hare JM. Inflammatory Cardiomyopathic syndromes. Circ Res. 2017;121(7):803–18.
4. Baboonian C, Davies MJ, Booth JC, McKenna WJ. Coxsackie B viruses and human heart disease. Curr Top Microbiol Immunol. 1997;223:31–52.
5. Badorff C, Lee GH, Lamphear BJ, Martone ME, Campbell KP, Rhoads RE, et al. Enteroviral protease 2A cleaves dystrophin: evidence of cytoskeletal disruption in an acquired cardiomyopathy. Nat Med. 1999;5(3):320–6.
6. Kuhl U, Pauschinger M, Seeberg B, Lassner D, Noutsias M, Poller W, et al. Viral persistence in the myocardium is associated with progressive cardiac dysfunction. Circulation. 2005;112(13):1965–70.
7. Lassner D, Siegismund CS, Kuhl U, Rohde M, Stroux A, Escher F, et al. CCR5del32 genotype in human enteroviral cardiomyopathy leads to spontaneous virus clearance and improved outcome compared to wildtype CCR5. J Transl Med. 2018;16(1):249.
8. Schultheiss HP, Kuhl U, Cooper LT. The management of myocarditis. Eur Heart J. 2011;32(21):2616–25.
9. Escher F, Kuhl U, Gross U, Westermann D, Poller W, Tschope C, et al. Aggravation of left ventricular dysfunction in patients with biopsy-proven cardiac human herpesvirus a and B infection. J Clin Virol. 2015;63:1–5.
10. Reddy S, Eliassen E, Krueger GR, Das BB. Human herpesvirus 6-induced inflammatory cardiomyopathy in immunocompetent children. Ann Pediatr Cardiol. 2017;10(3):259–68.

11. Pellett PE, Ablashi DV, Ambros PF, Agut H, Caserta MT, Descamps V, et al. Chromosomally integrated human herpesvirus 6: questions and answers. Rev Med Virol. 2012;22(3):144–55.
12. Kuhl U, Lassner D, Wallaschek N, Gross UM, Krueger GR, Seeberg B, et al. Chromosomally integrated human herpesvirus 6 in heart failure: prevalence and treatment. Eur J Heart Fail. 2015;17(1):9–19.
13. Verdonschot J, Hazebroek M, Merken J, Debing Y, Dennert R, Brunner-La Rocca HP, et al. Relevance of cardiac parvovirus B19 in myocarditis and dilated cardiomyopathy: review of the literature. Eur J Heart Fail. 2016;18(12):1430–41.
14. Schmidt-Lucke C, Zobel T, Schrepfer S, Kuhl U, Wang D, Klingel K, et al. Impaired endothelial regeneration through human parvovirus B19-infected circulating Angiogenic cells in patients with cardiomyopathy. J Infect Dis. 2015;212(7):1070–81.
15. Schmidt-Lucke C, Zobel T, Escher F, Tschope C, Lassner D, Kuhl U, et al. Human parvovirus B19 (B19V) up-regulates CXCR4 surface expression of circulating Angiogenic cells: implications for cardiac ischemia in B19V cardiomyopathy. J Infect Dis. 2018;217(3):456–65.
16. Hu HY, Wei SY, Huang WH, Pan CH. Fatal parvovirus B19 infections: a report of two autopsy cases. Int J Legal Med. 2019;133(2):553–60.
17. Kuhl U, Lassner D, Dorner A, Rohde M, Escher F, Seeberg B, et al. A distinct subgroup of cardiomyopathy patients characterized by transcriptionally active cardiotropic erythrovirus and altered cardiac gene expression. Basic Res Cardiol. 2013;108(5):372.
18. Duechting A, Tschope C, Kaiser H, Lamkemeyer T, Tanaka N, Aberle S, et al. Human parvovirus B19 NS1 protein modulates inflammatory signaling by activation of STAT3/PIAS3 in human endothelial cells. J Virol. 2008;82(16):7942–52.
19. Tschope C, Bock CT, Kasner M, Noutsias M, Westermann D, Schwimmbeck PL, et al. High prevalence of cardiac parvovirus B19 infection in patients with isolated left ventricular diastolic dysfunction. Circulation. 2005;111(7):879–86.
20. Greulich S, Kindermann I, Schumm J, Perne A, Birkmeier S, Grun S, et al. Predictors of outcome in patients with parvovirus B19 positive endomyocardial biopsy. Clin Res Cardiol. 2016;105(1):37–52.
21. Hjalmarsson C, Liljeqvist JA, Lindh M, Karason K, Bollano E, Oldfors A, et al. Parvovirus B19 in endomyocardial biopsy of patients with idiopathic dilated cardiomyopathy: foe or bystander? J Card Fail. 2019;25(1):60–3.
22. Pollack A, Kontorovich AR, Fuster V, Dec GW. Viral myocarditis--diagnosis, treatment options, and current controversies. Nat Rev Cardiol. 2015;12(11):670–80.
23. Dominguez F, Kuhl U, Pieske B, Garcia-Pavia P, Tschope C. Update on myocarditis and inflammatory cardiomyopathy: reemergence of endomyocardial biopsy. Rev Esp Cardiol (Engl Ed). 2016;69(2):178–87.
24. Maron BJ, Towbin JA, Thiene G, Antzelevitch C, Corrado D, Arnett D, et al. Contemporary definitions and classification of the cardiomyopathies: an American Heart Association scientific statement from the council on clinical cardiology, heart failure and transplantation committee; quality of care and outcomes research and functional genomics and translational biology interdisciplinary working groups; and council on epidemiology and prevention. Circulation. 2006;113(14):1807–16.
25. Friedrich MG. Tissue characterization of acute myocardial infarction and myocarditis by cardiac magnetic resonance. JACC Cardiovasc Imaging. 2008;1(5):652–62.
26. Caforio AL, Pankuweit S, Arbustini E, Basso C, Gimeno-Blanes J, Felix SB, et al. Current state of knowledge on aetiology, diagnosis, management, and therapy of myocarditis: a position statement of the European Society of Cardiology Working Group on Myocardial and Pericardial Diseases. Eur Heart J. 2013;34(33):2636–48.
27. Ferreira VM, Schulz-Menger J, Holmvang G, Kramer CM, Carbone I, Sechtem U, et al. Cardiovascular magnetic resonance in nonischemic myocardial inflammation: expert Recommendations. J Am Coll Cardiol. 2018;72(24):3158–76.
28. Van Linthout S, Tschope C. Viral myocarditis: a prime example for endomyocardial biopsy-guided diagnosis and therapy. Curr Opin Cardiol. 2018;33(3):325–33.

29. Kuhl U, Pauschinger M, Bock T, Klingel K, Schwimmbeck CP, Seeberg B, et al. Parvovirus B19 infection mimicking acute myocardial infarction. Circulation. 2003;108(8): 945–50.
30. Sisakian H. Cardiomyopathies: evolution of pathogenesis concepts and potential for new therapies. World J Cardiol. 2014;6(6):478–94.
31. Frustaci A, Russo MA, Chimenti C. Randomized study on the efficacy of immunosuppressive therapy in patients with virus-negative inflammatory cardiomyopathy: the TIMIC study. Eur Heart J. 2009;30(16):1995–2002.
32. Schultheiss HP, Piper C, Sowade O, Waagstein F, Kapp JF, Wegscheider K, et al. Betaferon in chronic viral cardiomyopathy (BICC) trial: effects of interferon-beta treatment in patients with chronic viral cardiomyopathy. Clin Res Cardiol. 2016;105(9):763–73.
33. Van Linthout S, Elsanhoury A, Klein O, Sosnowski M, Miteva K, Lassner D, et al. Telbivudine in chronic lymphocytic myocarditis and human parvovirus B19 transcriptional activity. ESC Heart Fail. 2018;5(5):818–29.
34. Sotiriou E, Heiner S, Jansen T, Brandt M, Schmidt KH, Kreitner KF, et al. Therapeutic implications of a combined diagnostic workup including endomyocardial biopsy in an all-comer population of patients with heart failure: a retrospective analysis. ESC Heart Fail. 2018;5(4):630–41.
35. But DY, Yuen MF, Fung J, Lai CL. Safety evaluation of telbivudine. Expert Opin Drug Saf. 2010;9(5):821–9.
36. Chan HL, Chen YC, Gane EJ, Sarin SK, Suh DJ, Piratvisuth T, et al. Randomized clinical trial: efficacy and safety of telbivudine and lamivudine in treatment-naive patients with HBV-related decompensated cirrhosis. J Viral Hepat. 2012;19(10):732–43.
37. Tschöpe C, Elsanhoury A, Schlieker S, Van Linthout S, Kühl U. Immunosuppression in inflammatory cardiomyopathy and parvovirus B19 persistence. Eur J Heart Fail. 2019;21:1468–9. https://doi.org/10.1002/ejhf.1560.
38. Merken J, Hazebroek M, Van Paassen P, Verdonschot J, Van Empel V, Knackstedt C, et al. Immunosuppressive therapy improves both short- and long-term prognosis in patients with virus-negative nonfulminant inflammatory cardiomyopathy. Circ Heart Fail. 2018;11(2):e004228.
39. Escher F, Kuhl U, Lassner D, Poller W, Westermann D, Pieske B, et al. Long-term outcome of patients with virus-negative chronic myocarditis or inflammatory cardiomyopathy after immunosuppressive therapy. Clin Res Cardiol. 2016;105(12):1011–20.
40. Frustaci A, Chimenti C, Calabrese F, Pieroni M, Thiene G, Maseri A. Immunosuppressive therapy for active lymphocytic myocarditis: virological and immunologic profile of responders versus nonresponders. Circulation. 2003;107(6):857–63.
41. Keam SJ. Telbivudine. Drugs. 2007;67(13):1917–29.
42. Agut H, Bonnafous P, Gautheret-Dejean A. Laboratory and clinical aspects of human herpesvirus 6 infections. Clin Microbiol Rev. 2015;28(2):313–35.
43. Matthews T, Boehme R. Antiviral activity and mechanism of action of ganciclovir. Rev Infect Dis. 1988;10(Suppl 3):S490–4.
44. Prichard MN, Whitley RJ. The development of new therapies for human herpesvirus 6. Curr Opin Virol. 2014;9:148–53.
45. Venturi C, Bueno J, Gavalda J, Tortola T, Pou L, Medina A, et al. Impact of valganciclovir on Epstein-Barr virus polymerase chain reaction in pediatric liver transplantation: preliminary report. Transplant Proc. 2009;41(3):1038–40.
46. Seeley WW, Marty FM, Holmes TM, Upchurch K, Soiffer RJ, Antin JH, et al. Post-transplant acute limbic encephalitis: clinical features and relationship to HHV6. Neurology. 2007;69(2):156–65.
47. Ishiyama K, Katagiri T, Ohata K, Hosokawa K, Kondo Y, Yamazaki H, et al. Safety of pre-engraftment prophylactic foscarnet administration after allogeneic stem cell transplantation. Transpl Infect Dis. 2012;14(1):33–9.
48. Ishiyama K, Katagiri T, Hoshino T, Yoshida T, Yamaguchi M, Nakao S. Preemptive therapy of human herpesvirus-6 encephalitis with foscarnet sodium for high-risk patients after hematopoietic SCT. Bone Marrow Transplant. 2011;46(6):863–9.

49. Watt T, Oberfoell S, Balise R, Lunn MR, Kar AK, Merrihew L, et al. Response to valganciclovir in chronic fatigue syndrome patients with human herpesvirus 6 and Epstein-Barr virus IgG antibody titers. J Med Virol. 2012;84(12):1967–74.
50. Troy SB, Blackburn BG, Yeom K, Caulfield AK, Bhangoo MS, Montoya JG. Severe encephalomyelitis in an immunocompetent adult with chromosomally integrated human herpesvirus 6 and clinical response to treatment with foscarnet plus ganciclovir. Clin Infect Dis. 2008;47(12):e93–6.
51. Paya C, Humar A, Dominguez E, Washburn K, Blumberg E, Alexander B, et al. Efficacy and safety of valganciclovir vs. oral ganciclovir for prevention of cytomegalovirus disease in solid organ transplant recipients. Am J Transplant. 2004;4(4):611–20.
52. Geddawy A, Ibrahim YF, Elbahie NM, Ibrahim MA. Direct acting anti-hepatitis C virus drugs: clinical pharmacology and future direction. J Transl Int Med. 2017;5(1):8–17.
53. Feld JJ, Foster GR. Second generation direct-acting antivirals—do we expect major improvements? J Hepatol. 2016;65(1 Suppl):S130–S42.
54. Danilau D, Malich N, Litvinchuk D, Karpov I. Ombitasvir/paritaprevir/ritonavir + dasabuvir +/– ribavirin for treatment of chronic hepatitis C 1 genotype in the Republic of Belarus. Clin Exp Hepatol. 2017;3(3):164–8.
55. Petruzziello A, Marigliano S, Loquercio G, Cacciapuoti C. Hepatitis C virus (HCV) genotypes distribution: an epidemiological up-date in Europe. Infect Agent Cancer. 2016;11:53.
56. Hussaini T. Paritaprevir/ritonavir-ombitasvir and dasabuvir, the 3D regimen for the treatment of chronic hepatitis C virus infection: a concise review. Hepat Med. 2016;8:61–8.
57. Matsumori A. Hepatitis C virus and cardiomyopathy. Herz. 2000;25(3):249–54.
58. Matsumori A, Matoba Y, Sasayama S. Dilated cardiomyopathy associated with hepatitis C virus infection. Circulation. 1995;92(9):2519–25.
59. Babiker A, Jeudy J, Kligerman S, Khambaty M, Shah A, Bagchi S. Risk of cardiovascular disease due to chronic hepatitis C infection: a review. J Clin Transl Hepatol. 2017;5(4):343–62.
60. Poller W, Kaya Z, Muche M, Kasner M, Skurk C, Kappert K, et al. High incidence of cardiac dysfunction and response to antiviral treatment in patients with chronic hepatitis C virus infection. Clin Res Cardiol. 2017;106(7):551–6.
61. Moradpour D, Grakoui A, Manns MP. Future landscape of hepatitis C research—translational and clinical perspectives basic. J Hepatol. 2016;65(1 Suppl):S143–S55.
62. Dustin LB, Bartolini B, Capobianchi MR, Pistello M. Hepatitis C virus: life cycle in cells, infection and host response, and analysis of molecular markers influencing the outcome of infection and response to therapy. Clin Microbiol Infect. 2016;22(10):826–32.
63. Kohli A, Shaffer A, Sherman A, Kottilil S. Treatment of hepatitis C: a systematic review. JAMA. 2014;312(6):631–40.
64. Wedemeyer H, Reimer J, Sandow P, Hueppe D, Lutz T, Gruengreiff K, et al. Long-term outcome of chronic hepatitis C virus infection in a real-world setting: the German LOTOS study. Liver Int. 2017;37(10):1468–75.
65. Poller W, Haghikia A, Kasner M, Kaya Z, Bavendiek U, Wedemeier H, et al. Cardiovascular involvement in chronic hepatitis C virus infections—insight from novel antiviral therapies. J Clin Transl Hepatol. 2018;6(2):161–7.
66. Gunthard HF, Saag MS, Benson CA, del Rio C, Eron JJ, Gallant JE, et al. Antiretroviral drugs for treatment and prevention of HIV infection in adults: 2016 recommendations of the international antiviral society-USA panel. JAMA. 2016;316(2):191–210.
67. Gunthard HF, Aberg JA, Eron JJ, Hoy JF, Telenti A, Benson CA, et al. Antiretroviral treatment of adult HIV infection: 2014 recommendations of the international antiviral society-USA panel. JAMA. 2014;312(4):410–25.
68. Dybul M, Fauci AS, Bartlett JG, Kaplan JE, Pau AK. Panel on clinical practices for the treatment of HIV. Guidelines for using antiretroviral agents among HIV-infected adults and adolescents. Recommendations of the panel on clinical practices for treatment of HIV. MMWR Recomm Rep. 2002;51(RR-7):1–55.
69. Sackoff JE, Hanna DB, Pfeiffer MR, Torian LV. Causes of death among persons with AIDS in the era of highly active antiretroviral therapy: new York City. Ann Intern Med. 2006;145(6):397–406.

70. Smith CJ, Ryom L, Weber R, Morlat P, Pradier C, Reiss P, et al. Trends in underlying causes of death in people with HIV from 1999 to 2011 (D:a:D): a multicohort collaboration. Lancet. 2014;384(9939):241–8.
71. Lorgis L, Cottenet J, Molins G, Benzenine E, Zeller M, Aube H, et al. Outcomes after acute myocardial infarction in HIV-infected patients: analysis of data from a French nationwide hospital medical information database. Circulation. 2013;127(17):1767–74.
72. Manga P, McCutcheon K, Tsabedze N, Vachiat A, Zachariah D. HIV and nonischemic heart disease. J Am Coll Cardiol. 2017;69(1):83–91.
73. Vachiat A, McCutcheon K, Tsabedze N, Zachariah D, Manga P. HIV and ischemic heart disease. J Am Coll Cardiol. 2017;69(1):73–82.
74. Ntusi NAB, Ntsekhe M. Human immunodeficiency virus-associated heart failure in sub-Saharan Africa: evolution in the epidemiology, pathophysiology, and clinical manifestations in the antiretroviral era. ESC Heart Fail. 2016;3(3):158–67.
75. Barbaro G, Di Lorenzo G, Grisorio B, Barbarini G. Cardiac involvement in the acquired immunodeficiency syndrome: a multicenter clinical-pathological study. Gruppo Italiano per lo Studio Cardiologico dei pazienti affetti da AIDS Investigators AIDS Res Hum Retroviruses. 1998;14(12):1071–7.
76. Cohen IS, Anderson DW, Virmani R, Reen BM, Macher AM, Sennesh J, et al. Congestive cardiomyopathy in association with the acquired immunodeficiency syndrome. N Engl J Med. 1986;315(10):628–30.
77. Belkin MN, Uriel N. Heart health in the age of highly active antiretroviral therapy: a review of HIV cardiomyopathy. Curr Opin Cardiol. 2018;33(3):317–24.
78. Group ISS. Lundgren JD, Babiker AG, Gordin F, Emery S, Grund B, et al. initiation of antiretroviral therapy in early asymptomatic HIV infection. N Engl J Med. 2015;373(9):795–807.
79. Pugliese A, Isnardi D, Saini A, Scarabelli T, Raddino R, Torre D. Impact of highly active antiretroviral therapy in HIV-positive patients with cardiac involvement. J Infect. 2000;40(3):282–4.
80. Lipshultz SE, Williams PL, Wilkinson JD, Leister EC, Van Dyke RB, Shearer WT, et al. Cardiac status of children infected with human immunodeficiency virus who are receiving long-term combination antiretroviral therapy: results from the adolescent master protocol of the multicenter pediatric HIV/AIDS cohort study. JAMA Pediatr. 2013;167(6):520–7.
81. Plebani A, Esposito S, Pinzani R, Fesslova V, Bojanin J, Salice P, et al. Effect of highly active antiretroviral therapy on cardiovascular involvement in children with human immunodeficiency virus infection. Pediatr Infect Dis J. 2004;23(6):559–63.
82. Bozkurt B, Colvin M, Cook J, Cooper LT, Deswal A, Fonarow GC, et al. Current diagnostic and treatment strategies for specific dilated cardiomyopathies: a scientific statement from the American Heart Association. Circulation. 2016;134(23):e579–646.
83. Currie PF, Goldman JH, Caforio AL, Jacob AJ, Baig MK, Brettle RP, et al. Cardiac autoimmunity in HIV related heart muscle disease. Heart. 1998;79(6):599–604.
84. Blaylock JM, Byers DK, Gibbs BT, Nayak G, Ferguson M, Tribble DR, et al. Longitudinal assessment of cardiac diastolic function in HIV-infected patients. Int J STD AIDS. 2012;23(2):105–10.
85. Cerrato E, D'Ascenzo F, Biondi-Zoccai G, Calcagno A, Frea S, Grosso Marra W, et al. Cardiac dysfunction in pauci symptomatic human immunodeficiency virus patients: a meta-analysis in the highly active antiretroviral therapy era. Eur Heart J. 2013;34(19):1432–6.
86. Onur I, Ikitimur B, Oz F, Ekmekci A, Elitok A, Cagatay AA, et al. Evaluation of human immunodeficiency virus infection-related left ventricular systolic dysfunction by tissue Doppler strain echocardiography. Echocardiography. 2014;31(10):1199–204.
87. Reinsch N, Kahlert P, Esser S, Sundermeyer A, Neuhaus K, Brockmeyer N, et al. Echocardiographic findings and abnormalities in HIV-infected patients: results from a large, prospective, multicenter HIV-heart study. Am J Cardiovasc Dis. 2011;1(2):176–84.
88. Lewis W, Simpson JF, Meyer RR. Cardiac mitochondrial DNA polymerase-gamma is inhibited competitively and noncompetitively by phosphorylated zidovudine. Circ Res. 1994;74(2):344–8.
89. Lewis W, Grupp IL, Grupp G, Hoit B, Morris R, Samarel AM, et al. Cardiac dysfunction occurs in the HIV-1 transgenic mouse treated with zidovudine. Lab Investig. 2000;80(2):187–97.

90. Jakeman B, Nasiri M, Ruth L, Morse C, Mahatme S, Patel N. Comparing the frequencies of contraindicated drug-drug interactions between differing antiretroviral regimens in HIV-infected patients. Ann Pharmacother. 2017;51(5):365–72.
91. Priyanka P, Varma DM, Immadisetti K, Rajesh R, Vidyasagar S, Guddattu V. Recognition of possible risk factors for clinically significant drug-drug interactions among Indian people living with HIV receiving highly active antiretroviral therapy and concomitant medications. Int J Risk Saf Med. 2017;29(1–2):25–55.
92. Semvua HH, Kibiki GS, Kisanga ER, Boeree MJ, Burger DM, Aarnoutse R. Pharmacological interactions between rifampicin and antiretroviral drugs: challenges and research priorities for resource-limited settings. Ther Drug Monit. 2015;37(1):22–32.
93. Durante-Mangoni E, Maiello C, Limongelli G, Sbreglia C, Pinto D, Amarelli C, et al. Management of immunosuppression and antiviral treatment before and after heart transplant for HIV-associated dilated cardiomyopathy. Int J Immunopathol Pharmacol. 2014;27(1):113–20.
94. McKimm-Breschkin JL. Influenza neuraminidase inhibitors: antiviral action and mechanisms of resistance. Influenza Other Respir Viruses. 2013;7(Suppl 1):25–36.
95. Birnkrant D, Cox E. The emergency use authorization of peramivir for treatment of 2009 H1N1 influenza. N Engl J Med. 2009;361(23):2204–7.
96. Greaves K, Oxford JS, Price CP, Clarke GH, Crake T. The prevalence of myocarditis and skeletal muscle injury during acute viral infection in adults: measurement of cardiac troponins I and T in 152 patients with acute influenza infection. Arch Intern Med. 2003;163(2):165–8.
97. Rezkalla SH, Kloner RA. Influenza-related viral myocarditis. WMJ. 2010;109(4):209–13.
98. Mamas MA, Fraser D, Neyses L. Cardiovascular manifestations associated with influenza virus infection. Int J Cardiol. 2008;130(3):304–9.
99. Bowles NE, Ni J, Kearney DL, Pauschinger M, Schultheiss HP, McCarthy R, et al. Detection of viruses in myocardial tissues by polymerase chain reaction. evidence of adenovirus as a common cause of myocarditis in children and adults J Am Coll Cardiol. 2003;42(3):466–72.
100. Caforio AL, Calabrese F, Angelini A, Tona F, Vinci A, Bottaro S, et al. A prospective study of biopsy-proven myocarditis: prognostic relevance of clinical and aetiopathogenetic features at diagnosis. Eur Heart J. 2007;28(11):1326–33.
101. Montcriol A, Wiramus S, Ribeiri A, Attard N, Nait-Saidi L, Kerbaul F, et al. Successful management of influenza a associated fulminant myocarditis: mobile circulatory support in intensive care unit: a case report. Cases J. 2008;1(1):46.
102. Moore DL, Vaudry W, Scheifele DW, Halperin SA, Dery P, Ford-Jones E, et al. Surveillance for influenza admissions among children hospitalized in Canadian immunization monitoring program active centers, 2003-2004. Pediatrics. 2006;118(3):e610–9.
103. Taremi M, Amoroso A, Nace HL, Gilliam BL. Influenza B-induced refractory cardiogenic shock: a case report. BMC Infect Dis. 2013;13:452.
104. Magnani JW, Dec GW. Myocarditis: current trends in diagnosis and treatment. Circulation. 2006;113(6):876–90.
105. Yoshimizu N, Tominaga T, Ito T, Nishida Y, Wada Y, Sohmiya K, et al. Repetitive fulminant influenza myocarditis requiring the use of circulatory assist devices. Intern Med. 2014;53(2):109–14.
106. Kounis NG, Zavras GM, Soufras GD, Kitrou MP. Hypersensitivity myocarditis. Ann Allergy. 1989;62(2):71–4.
107. Bratincsak A, El-Said HG, Bradley JS, Shayan K, Grossfeld PD, Cannavino CR. Fulminant myocarditis associated with pandemic H1N1 influenza a virus in children. J Am Coll Cardiol. 2010;55(9):928–9.
108. Miura M, Asaumi Y, Wada Y, Ogata K, Sato T, Sugawara T, et al. A case of influenza subtype a virus-induced fulminant myocarditis: an experience of percutaneous cardio-pulmonary support (PCPS) treatment and immunohistochemical analysis. Tohoku J Exp Med. 2001;195(1):11–9.

109. Morioka I, Nonoyama S, Tanaka-Taya K, Ihara T, Sugaya N, Ueta I, et al. Survey of Japanese infants younger than 3 months who were treated with oseltamivir for influenza: safety of oseltamivir treatment. Scand J Infect Dis. 2012;44(8):605–9.
110. Geladari EV, Kratimenos VN, Trigkidis K, Kokkinakis E. Myocarditis due to influenza B virus: the importance of early antiviral therapy. Cardiol Clin Res. 2016;4(6):1079.
111. Baik SH, Jeong HS, Kim SJ, Yoon YK, Sohn JW, Kim MJ. A case of influenza associated fulminant myocarditis successfully treated with intravenous Peramivir. Infect Chemother. 2015;47(4):272–7.
112. Hekimian G, Jovanovic T, Brechot N, Lebreton G, Leprince P, Trouillet JL, et al. When the heart gets the flu Fulminant influenza B myocarditis: a case-series report and review of the literature. J Crit Care. 2018;47:61–4.
113. Doll MK, Winters N, Boikos C, Kraicer-Melamed H, Gore G, Quach C. Safety and effectiveness of neuraminidase inhibitors for influenza treatment, prophylaxis, and outbreak control: a systematic review of systematic reviews and/or meta-analyses. J Antimicrob Chemother. 2017;72(11):2990–3007.
114. Lobo ML, Taguchi A, Gaspar HA, Ferranti JF, de Carvalho WB, Delgado AF. Fulminant myocarditis associated with the H1N1 influenza virus: case report and literature review. Rev Bras Ter Intensiva. 2014;26(3):321–6.
115. Samuel CE. Antiviral actions of interferons. Clin Microbiol Rev. 2001;14(4):778–809.
116. Brierley MM, Fish EN. Review: IFN-alpha/beta receptor interactions to biologic outcomes: understanding the circuitry. J Interf Cytokine Res. 2002;22(8):835–45.
117. Mark DF, Lu SD, Creasey AA, Yamamoto R, Lin LS. Site-specific mutagenesis of the human fibroblast interferon gene. Proc Natl Acad Sci U S A. 1984;81(18):5662–6.
118. Markowitz CE. Interferon-beta: mechanism of action and dosing issues. Neurology. 2007;68(24 Suppl 4):S8–11.
119. Keskinen P, Ronni T, Matikainen S, Lehtonen A, Julkunen I. Regulation of HLA class I and II expression by interferons and influenza a virus in human peripheral blood mononuclear cells. Immunology. 1997;91(3):421–9.
120. Swann JB, Hayakawa Y, Zerafa N, Sheehan KC, Scott B, Schreiber RD, et al. Type I IFN contributes to NK cell homeostasis, activation, and antitumor function. J Immunol. 2007;178(12):7540–9.
121. Urban SL, Berg LJ, Welsh RM. Type 1 interferon licenses naive CD8 T cells to mediate antiviral cytotoxicity. Virology. 2016;493:52–9.
122. Heim A, Stille-Seigener M, Pring-Akerblom P, Grumbach I, Brehm C, Kreuzer H, et al. Recombinant Interferons beta and gamma have a higher antiviral activity than interferon-alpha in coxsackievirus B3-infected carrier state cultures of human myocardial fibroblasts. J Interf Cytokine Res. 1996;16(4):283–7.
123. Deonarain R, Cerullo D, Fuse K, Liu PP, Fish EN. Protective role for interferon-beta in coxsackievirus B3 infection. Circulation. 2004;110(23):3540–3.
124. Kuhl U, Lassner D, von Schlippenbach J, Poller W, Schultheiss HP. Interferon-Beta improves survival in enterovirus-associated cardiomyopathy. J Am Coll Cardiol. 2012;60(14):1295–6.
125. Kuhl U, Pauschinger M, Schwimmbeck PL, Seeberg B, Lober C, Noutsias M, et al. Interferon-beta treatment eliminates cardiotropic viruses and improves left ventricular function in patients with myocardial persistence of viral genomes and left ventricular dysfunction. Circulation. 2003;107(22):2793–8.
126. Pauschinger M, Chandrasekharan K, Noutsias M, Kuhl U, Schwimmbeck LP, Schultheiss HP. Viral heart disease: molecular diagnosis, clinical prognosis, and treatment strategies. Med Microbiol Immunol. 2004;193(2–3):65–9.
127. Gran F, Martinez-Villar M, Soler-Palacin P, Fernandez-Polo A, Betrian P, Albert DC. Immunosuppressive therapy and interferon-1beta in acute myocarditis. Rev Esp Cardiol (Engl Ed). 2016;69(11):1106–7.
128. Nimmerjahn F, Ravetch JV. Anti-inflammatory actions of intravenous immunoglobulin. Annu Rev Immunol. 2008;26:513–33.

129. Anthony RM, Nimmerjahn F, Ashline DJ, Reinhold VN, Paulson JC, Ravetch JV. Recapitulation of IVIG anti-inflammatory activity with a recombinant IgG fc. Science. 2008;320(5874):373–6.
130. Gronwall C, Silverman GJ. Natural IgM: beneficial autoantibodies for the control of inflammatory and autoimmune disease. J Clin Immunol. 2014;34(Suppl 1):S12–21.
131. McNamara DM, Holubkov R, Starling RC, Dec GW, Loh E, Torre-Amione G, et al. Controlled trial of intravenous immune globulin in recent-onset dilated cardiomyopathy. Circulation. 2001;103(18):2254–9.
132. Maisch B, Hufnagel G, Kolsch S, Funck R, Richter A, Rupp H, et al. Treatment of inflammatory dilated cardiomyopathy and (peri)myocarditis with immunosuppression and i.v. immunoglobulins. Herz. 2004;29(6):624–36.
133. Pankuweit S, Maisch B. The heart in viral infections. Internist (Berl). 2010;51(7):836–43.
134. Trimpert C, Herda LR, Eckerle LG, Pohle S, Muller C, Landsberger M, et al. Immunoadsorption in dilated cardiomyopathy: long-term reduction of cardiodepressant antibodies. Eur J Clin Investig. 2010;40(8):685–91.
135. Dennert R, Velthuis S, Schalla S, Eurlings L, van Suylen RJ, van Paassen P, et al. Intravenous immunoglobulin therapy for patients with idiopathic cardiomyopathy and endomyocardial biopsy-proven high PVB19 viral load. Antivir Ther. 2010;15(2):193–201.
136. Selbing A, Josefsson A, Dahle LO, Lindgren R. Parvovirus B19 infection during pregnancy treated with high-dose intravenous gammaglobulin. Lancet. 1995;345(8950):660–1.
137. Guo Y, Tian X, Wang X, Xiao Z. Adverse effects of immunoglobulin therapy. Front Immunol. 2018;9:1299.
138. Duhem C, Dicato MA, Ries F. Side-effects of intravenous immune globulins. Clin Exp Immunol. 1994;97(Suppl 1):79–83.

Conventional Cardiological Therapies

18

Gianfranco Sinagra, Piero Gentile, Jessica Artico, Antonio Cannata', Enrico Fabris, and Merlo Marco

Myocarditis is an inflammatory disease of the myocardium characterized by a great heterogeneity of presentation and evolution. The main patterns of clinical presentation are chest pain, arrhythmias, and heart failure, and disease severity may range from asymptomatic or mild self-limiting syndromes to severe life-threatening scenarios requiring intensive hemodynamic support [1–4].

A deep etiological classification should be systematically performed approaching a clinically suspected myocarditis. In fact, although cardiotropic viruses are presumed to be the most frequent cause of myocarditis (about 90%) encountered in clinical practice, 10% of myocarditis can be triggered by different causes: bacteria, parasites, autoimmune diseases, hypersensitivity, high catecholamine states, drugs, toxic substances, or physical agents [5]. All possible etiologies should be considered because disease-specific therapy is mandatory in specific settings. Laboratory tests, apparently poorly useful in the management of viral myocarditis, are key to exclude other specific infective forms. Bacteria, such as diphtheria and Borrelia burgdorferi (Lyme disease), or parasites, such as Trypanosoma cruzi (Chagas disease), are very important in specific geographic regions [6, 7] and deserve specific antibiotic, such as tetracyclines for Lyme disease, or antiparasitic therapy, such as benznidazole or nifurtimox for Chagas disease. Furthermore, sarcoidosis, eosinophilic myocarditis, and giant cell myocarditis deserve prompt treatment with immunomodulatory and specific therapy.

Finally, in the setting of virus-negative myocarditis, specific therapies, like immunosuppression or immunomodulation therapies, should be generally reserved for patients presenting with major clinical syndromes (i.e., severe heart failure and/or life-threatening arrhythmias) that are refractory to conventional therapies.

G. Sinagra (✉) · P. Gentile · J. Artico · A. Cannata' · E. Fabris · M. Marco
Cardiovascular and Thoracic Department,
Azienda Sanitaria Universitaria Integrata di Trieste (ASUITS), Trieste, Italy

University of Trieste, Trieste, Italy
e-mail: gianfranco.sinagra@asuits.sanita.fvg.it; pierogentile.87@gmail.com; jessica.artico@hotmail.it; anto.cannata@gmail.com; enrico.fabris@hotmail.it; marco.merlo79@gmail.com

A. L. P. Caforio (ed.), *Myocarditis*, https://doi.org/10.1007/978-3-030-35276-9_18

Recently, a clinically oriented classification of myocarditis has been proposed based on event-risk derived by clinical and laboratory presentation and short-term evolution [1, 8]. This classification has essential implications in therapeutic strategies and prognostic stratification of those patients:

- *Low-risk myocarditis*: usually presenting with chest pain and/or supraventricular arrhythmias with preserved left ventricular function. This clinical scenario often has a rapid (1–4 weeks) and complete resolution of the electrocardiographic and echocardiographic abnormalities with excellent long-term prognosis.
- *Intermediate risk myocarditis*: characterized by mild-to-moderate ventricular dysfunction with persistent wall motion abnormalities, extensive late gadolinium enhancement (LGE) in the absence of severe left ventricular dysfunction, electrocardiographic changes, and non-sustained ventricular arrhythmias.
- *High-risk myocarditis*: usually presenting with recent-onset severe left ventricular dysfunction and refractory heart failure (HF) and/or life-threatening arrhythmias. Typically, the prognosis is highly dependent on the short-term response to therapy.

It appears that therapeutic regimens and intensity of treatment change according to initial presentation and severity of symptoms. However, the extent of left ventricular (LV) involvement, expressed as left ventricular ejection fraction (LVEF) reduction or LGE extension, has emerged as the main determinant of prognosis and helps in addressing a correct management algorithm.

Considering the great variability in clinical presentation and evolution, conventional therapy of myocarditis represents the first step and should be tailored on the basis of both pattern and severity of clinical presentation, amount of LV derangement (i.e., left ventricular dysfunction or LGE extent). The short-term response to conventional treatments should help in addressing further, specific therapeutic strategies (Fig. 18.1).

18.1 Chest Pain and Preserved LV Function

Patients presenting with chest pain and preserved left ventricular function often have a rapid (1–4 weeks) and complete clinical resolution with excellent long-term prognosis [1]. However, hospital admission and clinical monitoring are strictly recommended, since unstable clinical situation (e.g., life-threatening arrhythmias) might be presenting abruptly, despite the initially preserved systolic function [9].

Therefore, patients presenting with chest pain require no medical treatment in the absence of left ventricular dysfunction or major arrhythmias. In this subset of patients, a reasonable approach is to clinically reassess the patient after 1–2 weeks to ensure that troponin levels normalize and that symptoms of HF or arrhythmia do not develop [10]. In our experience, once all ECG and echocardiographic abnormalities have disappeared during the short-term follow-up, such patients may be considered fully recovered. However, in the presence of persistent subepicardial LGE at cardiac

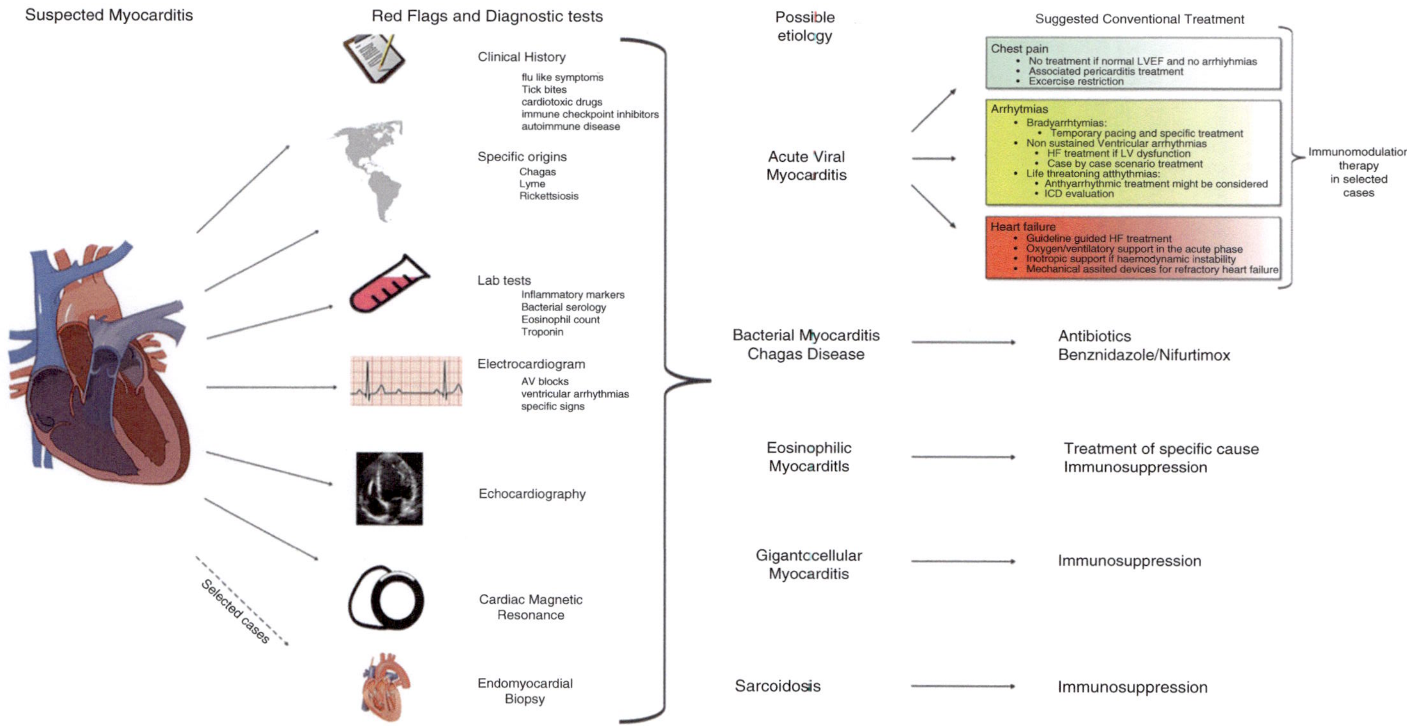

Fig. 18.1 Schematic representation of main clinical diagnostic and therapeutic pathways in patients with myocarditis

magnetic resonance, regardless of its extent, a noninvasive follow-up prolonged up to 2 years seems appropriate [1]. Recently, a multicenter Italian trial evaluated the role of cardiac magnetic resonance in patients with acute clinically suspected myocarditis and preserved left ventricular function. Patients with anteroseptal midwall LGE more frequently experienced arrhythmic events compared to other patterns of localization, such as the inferolateral pattern [11]. These patients, therefore, require individualized assessment to exclude possible specific causes such as sarcoidosis and to tailor possible antiarrhythmic strategies.

Exercise restriction should be maintained for at least 6 months after an acute myocarditis with normal left ventricular ejection fraction presenting with chest pain. The follow-up is pivotal: in case of resolution of ECG and/or echocardiographic abnormalities and in the absence of rest/effort significant arrhythmic burden or significant extent of LGE at CMR, physical activity could be allowed. In the other cases, even in the presence of apparently low-risk forms at presentation, exercise restriction and follow-up should be lifelong as intense physical activity may promote malignant arrhythmias or recurrences [1]. Patients presenting with persistent mild extent (i.e., 1–2 segments) LGE at the inferolateral wall in the absence of systolic dysfunction represent a grey scenario in this perspective. This issue should be further investigated in the future.

In the setting of myocarditis with associated pericarditis (i.e., concomitant minimal myocardial involvement in pericarditis, without left ventricular systolic dysfunction), management is similar to that recommended for pericarditis [12]. Colchicine is given at a dose of 1 mg per day for 3 months to prevent recurrence of pericarditis [13]. Non-steroidal anti-inflammatory drugs such as acetylsalicylic acid, ibuprofen, and indomethacin should be used with caution and generally be reserved for patients with normal ventricular function, because they worsen myocarditis in murine models [10].

Current medications used in heart failure (HF) such as beta-blockers, angiotensin converting enzyme inhibitors (ACE-I) or angiotensin receptor blockers (ARBs), and additional treatment with mineralocorticoid receptor antagonists (MRAs) and diuretics are not indicated in the absence of left ventricular dysfunction. However, the ITAMY study [11] suggested the need of further early predictors of adverse events in the very long-term follow-up of patients with persisting LGE. No data are available on additional cardiac MRI-related parameters (i.e., T1 and T2 mapping and feature tracking derived strain evaluation) in defining prognosis and in guiding therapy in this specific patient subgroup [14]. Future large studies are warranted.

18.2 Arrhythmias

The management of arrhythmias changes according to the type and severity of clinical presentation:

- *Bradyarrhythmia or advanced atrio-ventricular (AV) conduction defects* in the absence of LV dysfunction may be suggestive of infections by Borrelia or

Rickettsia, while in the presence of LV dysfunction may be suggestive of sarcoidosis or giant cell myocarditis [1]. Temporary pacing may be needed for a complete atrio-ventricular (AV) block, particularly if syncope or hemodynamic instability is present, while waiting for the effect of specific therapy. In patients with myocarditis caused by Borrelia burgdorferi or Rickettsia, antibacterial treatment in the early phases can prevent severe morbidity or death. Lyme disease treatment with ceftriaxone is safe and highly effective [15], while in the case of tickborne rickettsial disease, doxycycline is the drug of choice in children and adults. Empiric therapy should be promptly initiated in patients with a clinical presentation suggestive of Rickettsia or Lyme disease [16]. When bradyarrhythmia or advanced AV conduction defects are coexistent with LV dysfunction, cardiac sarcoidosis or giant cell myocarditis should be suspected. In such cases, an endomyocardial biopsy is useful in diagnosing and allowing planning of appropriate therapies [17].

– *Non-sustained ventricular arrhythmias*. This is considered a grey zone and a challenging scenario. Patients presenting with non-sustained ventricular tachycardia should be evaluated and treated according to the concomitant amount of LV derangement. When non-sustained ventricular tachycardia is iterative or frequent, associated with mild-to-moderate ventricular dysfunction and/or presence of LGE (even in the absence of LV dysfunction and remodeling) at cardiac MRI, they should be treated in line with current guidelines for heart failure management [18]. Non-sustained ventricular tachycardia reflects extensive myocardial derangement and increases in frequency with HF severity. Beta-blockers represent the first-line therapy. Angiotensin converting enzyme inhibitors (ACE-I) or angiotensin receptor blockers (ARBs) should be associated and could lead to an improvement in the arrhythmic profile, often due to LV reverse remodeling. However, there is no definite evidence of antiarrhythmic efficacy of beta-blockers, ACE-I/ARBs in this scenario. Moreover, there is no definite indication to MRAs in the absence of significant LV dysfunction, despite their known anti-fibrotic effect. Finally, there are no data on the efficacy of drugs such as amiodarone or sotalol in myocarditis patients without severe LV dysfunction. Thus, every patient should be specifically evaluated and the conventional, as well as specific treatment, should be based on the individualized assessment, LV derangement quantification, and a deep etiological classification.

Life-threatening ventricular arrhythmias, defined as sustained ventricular tachycardia or aborted sudden cardiac death (i.e., ventricular fibrillation or sustained ventricular tachycardia with successful resuscitation or cardioversion) represent a challenge in terms of diagnosis, clinical management, and arrhythmic risk stratification. Potential aggravating/precipitating factors (e.g., low serum potassium/magnesium) should be sought and corrected in patients with ventricular arrhythmias. Amiodarone (often in combination with a beta-blocker) may be used to suppress symptomatic ventricular arrhythmias, but it may adversely affect prognosis, especially in patients with more severe HF [19]. The indication for implantable cardioverter defibrillator (ICD) therapy is unclear and should be evaluated on an individual basis according to clinical presentation (e.g., aborted sudden cardiac death or syncope), the magnitude of structural–functional ventricular derangement (e.g., ventricular remodeling, presence of akinetic segments or aneurysmal deformation, and extent of LGE), the histopathologic substrate (e.g., cardiac sarcoidosis or giant cell myocarditis), and therapeutic response to standard care [2, 3]. Future multicenter and large studies are warranted in order to accurately identify ICD candidates among myocarditis patients presenting with malignant ventricular arrhythmias. Currently, a wearable ICD (an external defibrillator with leads and electrode pads attached to a wearable vest), that is able to recognize and interrupt VT/ventricular fibrillation, may be considered for a limited period of time as a bridge to the final decision to implant or to not implant an ICD. Likewise, referral for ablation should be considered in cases of persistent ventricular arrhythmias despite optimal medical (i.e., conventional and possibly specific) therapy and identification of a structured substrate, after excluding persisting inflammatory triggers.

18.3 Heart Failure

18.3.1 Presentation with Heart Failure and Severe LV Dysfunction

Patients with acute myocarditis presenting with HF, in particular when associated with severe LV dysfunction, can be classified in the scenario of "high-risk myocarditis" [1]. They have a consistent probability of major clinical events in the short- and long-term follow-up and their prognosis largely depends on the short-term response to conventional therapy.

Goals of treatment in this patient group are to improve their clinical status and to achieve hemodynamic stability. In fact, in active myocarditis associated with severe left ventricular dysfunction, major clinical decisions such as referral for heart transplantation, left ventricular assist device, or prophylactic ICD should be deferred and re-evaluated according to short-term evolution under optimal conventional medical treatment [2].

In the setting of acute HF, diagnostic workup and appropriate pharmacological and non-pharmacological treatments should be promptly and simultaneously started. The patient's vital cardiorespiratory functions including blood pressure, pulse oximetry, respiratory rate, and ECG should be continuously monitored; it is essential to evaluate whether oxygenation, heart rate, blood pressure, ventilation, peripheral perfusion, and urine output are adequate.

18.3.1.1 Oxygen Therapy and/or Ventilatory Support

Oxygen therapy is recommended in patients with HF and $SpO2 < 90\%$ or $PaO2 < 60$ mmHg to correct hypoxemia [18].

- Non-invasive positive pressure ventilation (CPAP, BiPAP) should be considered in patients with respiratory distress (respiratory rate >25 breaths/min, $SpO2 < 90\%$) and started as soon as possible in order to decrease respiratory distress and reduce the rate of mechanical endotracheal intubation [20]. In patients with cardiogenic shock with high filling pressures and high systemic vascular resistance, positive end-expiratory pressure (PEEP) can provide benefit if the RV is not compromised and the patient is not hypovolemic. In fact, RV perfusion can be compromised by elevated intra-pleural pressure from high PEEP or high airway pressure [21].

- Intubation is recommended, if respiratory failure, leading to hypoxemia ($PaO2 < 60$ mmHg (8.0 kPa)), hypercapnia ($PaCO2 > 50$ mmHg (6.65 kPa)), and acidosis ($pH < 7.35$), cannot be managed by non-invasive measures.

18.3.1.2 Pharmacological Therapy in the Acute Phase

Pharmacologic therapy in the acute phase aims to improve organ perfusion by increasing cardiac output and blood pressure. Treatment is guided by the continuous monitoring of organ perfusion and hemodynamic parameters [18].

- Intravenous loop diuretics are a cornerstone in the treatment of patients with acute HF and signs/symptoms of fluid overload and congestion. It is recommended to give diuretics either as intermittent boluses or as a continuous infusion, and the dose and duration should be adjusted according to patients' symptoms and clinical status [22].
- Intravenous vasodilators are the second most often used agents in acute HF for symptomatic relief. They provide dual benefit by decreasing venous tone (to optimize preload) and arterial tone (decreased afterload). Consequently, they may also increase stroke volume. In patients with systolic blood pressure (SBP) <90 mmHg (or with symptomatic hypotension) they should be avoided.
- Intravenous infusion of inotropes should be reserved for patients with a severe reduction in cardiac output, resulting in reduced systolic blood pressure (i.e., <90 mmHg) and/or signs/symptoms of hypoperfusion. Dobutamine is the most commonly used adrenergic inotrope. Levosimendan or PDE3 may also be used. Inotropes, especially those with adrenergic mechanisms, can cause sinus tachycardia and may induce myocardial ischemia and arrhythmias, thus ECG monitoring is required.
- A vasopressor (norepinephrine preferably) may be considered in patients who have cardiogenic shock, despite treatment with another inotrope to increase blood pressure and vital organ perfusion [23].
- Conventional heart failure treatment should be initiated as soon as possible, according to clinical presentation and hemodynamic stability. ACE-I/ARBs, beta-blockers, and MRAs are the first-line therapy for patients admitted with severe LV dysfunction. Up-titration to a maximal tolerated dosage is cautiously recommended in all patients to avoid severe life-threatening hypotension and side effects. Ivabradine should be considered in patients with contraindication or intolerance to beta-blockers or in which beta-blocker treatment is still insufficient to reduce rest heart rate. Angiotensin receptor-neprilysin inhibitors (ARNI) are recommended for still symptomatic patients after discharge; however, so far, there is no clear evidence to initiate ARNI treatment during hospital stay [18].

- Immunosuppressive and immunomodulation therapy appears suitable for patients with EMB-proven virus-negative active myocarditis with major clinical symptoms such as HF with severe ventricular dysfunction and/or life-threatening ventricular arrhythmias in whom conventional treatments have failed in the short term of 7–10 days [1]. The role of specific immunomodulating therapy will be treated in other chapters.

18.3.1.3 Mechanical Assist Devices

For patients presenting with acute HF who cannot be stabilized with medical therapy, mechanical assist devices systems can be used to unload the failing ventricle and maintain sufficient end-organ perfusion [18]. Typically, the use of these devices is restricted to a few days to weeks. However, in consideration of the potential reversibility of the disease, a frequent re-evaluation of clinical and instrumental parameters is crucial for the appropriate management of these patients that represent the typical scenario of mechanical assist device used as a bridge to recovery.

- To manage patients with acute HF or cardiogenic shock (INTERMACS level 1), extracorporeal membrane oxygenation (ECMO) may be used to stabilize hemodynamics and recover end-organ function, due to its broad spectrum of use and simplicity of implantation, although prognosis of these patients remains poor [24].
- Left ventricular or biventricular assist devices (VAD) are useful in this setting for patients admitted with fulminant myocarditis or with severe acute heart failure refractory to medical treatment. Bridge-to-recovery VAD implantation might be considered as a bail-out strategy and is able to improve survival (up to 60%) in patients with end-stage HF [25]. Evidence of efficacy of bridge-to-recovery LVAD in patients with myocarditis is anecdotal; in the future, more data are expected to be available for this interesting option.

Due to the high mortality rate of patients in cardiogenic shock requiring mechanical assist devices as bail-out strategy, these options should be performed at tertiary referral centers where the patients might be centralized.

18.3.1.4 Cardiac Transplantation

Cardiac transplantation should be deferred in the acute phase, because recovery may occur, but can be considered for hemodynamically unstable myocarditis patients if optimal pharmacological support and mechanical assistance cannot stabilize the patient [9].

18.3.1.5 Reducing the Risk of Sudden Cardiac Death

ICD implantation should be deferred until the resolution of the acute phase. In fact, an ICD is recommended to reduce the risk of sudden death and all-cause mortality in patients with symptomatic HF (NYHA Class II–III) and LVEF ≤35% despite ≥3 months of optimal medical therapy. Patients at high risk in the short term should be re-evaluated after an adequate period of conventional and possible immunosuppressive treatments. As for the major arrhythmic presentation, a wearable ICD may also be considered in this scenario (e.g., those with poor LVEF after acute myocarditis and with a high probability to recover in the short term). However, no prospective randomized clinical trials evaluating this device in the setting of acute myocarditis have been reported and the indication of a wearable ICD cannot extend to all patients with an HF onset [18]. New trials are needed to better identify ICD or wearable ICD indications.

18.3.1.6 Standard Treatment in the Chronic Phase (Dilated Cardiomyopathy)

Dilated cardiomyopathy (DCM) can be the modality of presentation of a previous subclinical and undiagnosed myocarditis. Conversely, approximately 50% of patients with myocarditis admitted with heart failure are likely to evolve in the so-called post-myocarditis DCM, despite optimal medical treatment [3]. Predictors of DCM evolution are still largely unknown. It is largely assumed that post-myocarditis DCM is due to the persistence of autoimmune-specific process that leads to LV dilatation and dysfunction. Furthermore, a possible interaction between environmental factors and specific genotypes has been hypothesized, although there is no solid evidence in the literature. Standard diagnostic tools, such as personal history, biochemical, ECG, echocardiographic, cardiac MRI, and in specific cases EMB, are the cornerstones to guide therapy. In fact, therapeutic regimens and intensity of treatment change according to initial presentation, severity of symptoms, and the amount of LV involvement, expressed by LVEF or LGE extension. Currently, conventional management of inflammatory cardiomyopathy focuses on reverse ventricular remodeling targeted by beta-adrenergic antagonists, ARBs/ACE-I, MRAs, and the novel agent ARNI [9]. ICD implantation is recommended to reduce the risk of sudden death and all-cause mortality in patients with symptomatic HF (NYHA Class II–III) and a left ventricular ejection fraction ≤35%, despite ≥3 months of optimal medical therapy. In patients with concurrent left bundle branch block, cardiac resynchronization therapy should be associated with the ICD. In patients with biopsy-proven myocarditis under immunosuppressive treatment, deferring ICD implantation after termination of immunosuppressive therapy should be considered.

The duration of conventional therapy in myocarditis and, mostly, post-myocarditis DCM is an open issue. Currently, it is suggested to continue life-long therapy, even in the presence of an apparently healing or healed process. Progression of the disease may occur in the very long term and there is a lack of specific prognostic predictors to address a possible downgrading of medical therapy [26, 27].

18.4 Acute Myocarditis in the Pediatric Population

Myocarditis can also affect children, in whom it is often characterized by a severe hemodynamic or arrhythmic scenario. The true prevalence and incidence of acute myocarditis in the pediatric population are not well established. Acute myocarditis accounts for 0.05% of all pediatric hospital admissions [19]. However, the true frequency is probably higher than reported, because of undiagnosed asymptomatic or mildly symptomatic cases. Suspected viral myocarditis in children often presents with more severe symptoms than in adults, perhaps due to an immature immune system, and is clinically challenging. Viral infection is considered the leading cause of myocarditis in children; enterovirus and adenovirus are the most frequently implicated viruses. Suspected viral myocarditis accounts for approximately 0.1% of all pediatric chest pain admissions and for approximately 5–10% of sudden cardiac deaths in children and adolescents, whereas approximately one-third of children admitted with a DCM phenotype are affected by myocarditis [28, 29].

A significant proportion of children with myocarditis undergoes spontaneous recover, while in other cases a supportive HF treatment can bridge these patients to recovery. Conventional treatment of pediatric myocarditis aims to achieve prompt hemodynamic stability and to control heart failure, if present. Therefore, when myocarditis is suspected, the young patient must be promptly hospitalized and monitored, mostly if HF is present. In fact, the clinical picture can be rapidly evolving towards deterioration. Conventional HF treatment is administered according to clinical presentation, including diuretics, ACE-I/ARBs, antiarrhythmic therapy if needed, and inotrope support in case of unstable hemodynamics. Circulatory mechanical support should be promptly considered to compensate HF and bridge patients to recovery or heart transplantation, when inotropic support, mechanical ventilation, and maximal medical management fail to restore hemodynamic stability.

Finally, although the pathophysiological mechanisms of acute myocarditis encourage the application of more specific therapies to target the immune response, large randomized biopsy-proven controlled trials are necessary to demonstrate the efficacy of specific immune-modulation, i.e., immunosuppression, intravenous immunoglobulins, or antiviral therapy in children [29].

References

1. Sinagra G, Anzini M, Pereira NL, Bussani R, Finocchiaro G, Bartunek J, et al. Myocarditis in clinical practice. Mayo Clin Proc. 2016;91(9):1256–66. https://doi.org/10.1016/j.mayocp.2016.05.013.
2. Anzini M, Merlo M, Sabbadini G, Barbati G, Finocchiaro G, Pinamonti B, et al. Long-term evolution and prognostic stratification of biopsy-proven active myocarditis. Circulation. 2013;128(22):2384–94. https://doi.org/10.1161/CIRCULATIONAHA.113.003092.
3. Anzini M, Merlo M, Artico J, Sinagra G. Arrhythmic risk prediction of acute myocarditis presenting with life-threatening ventricular tachyarrhythmias. Int J Cardiol. 2016;212:169–70. https://doi.org/10.1016/j.ijcard.2016.03.020.
4. Caforio AL, Calabrese F, Angelini A, Tona F, Vinci A, Bottaro S, et al. A prospective study of biopsy-proven myocarditis: prognostic relevance of clinical and aetiopathogenetic features at diagnosis. Eur Heart J. 2007;28(11):1326–33. https://doi.org/10.1093/eurheartj/ehm076.
5. Dennert R, Crijns HJ, Heymans S. Acute viral myocarditis. Eur Heart J. 2008;29(17):2073–82. https://doi.org/10.1093/eurheartj/ehn296.
6. Marin-Neto JA, Cunha-Neto E, Maciel BC, Simoes MV. Pathogenesis of chronic Chagas heart disease. Circulation. 2007;115(9):1109–23. https://doi.org/10.1161/CIRCULATIONAHA.106.624296.

7. Karatolios K, Maisch B, Pankuweit S. Suspected inflammatory cardiomyopathy. Prevalence of Borrelia burgdorferi in endomyocardial biopsies with positive serological evidence. Herz. 2015;40(Suppl 1):91–5. https://doi.org/10.1007/s00059-014-4118-x.
8. Pollack A, Kontorovich AR, Fuster V, Dec GW. Viral myocarditis—diagnosis, treatment options, and current controversies. Nat Rev Cardiol. 2015;12(11):670–80. https://doi.org/10.1038/nrcardio.2015.108.
9. Caforio AL, Pankuweit S, Arbustini E, Basso C, Gimeno-Blanes J, Felix SB, et al. Current state of knowledge on aetiology, diagnosis, management, and therapy of myocarditis: a position statement of the European Society of Cardiology Working Group on Myocardial and Pericardial Diseases. Eur Heart J. 2013;34(33):2636–48. https://doi.org/10.1093/eurheartj/eht210.
10. Sagar S, Liu PP, Cooper LT Jr. Myocarditis. Lancet. 2012;379(9817):738–47. https://doi.org/10.1016/S0140-6736(11)60648-X.
11. Aquaro GD, Perfetti M, Camastra G, Monti L, Dellegrottaglie S, Moro C, et al. Cardiac MR with late gadolinium enhancement in acute myocarditis with preserved systolic function: ITAMY study. J Am Coll Cardiol. 2017;70(16):1977–87. https://doi.org/10.1016/j.jacc.2017.08.044.
12. Adler Y, Charron P, Imazio M, Badano L, Baron-Esquivias G, Bogaert J, et al. 2015 ESC guidelines for the diagnosis and management of pericardial diseases: the task force for the diagnosis and Management of Pericardial Diseases of the European Society of Cardiology (ESC)endorsed by: the European Association for Cardio-Thoracic Surgery (EACTS). Eur Heart J. 2015;36(42):2921–64. https://doi.org/10.1093/eurheartj/ehv318.
13. Imazio M, Brucato A, Mayosi BM, Derosa FG, Lestuzzi C, Macor A, et al. Medical therapy of pericardial diseases: part I: idiopathic and infectious pericarditis. J Cardiovasc Med (Hagerstown). 2010;11(10):712–22. https://doi.org/10.2459/JCM.0b013e3283340b97.
14. Grun S, Schumm J, Greulich S, Wagner A, Schneider S, Bruder O, et al. Long-term follow-up of biopsy-proven viral myocarditis: predictors of mortality and incomplete recovery. J Am Coll Cardiol. 2012;59(18):1604–15. https://doi.org/10.1016/j.jacc.2012.01.007.
15. Shapiro ED. Lyme disease. N Engl J Med. 2014;371(7):684. https://doi.org/10.1056/NEJMc1407264.
16. Chapman AS, Bakken JS, Folk SM, Paddock CD, Bloch KC, Krusell A, et al. Diagnosis and management of tickborne rickettsial diseases: Rocky Mountain spotted fever, ehrlichioses, and anaplasmosis—United States: a practical guide for physicians and other health-care and public health professionals. MMWR Recomm Rep. 2006;55(RR-4):1–27.
17. Felker GM, Thompson RE, Hare JM, Hruban RH, Clemetson DE, Howard DL, et al. Underlying causes and long-term survival in patients with initially unexplained cardiomyopathy. N Engl J Med. 2000;342(15):1077–84. https://doi.org/10.1056/NEJM200004133421502.
18. Ponikowski P, Voors AA, Anker SD, Bueno H, Cleland JGF, Coats AJS, et al. 2016 ESC guidelines for the diagnosis and treatment of acute and chronic heart failure: the task force for the diagnosis and treatment of acute and chronic heart failure of the European Society of Cardiology (ESC)developed with the special contribution of the Heart Failure Association (HFA) of the ESC. Eur Heart J. 2016;37(27):2129–200. https://doi.org/10.1093/eurheartj/ehw128.
19. Towbin JA, Lowe AM, Colan SD, Sleeper LA, Orav EJ, Clunie S, et al. Incidence, causes, and outcomes of dilated cardiomyopathy in children. JAMA. 2006;296(15):1867–76. https://doi.org/10.1001/jama.296.15.1867.
20. Vital FM, Ladeira MT, Atallah AN. Non-invasive positive pressure ventilation (CPAP or bilevel NPPV) for cardiogenic pulmonary oedema. Cochrane Database Syst Rev. 2013;5:CD005351. https://doi.org/10.1002/14651858.CD005351.pub3.
21. Alviar CL, Miller PE, McAreavey D, Katz JN, Lee B, Moriyama B, et al. Positive pressure ventilation in the cardiac intensive care unit. J Am Coll Cardiol. 2018;72(13):1532–53. https://doi.org/10.1016/j.jacc.2018.06.074.

22. Felker GM, Lee KL, Bull DA, Redfield MM, Stevenson LW, Goldsmith SR, et al. Diuretic strategies in patients with acute decompensated heart failure. N Engl J Med. 2011;364(9):797–805. https://doi.org/10.1056/NEJMoa1005419.
23. de Backer D, Biston P, Devriendt J, Madl C, Chochrad D, Aldecoa C, et al. Comparison of dopamine and norepinephrine in the treatment of shock. N Engl J Med. 2010;362(9):779–89. https://doi.org/10.1056/NEJMoa0907118.
24. Nakamura T, Ishida K, Taniguchi Y, Nakagawa T, Seguchi M, Wada H, et al. Prognosis of patients with fulminant myocarditis managed by peripheral venoarterial extracorporeal membranous oxygenation support: a retrospective single-center study. J Intensive Care. 2015;3(1):5. https://doi.org/10.1186/s40560-014-0069-9.
25. Drakos SG, Kfoury AG, Stehlik J, Selzman CH, Reid BB, Terrovitis JV, et al. Bridge to recovery: understanding the disconnect between clinical and biological outcomes. Circulation. 2012;126(2):230–41. https://doi.org/10.1161/CIRCULATIONAHA.111.040261.
26. Halliday BP, Wassall R, Lota AS, Khalique Z, Gregson J, Newsome S, et al. Withdrawal of pharmacological treatment for heart failure in patients with recovered dilated cardiomyopathy (TRED-HF): an open-label, pilot, randomised trial. Lancet. 2019;393(10166):61–73. https://doi.org/10.1016/S0140-6736(18)32484-X.
27. Merlo M, Stolfo D, Anzini M, Negri F, Pinamonti B, Barbati G, et al. Persistent recovery of normal left ventricular function and dimension in idiopathic dilated cardiomyopathy during long-term follow-up: does real healing exist? J Am Heart Assoc. 2015;4(1):e001504. https://doi.org/10.1161/JAHA.114.000570.
28. Canter CE, Simpson KE. Diagnosis and treatment of myocarditis in children in the current era. Circulation. 2014;129(1):115–28. https://doi.org/10.1161/CIRCULATIONAHA.113.001372.
29. di Filippo S. Improving outcomes of acute myocarditis in children. Expert Rev Cardiovasc Ther. 2016;14(1):117–25. https://doi.org/10.1586/14779072.2016.1114884.

Arrhythmias in Myocarditis

19

Riccardo Vio, Alessandro Zorzi, and Domenico Corrado

19.1 Introduction

Myocarditis is caused by a broad variety of etiopathogenetic agents. The most common causes of infective myocarditis in North America and Europe are presumed to be viruses, whereas bacteria, fungi, and parasites are infrequent [1]. On the other hand, non-infective myocarditis, i.e., immune-mediated and toxic myocarditis, is also described. Whatever the cause, either infective or not, clinical presentation includes infarct-like symptoms, heart failure, and arrhythmias [2]. The presence of arrhythmias has diagnostic and prognostic implications, playing a crucial role in the decision-making of whether or not to perform an endomyocardial biopsy (EMB), which represents the gold standard for the diagnosis of myocarditis [3].

Virtually, all types of arrhythmias have been reported in patients with myocarditis, ranging from advanced heart block to ventricular fibrillation leading to sudden cardiac death [2, 4, 5]. The arrhythmic burden and the underlying mechanisms vary between the acute and chronic setting, depending on the relative impact of acute inflammation versus post-inflammatory myocardial fibrosis.

19.2 Acute Myocarditis

Pathogenetic mechanisms involved in myocarditis are not fully understood, remaining an open field of research. Most studies focus on viral and autoimmune myocarditis, postulating a three-phase process from acute injury to chronic dilated cardiomyopathy [2]. Acute injury leads to cardiac damage, exposure of intracellular

R. Vio · A. Zorzi · D. Corrado (✉)
Department of Cardiac, Thoracic, Vascular and Public Health Sciences,
University of Padua, Padua, Italy
e-mail: riccardo.vio.1@gmail.com; alessandro.zorzi@unipd.it; domenico.corrado@unipd.it

A. L. P. Caforio (ed.), *Myocarditis*, https://doi.org/10.1007/978-3-030-35276-9_19

Table 19.1 Prevalence of arrhythmias in patients with acute myocarditis

Arrhythmia	Prevalence (%)	Studies
Sustained supraventricular tachycardia	0.8	Anderson [9][a]
Atrial fibrillation/atrial flutter	2.5–14	Imazio [10], Anzini [8], Ukena [11]
Non-sustained ventricular tachycardia	28	Anzini [8]
Sustained ventricular tachycardia or ventricular fibrillation/flutter	7.3–9.7	Anzini [8], Anderson [9][a]
AV blocks (any degree)	10	Caforio [6]

[a]Pediatric population

antigens, and activation of the innate immune system, increasing the chance of developing arrhythmias. As a result, it has been reported that in up to 24% of cases the first clinical manifestation consists of arrhythmias (either tachy- or bradyarrhythmia), syncope, or sudden cardiac death [6–8]. Table 19.1 describes the prevalence of different arrhythmias in acute myocarditis (AM).

19.2.1 Supraventricular Arrhythmias

Sinus tachycardia is a common finding in AM secondary to the systemic inflammation and heart failure, whereas atrial inflammation is probably involved in the onset of atrial tachyarrhythmias [4]. In fact, the pathological process of AM often extends to the atria and atrial myocarditis in the absence of ventricular involvement has also been reported [12–15]. Since either local or systemic inflammation is associated with initiation and maintenance of atrial fibrillation (AF) in the general population [16, 17], it is not surprising that this arrhythmia represents a common complication in myocarditis, with a reported prevalence of 2.5–14% [8–11]. The postulated mechanism is that the inflammatory process promotes an increased automaticity of the atrial myocardium resulting in supraventricular ectopic beats, which may trigger AF [18]. In this regard, Basso et al. provided additional evidence, describing inflammatory cell foci in the myocardium around the pulmonary vein orifices in patients with Wolff-Parkinson-White syndrome who died suddenly because of pre-excited AF that converted into ventricular fibrillation [19]. The importance of these histological findings lies in the fact that ectopic activity arising from the pulmonary vein orifices, typically showing a short coupling interval (P-on-T ECG pattern), is a well-recognized trigger of AF (and target of catheter ablation) [18, 20–22]. The same increased automaticity can cause focal supraventricular tachycardias. Moreover, in patients with dual atrioventricular (AV) node pathways or accessory pathways, supraventricular ectopic beats may initiate paroxysmal supraventricular tachycardia [23]. Apart from increased automaticity, ongoing inflammation can lead to myocyte necrosis and fibrotic changes, perpetuating adverse electrical and structural remodeling and promoting disease chronicity [24].

19.2.2 Atrioventricular Blocks

Atrioventricular (AV) blocks are traditionally associated with myocarditis, being reported in 10% of biopsy-proven AM patients [6]. While first degree AV blocks are frequently encountered, advanced AV blocks are typical of specific forms of myocarditis, such as giant cell myocarditis, sarcoidosis, and bacterial AM.

Giant cell myocarditis is a rare and rapidly progressive inflammatory heart disease usually characterized by an ominous prognosis without heart transplantation [25], even if better outcomes were recently reported, thanks to earlier diagnosis and specific treatment [26–28]. Life-threatening arrhythmias such as advanced AV blocks and ventricular tachycardia or fibrillation represent a major challenge. In a recent series of patients diagnosed with giant cell myocarditis, distal AV conduction blocks were reported in 28% of them [29]. It seems reasonable to assume that the high proportion of observed advanced AV blocks may be related to inflammatory involvement of the cardiac conduction tissue, as documented with cardiac magnetic resonance [30].

Another disorder usually characterized by high-degree AV blocks is cardiac sarcoidosis (i.e., idiopathic granulomatous myocarditis). Arrhythmias such as AV block, ventricular tachycardia, or sudden cardiac death may represent the first clinical manifestation of the disease [31–33], or may precipitate the clinical condition of patients with known sarcoidosis. Of interest, autopsy studies reported myocardial granulomas in 20–30% of patients, with a patchy fashion distribution, although some regions are preferred including the interventricular septum and the atria, potentially justifying the conduction defects [34].

In addition to giant cell myocarditis and cardiac sarcoidosis, bacterial and protozoal infection may cause myocardial inflammation, typically associated with bradyarrhythmia. Lyme myocarditis results from the infection with Borrelia burgdorferi, particularly common in rural areas of Central and South America. It should be suspected in patients with a history of travel to endemic regions and AV conduction abnormalities [35]. Diphtheria myocarditis is another bacterial infection which is frequently associated with various degree of heart block [36].

On the other hand, Chagas disease, a protozoal infection caused by Trypanosoma cruzi, can present as AM with right bundle branch block or left anterior fascicular block [37], potentially leading to complete heart block.

19.2.3 Ventricular Arrhythmias

Ventricular arrhythmias vary from simple isolated ventricular ectopic beats to complex and life-threatening tachycardias. Anzini et al. documented the presence of non-sustained ventricular tachycardia in 28% of AM patients, whereas sustained ventricular tachycardia or ventricular fibrillation represented the first clinical manifestation in 6/82 patients [8].

Myocarditis accounts for 2–42% of sudden cardiac deaths among young people [38–58]. As shown in Table 19.2, older studies reported a higher prevalence of myocarditis among sudden death victims (22–42%) [38–41], whereas in more recent series the proportion of sudden cardiac deaths ascribed to myocarditis ranged from 2 to 20%, probably because of the improvements in differential diagnosis with other

Table 19.2 Proportion of sudden cardiac deaths due to myocarditis in young people (<40 years old) and/or athletes, according to different studies

Authors, year of publication	Period	Population	Age	SD	SCD	SCD due to myocarditis
Topaz and Edwards [38]	1960–1983	Minneapolis, Minnesota	7–35	50	43	12 (28%)
Neuspiel and Kuller [39]	1972–1980	Allegheny County, Pennsylvania	1–21	207	51	14 (27%)
Phillips et al. [40]	1965–1985	United States, air force recruits	17–28	–	19	8 (42%)
Drory et al. [41]	1976–1985	Israel	9–39	162	118	26 (22%)
Corrado et al. [42]	1979–1999	Veneto Region, Italy	12–35	300	259	32 (12%)
Eckart et al. [43]	1977–2001	US military training base	18–35	126	64	13 (20%)
Puranik et al. [44]	1995–2004	Sydney, Australia	5–35	427	241	28 (12%)
Corrado et al. [45]	1979–2004	Veneto Region, Italy	12–35	–	320	46 (14%)
Maron et al. [46]	1980–2006	United States, competitive athletes	<40	1866	690	41 (6%)
de Noronha et al. [47]	1996–2008	United Kingdom	<36	89	73	3 (4%)
Winkel et al. [48]	2000–2006	Denmark	1–35	–	470	– (7%)
Meyer et al. [49]	1980–2009	King County, Washington	0–35	–	361[a]	10[a] (3%)
Pilmer et al. [50]	2008	Ontario, Canada	2–40	–	174	9 (5%)
Harmon et al. [51]	2004–2008	United States	17–24	–	45	3 (7%)
Harmon et al. [52]	2007–2013	United States	14–18	–	50	7 (14%)
Maron et al. [53]	1980–2011	United States, competitive athletes	19 ± 6[b]	2406	842	57 (7%)
Grani et al. [54]	1999–2010	Switzerland	10–39	–	69	2 (3%)
Bagnall et al. [55]	2010–2012	Australia and New Zealand	1–35	–	490	– (7%)
Finocchiaro [56]	1994–2014	United Kingdom	7–35	–	258	– (2%)
Wisten et al. [57]	2000–2010	Sweden	1–35	–	552	75 (14%)
Thiene [58]	1980–2013	Veneto Region, Italy	[c]	–	650	– (12%)

SD sudden death, *SCD* sudden cardiac death

[a]Out of hospital cardiac arrests

[b]Mean age ± standard deviation

[c]Age not specified, but population described as "young and athletes"

diseases that may be associated with myocardial inflammation or fibrosis such as myocarditis [42–58]. The risk of sudden cardiac death is particularly remarkable for fulminant myocarditis that is characteristically associated with refractory malignant ventricular tachycardia and adverse short-term prognosis [5].

Several mechanisms have been proposed to explain the onset of ventricular arrhythmias in AM.

First, myocarditis may cause myocardial ischemia similar to coronary artery disease. Ischemic mechanisms include mural thrombi, coronary artery embolization, and arteritis [59]. In addition, vasoactive kinins and catecholamines produced during the acute phase of viral infection can cause coronary artery spasm [60].

Another mechanism contributing to the arrhythmic phenotype of AM is myocardial edema: local inflammation, cytokine release, and cell death constitute the basis for edema formation, resulting in some cases in increased left ventricular wall thickness (i.e., pseudoinflammatory hypertrophy) [61, 62]. A recent study demonstrated that the electrocardiographic expression of transmural edema consists in T-wave inversion, and interestingly such ECG abnormalities normalized completely during follow-up, underscoring its transient and acute nature [63]. The same author speculated that myocardial edema causes myocyte repolarization inhomogeneity and electrical instability through the dispersion of action potential duration (APD) between epicardium and endocardium of the left ventricular free wall. There is experimental evidence that electrical remodeling (i.e., the change in electrophysiological properties of the myocardium) occurs in myocarditis. Saito et al. found an APD prolongation in animal models of AM, owing to an imbalance between outward and inward currents caused by ion channel dysfunction [64]. The APD prolongation, which electrocardiographically translated into QT interval prolongation, predisposes to early afterdepolarization-triggered ventricular arrhythmias.

On the other hand, calcium overload secondary to increased catecholamine levels can cause delayed afterdepolarization triggering ventricular arrhythmias [65, 66]. In addition, altered calcium handling per se has been found in AM, contributing to the perturbation of normal cardiomyocyte function [67].

Animal models of coxsackievirus B3-induced myocarditis showed a downregulation of connexins expression, which are important components of gap junctions [68]. The resulting impairment of myocyte communication may further enhance electrical instability of the myocardial tissue.

Finally, AM has been associated with clinical deterioration of pre-existing cardiac diseases, such as hypertrophic cardiomyopathy [69]. Arrhythmogenic right ventricular cardiomyopathy patients suffering arrhythmic storms frequently display signs of acute inflammation at cardiac magnetic resonance or endomyocardial biopsy (so-called hot-phase), although the inflammatory mechanism (viral versus immune-mediated) remains to be established [70–72].

19.3 Acute Myocarditis and Sudden Death in Athletes

Athletes represent a group of individuals at-risk of developing AM because there is evidence that high-intensity exercise may depress the immune system [73]. Intensive training and competition periods have been shown to reduce salivary secretory immunoglobulin A [74, 75], which represents the first line of defense preventing colonization and replication of viruses and bacteria on the mucosal surface. Moreover, emerging evidence suggests an altered T-cell response in athletes, with the balance between T1 and T2 cells tipped to favor T2 immunity, putting them at increased risk of viral infections, particularly those affecting the upper respiratory tract [76, 77].

Previous studies in athletes who died suddenly showed that AM is the cause of death in 2–12% of cases [46, 56, 58, 78, 79]. Data from the Veneto region of Italy showed that the incidence rates of SD due to acute myocarditis in athletes did not significantly change after the introduction of systematic preparticipation screening (from 0.3/100.000 to 0.15/100.000, $p = 0.4$) [45]. The failure in identifying athletes with myocarditis by periodic screening is obviously caused by the acute nature of the disease. Moreover, the typical electrocardiographic changes of AM such as T-wave inversion are typically transient, potentially not leaving any sign of the process at the next visit [63]. However, even athletes showing a complete recovery (i.e., healed myocarditis) may later present ventricular arrhythmias due to myocardial scars (see below) [80].

For all the aforementioned considerations, athletes diagnosed with myocarditis should be restricted from exercise programs for 3–6 months, and before resuming competition left ventricular function must be normalized, without evidence of frequent or complex tachyarrhythmias and with normal troponin levels [81].

19.4 Post-inflammatory Myocardial Scar

Three arrhythmic mechanisms may explain the occurrence of life-threatening ventricular arrhythmias in patients who suffered AM: (1) recurrent myocarditis or persistent myocardial inflammation; (2) residual left ventricular dysfunction, and (3) post-inflammatory myocardial scar.

The healing process of AM can result in the formation of myocardial scars that may be the substrate for sustained ventricular tachycardia even in subjects with a normal left ventricular function. Post-inflammatory fibrosis typically shows a patchy or stria pattern and involves the subepicardial/midmyocardial layers of the infero-lateral left ventricular wall [61]. The lesions can be revealed by late enhancement on post-contrast cardiac magnetic resonance sequences while they are often undetectable by echocardiography. The reason of the low sensitivity of echocardiography is that the fibrosis involves a small myocardial area and is confined to the outer wall layers without reaching the subendocardium, which is the part of the left ventricle that contribute the most to myocardial thickening [82].

The role of myocardial fibrosis as a substrate for ventricular arrhythmias has been demonstrated by a study on 405 patients with clinically suspected myocarditis. During a mean follow-up of 4.4 years, ten major arrhythmic events occurred, all in patients with late gadolinium enhancement, suggesting myocardial scar on post-contrast cardiac magnetic resonance sequences [83].

Myocardial scar with a subepicardial/midmyocardial (i.e., non-ischemic) distribution has been increasingly reported as a myocardial substrate for life-threatening ventricular arrhythmias and cardiac arrest mostly in young people and athletes (Fig. 19.1) [80, 84–86]. Although the lesion is traditionally interpreted as a post-myocarditis scar [61, 87], there have been some cases with evidence of familial recurrence and positive genotyping for either desmosomal or non-desmosomal gene mutations [88, 89]. In these cases, the myocardial scar may represent an additional phenotypic variant of arrhythmogenic cardiomyopathy presenting as segmental and isolated involvement of the left ventricle (left-dominant arrhythmogenic cardiomyopathy).

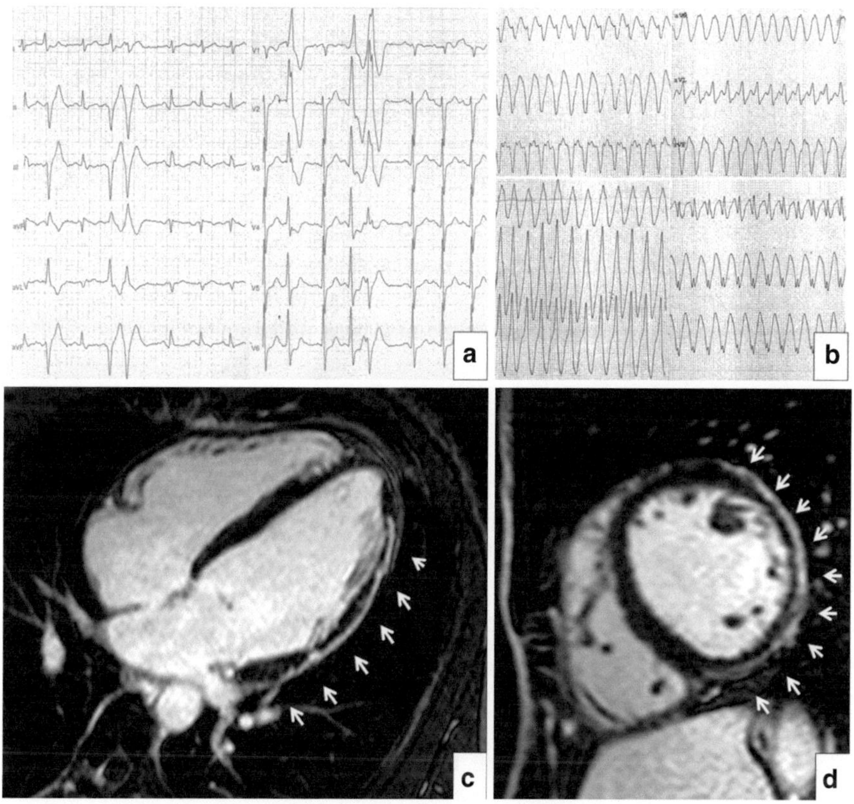

Fig. 19.1 Representative case of an athlete who suffered sustained ventricular tachycardia secondary to post-inflammatory myocardial fibrosis. A 42-year-old martial art player presented with frequent and coupled premature ventricular beats with right bundle branch block/superior axis morphology during exercise testing (**a**). The athlete experienced sustained ventricular tachycardia during follow-up (**b**). Post-contrast sequences on contrast-enhanced cardiac magnetic resonance, 4-chamber view (**c**) and short-axis view (**d**) revealed a subepicardial/midmyocardial "stria" of late-gadolinium enhancement involving the antero-lateral, lateral, and infero-lateral left ventricular wall consistent with post-inflammatory myocardial fibrosis. Reproduced with permission from [80]

19.5 Therapy

Given the absence of specific recommendations, management of arrhythmias in myocarditis should not differ from generally accepted clinical principles, based on current guidelines [5, 23, 90–92]. Patients presenting with symptomatic bradycardia or advanced heart block may require temporary pacemakers [93]. On the other hand, anti-arrhythmic drugs such as amiodarone could be indicated in case of symptomatic or sustained ventricular tachycardia. The therapy for ventricular fibrillation or hemodynamically unstable ventricular tachycardia is immediate electrical defibrillation/cardioversion. In patients who suffered cardiac arrest or with severe ventricular dysfunction resulting from myocarditis, the implantation of an ICD is indicated [5]. However, during the acute phase of the disease, ICD implantation may be deferred because the clinical status may significantly improve. In this context, the so-called wearable defibrillator (LifeVest, Zoll Medical Corporation) can represent a valid option as a bridge therapy, protecting the patients from life-threatening arrhythmias while observing the clinical course of the disease [94]. With regard to cardiac resynchronization therapy defibrillator (CRT-D) implantation, it is recommended for primary prevention in patients with reduced left ventricular function (<35%) and left bundle branch block in NYHA functional classes II–IV [95], bearing in mind the aforementioned timing considerations.

Finally, catheter ablation represents a symptomatic treatment for patients with recurrent ventricular tachycardia because of a post-inflammatory myocardial scar, particularly when anti-arrhythmic therapy is ineffective or not tolerated. However, because of the subepicardial distribution of myocardial fibrosis, an epicardial approach is often needed to achieve effective ablation of the arrhythmic substrate [85]. This technique should be performed in selected, highly experienced centers and since difficulties in the epicardial access have been described in patients with prior pericarditis, a careful risk-benefit evaluation should be performed in patients with documented pericardial involvement [96].

References

1. Caforio ALP, Marcolongo R, Basso C, Iliceto S. Clinical presentation and diagnosis of myocarditis. Heart. 2015;101(16):1332–44.
2. Caforio ALP, Pankuweit S, Arbustini E, Basso C, Gimeno-Blanes J, Felix SB, et al. Current state of knowledge on aetiology, diagnosis, management, and therapy of myocarditis: A position statement of the European Society of Cardiology Working Group on Myocardial and Pericardial Diseases. Eur Heart J. 2013;34(33):2636–48.
3. Cooper LT, Baughman KL, Feldman AM, Frustaci A, Jessup M, Kuhl U, et al. The role of endomyocardial biopsy in the management of cardiovascular disease. J Am Coll Cardiol. 2007;50(19):1914–31.
4. Baksi AJ, Kanaganayagam GS, Prasad SK. Arrhythmias in viral myocarditis and pericarditis. Card Electrophysiol Clin. 2015;7:269–81.
5. Priori SG, Blomström-Lundqvist C. 2015 European Society of Cardiology Guidelines for the management of patients with ventricular arrhythmias and the prevention of sudden cardiac death summarized by co-chairs. Eur Heart J. 2015;36(41):2757–9.

6. Caforio ALP, Calabrese F, Angelini A, Tona F, Vinci A, Bottaro S, et al. A prospective study of biopsy-proven myocarditis: prognostic relevance of clinical and aetiopathogenetic features at diagnosis. Eur Heart J. 2007;28(11):1326–33.
7. Grün S, Schumm J, Greulich S, Wagner A, Schneider S, Bruder O, et al. Long-term follow-up of biopsy-proven viral myocarditis. J Am Coll Cardiol. 2012;59(18):1604–15.
8. Anzini M, Merlo M, Sabbadini G, Barbati G, Finocchiaro G, Pinamonti B, et al. Long-term evolution and prognostic stratification of biopsy-proven active myocarditis. Circulation. 2013;128(22):2384–94.
9. Anderson BR, Silver ES, Richmond ME, Liberman L. Usefulness of arrhythmias as predictors of death and resource utilization in children with myocarditis. Am J Cardiol. 2014;114(9):1400–5.
10. Imazio M, Trinchero R. Myopericarditis: etiology, management, and prognosis. Int J Cardiol. 2008;127(1):17–26.
11. Ukena C, Mahfoud F, Kindermann I, Kandolf R, Kindermann M, BÖhm M. Prognostic electrocardiographic parameters in patients with suspected myocarditis. Eur J Heart Fail. 2011;13(4):398–405.
12. Begieneman MPV, Emmens RW, Rijvers L, Kubat B, Paulus WJ, Vonk ABA, et al. Ventricular myocarditis coincides with atrial myocarditis in patients. Cardiovasc Pathol. 2016;25(2):141–8.
13. Habara M, Fujieda H, Nakamura Y. Images in cardiology - atrial myocarditis: a possible cause of idiopathic enlargement of bilateral atria. Heart. 2006;92(6):842.
14. Larsen B, Maleszewski J, Edwards W, Cooper L Jr, Sobonya R, Thompson E, et al. Atrial giant cell myocarditis: a distinctive clinicopathologic entity. Circulation. 2013;127(1):39–47.
15. Frustaci A, Cameli S, Zeppilli P. Biopsy evidence of atrial myocarditis in an athlete developing transient sinoatrial disease. Chest. 1995;108(5):1460–2.
16. Schnabel RB, Larson MG, Yamamoto JF, Kathiresan S, Rong J, Levy D, et al. Relation of multiple inflammatory biomarkers to incident atrial fibrillation. Am J Cardiol. 2009;104(1):92–6.
17. Marcus GM, Smith LM, Ordovas K, Scheinman MM, Kim AM, Badhwar N, et al. Intracardiac and extracardiac markers of inflammation during atrial fibrillation. Heart Rhythm. 2010;7(2):149–54.
18. Haissaguerre M, Jais P, Shah D, Takahashi A, Hocini M, Quiniou G, et al. Spontaneous initiation of atrial fibrillation by ectopic beats originating in the pulmonary veins. N Engl J Med. 1998;339(10):659–66.
19. Basso C, Corrado D, Rossi L, Thiene G. Ventricular preexcitation in children and young adults: atrial myocarditis as a possible trigger of sudden death. Circulation. 2001;103(2):269–75.
20. Jais P, Haissaguerre M, Shah D, Chouairi S, Gencel L, Hocini M, et al. A focal source of atrial fibrillation treated by discrete radiofrequency ablation. Circulation. 1997;95(3):572–6.
21. Haissaguerre M, Jais P, Shah D, Garrigue S, Takahashi A, Lervegne T, et al. Electrophysiological end point for catheter ablation of atrial fibrillation initiated from multiple pulmonary venous foci. Circulation. 2000;101(12):1409–17.
22. Haissaguerre M, Shah D, Jais P, Hocini M, Yamane T, Deisenhofer I, et al. Electrophysiological breakthroughs from the left atrium to the pulmonary veins. Circulation. 2000;102(20):2463–5.
23. Katritsis DG, Boriani G, Cosio FG, Hindricks G, Jais P, Josephson ME, et al. European Heart Rhythm Association (EHRA) consensus document on the management of supraventricular arrhythmias, endorsed by Heart Rhythm Society (HRS), Asia-Pacific Heart Rhythm Society (APHRS), and Sociedad Latinoamericana de Estimulación Cardiaca y Elect. Eur Heart J. 2018;39(16):1442–5.
24. Frustaci A, Chimenti C, Bellocci F, Morgante E, Russo MA, Maseri A. Histological substrate of atrial biopsies in patients with lone atrial fibrillation. Circulation. 1997;96(4):1180–4.
25. Cooper LT, Berry GJ, Shabetai R. Idiopathic giant-cell myocarditis—natural history and treatment. N Engl J Med. 1997;336(26):1860–6.
26. Cooper LT, Hare JM, Tazelaar HD, Edwards WD, Starling RC, Deng MC, et al. Usefulness of Immunosuppression for giant cell myocarditis. Am J Cardiol. 2008;102(11):1535–9.
27. Maleszewski J, Orellana V, Hodge D, Kuhl U, Schultheiss H, Cooper L. Long-term risk of recurrence, morbidity and mortality in giant cell myocarditis. Am J Cardiol. 2015;115(12):1733–8.

28. Kandolin R, Lehtonen J, Salmenkivi K, Räisänen-Sokolowski A, Lommi J, Kupari M. Diagnosis, treatment, and outcome of giant-cell myocarditis in the era of combined immunosuppression. Circ Heart Fail. 2013;6(1):15–22.
29. Ekstrom K, Lehtonen J, Kandolin R, Raisanen-Sokolowski A, Salmenkivi K, Kupari M. Long-term outcome and its predictors in giant cell myocarditis. Eur J Heart Fail. 2016;18(12):1452–8.
30. Francone M, Chimenti C, Galea N, Scopelliti F, Verardo R, Galea R, et al. CMR sensitivity varies with clinical presentation and extent of cell necrosis in biopsy-proven acute myocarditis. JACC Cardiovasc Imaging. 2014;7(3):254–63.
31. Hamzeh N, Steckman DA, Sauer WH, Judson MA. Pathophysiology and clinical management of cardiac sarcoidosis. Nat Rev Cardiol. 2015;12:278–88.
32. Baughman RP, Grutters JC. New treatment strategies for pulmonary sarcoidosis: antimetabolites, biological drugs, and other treatment approaches. Lancet Respir Med. 2015;3:813–22.
33. Facco M, Cabrelle A, Teramo A, Olivieri V, Gnoato M, Teolato S, et al. Sarcoidosis is a Th1/Th17 multisystem disorder. Thorax. 2011;66(2):144–50.
34. Caforio ALP, Adler Y, Agostini C, Allanore Y, Anastasakis A, Arad M, et al. Diagnosis and management of myocardial involvement in systemic immune-mediated diseases: a position statement of the European Society of Cardiology Working Group on Myocardial and Pericardial Disease. Eur Heart J. 2017;38:2649–62.
35. HF MA, Klementowicz PT, Andrews C, Fisher JD, Feld M, Furman S. Lyme carditis: An important cause of reversible heart block. Ann Intern Med. 1989;110:339–45.
36. Celik T, Selimov N, Vekilova A, Kursaklioglu H, Iyisoy A, Kilic S, et al. Prognostic significance of electrocardiographic abnormalities in diphtheritic myocarditis after hospital discharge: a long-term follow-up study. Ann Noninvasive Electrocardiol. 2006;11(1):28–33.
37. Rassi A, Rassi A, Little WC, Xavier SS, Rassi SG, Rassi AG, et al. Development and validation of a risk score for predicting death in Chagas' heart disease. N Engl J Med. 2006;355(8):799–808.
38. Topaz O, Edwards JE. Pathologic features of sudden death in children, adolescents, and young adults. Chest. 1985;87(4):476–82.
39. Neuspiel DR, Kuller LH. Sudden and unexpected natural death in childhood and adolescence. JAMA. 1985;254(10):1321–5.
40. Phillips M, Robinowitz M, Higgins JR, Boran KJ, Reed T, Virmani R. Sudden cardiac death in air force recruits. JAMA. 1986;256(19):2696.
41. Drory Y, Kramer M, Lev B. Exertional sudden death in soldiers. Med Sci Sport Exerc. 1991;23(2):147–51.
42. Corrado D, Basso C, Rizzoli G, Schiavon M, Thiene G. Does sports activity enhance the risk of sudden death in adolescents and young adults? J Am Coll Cardiol. 2003;42(11):1959–63.
43. Eckart RE, Scoville SL, Campbell CL, Shry EA, Stajduhar KC, Potter RN, et al. Sudden death in young adults: a 25-year review of autopsies in military recruits. Ann Intern Med. 2004;141:829–34.
44. Puranik R, Chow CK, Duflou JA, Kilborn MJ, McGuire MA. Sudden death in the young. Heart Rhythm. 2005;2(12):1277–82.
45. Corrado D, Basso C, Pavei A, Michieli P, Schiavon M, Thiene G. Trends in sudden cardiovascular death in young competitive athletes after implementation of a preparticipation screening program. J Am Med Assoc. 2006;296(13):1593–601.
46. Maron BJ, Doerer JJ, Haas TS, Tierney DM, Mueller FO. Sudden deaths in young competitive athletes analysis of 1866 deaths in the united states, 1980–2006. Circulation. 2009;119(8):1085–92.
47. de Noronha SV, Sharma S, Papadakis M, Desai S, Whyte G, Sheppard MN. Aetiology of sudden cardiac death in athletes in the United Kingdom: a pathological study. Heart. 2009;95(17):1409–14.
48. Winkel BG, Holst AG, Theilade J, Kristensen IB, Thomsen JL, Ottesen GL, et al. Nationwide study of sudden cardiac death in persons aged 1–35 years. Eur Heart J. 2011;32(8):983–90.

49. Meyer L, Stubbs B, Fahrenbruch C, Maeda C, Harmon K, Eisenberg M, et al. Incidence, causes, and survival trends from cardiovascular-related sudden cardiac arrest in children and young adults 0 to 35 years of age: a 30-year review. Circulation. 2012;126(11):1363–72.
50. Pilmer CM, Porter B, Kirsh JA, Hicks AL, Gledhill N, Jamnik V, et al. Scope and nature of sudden cardiac death before age 40 in Ontario: a report from the cardiac death advisory committee of the office of the chief coroner. Heart Rhythm. 2013;10(4):517–23.
51. Harmon KG, Drezner JA, Maleszewski JJ, Lopez-Anderson M, Owens D, Prutkin JM, et al. Pathogeneses of sudden cardiac death in national collegiate athletic association athletes. Circ Arrhythm Electrophysiol. 2014;7(2):198–204.
52. Harmon KG, Asif IM, Maleszewski JJ, Owens DS, Prutkin JM, Salerno JC, et al. Incidence and etiology of sudden cardiac arrest and death in high school athletes in the United States. Mayo Clin Proc. 2016;91(11):1493–502.
53. Maron BJ, Haas TS, Ahluwalia A, Murphy CJ, Garberich RF. Demographics and epidemiology of sudden deaths in young competitive athletes: from the United States National Registry. Am J Med. 2016;129(11):1170–7.
54. Gräni C, Chappex N, Fracasso T, Vital C, Kellerhals C, Schmied C, et al. Sports-related sudden cardiac death in Switzerland classified by static and dynamic components of exercise. Eur J Prev Cardiol. 2016;23(11):1228–36.
55. Bagnall RD, Weintraub RG, Ingles J, Duflou J, Yeates L, Lam L, et al. A prospective study of sudden cardiac death among children and young adults. Supplementary appendix. N Engl J Med. 2016;374(25):2441–52.
56. Finocchiaro G, Papadakis M, Robertus JL, Dhutia H, Steriotis AK, Tome M, et al. Etiology of sudden death in sports insights from a United Kingdom Regional Registry. J Am Coll Cardiol. 2016;67(18):2108–15.
57. Wisten A, Krantz P, Stattin EL. Sudden cardiac death among the young in Sweden from 2000 to 2010: an autopsy-based study. Europace. 2017;19(8):1327–34.
58. Thiene G. Sudden cardiac death in the young: a genetic destiny? Clin Med J R Coll Phys Lond. 2018;18:s17–23.
59. Punja M, Mark DG, McCoy JV, Javan R, Pines JM, Brady W. Electrocardiographic manifestations of cardiac infectious-inflammatory disorders. Am J Emerg Med. 2010;28:364–77.
60. Yilmaz A, Mahrholdt H, Athanasiadis A, Vogelsberg H, Meinhardt G, Voehringer M, et al. Coronary vasospasm as the underlying cause for chest pain in patients with PVB19 myocarditis. Heart. 2008;94(11):1456–63.
61. Friedrich MG, Sechtem U, Schulz-Menger J, Holmvang G, Alakija P, Cooper LT, et al. Cardiovascular magnetic resonance in myocarditis: a JACC white paper. J Am Coll Cardiol. 2009;53:1475–87.
62. Pinamonti B, Alberti E, Cigalotto A, Dreas L, Salvi A, Silvestri F, et al. Echocardiographic findings in myocarditis. Am J Cardiol. 1988;62(4):285–91.
63. de Lazzari M, Zorzi A, Baritussio A, Siciliano M, Migliore F, Susana A, et al. Relationship between T-wave inversion and transmural myocardial edema as evidenced by cardiac magnetic resonance in patients with clinically suspected acute myocarditis: clinical and prognostic implications. J Electrocardiol. 2016;49(4):587–95.
64. Saito J, Niwano S, Niwano H, Inomata T, Yumoto Y, Ikeda K, et al. Electrical remodeling of the ventricular myocardium in myocarditis: studies of rat experimental autoimmune myocarditis. Circ J. 2002;66(1):97–103.
65. Eitel I, Lücke C, Grothoff M, Sareban M, Schuler G, Thiele H, et al. Inflammation in takotsubo cardiomyopathy: Insights from cardiovascular magnetic resonance imaging. Eur Radiol. 2010;20(2):422–31.
66. Akashi YJ, Goldstein DS, Barbara G, Ueyama T. Takotsubo cardiomyopathy a new form of acute, reversible heart failure. Circulation. 2008;118(25):2754–62.
67. Li Y, Ge S, Peng Y, Chen X. Inflammation and cardiac dysfunction during sepsis, muscular dystrophy, and myocarditis. Burn Trauma. 2013;1(3):109–21.

68. Zhang A, Zhang H, Wu S. Immunomodulation by atorvastatin upregulates expression of gap junction proteins in coxsackievirus B3 (CVB3)-induced myocarditis. Inflamm Res. 2010;59(4):255–62.
69. Frustaci A, Verardo R, Caldarulo M, Acconcia MC, Russo MA, Chimenti C. Myocarditis in hypertrophic cardiomyopathy patients presenting acute clinical deterioration. Eur Heart J. 2007;28(6):733–40.
70. Basso C, Ronco F, Marcus F, Abudureheman A, Rizzo S, Frigo AC, et al. Quantitative assessment of endomyocardial biopsy in arrhythmogenic right ventricular cardiomyopathy/dysplasia: an in vitro validation of diagnostic criteria. Eur Heart J. 2008;29(22):2760–71.
71. Chimenti C, Pieroni M, Maseri A, Frustaci A. Histologic findings in patients with clinical and instrumental diagnosis of sporadic arrhythmogenic right ventricular dysplasia. J Am Coll Cardiol. 2004;43(12):2305–13.
72. Bowles NE, Ni J, Marcus F, Towbin JA. The detection of cardiotropic viruses in the myocardium of patients with arrhythmogenic right ventricular dysplasia/cardiomyopathy. J Am Coll Cardiol. 2002;39(5):892–5.
73. Keaney LC, Kilding AE, Merien F, Dulson DK. The impact of sport related stressors on immunity and illness risk in team-sport athletes. J Sci Med Sport. 2018;21:1192–9.
74. Moreira A, Mortatti AL, Arruda AFS, Freitas CG, de Arruda M, Aoki MS. Salivary IgA response and upper respiratory tract infection symptoms during a 21-week competitive season in young soccer players. J Strength Cond Res. 2014;28(2):467–73.
75. Fahlman MM, Engels HJ. Mucosal IgA and URTI in American college football players: a year longitudinal study. Med Sci Sports Exerc. 2005;37(3):374–80.
76. Zhao G, Zhou S, Davie A, Su Q. Effects of moderate and high intensity exercise on T1/T2 balance. Exerc Immunol Rev. 2012;18:97–113.
77. Gleeson M, Pyne DB. Respiratory inflammation and infections in high-performance athletes. Immunol Cell Biol. 2016;94:124–31.
78. Maron BJ, McKenna WJ, Danielson GK, Kappenberger LJ, Kuhn HJ, Seidman CE, et al. American College of Cardiology/European Society of Cardiology clinical expert consensus document on hypertrophic cardiomyopathy: a report of the American College of Cardiology Foundation task force on clinical expert consensus documents and the European S. J Am Coll Cardiol. 2003;42:1687–713.
79. Harmon KG, Asif IM, Maleszewski JJ, Owens DS, Prutkin JM, Salerno JC, et al. Incidence, cause, and comparative frequency of sudden cardiac death in National Collegiate Athletic Association Athletes. Circulation. 2015;132(1):10–9.
80. Zorzi A, Marra MP, Rigato I, de Lazzari M, Susana A, Niero A, et al. Nonischemic left ventricular scar as a substrate of life-threatening ventricular arrhythmias and sudden cardiac death in competitive athletes. Circ Arrhythm Electrophysiol. 2016;9(7):e004229.
81. Pelliccia A, Solberg EE, Papadakis M, Adami PE, Biffi A, Caselli S, et al. Recommendations for participation in competitive and leisure time sport in athletes with cardiomyopathies, myocarditis, and pericarditis: position statement of the Sport Cardiology Section of the European Association of Preventive Cardiology (EAPC). Eur Heart J. 2019;40(1):19–33.
82. Rademakers FE, Rogers WJ, Guier WH, Hutchins GM, Siu CO, Weisfeldt ML, et al. Relation of regional cross-fiber shortening to wall thickening in the intact heart: three-dimensional strain analysis by NMR tagging. Circulation. 1994;89(3):1174–82.
83. Schumm J, Greulich S, Wagner A, Grün S, Ong P, Bentz K, et al. Cardiovascular magnetic resonance risk stratification in patients with clinically suspected myocarditis. J Cardiovasc Magn Reson. 2014;16(1):14.
84. Whyte G, Sheppard M, George K, Shave R, Wilson M, Prasad S, et al. Post-mortem evidence of idiopathic left ventricular hypertrophy and idiopathic interstitial myocardial fibrosis: is exercise the cause? Br J Sports Med. 2008;42(4):304–5.
85. Pilichou K, Mancini M, Rigato I, Lazzarini E, Giorgi B, Carturan E, et al. Nonischemic left ventricular scar sporadic or familial? Screen the genes, scan the mutation carriers. Circulation. 2014;130(21):e180–2.

86. d'Amati G, de Caterina R, Basso C. Sudden cardiac death in an Italian competitive athlete: pre-participation screening and cardiovascular emergency care are both essential. Int J Cardiol. 2016;206:84–6.
87. Friedrich MG, Marcotte F. Cardiac magnetic resonance assessment of myocarditis. Circ Cardiovasc Imaging. 2013;6(5):833–9.
88. Te Rijdt WP, Ten Sande JN, Gorter TM, van der Zwaag PA, van Rijsingen IA, Boekholdt SM, et al. Myocardial fibrosis as an early feature in phospholamban p.Arg14del mutation carriers: phenotypic insights from cardiovascular magnetic resonance imaging. Eur Heart J Cardiovasc Imaging. 2019;20(1):92–100.
89. Sen-Chowdhry S, Syrris P, Prasad SK, Hughes SE, Merrifield R, Ward D, et al. Left-dominant arrhythmogenic cardiomyopathy. an under-recognized clinical entity. J Am Coll Cardiol. 2008;52(25):2175–87.
90. Vardas PE, Auricchio A, Blanc JJ, Daubert JC, Drexler H, Ector H, et al. Guidelines for cardiac pacing and cardiac resynchronization therapy. The task force for cardiac pacing and cardiac resynchronization therapy of the European Society of Cardiology. Developed in collaboration with the European Heart Rhythm Association. Europace. 2007;9(10):959–98.
91. Dickstein K, Vardas PE, Auricchio A, Daubert JC, Linde C, McMurray J, et al. Focused update of ESC guidelines on device therapy in heart failure: an update of the 2008 ESC guidelines for the diagnosis and treatment of acute and chronic heart failure and the 2007 ESC Guidelines for cardiac and resynchronization therapy—Devel. Europace. 2010;12:1526–36.
92. Kirchhof P, Benussi S, Kotecha D, Ahlsson A, Atar D, Casadei B, et al. 2016 ESC guidelines for the management of atrial fibrillation developed in collaboration with EACTS. Eur Heart J. 2016;37(38):2893–962.
93. JCS Joint Working Group. Guidelines for diagnosis and treatment of myocarditis (JCS 2009). Circ J. 2011;75(3):734–43.
94. Prochnau D, Surber R, Kuehnert H, Heinke M, Klein HU, Figulla HR. Successful use of a wearable cardioverter-defibrillator in myocarditis with normal ejection fraction. Clin Res Cardiol. 2010;99:129–31.
95. Ponikowski P, Voors AA, Anker SD, Bueno H, Cleland JGF, Coats AJS, et al. ESC guidelines for the diagnosis and treatment of acute and chronic heart failure web addenda. Eur Heart J. 2016;37(27):2129–200.
96. Tschabrunn CM, Haqqani HM, Cooper JM, Dixit S, Garcia FC, Gerstenfeld EP, et al. Percutaneous epicardial ventricular tachycardia ablation after noncoronary cardiac surgery or pericarditis. Heart Rhythm. 2013;10(2):165–9.

Mechanical Assist Devices and Heart Transplantation

20

Gino Gerosa, Assunta Fabozzo, and Vincenzo Tarzia

Abbreviations

CE	European community certification
CRT	Cardiac resynchronization therapy
CS	Cardiogenic shock
DCM	Dilated cardiomyopathy
ecBiVAD	Extracorporeal biventricular assist device
ECLS	Extracorporeal life support
ECMO	Extracorporeal membrane oxygenator
FDA	Food and drug administration
HF	Heart failure
IABP	Intra-aortic balloon counterpulsation
ICD	Implantable cardioverter device
MCS	Mechanical circulatory support
MODS	Multiorgan dysfunction syndrome
SIRS	Systemic inflammatory response
TEE	Transesophageal echocardiogram

20.1 Introduction

Myocarditis is commonly identified as an inflammatory disease of the myocardium. It refers to clinical and histological manifestations of a broad range of pathological immune processes of the heart that ultimately can cause structural

G. Gerosa (✉) · A. Fabozzo · V. Tarzia
Department of Cardio-Thoracic and Vascular Science and Public Health,
Unit of Cardiac Surgery, Padova, Italy
e-mail: gino.gerosa@unipd.it; assunta.fabozzo@gmail.com; v.tarzia@gmail.com

A. L. P. Caforio (ed.), *Myocarditis*, https://doi.org/10.1007/978-3-030-35276-9_20

and functional cellular abnormalities, global or regional contractile impairment, and/or conduction system disease [1–3]. The actual incidence of myocarditis is difficult to determine as the confirmation of diagnosis depends upon histological and immunohistochemical analyses on endomyocardial biopsies [4–6]—gold diagnostic standard but frequently unavailable—or autoptic specimens. It is estimated that myocarditis contributes to the global burden of cardiovascular disease mainly through cardiogenic shock and heart failure, entailing sudden death (SD) and dilated cardiomyopathy (DCM), varying by age and region from approximately 0.5% and 4.0% [7]. Definition, thus diagnosis, are challenging due to heterogenicity of patients' presenting symptoms [8–10], although several attempts of classification have been proposed [11]. Frequently, myocarditis is determined by viral infections, but many other causes are also implicated, including toxins, medications, and autoimmune disease [12]. Several clinical scenarios are possible, ranging from flu-like to life-threatening states, requiring intensive care and a prompt surgical treatment. Clinical features and outcomes [13, 14] such as severity of clinical onset, recovery of heart function, development of chronic DCM, and mortality are certainly related to the etiological causes of myocarditis. Etiology, pathogenesis, diagnosis, and medical treatment are not described in detail in this chapter, as they were previously discussed. This section will focus on the surgical treatment of patients with myocarditis, describing both decision-making process and the available strategies, including extracorporeal, implantable ventricular mechanical supports, and heart transplant.

20.1.1 Mechanical Circulatory Support: An Overview

Mechanical circulatory supports (MCS) have dramatically changed the management of patients suffering from acute and chronic heart failure over the last three decades [15]. Primarily intended to support circulation during acute cardiogenic shock, in chronic settings, MCS have become an appealing solution also for organs' shortage-related issues and are currently accepted as effective therapeutic options for (1) patients requiring prompt hemodynamic stability for further clinical evaluation, such as those affected by acute or fulminant myocarditis, (2) patients waiting for organ transplantation, or as (3) destination therapy. Myocarditis may cause acute severe cardiac dysfunction, sometimes with fulminant clinical onset [16, 17]. To have a better understanding, the role of MCS in the management of patients with myocarditis can be classified according to the severity of symptoms and duration of intended support.

20.1.2 Acute or Fulminant Myocarditis Determining Cardiogenic Shock

Cardiogenic shock (CS)—due to any causes—is a dramatic clinical scenario that requires prompt patient's intensive care. Mechanical ventilation and administration of medications, such as inotropes and diuretics, are initial and valid therapeutic options for unstable patients. If medical treatment fails to achieve stable hemodynamic conditions, advanced strategies of cardio-pulmonary resuscitation, based on extracorporeal life support (ECLS), need to be soon established. Cardiogenic shock is not just a reduced cardiac contractile function but moreover a multiorgan dysfunction syndrome (MODS), which can result in peripheral hypoperfusion, systemic inflammatory response syndrome (SIRS), and sepsis [18].

The INTERMACS Registry identifies seven profiles (Table 20.1) to define the clinical severity of patients with heart failure [20]. This classification is universally accepted and its correlation to clinical outcomes is profusely described in the literature [21]. Following INTERMACS profiles, patients presenting with cardiogenic shock and requiring ECLS fall into the "crushing and burning" category (INTERMACS I).

Once MODS has developed, it is difficult to improve prognosis and reduce mortality by simply increasing cardiac output with a circulatory assist device. Prevention of MODS may depend on three critical factors: (1) optimal timing (i.e., early initiation) of mechanical circulatory support; (2) optimal level of mechanical circulatory support with reestablishment of adequate perfusion of critical organs, and (3) optimal prevention and management of potential device-related complications (i.e., device malfunction, infection).

In this critical scenario, MCS devices represent a "bridge to life" as they allow to keep the patient alive while the optimal therapeutic management is being determined ("bridge to decision").

The ideal device [22] to implant in this setting must

- be easy and quick to implant,
- enable hemodynamic support and myocardial protection,
- have low rate of complications.

Table 20.1 INTERMACS profiles [19]

Profile 1: Critical cardiogenic shock. "*Crash and burn*"	Definitive intervention needed within hours
Profile 2: Progressive decline. "*Sliding on inotropes*"	Definitive intervention needed within few days
Profile 3: Stable on inotropes. "*Dependent stability*"	Definitive intervention elective over a period of weeks to few months
Profile 4: Resting symptoms. "*Frequent flyer*"	Definitive intervention elective over period of weeks to few months
Profile 5: Exertion intolerant	Variable urgency depends upon maintenance of nutrition, organ function, and activity
Profile 6: Exertion limited. "*Walking wounded*	Variable depends upon maintenance of nutrition, organ function, and activity level
Profile 7: Advanced NYHA III	Transplantation or circulatory support may not currently be indicated

Therefore, devices that allow adequate support of blood circulation and that are implantable in a percutaneous fashion (through puncture of peripheral vessels—Seldinger technique) are preferable.

For this purpose, the devices currently available in clinic are:

1. *The Intra-Aortic Balloon counterpulsation* (IABP). It allows mechanical circulatory support by unloading the left ventricular pressure. It consists in a catheter-based (sheath size 8Fr) approach to insert a balloon into the descending aorta (pneumatic pump). Inflation of the balloon in diastole favors coronary perfusion and its deflation in systole determines pressure-unloading of the left ventricle. It is capable of supporting the circulation up to 1 L/min.
2. *TandemHeart* is a continuous flow centrifugal pump for short-term circulatory support (up to 6 h). It determines volume unloading of the left ventricle through a left atrial to femoral artery bypass. In detail, the inflow cannula (size 18–21 Fr) is inserted into a femoral vein and driven into the left atrium through transseptal puncture (femoral vein, inferior vena cava, right atrium, and left atrium), therefore unloading the LV. The outflow cannula (size 15–17 Fr) is percutaneously inserted into the femoral artery. This device can support circulation for about 4 L/min.
3. *The Impella* devices are micro-axial rotary pumps, meant to support circulation also for a short period of time (≤4 days for the Impella 2.5 and Impella CP, and ≤6 days for the Impella 5.0 and Impella LD). The Impella is positioned across the aortic valve to provide active support by transvalvular LV assistance, expelling aspirated blood from the left ventricle into the ascending aorta. The Impella Recover LP 2.5 and CP can provide up to 2.5 L/min and 4.3 L/min, respectively; it can be inserted percutaneously, whereas the Impella Recover LP 5.0 can deliver up to 5.0 L/min, but requires surgical incision of the femoral or axillary arteries. The Impella system is actually available also for RV support (Impella RP). From the combination of the two configurations, a *Bipella* support is also available.
4. *Veno Arterial ECMO/ECLS* guarantees extracorporeal circulatory support. The preferred configuration and most rapidly achievable procedural success, in an adult patient, are obtained through femoral vessels cannulation (percutaneously or after surgical isolation). Conversely, in pediatric patients (<15 kg), the carotid and the jugular vein are preferred as the diameter of other peripheral vessels is too small for a safe cannulation; alternatively, a median sternotomy may be performed to approach central vessels. The ECMO enables circulatory support up to 5 L/min.

In our experience, ECMO/ECLS represents the ideal device for refractory cardiogenic shock, as:

– It allows high cardiac output and adequate cardio-circulatory support.
– It is easy and rapid to implant ("at bedside").
– It is associated with low rate of complications (e.g., limb ischemia, embolization of atherosclerotic and/or thrombotic material, stroke, infection, and hemolysis).

In patients with acute myocarditis and CS, including children [23], once stable hemodynamic conditions are obtained, endomyocardial biopsies, 2D and 3D echocardiography, and other imaging modality (e.g., coronary angiogram) can be performed to complete diagnosis. Clarifying etiology and pathophysiology of the disease facilitates targeted pharmacological strategies.

Primary endpoints of this approach are *survival* and cardiac function *recovery*.

If a satisfying restoration (defined as a condition that allows clinical stability after weaning from MCS and ultimately hospital discharge) cannot be achieved, a long-term solution must be adopted. In our experience [24], among 64 patients with primary cardiogenic shock undergoing ECLS implantation (mainly ECMO, from January 2009 to March 2013), irrespective of the etiology, 30-day overall survival was 80% (51 of 64 patients), and 59% of patients were discharged, in whom survival at 48 months was 90%. Additionally, recovery was observed in 28% of the total population, whereas in the acute subgroup (that included patients with myocarditis and recent myocardial infarction) it was observed in almost 50%, confirming that in the context of acute etiologies, CS can be managed with a conservative approach (ECMO/ECLS is the only needed treatment). Finally, the duration of ECLS support was correlated to increased mortality.

Therefore, in our practice, if recovery is not achieved within 10 days (our selected threshold) from ECMO implantation, we prefer to shift it to longer-term solutions. Also, alternative ECLS configurations may be established to overcome concomitant matters, such as insufficient natural left ventricular venting through the aortic valve and inadequate organ perfusion.

In these cases, potential solutions are:

- implanting a cannula (20 Fr) into the apex of the left ventricle (also through an antero-lateral left thoracotomy) and its connection to the venous line of the ECMO.
- Impella (described before), EcPella (REF Pappalardo).
- Extracorporeal VAD.

After about 10 days, following our Institutional Protocols, we prefer to shift the ECMO support into the ecVAD (extracorporeal ventricular assist device, CentriMag Levitronix) to guarantee not only adequate ventricular venting and ventricular unloading but also optimal peripheral perfusion for longer period of assistance (up to 1 month). A right-, left-, or biventricular configurations are possible, based on patients' clinical needs. As mentioned, in acute and subacute settings, the evidence of a concomitant failure of the right ventricle compels biventricular circulatory support [25].

Surgical techniques for extracorporeal Bi-, L, or R- support may include median sternotomy to reach central vessels cannulation (aorta, pulmonary artery, or both) for outflow cannulae implantation and direct cardiac walls cannulation (e.g., left apical for LVAD). Alternatively, a minimally invasive approach (including femoral vessels cannulation, mini-thoracotomies for left and right supports, or dual lumen cannula—through jugular vein—for right ventricular support) may be performed.

Candidacy of patients with CS and ECMO to heart transplant must be soon taken into account. Once major contraindications (e.g., active infection) are excluded and a preserved neurological status is confirmed, urgent heart transplantation is indicated, and the evaluation of patient's immunological panel is determined. Shortage of compatible donors does not always guarantee the availability of transplantable grafts; therefore, long-term MCS may be used as bridge to it or as destination therapy (less frequently).

Figure 20.1 summarizes the procedural algorithm at our institution.

20.1.3 Surgical Strategies to Treat the Chronic Sequelae of Myocarditis

Almost 40% of all chronic patients with dilated cardiomyopathies (DCM) present immune-histological features compatible with myocarditis [26, 27]. In general, pharmacological treatment does not differ significantly from heart insufficiency due to other causes, except for those with an autoimmune mechanism, which can find relief also from specific immune-therapy (e.g., immunosuppression). Diuretics and ACE-inhibitors and—in selected cases—beta-blockers are commonly used in chronic settings to manage cardiac insufficiency. Patients with DCM and symptoms of congestive heart failure may also benefit from implantable cardioverter devices (ICD) or resynchronization therapy (CRT).

When all the medical options fail to adequately manage patients with HF after myocarditis, surgery may still offer an option.

Implantable mechanical assist devices are engaged in the treatment of patients with DCM after myocarditis as bridge to transplant or, rarely, as destination therapy. Appropriate timing for intervention and a correct choice of the optimal device to implant are crucial to improve survival and guarantee adequate systemic perfusion, avoiding multiorgan failure. The possibility of durable LVAD implantation depends primarily on the severity of other organs' failure as well as on possible recovery of ventricular function, and consequently determined by the underlying diagnosis of heart failure. The heterogeneous patient populations, the availability of multiple devices, and the lack of controlled studies make currently impossible to provide evidence-based recommendations on best timing and choice of durable LVAD [19, 28, 29]. First generation pulsatile devices (HeartMate XVE, Thoratec paracorporeal VAD; the latter still preferred for pediatric patients), although effective to support circulation, have demonstrated high rate of complications (i.e., thromboembolism, hemorrhagic events, infections, pump failure). More recently, continuous flow devices (Jarvik 2000, Heartware, Heartmate II and III) have greatly enhanced performance of first-generation pulsatile pumps. In particular the reduction of device's size and of the number of mobile parts, the limited contact surface between blood and device components have led to significant improvement of survival of patients, pump's durability, and hemocompatibility. Moreover, devices' miniaturization has allowed intrapericardial placement of the pump, minimizing surgical invasiveness [30, 31].

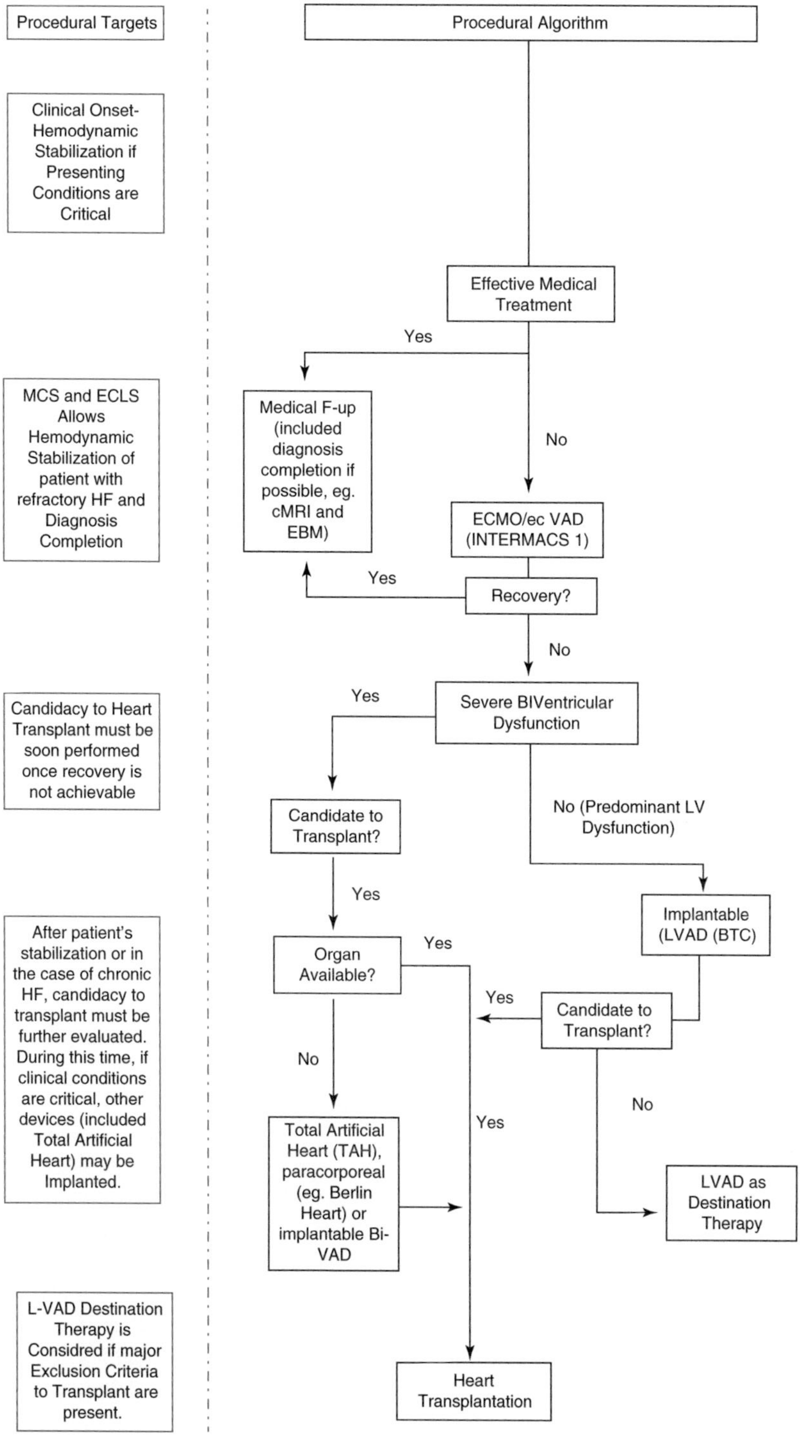

Fig. 20.1 Decisional algorithm and timing of intervention

Biventricular dysfunction during a myocarditis process is also rare. The association with a rare form of myocarditis, such as idiopathic hypereosinophilic syndrome, is described [32]. In these cases, if pharmacological treatments fail to achieve cardiac function recovery and candidacy to transplant is uncertain, a biventricular support becomes mandatory to guarantee patient's survival. Extracorporeal supports are feasible but limited in terms of durability of the treatment. To date, Syncardia Cardiowest Total Artificial Heart is the only FDA approved and CE marked device to temporarily replace the heart, while bridging the patient to transplant. It has the capability of supporting patients for long period of time with sufficient results in terms of survival [33–36]. Other devices, such as CARMAT, a totally implantable, electrically driven, biventricular device are available, also as destination therapy for compassionate use, but it is still under CE mark approval.

20.1.4 Heart Transplantation

Replacement of a persistent failing heart with a homologous compatible graft remains the optimal therapeutic option but, unfortunately, there are not enough donors to satisfy patients' request. Heart failure related to myocarditis carries mortality rates of 56% at 4.3 years and may lead to end-stage HF, requiring advanced therapies [37]. Heart transplantation is required in 1–8% of patients with myocarditis [38]. Surgery is performed following standard technique, and a bicaval anastomosis is mostly preferred at our institution. Literature data on clinical results of heart transplanted patients after myocarditis are sporadic and, for some extents, still controversial. It is still under debate if, compared to other forms of dilated cardiomyopathy, survival in transplanted patients after a myocarditis is associated with higher post-operative mortality. Children with myocarditis were more likely to be listed with the highest urgency compared with children with DCM [39]. More recently, it has been demonstrated that patients with myocarditis that do not recover from the acute event are generally younger, sicker, and more frequently require biventricular mechanical support compared to those who present with other myocarditis forms, but have comparable survival [40, 41]. Finally, the indication to transplant in cases of "Giant Cell-myocarditis" (GCs) remains controversial. It is an autoimmune and rare form of myocardial disease, having usually a dramatic onset (including sudden death and CS) that more often requires prolonged extracorporeal supports. Acute histological markers of the disease are extensive infiltrate of lymphocytes and eosinophils with macrophages giant cells associated with myocytic necrosis. After heart transplant, inflammatory infiltration seems to be able to invade the graft, compromising its performance and patients' clinical outcomes. Nevertheless, more recently, heart transplantation in patients with GCs-myocarditis seems not to differ in terms of post-operative survival compared to other forms of cardiomyopathies [17, 42]. Data on large cohorts of patients are mandatory to universally define the most efficient patients' therapeutic pathway.

20.2 Summary

- Cardiogenic shock after myocarditis, not responsive to medical treatment, can be surgically managed through mechanical circulatory support systems ("bridge to life").
- Optimal timing and strategies are essential to guarantee patients' survival and to possibly achieve cardiac recovery.
- While patients are mechanically supported, the diagnosis may be clarified, and targeted therapies instituted.
- In the acute setting, if recovery cannot be achieved, other surgical therapies must be adopted. They include implantable VAD, total artificial heart, and finally heart transplantation, once major contraindications, such as active infection, are excluded.
- In chronic settings, heart transplantation and implantable VAD are the most common and effective options to treat congestive heart failure due to the chronic sequelae of myocarditis.

References

1. Fung G, Luo H, Qiu Y, Yang D, McManus B. Myocarditis. Circ Res. 2016;118(3):496–514.
2. Cooper LT Jr. Myocarditis. N Engl J Med. 2009;360(15):1526–38.
3. Caforio ALP, Pankuweit S, Arbustini E, Basso C, Gimeno-Blanes J, Felix SB, Fu M, Heliö T, Heymans S, Jahns R, Klingel K, Linhart A, Maisch B, McKenna W, Mogensen J, Pinto YM, Ristic A, Schultheiss H-P, Seggewiss H, Tavazzi L, Thiene G, Yilmaz A, Charron P, Elliott PM. Current state of knowledge on aetiology, diagnosis, management, and therapy of myocarditis: a position statement of the European Society of Cardiology Working Group on Myocardial and Pericardial Diseases. Eur Heart J. 2013;34(33):2636–48.
4. Caforio AL, Calabrese F, Angelini A, Tona F, Vinci A, Bottaro S, Ramondo A, Carturan E, Iliceto S, Thiene G, Daliento L. A prospective study of biopsy-proven myocarditis: prognostic relevance of clinical and aetiopathogenetic features at diagnosis. Eur Heart J. 2007;28(11):1326–33.
5. Grün S, Schumm J, Greulich S, Wagner A, Schneider S, Bruder O, Kispert EM, Hill S, Ong P, Klingel K, Kandolf R, Sechtem U, Mahrholdt H. Long-term follow-up of biopsy-proven viral myocarditis: predictors of mortality and incomplete recovery. J Am Coll Cardiol. 2012;59(18):1604–15.
6. Cooper LT, Baughman KL, Feldman AM, Frustaci A, Jessup M, Kuhl U, Levine GN, Narula J, Starling RC, Towbin J, Virmani R, American Heart Association; American College of Cardiology; European Society of Cardiology; Heart Failure Society of America; Heart Failure Association of the European Society of Cardiology. The role of endomyocardial biopsy in the management of cardiovascular disease: a scientific statement from the American Heart Association, the American College of Cardiology, and the European Society of Cardiology. Endorsed by the Heart Failure Society of America and the Heart Failure Association of the European Society of Cardiology. J Am Coll Cardiol. 2007;50(19):1914–31.
7. Cooper LT Jr, Keren A, Sliwa K, Matsumori A, Mensah GA. The global burden of myocarditis: part 1: a systematic literature review for the global burden of diseases, injuries, and risk factors 2010 study. Global Heart. 2014;9:121–9.

8. Caforio ALP, Malipiero G, Marcolongo R, Iliceto S. Myocarditis: a clinical overview. Curr Cardiol Rep. 2017;19(7):63.
9. Caforio AL, Marcolongo R, Basso C, Iliceto S. Clinical presentation and diagnosis of myocarditis. Heart. 2015;101(16):1332–44.
10. McCarthy RE 3rd, Boehmer JP, Hruban RH, Hutchins GM, Kasper EK, Hare JM, Baughman KL. Long-term outcome of fulminant myocarditis as compared with acute (nonfulminant) myocarditis. N Engl J Med. 2000;342(10):690–5.
11. Sagar S, Liu PP, Cooper LT Jr. Myocarditis. Lancet. 2012;379:738–47. https://doi.org/10.1016/S0140-6736(11)60648-X.
12. Pollack A, Kontorovich AR, Fuster V, Dec GW. Viral myocarditis—diagnosis, treatment options, and current controversies. Nat Rev Cardiol. 2015;12(11):670–80.
13. Ammirati E, Cipriani M, Lilliu M, Sormani P, Varrenti M, Raineri C, Petrella D, Garascia A, Pedrotti P, Roghi A, Bonacina E, Moreo A, Bottiroli M, Gagliardone MP, Mondino M, Ghio S, Totaro R, Turazza FM, Russo CF, Oliva F, Camici PG, Frigerio M. Survival and left ventricular function changes in fulminant versus nonfulminant acute myocarditis. Circulation. 2017;136(6):529–45.
14. Ponikowski P, Voors AA, Anker SD, Bueno H, Cleland JGF, Coats AJS, Falk V, González-Juanatey JR, Harjola VP, Jankowska EA, Jessup M, Linde C, Nihoyannopoulos P, Parissis JT, Pieske B, Riley JP, Rosano GMC, Ruilope LM, Ruschitzka F, Rutten FH, van der Meer P, ESC Scientific Document Group. 2016 ESC Guidelines for the diagnosis and treatment of acute and chronic heart failure: The Task Force for the diagnosis and treatment of acute and chronic heart failure of the European Society of Cardiology (ESC). Developed with the special contribution of the Heart Failure Association (HFA) of the ESC. Eur Heart J. 2016;37(27):2129–200.
15. Pinney SP, Anyanwu AC, Lala A, et al. Left ventricular assist devices for lifelong support. J Am Coll Cardiol. 2017;69(23):2845–61.
16. Saito S, Toda K, Miyagawa S, Yoshikawa Y, Hata H, Yoshioka D, Domae K, Tsukamoto Y, Sakata Y, Sawa Y. Diagnosis, medical treatment, and stepwise mechanical circulatory support for fulminant myocarditis. J Artif Organs. 2018;21(2):172–9.
17. ElAmm CA, Al-Kindi SG, Oliveira GH. Characteristics and outcomes of patients with myocarditis listed for heart transplantation. Circ Heart Fail. 2016;9:e003259.
18. Stevenson LW, Pagani FD, Young JB, et al. INTERMACS profiles of advanced heart failure: the current picture. J Heart Lung Transplant. 2009;28:535–41.
19. Lahpor J, Khaghani A, Hetzer R, et al. European results with a continuous-flow ventricular assist device for advanced heart-failure patients. Eur J Cardiothorac Surg. 2010;37(2):357–61.
20. Werdan K, Gielen S, Ebelt H, et al. Mechanical circulatory support in cardiogenic shock. Eur Heart J. 2014;35:156–67.
21. Kirklin JK, Pagani FD, Kormos RL, Stevenson LW, Blume ED, Myers SL, Miller MA, Baldwin JT, Young JB, Naftel DC. Eighth annual INTERMACS report: special focus on framing the impact of adverse events. J Heart Lung Transplant. 2017;36:1080–6.
22. Ouwenee IDM, Henriques JPS. Percutaneous cardiac support devices for cardiogenic shock: current indications and recommendations. Heart. 2012;98:1246–54.
23. Morales DLS, Rossano JW, VanderPluym C, Lorts A, Cantor R, St Louis J, Koeh D, Sutcliffe DL, Adachi I, Kirklin JK, Rosenthal DN, Blume ED, Pedimacs Investigators. Third annual pediatric interagency registry for mechanical circulatory support (Pedimacs) report: pre-implant characteristics and outcomes. Ann Thorac Surg. 2019;107:993–1004.
24. Tarzia V, Bortolussi G, Bianco R, et al. Extracorporeal life support in cardiogenic shock: impact of acute versus chronic etiology on outcome. J Thorac Cardiovasc Surg. 2015;150(2):333–40.
25. Kuchibhotla S, Esposito ML, Breton C, Pedicini R, Mullin A, O'Kelly R, Anderson M, Morris DL, Batsides G, Ramzy D, Grise M, Pham DT, Kapur NK. Acute biventricular mechanical circulatory support for cardiogenic shock. J Am Heart Assoc. 2017;6:e006670. https://doi.org/10.1161/JAHA.117.006670.

26. Nagatomo Y, McNamara DM, Alexis JD, Cooper LT, Dec GW, Pauly DF, Sheppard R, Starling RC, Tang WH, IMAC-2 Investigators. Myocardial recovery in patients with systolic heart failure and autoantibodies against β(1)-adrenergic receptors. J Am Coll Cardiol. 2017;69(8):968–77.
27. Wojnicz R, Nowalany-Kozielska E, Wojciechowska C, et al. Randomized, placebo-controlled study for immunosuppressive treatment of inflammatory dilated cardiomyopathy: two-year follow-up results. Circulation. 2001;104:39–45.
28. Slaughter MS, Rogers JG, Milano CA, Russell SD, Conte JV, Feldman D, Sun B, Tatooles AJ, Delgado RM 3rd, Long JW, Wozniak TC, Ghumman W, Farrar DJ, Frazier OH, HeartMate II Investigators. Advanced heart failure treated with continuous-flow left ventricular assist device. N Engl J Med. 2009;361(23):2241–51.
29. den Uil CA, Akin S, Jewbali LS, dos ReisMiranda D, Brugts JJ, Constantinescu A, Arie Pieter Kappetein AP, Caliskan K. Short-term mechanical circulatory support as a bridge to durable left ventricular assist device implantation in refractory cardiogenic shock: a systematic review and meta-analysis. Eur J Cardiothorac Surg. 2017;52:14–25.
30. Carrozzini M, Bejko J, Guariento A, Rubino M, Bianco R, Tarzia V, Gregori D, Bottio T, Gerosa G. Minimally invasive implantation of continuous flow left ventricular assist devices: the evolution of surgical techniques in a single-center experience. Artif Organs. 2019;43:E41–52.
31. Tarzia V, Buratto E, Gallo M, Bortolussi G, Bejko J, Bianco R, Bottio T, Gerosa G. Implantation of the HeartWare HVAD: from full sternotomy to less invasive techniques. Ann Cardiothorac Surg. 2014;3(5):535–7.
32. Tarzia V, Buratto E, Gallo M, Bortolussi G, Bejko J, Dal Lin C, Torregrossa G, Bianco R, Bottio T, Gerosa G. Surgical implantation of the CardioWest total artificial heart. Ann Cardiothorac Surg. 2014;3(6):624–5.
33. Kawabori M, Kurihara C, Miller Y, Heck KA, Bogaev RC, Civitello AB, Cohn WE, Frazier OH, Morgan JA. Total artificial heart implantation for biventricular failure due to eosinophilic myocarditis. J Artif Organs. 2017;20(3):266–9.
34. El Banayosy A, Arusoglu L, Morshius M, et al. Cardiowest total artificial heart: bad Oeynhausen experience. Ann Thorac Surg. 2005;80:548–52.
35. Kirsch MEW, Nguyen A, Mastroianni C, et al. Syncardia temporary total artificial heart as bridge to transplantation: current results at la pitiè hospital. Ann Thoracic Surg. 2013;95:1640–6.
36. Torregrossa G, Morshuis M, Varghese R, et al. Results with syncardia total artificial heart beyond 1 year. ASAIO J. 2014;60:626–34.
37. Pietra BA, Kantor PF, Bartlett HL, Chin C, Canter CE, Larsen RL, Edens RE, Colan SD, Towbin JA, Lipshultz SE, Kirklin JK, Naftel DC, Hsu DT. Early predictors of survival to and after heart transplantation in children with dilated cardiomyopathy. Circulation. 2012;126: 1079–86.
38. Höyer S, Berglin E, Pettersson G, Edvardsson N, Waagstein F. Cardiac transplantation in patients with active myocarditis. Transplant Proc. 1990;22:1450.
39. Yoshizawa S, Kato TS, Mancini D, Marboe CC. Outcome of patients having heart transplantation for lymphocytic myocarditis. Am J Cardiol. 2013;112:405–10.
40. Garbern JC, Gauvreau K, Blume ED, Singh TP. Is myocarditis an independent risk factor for post-transplant mortality in pediatric heart transplant recipients? Circ Heart Fail. 2016;9(1):e002328.
41. Litovsky SH, Burke AP, Virmani R. Giant cell myocarditis: an entity distinct from sarcoidosis characterized by multiphasic myocyte destruction by cytotoxic T cells and histiocytic giant cells. Mod Pathol. 1996;9(12):1126–34.
42. Maleszewski JJ, Orellana VM, Hodge DO, et al. Long-term risk of recurrence, morbidity and mortality in giant cell myocarditis. Am J Cardiol. 2015;115:1733–8.

MIX
Papier aus verantwortungsvollen Quellen
Paper from responsible sources
FSC® C105338

If you have any concerns about our products,
you can contact us on
ProductSafety@springernature.com

In case Publisher is established outside the EU,
the EU authorized representative is:
Springer Nature Customer Service Center GmbH
Europaplatz 3, 69115 Heidelberg, Germany

Printed by Libri Plureos GmbH
in Hamburg, Germany